Advances in Equine Nutrition III

Edited by Joe D. Pagan Ph.D.
Kentucky Equine Research Inc., Versailles, Kentucky, USA

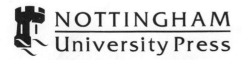
NOTTINGHAM
University Press

Nottingham University Press
Manor Farm, Main Street, Thrumpton
Nottingham, NG11 0AX, United Kingdom

NOTTINGHAM

First published 2005
© Kentucky Equine Research Inc. 2005

British Library Cataloguing in Publication Data
Advances in Equine Nutrition III
Pagan, J.D.

ISBN   1-904761-28-3

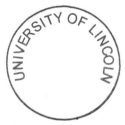

Disclaimer

Typeset by Nottingham University Press, Nottingham
Printed and bound by Hobbs the Printers Ltd., Hampshire, UK

CONTENTS

General Nutrition

Feeding Management

Performance Horses

Growth and Development

Pathological Conditions

GENERAL NUTRITION

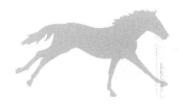

RECENT RESEARCH DEVELOPMENTS FROM KENTUCKY EQUINE RESEARCH

JOE D. PAGAN

Kentucky Equine Research, Inc., Versailles, Kentucky

Significant advances have been made over the past 30 years in the understanding of equine nutrition. Still, many questions remain unanswered about how to feed and manage horses. Over the past 12 years, Kentucky Equine Research has conducted numerous research studies that have addressed questions relevant to the horse feed industry. This paper will review five of the most recent studies.

Hay Intake and Performance

The amount of energy that a horse needs to run is directly related to the weight being moved (horse, rider, and tack) and the speed of running. Addition of weight increases the energy cost of locomotion. Diet can have a marked effect on body weight. Specifically, high-roughage diets increase the mass of ingesta in the equine large intestine, the result of greater water consumption and the ability of fiber to bind to water. High-fiber diets are desirable for horses engaged in endurance sports because the larger reservoir of fluid and electrolytes in the hindgut may lessen the severity of dehydration during prolonged exercise when compared with a low-fiber diet. On the other hand, the increase in body weight when horses consume a high-fiber diet will mandate an increase in energy expenditure at any given running speed and may be detrimental to performance, particularly during high-intensity exertion.

Traditionally, racehorse trainers restrict the amount of hay fed to horses before racing in an attempt to improve performance. However, no study has examined the effect of restricted hay intake on body weight, nor the effects of this dietary manipulation on exercise performance. Therefore, KER conducted a study to determine the effects of restricted hay intake on the metabolic responses of horses to high-intensity exercise (Rice et al., 2001). We hypothesized that, compared to ad libitum hay intake, a regimen of restricted hay feeding starting 3 days before a standardized exercise test would decrease body weight and reduce energy expenditure during running.

Four conditioned Thoroughbred horses were studied in a 2 x 2 crossover design. Initially, the length of time required for adaptation to ad libitum intake of grass hay was determined. Thereafter, the metabolic responses to sprint exercise (SPR) were examined in two dietary periods, each 5 days in duration: 1) Ad libitum (AL), where horses had free-choice access to hay; and 2) Restricted (RES), where hay intake was restricted (~1% of body weight) for 3 days before the exercise test. Feed and water were removed 4 h before the exercise test.

After measurement of body weight, horses completed a warm-up followed by 2 min at 115% of maximum oxygen uptake, then a 10-min walking recovery (REC). During the 3 days before SPR, hay intake in AL averaged (± SE) 10.1 ± 0.9 kg, whereas intake during RES was 4.3 ± 0.2 kg. Pre-exercise body weight was significantly lower in RES (528 ± 5 kg) than in AL (539 ± 4 kg). During SPR, total mass-specific VO_2 was higher (P=0.02) in RES (243 ± 8 ml/kg/2 min) than in AL (233 ± 10 ml/kg/2 min). Conversely, accumulated oxygen deficit was higher (P<0.01) in AL (89.4 ± 2.2 ml O_2/kg) than in RES (82.4 ± 1.7 ml O_2/kg). Peak plasma lactate was also higher in AL (22.2 ± 1.2 mM) than in RES (19.1 ± 2.1 mM), and VO_2 during recovery was 10% higher (P=0.12) in AL.

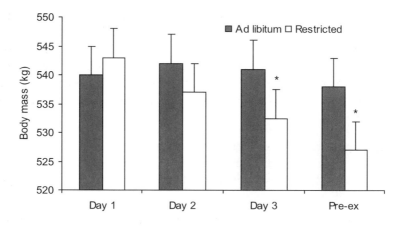

Figure 1. Body weight in the ad libitum and restricted hay intake groups for the 3-day period preceding the exercise test. Pre-ex = Body weight measured 5 min before the exercise test. *Significant (P<0.05) difference ad libitum vs. restricted.

The main findings of this study were: 1) compared to ad libitum hay feeding, 3 days of restricted (1% of body weight) hay intake was associated with an approximately 2% decrease in body weight; and 2) the reduction in body weight associated with restricted hay feeding resulted in an increase in the mass-specific rate of oxygen consumption during sprint exercise, with a corresponding decrease in anaerobic energy expenditure. The anaerobic contribution to energy expenditure during exercise was lower in RES than in AL as evidenced by lower values for accumulated oxygen deficit (Figure 2) and peak plasma lactate concentrations.

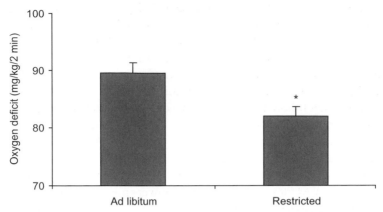

Figure 2. Accumulated oxygen deficit during 2 min of exercise at 115% of maximal oxygen uptake in the ad libitum and restricted treatments. *$P<0.05$ restricted vs. ad libitum.

Currently, it is recommended that performance horses receive hay at a minimum of 1% of body weight per day to satisfy requirements for long stem fiber and minimize digestive upsets. In this context, relative to the restriction protocol used in this study, more severe or longer-term restrictions of hay intake are not recommended. Nonetheless, on the basis of our results, further studies that examine the relationship between fiber intake, body weight, and exercise metabolism and performance are warranted.

Arabians vs. Thoroughbreds

Few studies have formally compared indices of athletic performance in different breeds of horses. Rose and colleagues (1995) described indices of exercise capacity in Thoroughbred and Standardbred racehorses that were examined because of poor performance. These researchers reported that aerobic capacity and total run time, measured during an incremental exercise test, were significantly greater in the Thoroughbreds compared to the Standardbreds. However, as these horses were examined for performance problems, it is difficult to apply the findings to normal racehorses.

In a recent KER study (Prince et al., 2001), we examined selected measures of exercise capacity and metabolism in a small group of Thoroughbred and Arabian horses of similar age, training background, and diet. Both breeds of horses are used for several athletic disciplines, ranging from sprint racing to endurance events. However, anecdotal evidence indicates that Thoroughbreds have superior high-intensity exercise capacity, whereas Arabian horses are regarded as superior performers during endurance exercise. We hypothesized that the facility of Thoroughbred horses for high-intensity exercise would be reflected in greater aerobic and anaerobic capacities when compared to the Arabian horses. We also hypothesized that respiratory exchange ratio (RER) would be lower in the Arabians during low-intensity exercise, reflecting a greater use of fat for energy.

The metabolic responses to low- and high-intensity exercise were compared in five Arabian (AR) and five Thoroughbred (Tb) horses. For 2 months before the study, horses were fed an identical diet and undertook a similar exercise training program. Horses then completed three treadmill (3° incline) trials: 1) an incremental test (MAX) for determination of aerobic capacity, V_{LA4}, and lactate threshold (LT; the percentage of VO_{2max} when plasma lactate = 4 mM); 2) a sprint test (SPR) for estimation of maximal accumulated oxygen deficit (MAOD) in which horses ran until fatigue at 115% VO_{2max}; and 3) a 90-min test at 35% VO_{2max} (LO). There was a minimum of 7 days between tests and the order of the SPR and LO trials was randomized. For all tests, VO_2, VCO_2, and RER were measured throughout exercise. For MAX, horses ran for 90 s at 4 and 6 m/s, with subsequent increases of 1 m/s every 60 s until fatigue. Blood samples were obtained during the last 10 s of each speed increment. In SPR, MAOD was calculated by subtracting actual VO from estimated O_2 demand. In LO, samples for measurement of plasma glucose and free fatty acids (FFA) were obtained at 0, 5, 15, 30, 45, 60, 75, and 90 min of exercise. Data were analyzed using Student's t-test or 2-way repeated measures ANOVA.

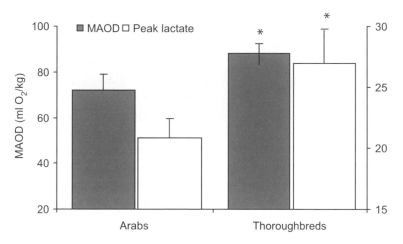

Figure 3. Maximum accumulated oxygen deficit and peak lactate concentrations for the Arabian and Thoroughbred horses during a single high-speed exercise test at 115% of maximum oxygen uptake.

VO_{2max} (P<0.001) and running speed (P<0.05) at VO_{2max} were higher in Tb (154 ± 3 ml/kg/min at 12.9 ± 0.5 m/s) than in AR (129 ± 2.5 ml/kg/min at 11.8 ± 0.2 m/s). Run time to fatigue during MAX was greater (P<0.05) in Tb (10.5 ± 0.5 min) than in AR (9.3 ± 0.3 min). However, V_{LA4} and LT were not different between groups. Run time during SPR (Tb 149 ± 16; AR 109 ± 11 s) and MAOD

(Tb 88 ± 4; AR 70 ± 6 ml O$_2$/kg) were higher (P<0.05) in the Tb group (Figure 3). During LO, FFA were higher (P<0.05) in AR than in Tb between 60 and 90 min, while RER was lower (P<0.05) from 60 to 90 min of exercise. The higher aerobic and anaerobic capacity of the Tb horses likely contributed to their superior high- intensity exercise performance. Conversely, the AR may be better adapted for endurance exercise as evidenced by the greater use of fat. These metabolic differences may reflect breed variation in muscle fiber types.

Glycemic Response with Beet Pulp

Previous studies in our laboratory demonstrated a marked glycemic response when horses were fed a fiber mix consisting of equal parts rice bran, soy hulls, wheat bran, and soaked beet pulp (Pagan et al., 1999a). We speculated that, in part, the beet pulp portion of this fiber mix was responsible for the increase in plasma glucose concentrations after meal ingestion. We further hypothesized that the magnitude of the glycemic response to beet pulp would depend on how the beet pulp was prepared. Therefore, KER conducted a study to determine how different preparations of shredded beet pulp affect glycemic response in Thoroughbred horses (Groff et al., 2001). In a 4 x 4 Latin square design, four mature geldings (mean age 12 yr, body weight 568 kg) were fed: 1) 0.75 kg rinsed beet pulp (Rinse); 2) 0.75 kg hydrated beet pulp (Hydrate); 3) 0.675 kg dry beet pulp and 0.075 kg molasses (BP/Molasses); and 4) 0.75 kg whole oats (Oats). Water was added to both the rinsed and hydrated beet pulp, which were then allowed to stand overnight. In the Rinse treatment, excess water was drained and the beet pulp was washed repeatedly until the concentration of glucose in the wash water was <1 mg/dl. In the Hydrate treatment, water was not removed before feeding the beet pulp. Each treatment period was 7 days. In each period, the diet consisted of the treatment meal (0700h), 2 kg of whole oats (1600h), and 6.8 kg alfalfa hay cubes, divided into three equal feedings, at 0700, 1600, and 2200. Horses were given access to free exercise on pasture during the day, although they were not allowed to graze. The glycemic response trials were performed on day 7 of each period after an overnight fast (10 h). The test meal was fed at 0700 h. Blood samples were taken before feeding to determine baseline glucose values and at 30-min intervals following feeding for 480 min. The morning allotment of alfalfa cubes was fed after completion of sample collection. Measurements included area under the curve, mean glucose (mg/dl), peak glucose (mg/dl), and time to peak glucose (min). Plasma glucose concentrations were statistically analyzed by the general linear model procedure for analysis of variance, with period, horse, and treatment included in the model. Statistical significance was set at P<0.05. Using area under the curve for whole oats as a standard of reference, a glycemic index was determined from area under the curve for the other treatments.

Ingestion of rinsed beet pulp resulted in significantly lower area under the curve, mean glucose, peak glucose, and time to peak glucose when compared to

Table 1. Area under the curve, mean glucose, peak glucose, and time to peak glucose concentration for all dietary treatments.

	Area under curve	MG (mg/dl)	PG (mg/dl)	TTP (min)	GI
Rinsed	1422[a]	91.2[a]	94.5[a]	195[b]	34.1
Hydrated	3017[b]	94.4[b]	105.4[b]	75[a]	72.2
Dry + molasses	3834[b]	95.1[b]	119.0[c]	83[a]	94.8
Whole oats	4175[b]	94.8[b]	114.6[c]	83[a]	100
SEM	406	0.41	2.72	37	
Statistical significance	0.01	0.05	0.01	0.01	

[abc] Treatments lacking a common superscript differ (P<0.05). MG, mean glucose; PG, peak glucose; TTP, time to peak glucose; GI, glycemic index

the other treatments (Table 1). Ingestion of Oats and BP/Molasses resulted in the highest glycemic response (Figure 4), while the plasma glucose response after Hydrate was intermediate between the Oats and BP/Molasses treatments and the Rinse treatment (Table 1, Figure 4). The estimated glycemic index was substantially lower for Rinse when compared to the other treatments (Table 1). The results of this study demonstrate that the glycemic response to a meal of beet pulp is markedly affected by preparation method. Removal of residual sugars by hydrating and rinsing dry beet pulp results in a negligible glycemic response, whereas the addition of 10% molasses to dry beet pulp results in a plasma glucose response that is indistinguishable from that observed after a meal of whole oats. These findings have important implications in the design of diets and feeding methods for horses that require diets low in hydrolyzable carbohydrate (e.g., horses with recurrent exertional rhabdomyolysis or polysaccharide storage myopathy).

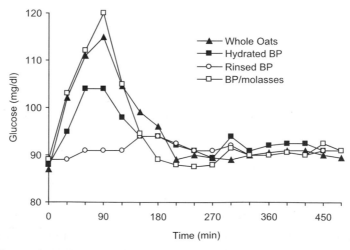

Figure 4. Plasma glucose concentrations after ingestion of whole oats, hydrated beet pulp, rinsed beet, and beet pulp and molasses in four horses.

Trace Mineral Requirements

Very little research has been conducted to determine the trace mineral requirements for athletic horses. In a previous KER study evaluating different forms of selenium (Se), horses supplemented with inorganic Se demonstrated a significant increase in urinary Se excretion after a single bout of exercise (Pagan et al., 1999b). These findings suggest that exercise increases the requirement for Se. Are the requirements for other microminerals also affected by exercise and training? To answer these questions, KER conducted a study (Hudson et al., 2001) to:

1. Determine the digestibility and retention of copper (Cu), zinc (Zn), and manganese (Mn) over four different levels of intake (basal, 50% of NRC added, 100% of NRC added, and 200% of NRC added);

2. Evaluate how regular exercise and training alters the requirements of these trace minerals.

Six mature Thoroughbred geldings [three sedentary (SED) and three horses in regular exercise training (EX)] were studied in a 16-week longitudinal experiment that consisted of 4 periods, each with a 23-day adaptation period followed by a 5-day complete collection digestion trial. In period 1, horses were fed an unfortified diet (basal intake – no supplementation), while in periods 2, 3 and 4 respectively, the diet included a supplement that provided 50, 100 and 200% of the NRC (1989) requirements for Cu, Zn, and Mn. For the basal diet, horses were fed unfortified sweet feed and timothy hay. This diet provided approximately 85%, 160% and 65% of the NRC recommendations for Cu, Mn and Zn, respectively. During the last week of this period, horses underwent a 5-day complete digestion trial. For the EX horses, a standardized exercise test was completed on the third day of the trial.

Table 2. Comparison of the true digestibility, endogenous loss, and estimated daily requirements for copper (Cu), zinc (Zn), and manganese (Mn) in sedentary (SED) horses (n = 3) and physically conditioned (EX) horses (n = 3). Data are mean ± SD.

		Cu	*Zn*	*Mn*
Digestibility (%)	SED	41.8 ± 17.6	25.4 ± 11.4	57.9 ± 10.0
	EX	54.5 ± 11.7	14.3 ± 3.9**	40.2 ± 11.8**
Endogenous loss (mg/day)	SED	15.7 ± 1.6	65.2 ± 25.6	304.8 ± 95.1
	EX	20.3 ± 18.0	69.6 ± 35.9	163.6 ± 67.9
Requirement (mg/day)	SED	44.2 ± 23.6	274.4 ± 87.5	528.6 ± 168.6
	EX	35.0 ± 24.6	461.3 ± 133.2*	408.3 ± 107.1

* $P < 0.05$ EX vs. SED
** $P < 0.1$ EX vs. SED

There was a significantly higher Zn requirement in EX than in SED horses (Table 2). Although there were no other significant differences between SED and EX, there were trends for lower true digestibility of Mn (P=0.059) and Zn (P=0.09) in EX. Results of this study suggest that exercise training results in a higher requirement for Zn but does not affect the true digestibility and maintenance requirements of Cu and Mn in mature Thoroughbred horses.

Corn Oil Affects Gastric Emptying

The ^{13}C-octanoic acid breath (or blood) test was recently developed as a noninvasive method for measuring the rate of solid-phase gastric emptying (GE). We used this method to test the hypothesis that GE is delayed following ingestion of a grain plus corn oil meal compared to a meal of grain alone (Geor et al., 2001). Four mature (10-12 yr) Arabian horses were studied in a 2 x 2 factorial design study. Factor A was the habitual diet, either a control (CON; hay plus sweet feed [SWF]) or an isocaloric fat-supplemented diet (FAT; hay, SWF, and corn oil). Factor B was the type of meal consumed for the GE test (SWF, 2 g/kg body weight vs. SWF 2 g/kg body weight plus 10% corn oil [OIL]). Each diet period lasted 10 weeks, with 6 weeks in between. GE studies were performed during the 4th and 8th weeks of each period. Within each dietary period, and in random order, horses were tested in both the SWF and OIL conditions with the following four treatment combinations: CON/SWF, CON/OIL, FAT/SWF, and FAT/OIL. For assessment of solid-phase GE, the test meals were labeled with 1 g of ^{13}C-octanoic acid. Blood samples for measurement of plasma glucose concentration and ^{13}C-enrichment were collected at 30 min and immediately before ingestion of the test meal and at frequent intervals thereafter for 7 h. Three indices of blood ^{13}C-enrichment were calculated: half-dose recovery time (t½), the time to peak blood ^{13}C-enrichment (t(max)), and the gastric emptying coefficient (GEC).

The glycemic response was markedly decreased in the OIL compared to the SWF trials (Figure 5). This effect of corn oil was not altered by habitual diet. The blood ^{13}C vs. time curve was altered such that it was not possible to calculate t½ and t(max) for one horse in both the CON/OIL and FAT/OIL trials. Excluding data from this horse, addition of corn oil to the meal of SWF was associated with a significant decrease in GEC and a significant increase in t½ and t(max), as shown (mean ± s.d.) in Table 3.

Based on this study, it was concluded that: 1) the addition of corn oil to a meal of sweet feed results in a delay in solid-phase GE; 2) the effect of oil on GE is not affected by short-term adaptation to a fat-supplemented diet; and 3) the slowing of GE may contribute to the blunted glycemic response following a grain meal containing corn oil. The delayed GE may be due to a direct effect of oil on motility or the resultant increased energy density of the test meal.

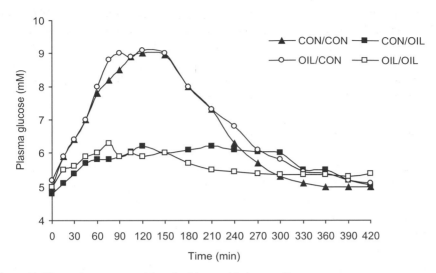

Figure 5. Glycemic response with and without added corn oil.

Table 3. Effect of adding corn oil on the gastric emptying coefficient (GEC), half-dose recovery time (t½), and the time to peak blood ^{13}C-enrichment (t(max)).

Treatment	GEC	$t½(h)$	$t(max)(h)$
CON/SWF	2.96 ± 0.15	2.25 ± 0.55	1.20 ± 0.21
CON/OIL	2.10 ± 0.14	3.87 ± 0.39	2.08 ± 0.30
FAT/SWF	3.02 ± 0.09	2.21 ± 0.45	1.24 ± 0.37
FAT/OIL	2.05 ± 0.21	4.11 ± 0.66	2.14 ± 0.28

Acknowledgments

Kentucky Equine Research wishes to thank the WALTHAM Centre for Pet Nutrition for providing funding for the studies related to Hay Intake and Performance, Arabians vs. Thoroughbreds, and Corn Oil Affects Gastric Emptying sections of this paper. Amanda Prince and Orlagh Rice were WALTHAM fellows while at KER.

References

Geor RJ, Harris PA, Hoekstra KE, Pagan JD. 2001. Effect of corn oil on solid-phase gastric emptying in horses. J Vet Int Med 2001 (abstract submitted).

Groff L, Pagan J, Hoekstra K, Gardner S, Rice O, Roose K, Geor R. 2001. Effect of preparation method on the glycemic response to ingestion of beet pulp in Thoroughbred horses. Proc. 17th Equine Nutr. and Physiol. Soc. Symp.

Hudson C, Pagan J, Hoekstra K, Prince A, Gardner S, Geor R. 2001. Effects of exercise training on the digestibility and requirements of copper, zinc and manganese in Thoroughbred horses. Proc. 17th Equine Nutr. and Physiol. Soc. Symp.

Pagan JD, Harris PA, Kennedy MAP, Davidson N, Hoekstra KE. 1999a. Feed type and intake affects glycemic response in Thoroughbred horses. Proc. 16th Equine Nutr. And Phys. Soc. Symp.149-150.

Pagan JD, Karnezos P, Kennedy MAP, Currier T, Hoekstra KE. 1999b. Effect of selenium source on selenium digestibility and retention in exercised Thoroughbreds. Proc. 16th Equine Nutr. and Physiol. Soc. Symp. 135-140.

Prince A, Geor R, Harris P, Hoekstra K, Gardner S, Hudson C, Pagan J. 2001. Comparison of the metabolic responses of trained Arabian and Thoroughbred horses during high and low intensity exercise Proc. 17th Equine Nutr. and Physiol. Soc. Symp.

Rice O, Geor R, Harris P, Hoekstra K, Gardner S, Pagan J. 2001. Effects of restricted hay intake on body weight and metabolic responses to high-intensity exercise in Thoroughbred horses. Proc. 17th Equine Nutr. and Physiol. Soc. Symp.

Rose RJ, King CM, Evans DL, Tyler CM, Hodgson DR. 1995. Indices of exercise capacity in horses presented for poor racing performance. Equine Vet J Suppl. 18:418-421.

PASTURE COUNTS: THE CONTRIBUTION OF PASTURE TO THE DIETS OF HORSES

NEVILLE GRACE
AgResearch Ltd., Grasslands Research Centre, Palmerston North, New Zealand

Introduction

The New Zealand livestock industry is based on pasture, and over the last 60 years considerable research has gone into (a) breeding more productive pasture species, (b) plants that respond to frequent grazing, (c) plants that are more resistant to disease (Tapper et al., 1999), and (d) the factors that influence pasture production (Korte et al., 1987). Associated with plant breeding programs have been fertilizer trials to improve plant nutrition (Roberts et al., 1996), the development of legumes (Caradus et al., 1996), particularly white clover, to fix atmospheric nitrogen, and grazing studies to improve pasture utilization (Clark and Brougham, 1979). In New Zealand, pasture is the major dietary component for broodmares and young horses. However, it is only recently that information on dry matter intakes (DMI) and digestible energy intakes (DEI) of pasture-fed Thoroughbred horses has become available, as well as observations on the influence that fresh herbage has on the growth and development of young horses.

Pasture Species

New Zealand pastures are usually a mixture of grasses and clovers with perennial ryegrass/white clover being the dominant pasture (Hunt, 1994). However, depending on climate, soil type, fertilizer applications, and livestock system, other grasses such as tall fescue, cocksfoot, phalaris, prairie grass, timothy, Yorkshire fog, and browntop are found in pastures, as well as red clover. When evaluating the feed value of grasses and clovers, in terms of lamb growth rates, it was found that the feed values of annual ryegrasses were greater than that of the perennial ryegrasses, while that of white clover was the highest (Ulyatt, 1971). The nutritive value or chemical composition of grasses change with season and plant maturity. Grasses in the leafy stage during late autumn, winter, and spring have the highest dry matter digestibilities, but this decreases as the seedhead emerges in late spring, because when the grass has become mature the soluble sugars and crude protein percentage decrease, while the cellulose and lignin percentage increase (Waghorn and Barry, 1987).

Seasonal Pattern of Pasture Dry Matter Production

The major determinants of plant growth are temperature and moisture, and these influence pasture dry matter (DM) production. Typically, in New Zealand the greatest pasture growth occurs during spring (October/November; 60 kg DM/ha/day), while the least growth occurs during winter (June/July; 14 kg DM/ha/day) (Milligan et al., 1987). This seasonal pasture production pattern influences livestock farming practices, with calving and lambing being planned for the spring when the quantity and quality of the pasture is at its best. In New Zealand mares foal from September to November with weaning occurring in March and April.

Relating Daily Pasture Dry Matter Production and Daily Dry Matter Requirements of the Horse

The supply of pasture DM and the DM requirements of the horse need to be matched in order to determine the number of horses that can be grazed per hectare, and to predict seasonal shortfalls in the supply of pasture DM. An example is illustrated in Figure 1 based on an annual mean pasture production of 11,500 kg DM/ha and a seasonal pattern of growth (kg DM/ha/day) of March 30, April 25, May 17, June 14, July 14, August 25, September 40, October 53, November 60, December 45, January 30, and February 25. The daily DM requirements for lactating mares, weanlings, and yearlings were 13.6, 5.5, and 6.8 kg DM/day, respectively, to ensure adequate milk yields and good growth rates.

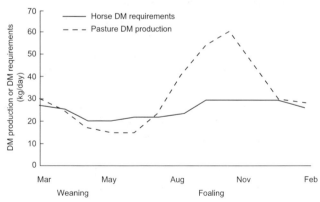

Figure 1. Relationship between daily pasture DM production and daily horse DM requirements. Stocking rate of 1.5 mares and their foals per hectare.

Foaling and mating occur in spring and weaning in autumn when pasture DM production is high, and therefore the horse's DM requirements are met. However, the pasture does not provide an adequate DM intake during mid to late pregnancy in winter (June-August), and supplementary feeding of pasture and legume hay is needed. Further, it is necessary that the surplus DM in spring and early summer (November-December) is conserved as good-quality hay for feeding during winter. The removal of the excess spring pasture also slows down the time period that the pasture becomes more mature, with its associated decrease in DM digestibility and digestible energy content. This is important in order to maintain pasture quality for lactating mares and their foals during the summer.

Feed Value of Pasture

The feed value of pasture for horses is determined by DM intake and its DM nutritive value, or chemical and mineral composition. Many factors such as the physiological state of the animal, its preferences, nutrient density, and environmental conditions can influence DM intakes, while other factors (e.g., pasture species, soil type, and fertilizer applications) can influence pasture chemical and mineral composition.

Determination of Dry Matter and Digestible Energy Intakes

The determination of the DM intakes of grazing animals is more difficult to measure than that for animals fed indoors, where the amounts of feed offered and refused can be accurately recorded. The technique to determine the DMI of grazing ruminants involves measuring the daily total fecal DM output, using indigestible markers such as chromium sesquioxide (Cr_2O_3), and dividing this by the indigestible fraction (1-digestibility) (Langlands, 1975). In many cases the digestibility of the pasture is determined using an in vitro technique.

In the case of the horse, the daily fecal DM outputs can be determined directly. Individual horses were placed behind electric fences on pasture areas of 50 m x 100 m, and each day all the fecal material was collected, weighed, and a subsample dried to determine the daily fecal DM output. The collection period was 8-9 days (Grace et al., 2002a). The indigestible fraction (1-digestibility) was determined immediately after the fecal collections by bringing at least 8 weanlings or yearlings indoors and placing them in sawdust-bedded loose boxes (3.5 m x 3.5 m). The digestibility study consisted of an eight-day preliminary period followed by a six-day collection period (Grace et al., 2002a; Grace et al., 2003). Each day the weanlings and yearlings were offered 50-60 kg of fresh pasture from the area they originally grazed, cut with a reciprocating mower to limit the damage to the fresh herbage, then packed in hay nets and fed as two meals (at 0800 and1730 h). All pasture not immediately fed was stored at 2-4° C to prevent deterioration of herbage quality. During the eight-day preliminary period all residual pasture and feces were collected and discarded. Water was available at all times. During the six-day collection period, the amounts of fresh pasture (50-60 kg) offered and the uneaten residual pasture were collected, weighed, and subsampled for DM determinations. The daily DM eaten was determined from the difference between the DM offered and the residual DM. Over the same period the feces were collected every hour, and the 24-hour fecal output was weighed and subsampled for DM determinations. Subsamples of pasture and feces were prepared for chemical and mineral analysis, as well as the determination of energy content.

A similar technique was used for the mares except they, with their foals, were placed in a bare 20 x 20 m corral fitted with a custom-made feeding station that ensured pasture was available to the mare, but not her foal. Each station consisted of a wall 1.2 m wide x 2.4 m high, a 1 m deep tray fitted to the wall 1.2 m from the ground, and a roof made of clear plastic sheeting to protect the cut pasture from the weather. The mares were offered 100-120 kg fresh pasture as two meals, while their foals were also provided with their own small amount of pasture not accessible to the mare (Grace et al., 2002b).

Dry Matter and Digestible Energy Intakes

The daily fecal DM output, DM digestibility, and pasture DE data used to calculate DM and DE intakes for pasture-fed horses in all our studies are summarized in Table 1 (Grace et al., 2002a,b; Grace et al., 2003).

The determined DE intakes of 146.9, 78.3, and 62.7 MJ DE/day for grazing mares, yearlings, and weanlings, respectively, are similar to the values of 134, 83, and 69 MJ DE/day recommended by the National Research Council (1989).

Table 1. Mean dry matter (DM) and digestible energy (DE) intakes of lactating mares, yearlings, and weanlings.

Parameter	Mare	Yearling	Weanling
Daily fecal DM output (kg/d)[1]	5.44	2.46	2.09
DM digestibility[2]	0.6	0.64	0.62
DM intake (kg/d)	13.6	6.8	5.5
DE of pasture (MJ/kg DM)[2]	10.8	11.5	11.4
DE intake (MJ DE/d)	146.9	78.2	62.7

[1]Determined in grazing horses.
[2]Determined in a subsequent indoor digestibility study.

Nutrient Value of Pasture

The nutritive value of a pasture is a reflection of its chemical and mineral composition.

Table 2. The chemical composition (g/kg DM) of pasture fed to mares, yearlings, and weanlings in the dry matter and digestible energy intake studies.

Nutrient	Spring Mare	Spring Yearling	Autumn Weanling
Crude protein	190	155	222
Soluble carbohydrate	112	71	72
Neutral detergent fiber	494	432	402
Acid detergent fiber	314	242	239
Lipid	25	28	33
DE content (MJ/kg DM)	10.8	11.5	11.4

CHEMICAL COMPOSITION

A summary of the mean crude protein, soluble carbohydrate, natural detergent fiber, acid detergent fiber, and lipid content (g/kgDM) of the pastures fed in the mare, yearling, and weanling intake studies (Grace et al., 2002a,b; Grace et al., Grace et al., 2003) is given in Table 2.

In general, the DE content of pasture is lower (11.2 v. 13.5 MJ/kg DM) and the crude protein is higher (190 v. 135 g/kg DM) than for grains.

There is a marked seasonal change in the chemical composition of pasture because as pasture plants mature, with head emergence and seed setting, the crude protein and soluble carbohydrate content decrease (30-50%), while the hemicellulose, cellulose, and lignin content (i.e., neutral and acid detergent fiber) increase (30-50%). This can result in about a 30% decrease in DM digestibility (Waghorn and Barry, 1987).

MINERAL COMPOSITION

The mineral content of pasture also shows a seasonal change, and this is illustrated in Table 3. The data presented are from the yearling study (Grace et al., 2002a).

Other factors influencing the mineral composition of pasture include pasture species, soil type, and fertilizer applications. In New Zealand some soils are low in Se and Co, and this is reflected in the need to supplement grazing livestock with Se and Co (vitamin B_{12}) in some areas (Grace, 1994).

A comparison of the daily mineral intakes of the pasture-fed horses in these studies and the mineral intakes recommended by the National Research Council (1989) and Duren (1996) would suggest that the intakes of Cu, Zn, Se, and Ca are not adequate to meet the daily requirements of horses (Table 4).

Table 3. Seasonal change in the mineral composition of pasture fed to yearlings (Grace et al., 2002a).

Month	Na	K	Ca	P	Mg	S	Cu	Fe	Mn	Zn	Se
	(g/kg DM)						(mg/kg DM)				
Aug	2.0	38.5	3.4	4.0	2.0	3.7	8.9	145	71	32	0.02
Sep	2.6	43.6	3.7	4.6	2.1	3.5	10.4	174	77	29	0.01
Oct	2.4	39.8	3.5	4.6	2.1	3.6	8.3	267	94	32	0.01
Nov	3.2	34.4	3.7	3.1	1.9	2.8	7.2	168	68	25	0.01
Dec	2.0	22.3	3.3	2.6	1.7	2.6	7.0	124	79	25	0.02
Jan	3.1	28.5	3.9	2.5	2.4	2.3	7.0	129	70	24	0.02
Feb	1.2	22.5	3.6	2.3	2.4	2.6	6.6	231	119	29	0.02

Table 4. Mineral intakes of New Zealand Thoroughbred yearlings, averaging 350-kg live weight and gaining 0.6 kg/day compared with recommended National Research Council (1989) dietary mineral intakes.

	Pasture-fed yearling[1]	National Research Council
Macroelements (g/day)		
Ca	24.5	34.0
P	24.0	19.0
Na	16.8	7.0
K	232.0	18.2
Mg	14.8	6.0
Microelements (mg/day)		
Cu	56	70
Zn	198	280
Mn	588	280
Fe	1249	350
Se	0.11	0.7

[1]Grace et al., 2002a.

Animal Performance

The most effective and informative approach used to detect a mineral deficiency is to compare animal performance such as growth, changes in tissue mineral concentrations, or the appearance and absence of clinical signs in mineral supplemented and unsupplemented control horses managed under the same conditions.

GROWTH

During all DM and DE studies the weanlings and yearlings were weighed at about monthly intervals, while the foals of the lactating mares were weighed weekly for about 8 weeks, and then at about monthly intervals. The observed growth rates were 0.70 kg/day for 280-kg weanlings and 0.60 kg/day for 350-kg yearlings fed only pasture. These growth rates were similar to those observed in North America (Hintz et al., 1979; Pagan, 1998). Likewise, the daily milk yields of the mares were satisfactory as the mean growth rate of their foals was 1.34 kg/day.

TISSUE MINERAL COMPOSITION

In the yearling grazing study (7 horses/group), one group was given extra Cu (185.7 v 55.7 mg/day), Zn (547.7 v 197.7 mg/day), Se (2.11 v 0.11 mg/day), P (34.0 v 24.0 g/day), and Ca (44.5 v 24.0 g/day), while the other group was unsupplemented. No mineral supplement treatment differences were observed in mean serum Cu (1.5 mg/L [23.8 μmol/L]), serum Zn (0.6 mg/L [9.2 μmol/L]), and liver Cu concentrations (20.2 mg/kg DM). Further, as there were no significant differences in animal growth rates between supplemented and unsupplemented horses, and the above tissue Cu and Zn values were within the normally expected ranges for horses (Frape, 1998), it was concluded that Cu and Zn intakes of the pasture-fed horses were adequate.

Table 5. Effect of Cu, Zn, and Se supplementation of young horses for 205 days on the liver Cu, serum Cu, serum Zn, and blood Se concentrations.

	Liver Cu mg/kg DM	Serum Cu mg/L	Serum Zn mg/L	Blood Se μg/L
Day 1				
Unsupplemented[1]	13.6 ± 2.5	1.6 ± 0.2	0.51 ± 0.03	41.3 ± 2.8
Supplemented	12.4 ± 0.8	1.7 ± 0.1	0.53 ± 0.04	41.6 ± 3.0
Day 150				
Unsupplemented	22.0 ± 2.8	1.5 ± 0.2	0.62 ± 0.05	40.5 ± 2.8[a]
Supplemented	18.2 ± 1.1	1.7 ± 0.2	0.61 ± 0.04	218.0 ± 8.3
Day 200				
Unsupplemented[1]	19.5 ± 2.7	1.4 ± 0.1	0.43 ± 0.01	73.6 ± 2.1[a]
Supplemented	19.4 ± 2.5	1.4 ± 0.1	0.47 ± 0.02	267.0 ± 8.5

[a]Unsupplemented and supplemented significantly different (p < 0.001).
[1]The pasture provided 55.7, 197.7, and 0.11 mg/day Cu, Zn, and Se, respectively. The supplement provided an extra 130, 350, and 2 mg/day of Cu, Zn, and Se, respectively.

In contrast, Se supplementation, in this study, resulted in the blood Se concentrations being increased from 40.5 to >218 µg/L (500 to >2760 nmol/L) but had no significant effect on the growth rates of the yearlings (0.6 v 0.59 kg/day) over the 205 days of the trial (Grace et al., 2002a). However, the Se status of the unsupplemented yearlings was considered to be too low, as the accepted blood Se concentration range is 1600-3200 nmol/L (Caple et al., 1991) and given that white muscle disease has been observed in foals from mares with blood Se concentrations <27 µg/L (<350 nmol/L) (Caple et al., 1978). Therefore, horses grazing New Zealand pastures containing 0.01-0.05 mg Se/kg DM should be supplemented with Se to ensure that their Se status is always adequate. The National Research Council (1989) dietary Se requirement for horses is 0.1 mg Se/kg DM.

CLINICAL SIGNS

In the yearling mineral supplementation study (Grace et al., 2002a), physitis was observed and the condition was scored by the same observer in December, January, and February. The medial and lateral aspects of the distal radial physis were scored separately by the observer standing directly in front of the standing horse. Score 0 was considered normal, having no significant prominence in the region of the distal radial physis, 1 indicated some prominence, 2 indicated distinct enlargement, and 3 indicated gross enlargement. Medial and lateral scores were combined to give an overall score. The limbs were palpated to determine if pain in the radial physical area was present or not. The mineral supplementation had no significant effect on the condition while the mean physis scores (of unsupplemented and supplemented horses) were 2.6, 5.1, and 3.2 for December, January, and February, respectively. These reflected a mild to moderate distal radial physical swelling which was not associated with any painful response to palpation. In this study the above condition should be regarded as a physiological "normal," probably a growth-related physical prominence which resolved completely without treatment.

Overseas studies have reported a decrease in the incidence of developmental orthopedic disease (DOD) lesions when the dietary Cu was increased to 25 mg Cu/kg DM (Knight et al., 1990; Hurtig et al., 1993). The dietary Cu requirement recommended by the National Research Council (1989) is 10 mg/kg DM. The effect of Cu status on the evidence of bone and cartilage lesions was investigated in 21 Thoroughbred foals, where foals and their dams grazed pasture containing 4.4-8.6 mg Cu/kg DM (Pearce et al., 1998). Four treatment groups were set up by randomly allocating mares and their foals to either Cu-supplemented (0.5 mg Cu/kg live weight; equivalent to pasture containing 25 mg Cu/kg DM) or unsupplemented control groups. The design allowed the effect of Cu supplementation of the mare and foal to be examined independently. Mare Cu supplementation increased foal liver Cu concentrations (253.9 v 423.8 mg/kg DM). At euthanasia at 150 days of age, a detailed examination was made of all limb and cervical spine articulations, as well as an examination of the physes from the proximal humerus, proximal and distal radius and tibia, distal femur, third metatarsus, and third metacarpus. Articular cartilage lesions were minor in all foals, with no evidence of clinical DOD in vivo, with the exception of minor radiographic changes assessed at postmortem. Copper supplementation of the foals had no effect on any of the bone and cartilage parameters. Copper supplementation of the mares did not abolish DOD in growing foals in the New Zealand pastoral situation, emphasizing the likely multifactorial nature of this condition (Pearce et al., 1998).

To determine whether New Zealand pastures provide an adequate Ca intake to ensure optimum bone growth and development in weanlings, a Ca supplementation trial was carried out (Grace et al., 2003). Seventeen weanlings were randomly divided into three groups and fed pasture containing 3.5 g Ca/kg DM, and fed none or calcium carbonate ($CaCO_3$) supplement for 84 days. Group 1 was on a low-Ca diet (3.5 g/kg DM); Group 2 medium-Ca diet (6.3 g/kg DM), and Group 3 high-Ca diet (12.0 g/kg DM). Just before and after Ca supplementation, the horses were anesthetized and the left radius, third metacarpus, and first phalanx were scanned using a peripheral quantitative computed tomography scanner to determine cortical Ca content, cortical density, cortical area, periosteal circumference, and bone strength (strain stress index). A significant increase in bone strength was observed with time, but the changes in bone strength were not associated with increased Ca intakes, showing that the pasture provided an adequate Ca intake.

In summary, the various mineral supplementation studies to date show that New Zealand pastures (Table 3) with the exception of Se, provide adequate intakes of minerals including Ca, P, Cu, and Zn to ensure optimum growth and development in young horses, as well as satisfactory milk yields in mares.

Other Considerations

Pastures must be well managed to maintain their feed value, because once they become long and mature, various plant components change and feed value of the pasture decreases. For example, crude protein and soluble sugars decrease, while cellulose, hemicellulose, and lignin increase, and this is associated with a decrease in DM digestibility (Waghorn and Barry, 1987). Horses have a preference for prairie grass and ryegrasses compared with timothy, tall fescue, and white clover (Hunt, 1994). The selective grazing behavior of horses results in uneaten pasture plants eventually becoming the dominant species in the sward, thereby greatly reducing the value of the pasture for horses. Grazing these pastures with sheep and cattle helps to maintain the sward at an even height, and grass species that are unpalatable to horses do not become dominant. Soil fertility must be maintained with regular applications of fertilizer, and pastures may have to be resown every 4-5 years to maintain the presence of grass and clover species that are palatable and are of high nutritive value.

Acknowledgements

To Professor Elwyn Firth, Drs. Simon Pearce, Chris Rogers, Erica Gee, and Peter Fennessy, and Ms. Hilary Shaw for their assistance with the various studies.

References

Caple, I.W. 1991. Disorders of mineral nutrition in horses in Australia. In: Equine Nutrition. p. 3-12. Nutrition Society of Australia and Post Graduate Committee in Veterinary Science, University of Sydney.

Caple, I.W., S.J.A. Edwards, W.M. Forsyth, P. Whiteley, R.H. Selth, and L.J. Fulton. 1978. Blood glutathione peroxidase activity in horses in relation to muscular dystrophy and selenium nutrition. Aust. Vet. J. 54:57-60.

Caradus, J.R., R.J.M. Hay, and D.R. Woodfield. 1996. The positioning of white clover cultivars in New Zealand. In: Woodfield, D.R. (Ed). White clover: New Zealand's Competitive Edge. Proceedings of a joint symposium between Agronomy Society of New Zealand and New Zealand Grassland Association. Lincoln University, New Zealand. p. 45-50.

Clark, D.A., and R.W. Brougham. 1979. Feed intake of grazing Friesian bulls. Proc. NZ Soc. Anim. Prod. 39:265-274.

Duren, S. 1996. Delivering essential nutrients to young, growing horses. In: Focus on Equine Nutrition: Mineral Requirements and Management of the Growing Horse. p. 23-52. Kentucky Equine Research Inc., Versailles.

Frape, D. 1998. Equine Nutrition and Feeding. (2nd Ed.). Blackwell Science, London. p. 43-71.

Grace, N.D. 1994. Managing trace element deficiencies. New Zealand Pastoral Agriculture Research Institute, Palmerston North.

Grace, N.D., E.K. Gee, E.C. Firth, and H.L. Shaw. 2002a. Digestible energy intake, dry matter digestibility and mineral status of grazing New Zealand Thoroughbred yearlings. NZ Vet. J. 50:63-69.

Grace, N.D., H.L. Shaw, E.K. Gee, and E.C. Firth. 2002b. Determination of the digestible energy intake and apparent absorption of macroelements in pasture-fed lactating Thoroughbred mares. NZ Vet. J. 50:182-185.

Grace, N.D., C.W. Rogers, E.C. Firth, T.L. Faram, and H.L. Shaw. 2003. Digestible energy intake, dry matter digestibility and effect of increased calcium intake on bone parameters of grazing Thoroughbred weanlings in New Zealand. NZ Vet. J. (In press).

Hintz, H.F., R. Hintz, and L.D. van Vleck. 1979. Growth rate of Thoroughbreds: Effect of age of dam, year and month of birth and sex of foal. J. Anim. Sci. 48:480-487.

Hunt, W.F. 1994. Pastures for Horses. New Zealand Equine Research Foundation, Palmerston North.

Hurtig, M.B., S.L. Green, H. Dobson, Y. Mikuni-Takagaki, and J. Choi. 1993. Correlative study of defective cartilage and bone growth in foals fed a low-copper diet. Eq. Vet. J. Supp. 16:66-73.

Knight, D.A, S.E. Weisbrode, L.M. Schmall, S.M. Reed, A.A. Gabel, L.R. Bramlage, and W.I. Tyznik. 1990. The effects of copper supplementation on the prevalence of cartilage lesions in foals. Eq. Vet. J. 22:426-432.

Korte, C.J., A.C.P. Chu, and T.R.O. Field. 1987. Pasture production. In: A.M. Nicol (Ed.) Livestock Feeding on Pasture. NZ Soc. Anim. Prod. Occ. Pub. No. 10:7-20.

Langlands, J.P. 1975. Techniques for estimating nutrient intake and its utilization by grazing ruminants. In: I.W. McDonald and A.C.I. Warner (Eds.) Digestion and Metabolism in the Ruminant. p. 320-322. The University of New England Publishing Unit, Armidale, Australia.

Milligan, K.E., I.M. Brookes, and K.F. Thompson. 1987. Feed planning on pasture. In: A.M. Nicol (Ed.) Livestock Feeding on Pasture. NZ Soc. Anim. Prod. Occ. Pub. No. 10:75-88.

National Research Council. 1989. Nutrient Requirements of Horses. National Academy Press, Washington DC.

Pagan, J.D. 1998. A summary of growth rates of Thoroughbreds in Kentucky. In: J.D. Pagan (Ed.) Advances in Equine Nutrition. p. 449-455. Kentucky Equine Research Incorporated, Nottingham University Press, Nottingham.

Pearce, S.G, E.C. Firth, N.D. Grace, and P.F. Fennessy. 1998. Effect of copper supplementation on the evidence of developmental orthopaedic disease in pasture-fed New Zealand Thoroughbreds. Eq. Vet. J. 30:211-218.

Roberts, A.H.C., J.D. Morton, M.B. O'Connor, and D.C. Edmeades. 1996. Building a solid foundation for pasture production in Northland: P, K, S and lime requirements. Proc. NZ Grassland Assoc. 57:119-126.

Tapper, B.A., and G.C.M. Latch. 1999. Selection against toxin production in endophyte-infected perennial ryegrass. In: D.R. Woodfield and C. Matthew (Eds.) Ryegrass Endophyte: An Essential New Zealand Symbiosis. Proc. NZ Grassland Assoc. Symposium, Napier, New Zealand.

Ulyatt, M.J. 1971. Studies on the causes of the differences in pasture quality between perennial ryegrass, short rotation ryegrass, and white clover. NZ J. Agr. Res. 14:352-367.

Waghorn, G.C., and T.N. Barry. 1987. Pasture as a nutrient source. In: A.M. Nicol (Ed.) Livestock Feeding on Pasture. NZ Soc. Anim. Prod. Occ. Pub. No 10:21-37.

NUTRITION AND THE EQUINE FOOT

PETER HUNTINGTON[1] AND CHRIS POLLITT[2]
[1]*Kentucky Equine Research Australasia*
[2]*Australian Equine Laminitis Research Unit, Queensland, Australia*

Many performance and racehorses cannot perform to their potential because of hoof problems. The old adage "no hoof, no horse" still applies today and this article examines some of the nutritional factors that impact the hoof. There are many factors that can influence development of the hoof, and this article will discuss some of these variables that can aid the search for increased hoof growth and improved hoof quality. Unfortunately, rapid hoof wall growth may not be synonymous with top hoof quality.

Despite recent advances in the prevention or treatment of equine disease, laminitis remains high on the list of potentially crippling or life-threatening diseases. The second part of the article will summarize new research findings in the cause, pathogenesis, prevention, and treatment of laminitis.

Factors Affecting Hoof Growth

Hoof growth is influenced by several factors. These include age, breed, genetics, metabolic rate, exercise, external temperature, environmental moisture, illness, trimming, and shoeing. Nutritional influences include energy intake, protein and amino acid intake and metabolism, minerals such as zinc and calcium, and vitamins such as biotin and vitamin A.

Moisture has an influence on both hoof growth and strength of hoof horn. Growth is often increased in wet conditions, and this could be a primary effect from increased hoof moisture or a secondary effect of greater pasture growth and energy intake. However, it has been demonstrated that poor-quality, softer horn has a higher water content (Coenen and Spitzlei, 1997). Butler and Hintz (1977) showed that hoof moisture in growing ponies dropped from 29% at the coronary border to 27% at the tip of the toe, and this was associated with, but not necessarily responsible for, a 30% increase in hoof strength between the two areas.

Energy Intake

When faced with bad feet, the first thing to consider when evaluating a feed program is total feed (energy) intake. Meeting energy requirements may be the first and most important step in ensuring hoof growth and integrity. A horse in negative energy balance will utilize protein in the diet or body to make up energy needs for maintenance or growth. This may create a secondary protein or amino acid deficiency.

Butler and Hintz (1977) showed that hoof wall growth was 50% greater in growing ponies in positive energy balance than in ponies on restricted diets with reduced body growth rate. But the restriction in energy, protein, and mineral intake did not reduce hoof wall strength. It is a common observation that when horses gain weight on lush spring grass they also grow hoof faster.

Hoof tissue contains about 3-6% fat to bind some of the cells together and to help repel water. Recent research has shown that increasing the dietary intake of fat has little effect on hoof growth rate or strength (Lewis, 1995; Ott and Johnson, 2002), but fat can be a valuable addition to the diet for other reasons such as maintaining positive energy balance or coat conditioning.

Protein and Amino Acids

The hoof wall is about 93% protein on a dry matter basis. Because of the composition of the hoof wall, most of the commercially available hoof supplements contain methionine. However, methionine is just one of the amino acids contained in the protein of the hoof, and deficiencies of any essential amino acid can be as detrimental as a deficiency of methionine. Hoof contains high levels of cystine, arginine, leucine, lysine, proline, serine, glycine, and valine, and lower levels of methionine, phenylalanine, and histidine (Samata and Matsuda 1988; Coenen and Spitzlei, 1997). Coenen and Spitzlei compared the amino acid content of normal hoof and horn of poor quality. They found a linear correlation between cystine content and hardness in normal horn but not in poor-quality horn. The protein of normal horn contained higher levels of threonine, phenylalanine, and proline and lower levels of arginine than poor-quality horn.

Ekfalck et al. (1990) showed there was a clear difference between the distribution of the two sulfur-bearing amino acids in the keratinizing epidermis of the hoof. Cystine was located mainly in keratinocytes of the keratogenous zone in the matrix and in the nucleated keratinocytes that formed the incompletely keratinized basal part of the primary epidermal laminae and covered the lateral surface of the outer, fully keratinized part of those laminae. Methionine was located primarily in the stratum basale and in the stratum spinosum of the matrix and in the secondary epidermal laminae of the laminar layer. The pathway that converts methionine to cysteine is thought to be imperative in the production of quality hoof.

Protein-deficient diets lead to reduced hoof growth and splitting and cracking of the hoof (Lewis, 1995). However, Richardson and Ott (1977) looked at the influence of amino acid intake and found that diets intended to support more rapid growth of young horses did not necessarily maximize hoof growth. They showed that brewer's dried grains, a protein source with a lysine content low enough to restrict growth in young horses, led to significantly increased hoof growth compared to diets based on soybean meal. In another study at the University of Florida, 39 Thoroughbred and Quarter Horse yearlings were used in two 112-day experiments to determine the effect of lysine and threonine supplementation on growth and development (Graham et al., 1994). The addition of 0.2% lysine to a basal diet led to an increase in growth, and this effect was enhanced by an extra 0.1% threonine; however, no changes were seen in hoof growth due to diet. This suggests that the amino acid needs for body growth and hoof growth are different.

Gelatin is a protein source used to treat fingernail growth abnormalities in man. Research has revealed that gelatin supplementation has no influence on hoof growth or quality. Butler and Hintz (1977) also examined the effects of gelatin in the diet of growing ponies and found no impact on hoof growth or quality. Goodspeed et al. (1970) reported that the addition of 114 g of gelatin per day added to a growing ration reduced hoof specific gravity but had little effect on hoof tensile strength.

Minerals

Current thinking on the relationship of diet and hoof integrity puts too much emphasis on zinc and too little emphasis on the other minerals necessary for metabolism. The health of the foot is an extension of the health of the horse, and if mineral deficiencies compromise horse health in general, then the health of the foot is going to be negatively impacted as well. There is justification for looking specifically at zinc when trying to put together the "hoof healthy" diet. Zinc is involved in the health and integrity of hair, skin, and hoof, but adding additional zinc to a diet that is already adequate in zinc is not going to automatically result in any dramatic increases in hoof quality or growth rate.

Coenen and Spitzlei (1997) have shown that 25 horses with poor horn quality have lower blood and hoof zinc levels than 38 horses with normal feet. There was no difference in the levels of copper and selenium in the same horses. This may be due to individual zinc absorption, metabolism, or retention abnormalities. The same study showed that supplementation with 300-500 mg zinc per day led to an increase in the zinc content of the horn. Butler and Hintz (1977) found that limit-fed ponies with reduced hoof growth had significantly higher zinc levels in hoof horn, but there was no correlation with strength or elasticity. A recent study in Japan reported that horses consuming diets low in zinc and copper were more likely to have white line disease than horses that were supplemented with higher levels of these trace minerals (Hihami, 1999). The form of zinc in the diet may have some relevance to the poor-footed horse as chelated zinc may produce results when inorganic zinc does not work. Chelated zinc contains zinc bound to an animo acid, and the zinc is absorbed with the protein, which potentially enhances absorption. Chelated zinc is used widely in dairy cattle to improve hoof strength, and most hoof supplements contain chelated zinc.

Ott and Johnson (2001) examined the effect of mineral source on growth and hoof development of yearling horses. Fifteen yearlings were fed one of two diets for 112 days. Diet A provided NRC or higher levels of all of the nutrients with trace minerals provided in an inorganic form. Diet B provided the same amount of each mineral except that supplementary zinc, manganese, and copper were added as proteinates. Trace mineral source had no effect on feed intake, nutrient intake, or feed efficiency. Growth of the yearlings was generally not influenced by source of mineral except for hip height, which was greater for the proteinate-supplemented yearlings. Hoof growth was significantly greater for colts when compared to fillies and for proteinated minerals compared to inorganic minerals. The increase in hoof growth due to the proteinated minerals was about 4%. Breaking strength of the hoof was greater for Quarter Horses than Thoroughbreds but was not influenced by sex or feeding.

In another study, Siciliano et al. (2001) compared supplementation with inorganic and organic sources of manganese, zinc, and copper in adult mares where 50% of the trace mineral needs were supplied by chelated minerals. No differences in hoof growth rate, hoof hardness, and tensile strength were detected. Hoof wall trace mineral content was not influenced by the diets. The differences between these two variable results may be due to the age of the animals or the amount of chelated minerals used. Growing animals are likely to exhibit a greater demand for nutrients needed for growth and may not have the option of providing extra minerals for hoof development.

Although calcium is only present at 300-350 mg/kg hoof wall, it is involved in creating the sulfur cross-links between the hoof proteins and in the cohesion of cells to each other. Kempson (1987) reported that 31 of 33 horses with brittle feet had a loss of the tubular structure in the stratum medium and internum. Twenty of these horses had failed to respond to biotin supplementation, but the majority showed an improvement when the protein and calcium intakes were increased. These horses were reported to be on diets of oats or bran and chaff or grass hay. Supplementation with lucerne supplied extra calcium and boosted protein and amino acid intake, so the exact cause of the improvement cannot be determined. If calcium levels in the diet are low, then supplying extra calcium may positively impact hoof quality as well as bone quality.

Selenium is the mineral with the narrowest safety margin between the requirement and toxic levels. Signs of toxicity include loss of hair, lameness, hoof rings and cracks, and separation of hoof walls (Lewis, 1995). This can be due to pastures that accumulate selenium such as those found in areas of the western United States or central Queensland. There are also reports of selenium toxicity due to inadvertent overdoses from premixes in feed in England or oral and injectable supplements in New Zealand.

Biotin

Most of the emphasis on research on hoof growth and hoof wall quality has involved the vitamin biotin. It is thought that the normal horse has a biotin requirement of 1-2 mg per day, and this can be supplied in certain feedstuffs as a component of commercial vitamin and mineral premixes or by intestinal synthesis by micro-organisms in the large intestine. Biotin is a cofactor in a number of enzyme systems. In other animals, chronic biotin deficiencies lead to lesions of the skin and other keratinized structures, and supplementary biotin was first used in pigs to treat hoof problems. Studies have shown that supplemental biotin at levels of 15-20 mg per day has had positive effects on hoof quality in some horses and may increase hoof growth but does not assist all horses. Biotin is the most expensive vitamin to supplement and patience is necessary as it takes 9-12 months to grow an entire new hoof.

Comben et al. (1984) published one of the first case studies after having extrapolated the dose of biotin from the breeding sow. They used 15 mg for Thoroughbreds and 15-30 mg for draft horses with poorly shaped hooves, cracks in the hoof wall, and soft and crumbling horn. After five months of treatment, the hoof horn was thicker and harder, and improvement continued when the horses were examined another four months later. Shoeing was easier and shoes lasted longer as there was more strong horn onto which the shoe could be nailed.

Josseck et al. (1995) reported a controlled, double-blind study in which 42 600-700-kg Lipizzaner stallions with poor-quality hooves were treated with 20 mg biotin per day for over three years. Assessments of hoof quality were made and compared to control horses. This study showed that it took six months for appreciable differences between treated and control horses and nine months to achieve a statistically significant difference. Some horses did not improve until more than one year after treatment began, but hoof horn quality continued to improve as the period extended beyond 18 months. Biotin treatment reduced the incidence and severity of hoof horn defects, increased tensile strength, and improved condition of the white line. Significant changes in tensile strength were not seen until 33 months after treatment began. Treated horses had plasma biotin levels of over 1000 ng/ml compared to a mean level of 350 ng/ml in untreated horses. In this experiment, however, biotin supplementation did not increase hoof growth rate. Zenker et al. (1995) reported histological findings from the Lipizzaner study and found a significant reduction in the horn abnormalities in treated horses only after 19 months of treatment. The major pathological changes were microcracks in the transition from the middle to the inner zone of coronary horn and separation of the sole from the coronary horn in the white line.

Buffa et al. (1992) gave differing doses of biotin to horses and compared the effect on hoof growth rate and hardness in groups of eight horses. Horses were treated for 10 months with a placebo, 7.5 mg per day, 15 mg per day, or 15 mg daily in alternate months. All treatment groups had significantly greater hoof growth and hardness than control horses, with best results in the horses getting 15 mg per day. The increase in hardness was more apparent at the toe and quarters than at the heel. Seasonal influences were seen in hoof hardness, and all hooves were harder in the dry season.

Geyer and Schulze (1994) conducted a long-term study on the influence of dietary biotin in horses with brittle hoof horn and chipped hooves. The study was performed over periods from one to six years. Ninety-seven horses received 5 mg of biotin per 100 to 150 kg of body weight daily; 11 horses were not supplemented with biotin and served as controls. The hooves of all horses were evaluated macroscopically every three to four months and horn specimens of the proximal wall were examined histologically and physically in 25 horses. The hoof horn condition of the biotin-supplemented horses improved after eight to 15 months of supplementation, but the hoof horn condition of most control horses remained constant throughout the study. The hoof horn condition deteriorated in seven of 10 horses after biotin supplementation was reduced or terminated. The horn growth rate of treated horses and of control horses was the same.

Reilly et al. (1998) used a higher dose rate of biotin in a controlled feeding trial. They examined the effect of 0.12 mg/kg body weight on growth and growth rate of the hooves of eight paired ponies. After five months, treated ponies had a significantly faster mean hoof growth at the midline of 35.34 mm, compared to control animals' 30.69 mm. Comparison of regression analysis also showed that biotin supplementation produced a significantly higher growth rate of hoof horn in this trial. Treatment animals had a 15% higher growth rate of hoof horn and 15% more hoof growth at the midline. The positive effect on hoof growth seen in this study may be due to the higher dose of biotin used, which equates to 60 mg per day in a 500-kg Thoroughbred horse.

There is evidence that adequate amounts of vitamin A in the diet may be important in promoting normal hoof wall growth. Vitamin A is involved in maintaining epithelial integrity and may have an important role in cell maturation and differentiation in the foot. Vitamin A is present in green grass, new hay, commercial feeds, and supplements. Deficiencies are unlikely given that vitamin A is present in many feeds and is stored in the body for some time but can occur in dry conditions or in horses on an unsupplemented diet.

The Bottom Line on Improving Hoof

Even though most poor feet are a result of genetic factors and bad mechanics, there is a piece of the riddle that can be solved with good nutrition. Use a feed that is designed for the class of horse you are feeding, and feed enough of it to get the desired body condition. Look for feeds that are balanced for macro- and microminerals. Zinc and calcium are critical for hoof growth and strength. Apart from special feed concentrates which are designed to be fed with oats, commercial feeds should not be cut with oats as this wrecks the nutrient balance the nutritionist has attempted to achieve. In addition to a good feed, emphasis should be placed on high-quality hay such as lucerne (alfalfa). Sometimes it is necessary to restrict energy intake in specific diets. In these cases, it is important to make sure requirements for the other nutrients are met.

If everything is being done from nutritional and farriery (shoeing/trimming/ hoof dressing) angles and hoof quality is still poor, it is worth experimenting with supplemental biotin, methionine, and zinc. Unfortunately, there is no quick fix and maintaining a good foot on a horse is a combined result of good farriery, good nutrition, good health care, and selecting for horses that genetically have healthy hooves.

Laminitis

Laminitis is the most serious disease of the equine foot and causes pathological changes in anatomy that lead to long-lasting, crippling changes in function. It is the second biggest killer of horses after colic. In the National Animal Health Monitoring System (NAHMS) report for the year 2000 in the United States, 13% of all horse operations (excluding racetracks) had a horse with laminitis in the previous year and 4.7% of these animals died or were euthanatized. More horses were affected by laminitis in spring and summer than in winter. Grazing lush pasture and grain overload was the cause of 50% of the laminitis cases reported. The report concluded that proper grazing and feed management could prevent approximately 50% of laminitis cases. Grass founder is thus a major cause of laminitis in the United States, and the same is probably true of most temperate regions of the world. There is anecdotal evidence that selective breeding for high fructan concentration in pastures designed for ruminants is increasing the incidence of grass founder in horses in the United States (Watts, 2001) At the Australian Equine Laminitis Research Unit, we have been studying how fructan from plants induces laminitis, discovering how and when pasture species produce dangerous levels of fructan, and pinpointing which pasture species produce the most fructan.

Laminitis has a developmental phase, during which lamellar separation is triggered. This precedes the appearance of the foot pain of laminitis (Moore et al., 1989). The developmental period lasts 40-48 hours in the case of laminitis caused by excessive ingestion of nonstructural carbohydrates such as starch or fructan. Sometimes no clinical developmental phase can be recognized, and the horse or pony is discovered in the acute phase of laminitis with no apparent ill health or inciting problem occurring beforehand. This appears to be the case with grass founder or laminitis resulting from the ingestion of pasture. Recently, Longland and Cairns (1998), researching the metabolism of grass in Great Britain, have shown that under certain climate conditions, fructan may reach very high concentrations in the stem of grass (<50% DM).

Fructan in Pasture

Trials on pasture consumption by horses in southeast Queensland (McMeniman, 2000) showed that during one warm, wet summer month pasture intake went from 5 kg/day to 15 kg/day. If fructan concentration during that month was 30%, then an intake of 3-4 kg fructan/horse/day was theoretically possible. However, none of the horses developed any health problems, so fructan accumulation was probably not occurring. If consumption of 3-4 kg of pasture fructan had occurred, laminitis was likely as dosing horses with 3-4 kg of pure commercial grade fructan (extracted from plants) causes experimental induction of laminitis almost without fail. The slower rate of intake of fructan from pasture may explain the difference between field intake from pasture and experimental boluses by stomach tube.

Horses and other herbivores in general are quite selective about what they eat, and there is a positive correlation between total nonstructural carbohydrate (TNC) content and plant selection. In other words, if one pasture species is in a sugar accumulation phase it will be sought out and consumed (Mayland et al., 2000).

Domestic horses encounter fertilized, irrigated, monocultured pastures across all seasons and may have little choice in what they consume. Under certain and yet ill-defined circumstances, fructans are produced by such grasses and are consumed by horses in high enough quantities to cause laminitis. Although starch is the major carbohydrate (CHO) contained in the seeds of pasture species, for much of the growing season it forms only a minor component of the total reserve of CHO within the plant. Prior to flowering, the leaves, stems, and tips of grasses accumulate a mixture of sucrose (glucose and fructose) and polymers of fructose (fructans), often to extremely high concentrations. Fructans function as reserve carbohydrates and are stored at different sites within the plant. A range of different internal and external factors influences patterns of fructan synthesis and storage. During flower development, fructan accumulation is high and can reach 50% of dry matter (Pollock and Cairns, 1991). Fructan concentration falls to insignificance when seed formation is complete and when drought and summer dieback occurs. With the advent of cooler, moister conditions, however, the formation of vegetative tillers occurs, and these are high in fructan. There is sound experimental evidence that chilling grass in the face of prolonged periods of radiant light stimulates a dramatic increase in fructan production (Pollock and Cairns, 1991). This is explained by photosynthesis driving sugar production (stored as fructan) while a reduction in the demand for carbon (less growth and metabolism) occurs because of chilling. Total tissue CHO content can reach 60-70% DM with up to 50% of this as fructan. It seems likely that horse pastures exposed to low nocturnal ground temperature and bright sunny days, as occurs in spring and autumn in most temperate regions, could accumulate dangerously high fructan levels, sufficient to trigger laminitis.

Pathophysiology of Laminitis

Inulin is a term applied to a heterogeneous blend of fructose polymers found widely distributed in nature as plant storage carbohydrates. Oligofructose is a subgroup of inulin, consisting of polymers with a degree of polymerization (DP) less than or equal to 10 (Niness, 1999). Inulin and oligofructose are fructans extracted on a commercial basis from the chicory root. Native chicory inulin has an average DP of 10 to 20, whereas oligofructose contains chains of DP of 2 to 10, with an average DP of 4 (Flamm et al., 2001). Inulin and oligofructose are not digested in the upper part of the gastrointestinal tract nor are they absorbed and metabolized in the glycolytic pathway or directly stored as glycogen. None of the molecules of fructose and glucose that form inulin and oligofructose appear in portal blood. They do not lead to a rise in serum glucose or stimulate insulin secretion. These materials are fermented by the microflora of the colon where they stimulate the growth of intestinal bifidobacteria. This fermentation produces D-lactate and a rapid drop in pH in the large intestine.

Enzymes capable of destroying key components of the hoof lamellar attachment apparatus (Pollitt and Daradka, 1998) have been isolated from normal lamellar tissues and in increased quantities from lamellar tissues affected by laminitis (Pollitt et al., 1998). The enzymes are metalloproteinase-2 and metalloproteinase-9 (MMP-2 and MMP-9). Lamellar tissues affected by laminitis upregulate their MMP gene (Kyaw-Tanner and Pollitt, unpublished), and increased amounts of MMP, in its active form, are found in laminitis affected tissues (Pollitt et al., 1998). Our evidence suggests that laminitis is triggered as increasing quantities of microbial substances manufactured in the large bowel from excess carbohydrate substrate are delivered to lamellar tissues via a vasodilated foot circulation (Pollitt and Davies, 1998). Testing a wide range of putative laminitis trigger factors (e.g., cytokines, eicosanoids, gram-negative bacterial endotoxins) with the in vitro laminitis model developed at the Australian Equine Laminitis Research Unit (AELRU), only the supernatants of cultured hindgut bacteria readily induced in vitro laminitis via the MMP activation pathway (Mungall et al., 2001).

Key pathologic changes include loss of cellular shape of the secondary epidermal lamellae and loss of attachment of the basement membrane of the lamellae, which is then lysed by MMP. The basement membrane is the key structure bridging the epidermis of the hoof to the connective tissue of the third phalanx, so it follows that the loss and disorganization of basement membrane leads to the failure of hoof anatomy seen in laminitis. Another component is loss of the lamellar capillaries, which may explain increased resistance to blood flow and the bounding digital pulse seen during early laminitis. The enzymatic theory of laminitis etiology challenges the existing view that laminitis develops from vascular changes to the circulation of the hoof. There is strong evidence that the foot circulation is vasodilated during the developmental phase of laminitis. This vasodilation is important to allow a high enough concentration of trigger factors to reach the lamellar tissues.

Laminitis Induction Model

When consumed by horses, oligofructose is rapidly fermented in the hindgut. If the amount of oligofructose exceeds 7.5 g/kg live weight a gastrointestinal disturbance is triggered that somehow leads to laminitis. In the presence of excess oligofructose substrate, gram-positive microorganisms proliferate preferentially and become the dominant microflora. This altered population of hindgut microflora liberates substances that compromise the normally impervious epithelial mucosal barrier lining the lumen of the large bowel and causes it to leak. Permeability of the equine hindgut during the developmental stage of carbohydrate-induced laminitis has been demonstrated (Weiss et al., 1998).

In preliminary trials, we have induced mild laminitis by administering a bolus of commercially available fructan (Raftilose) into the stomach of horses. A dose of 7.5 g/kg results in laminitis 48 hours later, half the amount of starch required in the starch-induction model to induce laminitis. Because fructan is a soluble sugar, the bolus was easily dissolved in water and could be administered as a single dose via stomach tube. The animals developed a fever and projectile, acid diarrhea just as they do with the starch-induction model, but *without colic*. By 36 hours, the animals had normal feces, their appetite had returned, and they were returning to metabolic normality, but they had laminitis confirmed by histopathology (Pollitt, 1996). Higher doses of fructan led to more severe clinical laminitis. This is a new, more humane model for laminitis induction unique to our laboratory. At 24 hours, the feces were very acid and contain no gram-negative organisms and consisted of gram-positive rods and diplococci, thus supporting our contention that it is gram-positive organisms, rapidly proliferating on excess substrate, that are responsible for laminitis.

Cryotherapy as a Preventative Agent

Cryotherapy is an effective first aid strategy for a range of conditions, particularly in human medicine (Swenson et al., 1996). Anecdotal evidence suggests that it may be useful during the developmental phase of laminitis; several early texts recommend placing horses in cold streams to cool the feet. Indeed, digital vasoconstriction during the developmental stage appeared to protect horses against laminitis (Pollitt and Davies, 1998) and led Pollitt (1999) to suggest that cryotherapy may be an effective strategy to prevent laminitis. Support for the concept of laminitis cryotherapy came from the scintographic studies of Worster et al. (2000) that showed digital soft tissue perfusion was significantly reduced after the application of cold water for 30 minutes.

Six Standardbred horses were dosed with 10 g/kg oligofructose using the method described previously by Pollitt and van Eps (2002). Each horse had one front limb placed in a rubber boot containing a mixture of 50% cubed ice and 50% water for the duration of the 48-hour experimental period. The boot was continually replenished with ice to maintain a level just below the carpus. Clinical observations, including surface temperature of the hind feet, were made every two hours. Internal hoof temperature of the forefeet was monitored continuously with data-logging devices attached to temperature probes inserted 8 mm into the hoof wall on the dorsal midline. Internal boot temperature and ambient temperature were also monitored constantly with data-logging devices. All horses were euthanatized at 48 hours, and stained sections of the hoof wall lamellae were examined with a light microscope. The severity of the laminitis was graded using the scoring system of Pollitt (1996).

Internal hoof temperature of the iced foot was maintained at less than 5° C at all times. During the last 12-15 hours of the experiment, hoof temperatures of the untreated feet exhibited a prolonged period of raised temperature consistent with digital vasodilation. All horses tolerated the ice boot well. Skin sensation and function of the iced limb was not impaired upon removal of the boot prior to euthanasia. All horses exhibited a degree of lameness associated with one or more of the untreated limbs. There was no significant histological evidence of laminitis in the treated hooves, but all of the untreated hooves had histological laminitis ranging from grade 1 (mild) to grade 3 (severe). Molecular biology performed on hoof tissue samples consistently showed normal expression of MMP2 RNA in the iced feet, with markedly increased expression in the nontreated feet.

Cryotherapy, when applied to one foot, was effective in preventing the development of acute laminitis in the face of a challenge that caused laminitis in the remaining three untreated feet ($p<0.05$). We propose that vasoconstriction of the digital circulation during the developmental stage of acute laminitis prevents delivery of hematogenous laminitis trigger factors, probably of hindgut microbial origin (Mungall et al., 2001) to the lamellar tissue. The low temperatures achieved by the application of iced water to horses' distal limbs may also act to inhibit MMP enzymatic activity even if triggering factors were present. For ethical reasons, the laminitis induction experiments were terminated at 48 hours when the foot pain of laminitis appeared. What has not been determined by these experiments is whether laminitis could still develop after the period of cryotherapy had ceased. Cryotherapy is a potentially effective prophylactic strategy in horses with conditions placing them at risk of developing acute laminitis. By the time foot pain is apparent, lamellar pathology is underway, thereby missing an opportunity to prevent or ameliorate lamellar pathology.

Thus, we have discovered a pathway that links the metabolism of pasture grass (fructan production) to fermentative activity in the equine large bowel (gram-positive bacterial proliferation) that leads to laminitis (the triggering of uncontrolled

MMP activation and lamellar basement membrane destruction). Domestic horses encounter fertilized, irrigated, monocultured pastures across the seasons and have little choice in what they consume. Under certain, ill-defined circumstances, fructans are produced by such grasses and are consumed by horses in high enough quantities to cause laminitis. The task ahead is to devise ways of managing horse pastures to reduce fructan production, find a means of measuring fructan levels so dangerous pasture can be identified, find ways of managing horses to reduce pasture fructan consumption, and manage fructan-fermenting hindgut bacteria to prevent formation of laminitis trigger factors. Cryotherapy is a promising preventative agent in horses at risk of developing laminitis.

References

Buffa, E.A., S.S. van den Berg, F.J.M. Verstraete, and N.G.N. Swart. 1992. Effect of dietary biotin supplement on equine hoof horn growth rate and hardness. Equine Vet. J. 24:472-474.

Butler, K.D., Jr., and H. F. Hintz. 1977. Effect of level of feed intake and gelatin supplmentation on growth and quality of hoofs of ponies. J. Anim. Sci. 44:257-261.

Coenen, M., and S. Spitzlei. 1997. The composition of equine hoof horn with regard to its quality (hardness) and nutrient supply of horses. Proc. 15th Equine Nutr. Physiol. Symp. p. 209-212.

Comben, N., R.J. Clark, and D.J.B. Sutherland. 1984. Clinical observations on the response of equine hoof defects to dietary supplementation with biotin. Vet. Rec. 115:642-645.

Ekfalck, A., L.E. Appelgren, B. Funkquist, B. Jones, and N. Obel. 1990. Distribution of labelled cysteine and methionine in the matrix of the stratum medium of the wall and in the laminar layer of the equine hoof. J. Vet Med. Series A 37:481-491.

Flamm G., W. Glinsmann, D. Kritchevsky, L. Prosky, and M. Roberfroid. 2001. Inulin and oligofructose as dietary fiber: A review of the evidence. Critical Rev. Food Science and Nutrition. 41:353-362.

Geyer, H., and J. Schulze. 1994. The long-term influence of biotin supplementation on hoof horn quality in horses. Schweiz. Arch. Tierheilkd. 136:137-49.

Goodspeed, J., J.P. Baker, H.J. Casada, and J.N. Walker. 1970. Effects of gelatin on hoof development in horses. J. Anim. Sci. 31:201 (abstr).

Graham, P.M., E.A. Ott, J.H. Brendemuhl, and S.H. TenBroeck. 1994. The effect of supplemental lysine and threonine on growth and development of yearling horses. J Anim. Sci. 72:380-6.

Hihami, A. 1999. Occurrence of white line disease in performance horses fed low-zinc and low-copper diets. J. Equine Sci. 10:1-5.

Josseck, H., W. Zenker, and H. Geyer. 1995. Hoof horn abnormalities in Lipizzaner horses and the effect of dietary biotin on macroscopic aspects of hoof horn quality. Equine Vet. J. 27:175-182.

Kempson, S.A. 1987. Scanning electron microscope observations of hoof horn from horses with brittle feet. Vet. Rec. 120:568.

Lewis, L.D. 1995 In: Equine Clinical Nutrition. Williams and Wilkins, Philadelphia.

Longland, A., and A. Cairns. 1998. Sugars in grass: An overview of sucrose and fructan accumulation in temperate grasses. In: Proceedings of the Dodson and Horrell International Research Conference on Laminitis. Stoneleigh, Warwickshire, England. pp 1-3.

Mayland, H.F., G.E. Shewmaker, P.A. Harrison, and N.J. Chatterton. 2000. Nonstructural carbohydrates in tall fescue cultivars: Relationship to animal preference. Agron. J. 92:1203-1206.

McMeniman, N.P. 2000. Nutrition of grazing broodmares, their foals and young horses. RIRDC publication 00/28. http://www.rirdc.gov.au/reports/HOR/00-28.pdf.

Moore, J.M., D. Allen, and E.S. Clark. 1989. Pathophysiology of acute laminitis. In: Vet. Clinics North Amer. Equine Practice 5:67-72.

Mungall, B.A., M. Kyaw-Tanner, and C.C. Pollitt. 2001. In vitro evidence for a bacterial pathogenesis of equine laminitis. Vet. Microbial. 79:209-223.

Niness, K.R . 1999. Inulin and oligofructose: What are they? J. Nutr. 129(7): 1402S1406S, Suppl. S.

NRC. 1989. Nutrient Requirements of Horses, 5th Rev. Ed. National Academy Press, Washington, DC.

Ott, E.A., and E.L. Johnson. 2001. Effect of trace mineral proteinates on growth and skeletal development in yearling horses. J. Equine Vet. Sci. 21:287-292.

Ott, E.A., and E.L. Johnson. 2002. Nutritional factors influencing hoof development in horses. In: Proc. Bluegrass Laminitis Symposium.

Pollitt, C.C. 1996. Basement membrane pathology: A feature of acute laminitis. Equine Vet. J. 28:38-46.

Pollitt, C.C. 1999. Equine laminitis: Current concepts of inner hoof wall anatomy, physiology and pathophysiology. In: Large Animal Proc. of the 9th Ann. Amer. College of Vet. Surgeons Symp., pp. 175-180. San Fransisco.

Pollitt, C.C., and M. Daradka. 1998. Equine laminitis basement membrane pathology: Loss of type IV collagen, type VII collagen and laminin immunostaining. The Equine Hoof. Equine Vet. J. Suppl. 27:139-144.

Pollitt, C.C., and Davies, C.L. 1998. Equine laminitis: Its development post alimentary carbohydrate overload coincides with increased sublamellar blood flow. The Equine Hoof. Equine Vet. J. Suppl. 26:125-132.

Pollitt, C.C., M.A. Pass, and S. Pollitt. 1998. Batimastat (BB-94) inhibits matrix metalloproteinases of equine laminitis. The Equine Hoof. Equine Vet. J. Suppl. 26:119-124.

Pollitt, C.C., and van Eps, A.W. 2002. Equine laminitis: A new induction model based on alimentary overload with fructan. In: Proc. Austr. Equine Vet. Assoc. Bain-Fallon Memorial Lectures (Abstr.).

Pollock, C.J., and A.J. Cairns. 1991. Fructan metabolism in grasses and cereals. Annu. Rev. Plant Physiol. Plant Mol. Biol. 42:77-101.

Reilly, J.D., D.F. Cottrell, R.J. Martin, and D.J. Cuddeford. 1998. Effect of supplementary dietary biotin on hoof growth and hoof growth rate in ponies: A controlled trial. The Equine Hoof. Equine Vet. J. Suppl. 26:51-57.

Richardson, G.L., and E.A. Ott. 1977. Influence of protein source and lysine intake on growth and composition of hoofs of yearling foals. In: 69th Ann. Meeting Amer. Soc. Anim. Sci. p. 105 (Abstr.).

Samata, T., and M. Matsuda. 1988. Studies on the amino acid compositions of the equine body hair and the hoof. Jpn. J. Vet. Sci. 50:333-340.

Siciliano, P.D., K.D. Cully, T.E. Engle, and C.W. Smith. 2001. Effect of trace mineral source (inorganic vs organic) on hoof wall-growth rate, -hardness, and -tensile strength. In: Proc. 17th Equine Nutr. Physiol. Sym., p. 143-144.

Swenson, C., L. Sward, J. Karlsson. 1996. Cryotherapy in sports medicine. Scan. J. Med. Sci. Sports 6:193-200.

USDA. 2000. Lameness and Laminitis in US horses. National Animal Health Monitoring System. Fort Collins, CO. #N318.0400.

Weiss, D.J., O.A. Evanson, J. MacLeay, and D. Brown. 1998. Transient alteration in intestinal permeability to technetium Tc99m diethylene triamino-pentaacetate during the prodromal stages of alimentary laminitis in horses. Am. J. Vet. Res. 59:1431-1433.

Worster, A.A., E.M. Gaughan, J.J. Hoskinson, J. Sargeant , and J.H. Erb. 2000. Effects of external thermal manipulation on laminar temperature and perfusion scintigraphy of the equine digit. N. Z. Vet. J. 48:111-116.

Zenker, W., H. Josseck, and H. Geyer. 1995. Histological and physical assessment of poor hoof horn quality in Lipizzaner horses and a therapeutic trial with biotin and a placebo. Equine Vet. J. 27:183-191.

DIETARY LIPID FORM AND FUNCTION

CATHERINE E. DUNNETT
Independent Equine Nutrition, Newmarket, UK

Lipids are a diverse group of chemical compounds that share the common characteristic of being insoluble in water but soluble in organic solvents. The term lipid encompasses triglycerides, the most abundant lipid in the body, and their constituent fatty acids as well as cholesterol, phospholipids, and sterols. This review will focus upon fats and oils, which are the most significant dietary lipids. Lipids that are solid at room temperature are known as fats, and those that are liquid at room temperature are known as oils, although they are also generically referred to as fats.

The fatty acid molecule, which is common to most lipids, consists of a chain of carbon atoms (C3-C24). At one end of the molecule, designated the alpha end, is a carboxyl group (COOH), and at the other end, the omega end, there is a methyl group. When all of the bonds between the carbon atoms are single bonds, the fatty acid is said to be saturated (e.g., stearic acid). In contrast, when one or more of the carbon to carbon (C-C) bonds is a double bond, it is said to be unsaturated. While a fatty acid molecule with a single double bond is known as a monounsaturated fatty acid (e.g., oleic acid), one with two or more double bonds is said to be a polyunsaturated fatty acid (PUFA) (e.g., linoleic acid).

Fats and oils are not made up from a single type or category of fatty acid but are complex mixtures of many different fatty acids. Fatty acids combine with glycerol to form triglycerides (three fatty acids plus one glycerol), which are the main component of both fats and oils. Fats are usually high in triglycerides containing predominantly saturated fatty acids and are less affected by heat, so they tend to be solid at room temperature. In contrast, oils are usually high in triglycerides, containing predominantly monounsaturated or polyunsaturated fatty acids. Oils are susceptible to the effects of heat and, as a result, are usually liquid at room temperature.

Saturated fatty acids have a very ordered, straight-chain structure, which allows them to pack together very tightly; unsaturated fatty acids tend to be less orderly and only loosely packed. This arrangement makes the latter more susceptible to the effects of heat, so they tend to become liquid or melt at lower temperatures. The other factor that affects the characteristics of fat, which contains predominantly saturated fatty acids, is C-C chain length. Long-chain saturated fatty acids tend to produce fats that are solid at room temperature, yet those containing a predominance of medium- (C6–C10) or short-chain (up to C6) fatty acids prove to be the exceptions, remaining liquid at room temperature.

Table 1. Comparison of dietary fats and oils in terms of saturated fatty acid and the most common unsaturated fatty acids (Wardlaw, 1999).

Fats and Oil	Saturated fatty acid %	Linoleic acid %	Alpha-linolenic acid %	Mono-unsaturated fatty acids %
Olive Oil	14	8	1	77
Canola (Rapeseed) Oil	6	22	10	62
Corn Oil	13	61	—	25
Sunflower Oil	11	69	—	20
Soybean Oil	15	54	7	24
Safflower Oil	10	77	trace	13
Coconut Oil	92	2	—	6
Tallow	41	11	1	47

Omega-3 and Omega-6 Series

The position of the first C-C double bond within an unsaturated fatty acid affects its metabolism by the body, and this feature is used to further classify unsaturated fatty acids. Omega-3 fatty acids are those that have their first C-C double bond between the third and fourth carbon atom from the methyl group or omega end. Similarly, omega-6 fatty acids are those that have their first C-C double bond between the sixth and seventh carbon atom from the omega end, and omega-9 fatty acids are those with their first C-C double bond between the ninth and tenth carbon atoms from the omega end.

In feed ingredients, alpha-linolenic acid, which is found in high concentrations in linseed oil and cod liver oil, is the major omega-3 fatty acid; linoleic acid, which is found in high concentrations in corn and soya oil, is the primary omega-6 fatty acid; and oleic acid, which is found in high concentrations in olive and many other vegetable oils, is the major omega-9 fatty acid.

As with humans (Wardlaw, 1999), horses are unlikely to be able to synthesize fatty acids, which have their first C-C double bond before the ninth carbon atom from the omega end. In other words, the omega-3 and omega-6 fatty acids must be provided by the diet and are termed essential fatty acids (EFA). Fatty acids from the omega-3 and omega-6 series perform numerous important functions within the body: parts of vital body structures, components of phospholipids, roles in immune function, roles in vision, and integration into cell membranes.

Additionally, both alpha-linolenic and linoleic acids are metabolized further by cells and used in the synthesis of hormone-like substances called eicosanoids.

Omega-6 fatty acids are converted primarily to arachadonic acid, and omega-3 fatty acids are converted to eicosapentaenoic acid (EPA) and docosahexaenoic acid (DHA). Further biochemical modification results in the production of eicosanoids, including substances called prostaglandins, prostacyclin, thromboxanes, and leukotrienes. Unlike regular hormones such as insulin or the thyroid hormones, these "local hormones" are used where they are produced and are not transported to their site of action in the blood.

The omega-3 and omega-6 fatty acids follow different biochemical pathways to produce distinct types of prostaglandins and thromboxanes, each of which has very different effects in the body. The eicosanoids are potent regulators of vital body functions such as blood pressure, blood clotting, and immune and inflammatory responses. In general terms, the eicosanoids produced from omega-6 fatty acids tend to increase inflammatory processes and blood clotting. Eicosanoids produced from omega-3 fatty acids tend to decrease blood clotting and inflammatory response, although this is a gross simplification as the mechanisms involved are very complex. The physical and functional properties of cell membranes are affected by the relative fatty-acid composition of membrane-bound phospholipids, which can be altered according to the fatty-acid composition of dietary triglycerides. The different biochemical pathways involved in eicosanoid production utilize and therefore compete for the same enzymes, so the degree of inflammation, for example, is influenced by the relative proportions of omega-6 and omega-3 fatty acids present in cell membranes (Baur, 1994).

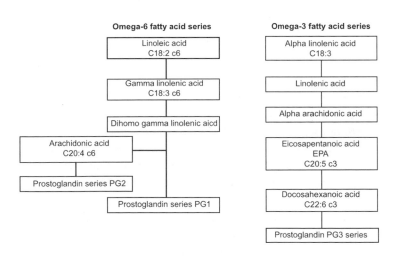

Figure 1. Biochemical pathways involved in eicosanoid production.

The reputed beneficial effects of the omega-3 fatty acids are largely due to the conversion of EPA and DHA to the prostaglandin PG3 series. However, the conversion of the parent precursor alpha-linolenic acid to both EPA and DHA is relatively innefficient due to low activities of the enzyme delta-6 desaturase (Baur, 1994). In domestic animals, dietary supplementation with omega-3 fatty acids may be a useful adjunct to treatment of renal disease, rheumatoid arthritis, cutaneous inflammatory disorders, autoimmune disease, and possibly cancer (Baur, 1994). While there are few studies on dietary omega-3 fatty acids in horses, Henry et al. (1991) reported that dietary intervention with rations rich in alpha-linolenic acid in the form of linseed oil were potentially useful in preventing some of the deleterious effects of endotoxemia in horses. Recently, a double-blind crossover trial using Icelandic ponies predisposed to recurrent seasonal pruritis (sweet itch) revealed that supplementation with linseed (flax), a rich source of alpha-linolenic acid, improved the average skin-test response to *Culicoides*, the biting fly implicated in the condition (Pearson-O'Neill et al., 2002).

A minimum requirement for linolenic acid of 0.1% has been recommended for horses (Vitec, 1987), where the requirement for linoleic acid is considered to be close to 1-4% of the total dry matter intake (Vitec, 1987). Although there are no published guidelines for horses regarding the optimum ratio of C6 to C3 fatty acids in the diet, the consensus in other animals seems to be a ratio of about 10:1 (Vitec, 1987). An EFA deficiency in other species is characterized by a dry lusterless coat, scaly skin, and predisposition to skin infections. However, a true EFA deficiency with similar symptoms has not been documented in horses, despite diets with a very low total fat and linoleic acid content being fed (0.05% and .03%, respectively) (Sallmann et al., 1991). The only finding linked to this low intake of fat was a reduction in the plasma and tissue levels of vitamin E, which may reflect reduced absorption from the diet.

The number and position of the double bonds in omega-3 fatty acids makes them particularly susceptible to oxidation, leading to the formation of hydroperoxides, which are at best unpalatable but will also contribute to cell membrane destruction in vivo. These oils should be protected from rancidity by suitable antioxidant products, and additional vitamin E is needed to protect them once they have been ingested.

EFA nutrition in the horse is of great interest due to its clinical relevance, and the lack of research in this area offers great scope for future investagations. However, the relationship between eicosanoids and their essential fatty acid precursors is complex and requires thorough investigation before dietary recommendations can realistically be made.

Fat or Oil Supplementation

Fats and oils are regularly added to the diets of horses and have proven to be both palatable and highly digestible. They are usually added to the diet to increase energy density, which offers an advantage when appetite limits the provision of adequate energy to maintain condition or when a reduced intake of hydrolyzable carbohydrate (CHO-H) is advocated from a clinical standpoint. Diets characterized by high fiber content, oil supplementation, and reduced levels of CHO-H have been recommended for horses with a predisposition to equine rhabdomyolysis syndrome (ERS) and have also been advocated as being safer for laminitic horses (Harris and Naylor, 2001). The recent implication of high-glycemic diets in developmental orthopedic disease has initiated interest in fat supplementation as a means of restricting CHO-H intake to reduce the glycemic nature of feeds, thus making them suitable for young stock (Ralston, 1995; Pagan et al., 2001). Additionally, it is common practice for horse owners or trainers to supplement the diet with oil in order to gain from its reputed benefits on exercise performance, both for endurance and sprint exercise.

Low levels of oil have been added to commercial formulations for many years, acting as a dust suppressant and easing the passage of ingredients through manufacturing plants, which reduces the buildup of debris on plant machinery. Likewise, horse owners have fed oil for many years, prior to the current fashion for fat supplementation, in the form of cod liver oil or boiled linseed with the premise of improving coat condition and promoting weight gain. The maximum level at which fat or oil can be added to the diet is largely dependent on the physical restraints of feed manufacture, such as if it is fed as part of a cube or mix. Top-dressing allows much larger quantities of oil to be added to the diet as does the use of straight feedstuffs such as cooked linseed or rice bran; however, feed refusal may become an issue at very high levels of inclusion.

Palatability

Both vegetable oil and animal fats have proven to be palatable in horses. Bowman et al. (1979) compared the palatability of 10 different types of fat and oil using a cafeteria-style palatability test. In each palatability trial, corn oil was used as a control feed and was tested against three blends of either vegetable and animal fat, vegetable oils only, or animal fats only. In each case, the oil or fat source was added to a concentrate feed at a level of 15% (by weight). Corn oil was found to be the most palatable when compared to either of the other three sources offered. In an extension of this trial, the relative palatability of each fat or oil was calculated by comparison against the acceptability of corn oil using multiple measurements taken over 7-10 days. During each trial, corn oil was found to be the most acceptable followed in relative terms by a vegetable and animal fat blend with a linoleic acid content of 30.8% (Holland et al., 1998). Please refer to Figure 2. This trial looked at palatability over a relatively short period of time (10 days), but other digestibility and exercise-oriented studies over the years have fed oil- or fat-supplemented diets for periods of between three weeks and 16 months with few reported palatability issues. Harris et al. (1999) reported good feed intake during a 16-month trial where horses were fed a basal diet (7% of digestible energy [DE] as oil) supplemented with either a highly unsaturated (soya) or saturated (coconut) vegetable oil providing a final level of 27% of the total DE intake as oil.

Furthermore, there were no references made to any significant palatability problems during this trial. Care should be taken when extrapolating palatability data for specific oil sources from country to country as different processing techniques can affect palatability.

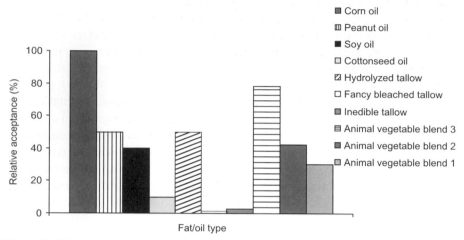

Figure 2. Relative acceptance of fats used in palatability experiments compared to corn oil (Holland et al., 1998).

Digestibility

Both DE and metabolizable energy (ME) have consistently been reported to increase as a result of the addition of fat or oil to the diet (Hollands and Cuddeford, 1992; McCann et al., 1987; Rich et al., 1981). However, the form in which the fat is available (i.e., free in the form of oil or animal fat, or encapsulated in cereal grains or oilseeds) may affect its digestibility (McCann et al., 1987). Fat is digested predominantly in the small intestine, whereas cell wall material is fermented in the hindgut. The encapsulation of oil in cereal grains or oilseeds may affect its digestibility, as some fiber may have to be digested to free the integral oil. Kronfeld et al. (2001) suggested that the lower apparent digestibility of this endogenous oil as opposed to supplemental oil may indeed be related to differences in the nature of ether extract; alternatively, the authors proposed a rate-limiting effect of lipase activity related to the oil content of the diet or even the presence of a lipase inhibitor in an ingredient of the endogenous oil source. In ruminants, the addition of vegetable oils to the diet has been shown to have a negative impact on fiber digestibility. Free vegetable oil coats the fiber fraction, disrupting ruminal fermentation. Integral oil does not appear to have the same effect, probably because the oil is released more slowly (Coppock and Wilks, 1991). In contrast, no apparent adverse effect on neutral detergent fiber (NDF) or acid detergent fiber (ADF) was reported in horses fed a high-fiber diet supplemented with oil (4-17% of DM)

(Hollands and Cuddeford, 1992). Likewise, Kronfeld et al. (2001) reported that fat and oil had no associative effect on fiber digestibility when hay- and grain-based diets were supplemented with various sources and levels of oil. Recent work by Jansen et al. (2001), however, has suggested that total tract fiber digestibility is in fact affected by oil supplementation.

In contrast to the work of Hollands and Cuddeford (1992), Kronfeld et al. (2001) reported a substantial negative associative effect of fat or oil supplementation on crude protein digestibility in a high proportion of digestibility trials recently reviewed.

Apparent absorption of calcium and magnesium are reportedly unchanged by the addition of fat or oil to the diet (Rich et al., 1981; McCann et al., 1987). This is in contrast to work in other species where fat-supplemented diets have been associated with reduced calcium absorption, possibly due to the formation of calcium soaps in the small intestine as discussed by Hollands and Cuddeford (1992). These authors also reported an increase in the apparent digestibility of phosphorus in response to oil supplementation, which they suggest may be due to enhanced absorption of phosphorus in the small intestine.

Glycemic Response

The energy density of feeds can be increased through the addition of oil, making the inclusion of high levels of cereal grains unnecessary. Diets that are high in fiber and low in nonstructural carbohydrates (sugar and starch) are now more common. The energy density in these feeds is increased through the addition of supplemental oil. Glycemic response and insulin release is significantly lower in response to diets that are high in fiber and oil in comparison to more traditional grain-based feeds (Williams et al., 2001) and also for grain-based feeds that are top-dressed with oil (Pagan et al., 1999). The reduction in glycemic response to feeding is partly due to the lower starch and sugar content of these former feeds but is also likely to be influenced by the presence of oil in the latter. The presence of fats and oils in the small intestine stimulates the secretion of a hormone called cholecystokinin. This hormone decreases gastric motility and delays gastric emptying, thus affecting transit time and the rate of prececal starch digestibility. Additionally, the increased energy density achieved through the addition of oil often means that meal size can be reduced, which again will affect transit time and hence glycemic response.

Behavior

Fat or oil supplemented diets have been reputed to modify behavior in excitable horses. Holland et al. (1996) provided the first quantitative evidence of this by reporting that spontaneous activity and reactivity, evaluated as response to pressure, loud noise, and sudden visual stimuli, was reduced in horses fed a diet supplemented with soy lecithin and corn oil. Lecithins are a group of phospholipids that contain two fatty acids, a phophate group, and a choline molecule. They function as emulsifiers of fat by breaking it down into small droplets or micelles. They form a bridge between the fat and water, allowing mixture with water. Lecithins are produced by the liver and are released into the small intestine, where they emulsify dietary fats and oils and enlarge the surface area over which digestive enzymes can act. The reputed effect of soy lecithin and corn oil on behavior is relevant not only for leisure horses but also for those with a predisposition towards ERS. Stress and nervousness are two factors that increase the likelihood that a horse susceptible to ERS will develop muscle damage (MacLeay et al., 1999a).

Metabolic Effects of Fat or Oil Supplementation

The effect of fat or oil supplementation on resting muscle glycogen concentration and its subsequent rate of use during exercise is a controversial topic. Many researchers reported an increase in resting muscle glycogen concentration and subsequent utilization during moderate- to high-intensity exercise, despite a reduction in the nonstructural carbohydrate (NSC) content of the fat-supplemented versus control diets (Meyers et al., 1989; Oldham et al., 1990; Harkins et al., 1992; Scott et al., 1992). Equally, however, several authors have found no such increase in resting muscle glycogen concentration or subsequent utilization during exercise in horses fed diets providing comparable levels of fat (Pagan et al., 1987; Greiwe et al., 1989; Eaton et al., 1995; Orme et al., 1997; Hyyppa et al., 1999). In the former studies, the muscle glycogen concentrations measured were often very low in comparison to previously established levels and the effect of differences in the energy and protein content of the control and fat-supplemented diets, as well as the presence of any training effect, cannot be overlooked. Additionally, differences in the content and source of NSC in the fat- or oil-supplemented diets may also offer some explanation of the contradictory results reported between study groups. Prececal digestibility, glycemic response, and postprandial insulin concentration will affect glycogen synthesis.

Glycogen repletion rates following moderate-intensity exercise were reduced in horses fed a basal diet supplemented with rapeseed oil (7.5% of total DM, 14% DE) compared to the basal diet alone. However, this effect was abolished once these horses were adapted to an oil-supplemented diet (5% of total DM) for a period of three weeks (Hyyppa et al., 1999). Pre-exercise muscle glycogen concentrations were not significantly different when both normal horses and those suffering from recurrent equine rhabdomyolysis (RER) were fed either a high-oil diet (20% of total DE), a low-oil, low-carbohydrate control diet, or a high-carbohydrate diet. However, there was a trend towards lower muscle glycogen concentrations in the horses fed the high-oil diet and, in contrast, higher concentrations in the horses fed the high-carbohydrate diet compared to the control diet (MacLeay et al., 1999b).

It would seem that horses are able to maintain normal muscle glycogen levels in the face of moderate levels of fat supplementation (7.5% of total DM, 14% DE), despite reduced CHO-H intake, provided that a period of adaptation is undertaken. This has obvious advantages for certain types of performance horses in which muscle glycogen availability is important but high intake of grain rich in CHO-H is undesirable. In contrast, there is some suggestion that high intakes of supplemental oil may reduce muscle glycogen, which could be detrimental to performance in some instances but may be advantageous with respect to certain clinical conditions such as ERS.

Metabolic Adaptation

Fat or oil supplementation of the diet is characterized by an increase in plasma cholesterol and phospholipids and a reduction in plasma triglyceride (Orme et al., 1997; Geelen et al., 1999). Enzymatic studies suggest that the fat-adapted horse has an increased capacity for uptake of free fatty acids from circulating triglycerides into muscle (Orme et al., 1997; Geelen et al., 1999, 2000). Artificial elevation of plasma FFA prior to the onset of low-intensity exercise indicates that horses have the capacity to increase the contribution of fat to energy generation when substrate availability allows (Orme et al., 1995). Furthermore, it has been suggested by Orme et al. (1997) that the capacity for oxidation of FFA and carbohydrate may be increased in response to oil supplementation as indicated by an increase in the activity of key oxidative enzymes. However, this effect was not repeated in a similar study by Geelen et al. (2000).

This higher capacity for fat oxidation is confirmed by a lower observed respiratory exchange ratio in fat-adapted horses exercising at low to moderate intensities (Dunnett et al., 2002). This finding allows for a glycogen-sparing effect with a potentially positive outcome on performance during exercise, where the intensity and duration are compatible with increased fat utilization. Despite these treadmill-based studies, no endurance-type performance trials have been reported to date. However, fat supplementation (up to 20% of the total DE) is common in the diets of competitive endurance horses.

The concentration of insulin, a potent antilipolytic hormone, has been reported to be lower both postprandially (Williams et al., 2001) and during exercise following oil supplementation (Pagan et al., 1994). The metabolic response to oil supplementation, in terms of FFA oxidation, increase in lipoprotein lipase activity, and muscle oxidative capacity, could be mediated in part via characteristic changes in postprandial and exercise-induced insulin concentrations. In other words, these adaptive effects may not be directly attributable to the oil supplementation per se. They may simply reflect differences in the hormonal response to test and control diets, changes in the level of CHO-H, and any associative effects of the oil on the rates of gastric emptying and transit time.

The metabolic response to oil supplementation occurs rapidly and is apparent after just three weeks of supplementation (Hughes et al., 1995; Orme et al., 1997).

These supplementation effects are, however, transient and dependent on continued use, with the response being abolished within five weeks of withdrawal of the oil-supplemented diet (Orme et al., 1997). The response to oil supplementation may also vary between individual horses, depending on their inherent ability to utilize fat as a fuel source during exercise (Dunnett et al., 2002).

Performance Effects

The effect of fat or oil supplementation on exercise performance is not unequivocal. Some researchers report improvements and others indicate no changes (Topliff et al., 1983; Essen-Gustavsson et al., 1991; Moser et al., 1991). It was expected that any positive effect of fat or oil supplementation would be dependent on the intensity and duration of exercise as well as the training status of the horses. Improvement in performance in response to fat or oil supplementation is feasible where either a glycogen-sparing effect occurs, mediated by an increase in fat oxidation either during training or during the competition, or where resting muscle glycogen concentration is increased by an unidentified mechanism. Meyers et al. (1989) and Oldham et al. (1990) reported a greater capacity for exercise during a standardized treadmill exercise test, and Harkins et al. (1992) demonstrated improved racetrack performance. These performance effects were suggested to have been mediated via an observed increase in resting muscle glycogen concentration and associated increase in glycogen utilization rates during exercise. Latterly, however, Eaton et al. (1995) reported an increased capacity for high-intensity exercise and a greater mean accumulated oxygen debt in fat-supplemented horses with no corresponding change in resting muscle glycogen concentration or subsequent utilization during exercise. It is unlikely that any positive effect on high-intensity exercise is due to increased fat oxidation during exercise because the contribution of FFA oxidation to energy generation during this type of exercise is likely to be low. An increased flux through glycolysis, characteristic of high-intensity exercise, would lead to an accumulation of acetyl CoA, which may inhibit the carnitine transport system needed for FFA uptake into mitochondria. It is, however, possible that chronic fat supplementation may lead to improvements in carbohydrate oxidation rates due to increases in key Krebs cycle enzymes such as citrate synthase (Orme et al., 1997).

Thermal Load

A further advantage to fat or oil supplementation is a reduction in thermal load. Physiological processes including ingestion, fermentation, and assimilation, as well as the metabolic process of energy generation, are not completely efficient and heat is produced as a consequence, giving rise to a thermal load. The total amount of heat produced as a consequence of maintenance processes is referred to as the heat of maintenance (Hm), and additional heat produced as a consequence of exercise or work is known as heat of work (Hw). A horse's thermal load is equivalent to the total of Hm and Hw, which must be dissipated in order to maintain normal body temperature. Exercise in hot environments presents a greater challenge to the horse's thermoregulatory system, and measures that are effective in reducing the thermal load could confer a performance advantage.

Diets supplemented with fats or oil have been suggested to reduce thermal load by a number of different mechanisms. An increase in the energy density of the diet (e.g., through the addition of fat or oil) reduces the work of feeding or the heat of ingestion, and when accompanied by a lowered forage to concentrate ratio, this would be additive to a reduced heat of fermentation. Reduced gut fill or ballast as a result of the increase in energy density may also have an effect on Hw. In addition, the heat produced per molecule of ATP generated was calculated to be least during the direct oxidation of long-chain fatty acids (stearic and linoleic acids) compared to carbohydrates (glucose), amino acids (leucine), or volatile fatty acids (propionic or acetic acid) (Kronfeld, 1996). This premise is also apparent when each of these energy sources is oxidized indirectly following storage as glycogen, triglyceride, or lactate in the case of glucose or as triglyceride in the case of stearic acid or acetic acid.

McCann et al. (1987) reported that heat production, expressed as a percentage of total DE, was lower for three types of fat-supplemented diets in comparison to a control diet. Calculation of energy balance (ME - heat production) by calorimetry revealed a significant increase over the control diet. Using a model to compare energetic efficiencies and heat production of three diets that provided varying proportions of fermentable carbohydrate (CHO_f), hydrolyzable carbohydrate (CHO_h), fat, and protein, Kronfeld (1996) calculated that the high-fat diet (which also provided the lowest levels of CHO_f and CHO_h) would result in the lowest total heat production, equivalent to the sum of Hm and Hw.

Fatty Acid Chain Length

Little work has been carried out to investigate the effect of fatty acid chain length or degree of saturation on exercise metabolism. Oils such as coconut and palm contain a high proportion of medium-chain fatty acids (MCFA) (C6-C10). The mechanism by which these fatty acids are absorbed from the intestinal lumen is somewhat different than their long-chain counterparts. As a result of their greater solubility in water, MCFA are absorbed much more quickly from the small intestine and unlike long-chain fatty acids are not re-esterified in the intestinal epithelial cells. MCFA are absorbed intact and are transported from the intestine to the liver, via the portal circulation, in association with albumin. Furthermore, oxidation of the former can occur either with or without the involvement of the carnitine-dependent mitochondrial transport system. These differences in the mechanism of absorption and oxidation for MCFA make their metabolism more rapid than long-chain sources. There has been a suggested beneficial effect of MCFA on performance reported in horses fed coconut oil (10% of a grain-based concentrate pellet) during exercise of moderate speed and duration (8-9 m/s, 8 minutes) (Pagan et al., 1993). Horses exhibited lower plasma lactate or ammonia concentrations in response to this exercise when fed the coconut oil in comparison to a traditional grain-based control diet or a soya oil-supplemented diet, respectively. The authors suggest that the fatty acid composition of the coconut oil may have allowed more rapid mobilization and oxidation of fatty acids, permitting a significant contribution to energy release during moderately intense exercise. However, subsequent trials have failed to support these findings. A field-based trial by Jackson et al. (2001) failed to repeat these observed changes in lactate response to exercise when feeding MCFA; however, an increase in pre-exercise plasma betahydroxybutyrate concentration was observed. As these authors suggest, this may provide evidence of increased oxidation of medium-chain fatty acids to ketones in the group supplemented with MCFA. A subsequent long-term fat acclimation trial, which involved horses being fed a diet supplemented with predominantly saturated (MCFA) or unsaturated oils, revealed no significant change in insulin or lactate response to exercise. This was apparent following the first nine months of the trial, where the saturated or unsaturated supplemental oil contributed 12% of the total DE, and following a further six months of supplementation, where the level of oil fed was increased to provide a total of 20% of DE (Harris et al., 1999). There is no clear evidence to support the use of MCFA in performance horses.

Vitamin E

Supplementation of the equine diet with oil may bring with it an increased requirement for antioxidant provision, including vitamin E, because enhanced fat oxidation increases the production of peroxyl free radicals. This may in part be satisfied by the natural tocopherol content of the oil, which is dependent on its source and is related to its polyunsaturated fatty acid content.

The term vitamin E refers to a group of compounds known as tocopherols, with the most biologically active form being alpha-tocopherol. Vegetable oils are the richest dietary sources of natural vitamin E, a fat-soluble vitamin that functions as a membrane-bound antioxidant. Vitamin E traps lipid peroxyl free radicals produced from unsaturated fatty acids when oxidative stress arises. The orientation of vitamin E within cell membranes appears to be critical to its functionality. Vitamin E is an amphipathic molecule, a structure that incorporates hydrophobic (water-hating) and hydrophilic (water-loving) properties. This characteristic facilitates its orientation and retention within the lipid bilayer of cell membranes, probably giving it an ideal position for free-radical scavenging and thus protection of cell membranes.

The level and type of tocopherol in vegetable oil vary among different oil sources. Natural tocopherols largely act as an internal antioxidant to prevent oxidation of unsaturated fatty acids that make up the constituent triglyceride and hence prevent rancidity of the oil. The level of vitamin E in an oil appears to be related to its polyunsaturated fatty acid content, specifically the combined amounts of linoleic and alpha-linolenic fatty acids. Horses appear to absorb natural forms of vitamin E to a much greater extent than synthetic versions (Gansen et al., 1995). Additionally, when the absorption of different sources of vitamin E was compared in Thoroughbred yearlings, higher plasma concentrations were reported with the d-forms compared to equivalent amounts of the dl-form (Wooden et al., 1991).

Early studies in human subjects suggested that requirement for vitamin E increased with increasing dietary polyunsaturated fatty acid content (Wardlaw, 1999). Looking at both human and animal studies, the requirement for vitamin E was estimated to be 0.6 mg of alpha-tocopherol per gram of linoleic acid, which equates to an additional 36 mg of vitamin E per 100 g of vegetable oil added. For most animal species 3 mg of alpha-tocopherol is recommended for each 1 g of omega-3 polyunsaturated fatty acid (Vitec, 1987). For soya or corn oil, this would equate to 180 mg per 100 g of oil. However, both soya and corn oil have an endogenous tocopherol content of about 60 mg per 100g, leaving a net requirement for 120 mg per 100g of oil or 108 mg vitamin E per 100 ml of oil. Care should, however, be taken to ensure that vitamin E levels are adequate to take into account the shelf life of the product as endogenous tocopherol levels may be substantially reduced during storage without additional antioxidant support.

Table 2. Typical vitamin E content of fats and oils (mg/100 g oil). Total tocopherol is the sum of alpha-tocopherol and gamma-tocopherol (Dupont et al., 1990).

Oil or fat	α-tocopherol	γ-tocopherol	Total
Lard	1.20	0.70	1.90
Olive	7.94	trace	7.94
Sunflower	48.70	5.10	53.80
Rapeseed	25.82	30.01	55.83
Soybean	10.25	50.48	60.73
Corn	11.28	50.76	62.04

Horses fed a diet supplemented with 6.4% soya oil and containing current NRC recommended levels of vitamin E (80 IU/kg DM) showed no significant change in the ratio of alpha-tocopherol to total lipid (serum cholesterol and triglyceride) compared to an isoenergetic control diet (Siciliano and Wood, 1993). This may indicate that either the current requirements for vitamin E were high enough to cope with the level of addition of PUFA-containing oil or that the endogenous tocopherol content of the oil itself diminished the need for further supplementation. Likewise, McMeniman et al. (1992) reported no reduction in plasma or muscle vitamin E status in ponies fed a diet in which 10% of the total DE was provided in the form of corn oil. However, in the same study plasma thiobarbituric acid reactive substances (TBARS) and breath pentone, which are indicative of "oxidative stress," were increased during exercise, especially in those horses with a relatively low plasma vitamin E concentration.

Added vegetable oils and animal fats have previously been used in the commercial manufacture of horse feed. Additionally, ingredients such as linseed meal, soya, rice bran, peanuts, and sunflower meal have been utilized for their endogenous oil content. In the post BSE era, however, it is now the vegetable oils and oilseed products which largely prevail as raw materials. Supplementation of the equine diet with fat or oil offers many potential advantages, ranging from effects on behavior to those on performance. Oil is readily accepted by horses; however, care should be taken in introducing it into the diet and the level of supplementation should be increased gradually in order to avoid digestive problems. For performance effects, the adaptive response to fat supplementation is long-term and measured in weeks rather than days. Care should also be taken to provide an overall balance of protein as well as minerals and trace elements when integrating oil into the diet, as oil will not contribute to the provision of these latter nutrients.

References

Baur, J.E., 1994. The potential for dietary polyunsaturated fatty acids in domestic animals. Aust. Vet. J. 71:342-345.

Bowman, V.A., J.P. Fontenot, T.N. Meacham, K.E., and Webb. 1979. Acceptability and digestibility of animal vegetable and blended fats by equine. In: Proc. 6th Equine Nutr. Physiol. Symp., p. 74.

Coppock, C.E., and D.L. Wilks. 1991. Supplemental fat in high energy rations for lactating cows: Effects on intake, digestion, milk yield and composition. J. Anim. Sci. 69:3826-3837.

Dunnett, C.E., D. Marlin, and R.C. Harris. 2002. Effect of dietary lipid on response to exercise: Relationship to metabolic adaptation. Equine Vet. J. Suppl. 34.

Dupont, J., P.J. White, M.P. Carpenter, E.J. Schaefer, S.N. Meydani, C.E. Elson, M. Woods, and S.L. Gorbach. 1990. Food uses and health effects of corn oil. J. Amer. Coll. Nutr. 9:438- 470.

Eaton, M.D., D.R. Hodgson, D.L. Evans, W.L. Bryden, and M.W. Ross. 1995. Effect of a diet containing supplementary fat on the capacity for high intensity exercise. Equine Vet. J. Suppl. 18:353-356.

Essen-Gustavsson, B., E. Blomstrand, K. Karlstrom, A. Lindholm, and S.G.B. Persson. 1991. Influence of diet on substrate metabolism during exercise. In: S.G.B. Persson, A. Lindholm, and L.B. Jeffcott (Eds.). Equine Exercise Physiology: Proc. 3rd International Conf. pp. 288-298. ICEEP Publications.

Gansen, S., A. Lindener, and A. Wagener. 1995. Influence of a supplementation with natural and synthetic vitamin E on serum alpha-tocopherol content and v4 of Thoroughbred horses. Proc. 14th Equine Nutr. Physiol. Soc. Symp., p. 68.

Geelen, S.N., W.L. Jansen, M.J. Geelen, M.M. Sloet van Oldruitenborgh-Oosterbaan, and A.C. Beynen. 2000. Lipid metabolism in equines fed a fat-rich diet. Int. J. Vitam. Nutr. Res. 70:148-152.

Geelen, S.N., M.M. Sloet van Oldruitenborgh-Oosterbaan, and A.C. Beynen. 1999. Dietary fat supplementation and equine plasma lipid metabolism. Equine Vet. J. Suppl. 30:475-478.

Greiwe, K.M., T.N. Meacham, G.F. Fregin, and J.L. Walberg. 1989. Effect of added dietary fat on exercising horses. In: Proc. 11th Equine Nutr. Physiol. Sym., pp. 101-106.

Harkins, J.D., G.S. Morris, R.T. Tulley, A.G. Nelson, and S.G. Kamerling. 1992. Effect of added dietary fat on racing performance in Thoroughbred horses. J. Equine Vet. Sci. 12:123-129.3

Harris, P.A, and J.M. Naylor. 2001. Clinical Nutrition. In: K. Coumbe (Ed.) Equine Veterinary Nursing Manual. pp. 126-139. Blackwell Science, Oxford.

Harris, P.A., J.D. Pagan, K.G. Crandell, and N. Davidson. 1999. Effect of feeding Thoroughbred horses a high unsaturated or saturated vegetable oil supplemented diet for 6 months following a 10 month fat acclimation. Equine Vet. J. Suppl. 30:468-474.

Henry, M.M., J.N. Moore, and J.K. Fischer. 1991. Influence of an omega-3 fatty acid enriched ration on in vivo responses of horses to endotoxin. Am. J. Vet. Res. 52:523-527.

Holland, J.L., D.S. Kronfeld, and T.N. Meacham. 1996. Behavior of horses is affected by soy lecithin and corn oil in the diet. J. Anim. Sci 74:1252-1255.

Holland, J.L., D.S. Kronfeld, G.A. Rich, K.A. Kline, J.P. Fontenot, T.N. Meacham, and P.A. Harris. 1998. Acceptance of fat and lecithin containing diets by horses.Appl. Anim. Behav. Sci. 56:91-96.

Hollands, T., and D. Cuddeford. 1992. Effect of supplementary soya oil on the digestibility of nutrients contained in a 40:60 roughage/concentrate diet fed to horses. Europaische Konferenz uber die Ernahrung des Pferdes . 8:128-132.

Hughes, S.J., G.D. Potter, L.W. Greene, T.W. Odom, and M. Murray-Gerzik. 1995. Adaptation of Thoroughbred horses in training to a fat supplemented diet. Equine Vet. J. Suppl. 18:349-352.

Hyyppa, S., M. Saastamoinen, and A. Reeta Poso. 1999. Effect of a post exercise fat-supplemented diet on muscle glycogen repletion. Equine Vet. J. Suppl. 475-493.

Jackson, C.A., E.A. Ott, M.B. Porter, and J. Kivipelto. 2001. The effect of medium chain triglycerides in exercising Thoroughbred horses. Proc. 17th Equine Nutr. Physiol. Soc. Sym., pp. 150-152.

Jansen, W.L., J. van der Kuilen, S.N. Geelen, and A.C. Beynen. 2001. The apparent digestibility of fiber in trotters when dietary soybean oil is substituted for an isoenergetic amount of glucose. Arch Tierernahr 54(4):297-304.

Kronfeld, D.S. 1996. Dietary fat affects heat production and other variables of equine performance under hot and humid conditions. Equine Vet. J. Suppl. 22:22-34.

Kronfeld, D.S., J.L. Holland, G.A. Rich, S.E. Custalow, J.P. Fontenot, T.N. Meacham, D. Sklan, and P. Harris. 2001. Digestibility of fat. Proc.17th Equine Nutr. Physiol. Symp., pp. 156-158.

MacLeay, J.M., S.A. Sorum, S.J. Valberg, W.E. Marsh, M.D. Sorum. 1999. Epidemiologic analysis of factors influencing exertional rhabdomyolysis in Thoroughbreds. Am. J. Vet. Res. 60(12):1562-1566.

MacLeay, J.M., S. Valberg, J.D. Pagan, F. De La Corte, J. Roberts, J. Billstrom, J. McGinnity, and H. Kaese. 1999. Effect of diet on Thoroughbred horses with recurrent exertional rhabdomyolysis performing a standardised exercise test. Equine Vet. J. Suppl. 30:458-462.

McCann, J.S., T.N. Meacham, and J.P. Fontenot. 1987. Energy utilization and blood traits of ponies fed fat-supplemented diets. J. Anim. Sci. 65:1019-1026.

McMeniman, N.P., and H.F. Hintz. 1992. Effect of vitamin E status on lipid peroxidation in exercised horses. Equine Vet. J. 24:482.

Meyers, M.C., G.D. Potter, J.W. Evans, L.W. Greene, and S.F. Crouse. 1989. Physiologic and metabolic response of exercising horses to added dietary fat. J. Equine Vet. Sci. 9:218-223.

Moser, L.R., L.M. Lawrence, J. Novakofski, D.M. Powell, and M.J. Biel. 1991. The effect of supplemental fat on exercising horses. Proc. 12th Equine Nutr. Physiol. Symp., pp. 103-108.

Oldham, S.L., G.D. Potter, J.W. Evans, S.B. Smith, T.S. Taylor, and W.S. Barnes. 1990. Storage and mobilization of muscle glycogen in exercising horses fed a fat-supplemented diet. J. Equine. Vet. Sci. 10:353-359.

Orme, C.E., R.C. Harris, and D. Marlin. 1995. Effect of elevated plasma FFA on fat utilization during low intensity exercise. Equine Vet. J. Suppl. 18:199-204.

Orme, C.E., R.C. Harris, D.J. Marlin, and J. Hurley. 1997. Metabolic adaptation to a fat-supplemented diet by the Thoroughbred horse. Br. J. Nutr. 78:443-458.

Pagan, J.D., I. Burger, and S.G. Jackson. 1994. The long-term effects of feeding fat to 2-year-old Thoroughbreds in training. Equine Vet. J Suppl. 18:343-348.

Pagan, J.D., B. Essen-Gustavsson, A. Lindholm, and J. Thornton. 1987. The effect of dietary energy source on exercise performance in Standardbred horses. In: Gillespie JR, Robinson NE (Eds.). Equine Exercise Physiology: Proc. 2nd International Conf. pp. 686-700. ICEEP Publications.

Pagan, J.D., R.J. Geor, S.E. Caddel, P.B. Pryor, and K.E. Hoekstra. 2001. The relationship between glycemic response and the incidence of OCD in Thoroughbred weanlings: A field study. In: Proc. 47th AAEP Conv., pp. 322-325.

Pagan, J.D., P.A. Harris, M.A.P. Kennedy, N. Davidson, K.E. Hoekstra. 1999. Feed type and intake affects glycemic response in Thoroughbred horses. In: Proc. 13th Equine Nutr. Physiol. Symp., pp. 149-150.

Pagan, J.D., W. Tiegs, S.G. Jackson, and H.Q. Murphy. 1993. The effect of different fat sources on exercise performance in Thoroughbred racehorses. In: Proc. 13th Equine Nutr. and Physiol. Symp., pp. 125-129.

Pearson-O'Neill, W., S. McKee, and A.F. Clarke. 2002. Flaxseed as a potential treatment for allergic skin disease in horses. www.nutraceuticalalliance.com.

Ralston, S.L. 1995. Postprandial hyperglycemia/hyperinsulinemia in young horses with osteochondritis dissecans. J. Anim. Sci. 73:184.

Rich, G.A., J.P. Fontenot, and T.N. Meacham, 1981. Digestibility of animal, vegetable and blended fats by equine. In: Proc. 7th Equine Nutr. Physiol. Soc. Symp., pp. 30-36.

Sallmann, H.P., E. Kienzel, and H. Fuhrmann. 1991. Metabolic consequence of feeding ponies with marginal amounts of fat. In: Proc. 12th Equine Nutr. Physiol. Symp., pp. 81-82.

Scott, B.D., G.D. Potter, L.W. Greene, P.S. Hargis, and J.G. Anderson. 1992. Efficacy of a fat-supplemented diet on muscle glycogen concentrations in exercising Thoroughbred horses maintained in varying body conditions. J. Equine Vet. Sci. 12:109-113.

Siciliano, P.D., and C.H. Wood. 1993. The effect of added dietary soybean oil on vitamin E status of the horse. In: Proc. 13th Equine Nutr. Physiol. Soc. Symp., p. 3.

Topliff, D.R., G.D. Potter, T.R. Dutson, J.L. Kreider, and G.T. Jessup. 1983. Diet manipulation and muscle glycogen in the equine. In: Proc. 8th Equine Nutr. Physiol. Symp., pp. 119-124.

Vitec, 1987. Omega-3 fatty acids. Roche Report. A5, pp. 1-5.

Wardlaw, G.M. 1999. Perspectives in Nutrition (4th Ed.). pp. 113-156. McGraw-Hill Publishing, New York.

Williams, C.A., D.S. Kronfeld, W.B. Staniar, and P.A. Harris. 2001. Plasma glucose and insulin responses of Thoroughbred mares fed a meal high in starch and sugar or fat and fiber. J. Anim. Sci. 79:2196-2201.

Wooden, G.R., and A.M. Papas. 1991. Utilization of various forms of vitamin E by horses. In: Proc. 12th Equine Nutr. Physiol. Soc. Symp., p. 265.

THE GLYCEMIC AND INSULINEMIC INDEX IN HORSES

INGRID VERVUERT AND MANFRED COENEN
Institute of Animal Nutrition, School of Veterinary Medicine, Hannover, Germany

Introduction

In horses, the total tract apparent digestibility of starch for various types of grain is usually very high. Arnold et al. (1981) reported values of 97.0, 96.7, and 97.0% respectively for corn, oats, and sorghum starch. On the other hand, considerable differences in prececal starch digestibility were observed between the different starch sources. In general, the prececal digestibility of oat starch exceeds that of corn starch or of barley starch (Kienzle et al., 1992; Potter et al., 1992; Meyer et al., 1995). Prececal starch digestibility of grains is improved by different processing techniques. The granular structure of starch might be destroyed mechanically (e.g, rolling, crushing, or grinding) or by heat and pressure in combination with moisture (Kienzle et al., 1992; Potter et al., 1992; Meyer et al., 1995). The effect of thermal processing such as micronizing, steam-flaking, or popping is an irreversible swelling and destruction of the internal crystalline structures of the starch granules; this transformation is termed gelatinization (Holm et al., 1988; Selmi et al., 2000). Thus, the extent of prececal digestion influences the proportion of cereal carbohydrates absorbed as glucose in the small intestine and that are fermented and absorbed as volatile fatty acids or lactic acids in the large intestine.

Consequently, an increase in availability of starch for enzymatic digestion in the small intestine might alter the metabolic response as more substrate will be absorbed. In humans, the measurement of blood glucose and insulin response is known as a suitable tool for assessing the effects of food processing on starch digestion (Jenkins et al., 1981; Brand et al., 1985; Granfeldt et al., 1994). In human subjects, starchy foods have been classified over the entire range from restrained, or low glycemic and insulin response, to rapid with respect to effects on blood glucose and insulin responses after a meal (Jenkins et al., 1988; Granfeldt et al., 1994). The resulting glycemic or insulinemic index utilized white bread as the standard source and all foods were ranked accordingly (Jenkins et al., 1981).

Influence of Grain Source and Processing Techniques on the Glycemic and Insulinemic Responses in Horses: Recent Work

Information is available regarding the influence of various grain sources on glucose and insulin response in horses, but no such glycemic or insulinemic index has yet been formulated for horses.

Stull and Rodiek (1988) noticed a significant increase in plasma glucose concentration after corn feeding as well as after a combined diet of corn and alfalfa (50% corn and 50% alfalfa) in two-year-old Quarter Horse geldings. Insulin concentrations closely followed the glucose curves. However, postprandial response area for glucose did not differ between alfalfa feeding (100%), corn feeding (100%), and combined corn and alfalfa feeding (50% corn and 50% alfalfa).

In ponies (age 3 to 18 years), oat feeding caused higher blood glucose concentrations in comparison to whole corn or barley. The addition of roughage to the diet blunted the postprandial rise in blood glucose, while the increase in starch intake (2 g starch/kg BW per meal and 4 g starch/kg BW per meal, respectively) did not influence blood glucose response (Radicke et al., 1994). The higher glycemic response to oat feeding was accompanied by a higher prececal starch digestibility rate of oats. However, in the study by Radicke et al. (1994), mean peak plasma glucose concentrations after oat feeding were lower (<5.55 mmol/L) when compared to the mean peak plasma glucose concentrations following corn feeding (7.85 ± 1.03 mmol/L) measured by Stull and Rodiek (1988), although starch intake was comparable between these two studies. No differences in mean postprandial peak plasma glucose concentrations were observed for sweet feed (45% cracked corn, 45% whole oats, and 10% molasses), whole oats, and cracked corn by Pagan et al. (2001) in six Thoroughbred geldings. Furthermore, area under the postprandial glucose curve did not differ for whole oats and cracked corn, but mean glucose concentrations were higher for whole oats (5.51 mmol/L) when compared to cracked corn (5.4 mmol/L).

The effect of corn processing on glycemic response was investigated by Hoekstra et al. (1999) in 6 horses (four Arabians, two Thoroughbreds; age 6 to 10 years). This experiment was conducted to evaluate how cracking, grinding, or steam processing affects starch digestibility of corn using glycemic response as an indirect measure of prececal starch digestibility. The glycemic response of each grain was compared using a glycemic index in which each feed´s glucose area under the curve (AUC) was expressed relative to cracked corn. The highest glycemic index was noticed for the steam-flaked corn (2 g starch/kg BW in a single meal; Figure 1). It is speculated that the high glycemic response reflects changes in prececal starch digestibility by thermal corn processing.

In a recent study by our own research group, mechanical or thermal processing of oats, barley, or corn did not clearly influence glycemic or insulinemic response in horses (Bothe 2001; Vervuert et al., 2002; Coenen et al., 2002). In a crossover design, six Standardbred horses (age 4 to 15 years, mean body weight 450 ± 37

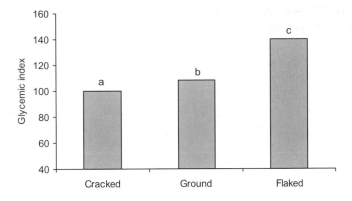

Figure 1. Glycemic index for processed corn (starch intake is 2 g/kg BW in a single meal) (Hoekstra et al., 1999).

kg) were fed in random order: untreated, finely ground, steam-flaked, and popped grain. All diets were adjusted to a starch content of 630 g starch per day from oats, barley, or corn (1.2-1.5 g starch/kg BW in a single meal). Grain feeding resulted in a significant increase in plasma glucose and insulin concentrations, but glucose and insulin peaks as well as AUC were not clearly influenced by grain processing of oats, barley, and corn (Table 1).

Table 1. Peak glucose (mmol/L), peak insulin (μU/ml), and area under the curve (AUC) for all diets.

Dietary treatment	Horses (N)	Glucose peak (mmol/L)	Glucose AUC	Insulin peak (μU/ml)	Insulin AUC
oats, untreated	6	6.7 ± 1.3	1659 ± 254	31.9 ± 22.9	6052 ± 4623
finely ground	6	6.6 ± 0.9	1697 ± 318	49.3 ± 54.1	9946 ± 11415
steam-flaked	6	6.1 ± 0.2	1549 ± 67	22.9 ± 6.7	4662 ± 1351
popped	3	6.0 ± 1.2	1577 ± 187	27.2 ± 21.6	4998 ± 3166
barley, untreated	6	6.1 ± 0.5	1564 ± 160[a]	19.1 ± 6.5[ab]	3792 ± 1713[a]
finely ground	6	5.7 ± 0.7	1494 ± 144[bc]	19.9 ± 8.2[a]	3766 ± 1565[ac]
steam-flaked	6	6.5 ± 0.6	1541 ± 116[ac]	29.4 ± 11.9[a]	5135 ± 2012[bc]
popped	3	6.1 ± 0.4	1563 ± 132[ac]	21.5 ± 8.1[b]	3840 ± 2164[a]
corn, untreated	6	6.6 ± 0.8	1630 ± 170	23.6 ± 12.9	4333 ± 2129
finely ground	6	6.2 ± 1.2	1527 ± 175	30.4 ± 22.9	4539 ± 2455
steam-flaked	4	5.9 ± 0.3	1513 ± 48	24.6 ± 10.6	4674 ± 1889
popped	3	6.3 ± 1.2	1691 ± 283	18.8 ± 10.8	3511 ± 1929

Treatments lacking a common superscript differ (P<0.05) within a column.

Insulin concentrations followed the glucose curves, but the correlation of mean plasma glucose and plasma insulin concentrations was not as close as expected and best described by the following equation: $y = 12.6 \, x - 49.24$, where y = mean plasma insulin and x = mean plasma glucose ($r^2 = 0.47$, $p<0.001$).

The glycemic index where each feed's glucose area under the curve was expressed relative to untreated oats varied between $90.44 \pm 13.55\%$ (steam-flaked corn) and $112.02 \pm 18.71\%$ (popped corn, $P< 0.05$.). The insulin index where each feed's insulin area under the curve was expressed relative to untreated oats ranged between $78.06 \pm 33.75\%$ (untreated barley) and $114.76 \pm 34.06\%$ (popped corn, n.s.). The glycemic and insulinemic indexes of oat, barley, and corn processing are shown in Figure 2.

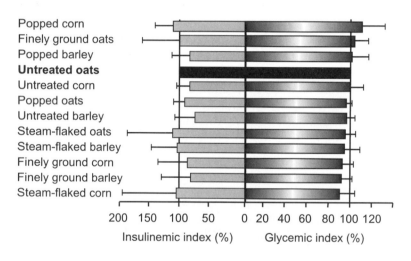

Figure 2. Glycemic and insulinemic indexes for processed oats, barley, and corn (starch intake is 1.2 1.5 g/ kg BW in a single meal).

In our study one striking feature was the high variation in plasma glucose and insulin response between the horses (e.g., peak plasma insulin concentrations for oat treatment; Figure 3). The reasons for the great individual variation are not fully understood. Ralston (1992) noticed a similar individual reaction in horses after feeding pelleted concentrates with a high or low level of soluble carbohydrates. In accordance, a high variation in glycemic response was monitored by Venner and Ohnesorge (2001) after an oral glucose load in healthy horses. A great variation in behavioral response to grain feeding is monitored by several horse owners and might be related to the variable glycemic and insulinemic responses to starch feeding.

In contrast to the investigation by Hoekstra et al. (1999), the effects of mechanical or thermal grain processing seemed to be of minor importance for the metabolic reaction and were not reflected in a raised glycemic or insulinemic response. However, untreated barley or corn was known to have a low prececal starch digestibility, and thermal treatment enhanced starch digestibility in the small intestine about threefold (Kienzle et al., 1992; Potter et al., 1992; Meyer et al., 1995). On the other hand, the improvement in prececal starch digestibility by grain processing and the increase in substrate availability might have been masked by other factors. Some of these factors include the chemical nature of the grain (amylose-amylopectin ratio), interactions with proteins and fat, the presence of dietary fiber, the rate of gastric emptying, and amylase availability in the small intestine (Rooney and Pflugfelder, 1986; Granfeldt et al., 1994).

Several studies have been conducted in humans to compare the amylose-amylopectin content of starch and its effect on glycemic and insulinemic response. The glucose and insulin response to high-amylose starch is significantly lower when compared to starch with moderate levels of amylose (Byrners et al., 1995; Kabir et al., 1998). More research is necessary to compare the digestibility of and metabolic reaction to different varieties of oats, barley, and corn.

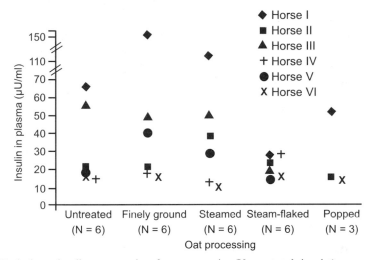

Figure 3. Peak plasma insulin concentrations for oat processing (Vervuert et al., in print).

Clinical Application of the Glycemic and Insulinemic Index in Horses

The nutritional importance of postprandial glucose and insulin response with regard to different sources of cereals and processing techniques is gaining greater awareness. On one hand, a high prececal starch digestibility is important to minimize starch flow into the large intestine, which might lead to considerable alterations in the microbial fermentation. On the other hand, exaggerated plasma glucose and insulin responses after carbohydrate intake have been associated with noninsulin-dependent diabetes and cardiovascular diseases in humans. Foods that elicit low postprandial glycemic responses are considered beneficial in subjects with metabolic diseases as well as in healthy human subjects. In horses, glucose and insulin control may be impaired in a number of life stages and/or conditions such as diabetes, obesity, gestation, pituitary dysfunction, laminitis, and aging. In horses with impaired glucose metabolism, plasma glucose concentration remains higher for longer periods of time, and horses were less sensitive to insulin than control individuals.

Table 2. Plasma glucose (mmol/L) in OCD-negative (OCD -) and OCD-positive (OCD +) horses after feeding meals of sweet grain mix plus hay (Ralston, 1996).

| | *Time after feeding (hours)* | | | | | | |
	0	*1*	*2*	*3*	*4*	*5*	*6*
OCD -	6.89 ± 0.13	9.12 ± 0.20	8.85 ± 0.26	8.29 ± 0.18	7.78 ± 0.12	7.29 ± 0.11	7.04 ± 0.11
OCD +	6.22 ± 0.17	10.3 ± 0.52	11.4 ± 0.06	10.2 ± 0.69	8.59 ± 0.50	7.01 ± 0.36	6.36 ± 0.27

These results by Ralston (1996) were supported in a field study with 218 Thoroughbred weanlings where a high glucose and insulin response to a concentrate meal was associated with an increased incidence of OCD (Pagan et al., 2001). At Rutgers University a patented glucose challenge test has been developed to identify foals with a high risk of developing OCD by their glycemic and insulinemic response (Ralston, 2001). Based on these results it would be beneficial to feed young growing horses feedstuffs that are known to elicit a moderate or low glycemic and insulinemic response.

METABOLIC DYSFUNCTIONS AND THE GLYCEMIC AND INSULINEMIC INDEX

Ponies that were fat or had previously suffered laminitis were found to be more intolerant to oral glucose loads than healthy ponies or Standardbred horses (Jeffcott et al., 1986). These ponies exhibited a far greater response in plasma glucose and insulin levels after glucose loading (1 g glucose/kg BW). Furthermore, aged horses often exhibit a relative glucose intolerance characterized by hyperglycemia and hyperinsulinemia following a glucose challenge (Ralston et al., 1988).The glucose intolerance in old horses is caused by a high incidence of pituitary adenomas. The pituitary adenomas cause excess corticosteroid secretion and impaired glucose metabolism.

The dietary management of glucose intolerance in horses is not well defined. However, there are two different ways of influencing dietary glycemic load:

reducing carbohydrate intake or using feedstuffs with a low glycemic index. However, in humans there is good evidence that a high-carbohydrate intake with a low glycemic index improved pancreatic b -cell function in subjects with impaired glucose tolerance in comparison to a low-carbohydrate and high monounsaturated fat diet (Wolever et al., 2002). In consequence, diets with a low glycemic index might be preferable in dietary prevention and management of glucose intolerance in horses.

GLYCEMIC AND INSULINEMIC RESPONSE PRIOR TO EXERCISE AND TRAINING

Dietary management prior to exercise may affect performance by altering energy metabolism during exercise in horses. In several investigations, corn feeding one, two, three, or four hours prior to exercise resulted in a marked drop in plasma glucose and insulin concentration below pre-feeding levels during exercise (Rodiek et al., 1991; Lawrence et al., 1995; Stull and Rodiek 1995; Pagan and Harris,1999). In general, horses that began exercise with high blood glucose and insulin levels (e.g., after corn feeding) showed a transient hypoglycemia during exercise, but the size of the meal (1, 2, or 3 kg) did not affect the response, although higher pre-exercise glucose levels were observed when the horses received 3 kg of corn (Lawrence et al., 1993). In contrast, horses with lower pre-exercise blood glucose and insulin concentrations (e.g., after alfalfa feeding) maintained steady glucose and insulin levels throughout exercise.

A drop in blood glucose concentration may indicate a lack of glucose availability for the muscle or brain and might have a deleterious effect on performance. In addition, FFA concentrations during exercise as a major substrate for energy metabolism were very low when horses received a pre-exercise meal of corn (Lawrence et al., 1993; Pagan and Harris 1999). In the performance horse, it might be useful to develop feeding strategies that include feedstuffs with a high carbohydrate content and low glycemic index.

Conclusion

In humans, starchy foods have been classified over the entire range from restrained to rapid with respect to effects on blood glucose and insulin responses after a meal. The resulting glycemic or insulinemic index utilized white bread as the standard source, and all foods were ranked accordingly. In horses, the classification of starchy foods with respect to their effects on blood glucose and insulin responses after a meal might prove useful in developing appropriate feeding strategies for horses with impaired glucose control or for performance horses. The glycemic or insulinemic index for horses should use untreated oats as the standard source. Nutritional factors like amylose-amylopectin ratio, interactions with proteins, or the presence of dietary fiber that might influence the glycemic and insulinemic index should be developed, and the great individual differences in response to starch feeding need further investigation. Furthermore, research is necessary to investigate the relationship between prececal starch digestibility and the glycemic and insulinemic index as an indirect measurement of prececal starch digestibility in horses.

References

Arnold, F. F., G. D. Potter, J. L. Schelling, and W. L. Jenkins. 1981. Carbohydrate digestion in the small and large intestine of the equine. In: 7th Equine Nutr. Physiol. Sym., p. 19.

Bothe, C., 2001. Effekte unterschiedlicher Stärketräger und deren Bearbeitung auf die postprandiale Glucose- und Insulinreaktion beim Pferd. Hannover, Tierärztl. Hochschule, Diss.

Brand, J. C., P. L. Nickolson, A. W. Thorburn, and A. S. and Truswell. 1985. Food processing and the glycemic index. Am. J. Clin. Nutr. 42:1192.

Byrners, S. E., J. C. Brand, and G. S. Denyer. 1995. Amylopectin starch promotes the development of insulin resistance in rats. J. Nutr. 125:1430.

Coenen, M., I. Vervuert, and C. Bothe. 2002. Effects of barley processing on the glycemic and insulin responses in horses. J. Appl. Physiol. Nutr.

Granfeldt, Y., H. Liljeberg, A. Drews, R. Newman, and I. Björck. 1994. Glucose and insulin responses to barley products. Influence of food structure and amylose-amylopectin ratio. Am. J. Clin. Nutr. 59:1075.

Hoekstra, K. E., K. Newman, M. A. Kennedy, and J. D. Pagan. 1999. Effect of corn processing on glycemic responses in horses. In: 16th Equine Nutr. Physiol. Sym., p. 144.

Holm, J., I. Lundquist, I. Björck, A. C. Eliasson,, and N. G. Asp. 1988. Degree of starch gelatinization, digestion rate of starch in vitro, and metabolic response in rats. Am. J. Clin. Nutr. 47:1010.

Jeffcott, l. B., J. R. Field, J. G. McLean, and K. O'Dea. 1986. Glucose tolerance and insulin sensitivity in ponies and Standardbred horses. Equine Vet. J. 18:97.

Jenkins, D. J. A., T. M. S. Wolever, R. H. Taylor, H. Barker, H. Fielden, J. M. Baldwin, A. C. Bowling, H. C. Newmann, A. L. Jenkins, and D. V. Goff. 1981. Glycemic index of foods: A physiological basis for carbohydrate exchange. Am. J. Clin. Nutr. 34:362.

Jenkins, D. J., T. M. Wolever, and A. L. Jenkins. 1988. Starchy foods and glycemic index. Diabetes Care 11:149-159.

Kabir, M., S. W. Rizkalla, M. Champ, J. Luo, J. Boillot, F. Bruzzo, and G. Slama. 1998. Dietary amylose-amylopectin starch content affects glucose and lipid metabolism in adipocytes of normal and diabetic rats. J. Nutr. 128:35.

Kienzle, E., S. Radicke, S. Wilke, E. Landes, and H. Meyer. 1992. Praeileale Stärkeverdauung in Abhängigkeit von Stärkeart und -zubereitung. 1. Europ. Conf. Horse Nutr., Pferdeheilkunde, 103.

Lawrence, L. M., L. V. Soderholm, A. Roberts, J. Williams, and H. Hintz. 1993. Feeding status affects glucose metabolism in exercising horses. J. Nutr. 123:2152.

Lawrence, L. M., J. Williams L. V. Soderholm, A. Roberts, and H. Hintz. 1995. Effect of feeding state on the response of horses to repeated bouts of intense exercise. Equine Vet. J. 27:27.

Meyer, H., S. Radicke, E. Kienzle, S. Wilke, D. Kleffken, and M. Illenseer. 1995. Investigations on preileal digestion of starch grain, potato and manioc in horses. J. Vet. Med. A 42:371.

Pagan, J. D., R. J. Geor, S. E. Caddel, P. B. Pryor, and K. E. Hoekstra. 2001. The relationship between glycemic response and the incidence of OCD in Thoroughbred weanlings: A field study. In: Proc. 47th AAEP Conv., pp. 322-325.

Pagan, J. D. and P. A. Harris. 1999: The effects of timing and amount of forage and grain on exercise response in Thoroughbred horses. Equine Vet. J. Suppl. 30:451.

Potter, G. D., F. F. Arnold, D. D. Householder, D. H. Hansen and K. M. Brown. 1992. Digestion of starch in the small or large intestine of the equine. 1. Europ. Conf. Horse Nutr., Pferdeheilkunde, 107.

Radicke, S., H. Meyer, and E. Kienzle. 1994. Über den Einfluß von Futterart und Fütterungszeitpunkt auf den Blutglucosespiegel bei Pferden. Pferdeheilkunde 10:187.

Ralston, S. L. 1992. Effect of soluble carbohydrate content of pelleted diets on postprandial glucose and insulin profiles in horses. 1. Europ. Conf. Horse Nutr., Pferdeheilkunde, 112.

Ralston, S. L. 1996. Hyperglycemia/hyperinsulinemia after feeding a meal of grain to young horses with osteochondritis dissecans (OCD) lesions. 2. Europ. Conf. Horse Nutr., Pferdeheilkunde, 320.

Ralston, S. L. 2001. Glucose intolerance and developmental orthopedic disease in foals–A connection? In: J.D. Pagan and R.J. Geor [Eds.] Advances in Equine Nutrition II. p. 397-401. Nottingham University Press, Nottingham, UK.

Ralston, S. L., C. F. Nockels, and E. L. Squires. 1988. Differences in diagnostic test results and hematologic data between aged and young horses. Am. J. Vet. Res. 49:1387.

DOES IT WORK? TESTING THE EFFICACY OF FEED SUPPLEMENTS

KENNETH H. MCKEEVER
Rutgers - The State University of New Jersey, New Brunswick, New Jersey

Advancements in equine nutrition have boomed in the last several years. In the past, nutritional research focused on the nutritional content and availability of various feedstuffs with an eye on providing a balanced ration to meet the energy and nutrient needs of the equine athlete. More recent research has followed the example of human sports nutrition and has examined the physiology of energy homeostasis with the goal of understanding how to improve the delivery of metabolic substrates to increase performance and to speed recovery from exercise. To that end a whole new industry has grown up around dietary supplements that purportedly alter metabolic pathways to improve nutrient utilization and to ultimately enhance performance.

The blitz of advertising that usually accompanies such miracle ergogenic (i.e., performance-enhancing) products would make one think that a great deal of scientific research has been published to support those claims. Unfortunately, many of the new dietary supplements and other products that have come on the market are being pushed with little scientific basis for the assertions made on their labels. In many cases, horses were not used in trials to demonstrate efficacy of these new and often expensive avant-garde dietary supplements and nutraceuticals. So how can we determine if a new supplement improves performance or has true potential to improve athletic capacity? This paper will outline some basic principles that can guide future research. These same guidelines can also be used to evaluate the soundness of information touted on new products designed for the equine athlete.

One recently published source suggests that a series of questions should guide the decision to use new dietary and other supplements in human athletes (Robertson, 1991). Robertson (1991) asks, "Is the purported performance-enhancing product safe or unsafe? Is it legal or illegal? And lastly, is it effective or ineffective?" All are valid questions that should be asked by horse owners and trainers. Unfortunately, many of the nutritional products being given to horses have not been tested for safety. Some may actually be "natural" sources of banned substances and thus illicit according to rules of competition. However, if a product is safe and legal, the last question is the one most horse owners want to have answered before they buy a product. So, how do we know if a product can help a horse perform better?

The best way to answer this question is to collect data during a competition or race against peers. However, those types of field studies have a great deal of experimental variation and require large numbers of subjects to determine if there are beneficial effects. Furthermore, how many horse owners are going to volunteer to have their animal placed in the group that gets the control if the treatment is going to help them win? Also, most racing jurisdictions are not going to allow the administration of a supplement to only a fraction of the competitors. Therefore, most recent research involves experiments conducted using smaller representative populations or studies conducted in a treadmill lab where experimental variation can be minimized. Nevertheless, planning for those types of studies and evaluation of the resulting data should be done after asking a series of questions:

1.   Is there a sound biochemical or physiological basis for claims that a product can improve performance?

   a. Does the claim make physiological sense?

   b. Or does the claim contradict what we already know from basic metabolic physiology and nutrition?

   c. Are there sound peer-reviewed studies from other species that suggest that the product may have an effect when used in an athletic horse?

2.   Does the horse utilize the substance in the same way as other species?

   a. Do we know the pharmacokinetics of the substance?

      i. Do we know the best route of administration?

      ii. Do we know the bioavailability of the substance?

   b. Do we know the pharmacodynamics of the substance? How much do we need to produce a beneficial effect?

   c. Is there a dose-dependent relationship?

3.   Has the product been tested in horses using properly designed studies?

   a. Is there a sound rationale for the efficacy of the product?

   b. Are the studies hypothesis-driven?

   c. Are the methods acceptable, accurate, and repeatable?

   d. Are there proper controls?

   e. In field studies (or even controlled treadmill studies), is the number of subjects large enough to ensure proper statistical power to detect a difference?

   f. Were the studies conducted in a blind fashion?

g. Were the treatments assigned in a random fashion?

h. Were there environmental controls?

i. Were the horses in the same state of fitness?

j. Were the horses familiar with the experimental surroundings?

k. Does the study measure physiological capacity or athletic performance?

l. Are the measured parameters really appropriate? Do they really serve as markers of aerobic or anaerobic capacity or athletic performance?

4. Is there specificity as far as the types of tests used to evaluate the effect on performance?

a. The concept of specificity dictates that the test used to evaluate performance and the training used to condition the horse should match the type of competition to be performed. Thus, do the tests simulate the specific type of competition?

b. Is the breed of horse used in the experiment appropriate?

   i. Thoroughbreds and Standardbreds vs. Quarter Horses vs. Arabians, etc.?

   ii. Are the animals middle-distance athletes vs. sprint athletes vs. endurance athletes?

c. Are the physiological markers to be measured appropriate? Are those markers representative of the physiological processes that limit the ability to win in a specific type of competition?

5. Are proper statistical methods being used, and are they interpreted correctly?

6. If the studies have been designed and conducted properly, have the results been interpreted properly?

a. Are the results being applied to the correct type of activity (sprint, jumping, endurance, etc.)?

b. Is the interpretation applied correctly to metabolic action of a substance and how it should affect pathways that impact performance?

These are just a few of the questions that should be asked when designing a study and/or interpreting scientific results used in an efficacy claim for a new nutritional product. Too often, the research that serves as the basis for efficacy claims does not follow even the basic rules of experimental design. For example, one product insert that I have used to teach students at Rutgers lists only one subject per treatment group. Some studies have even tried to apply data in an inappropriate manner. In one instance, a product claimed to benefit the performance of racehorses when the efficacy of the product was established using endurance horses. However, the most common problem associated with the marketing of these products is an excessive reliance on anecdotal information gained from testimonials. Research on the use of ergogenics and nutraceuticals in human sports medicine has shown efficacy for many of the most popular products on the market. The most classic examples are the long list of ubiquitous nutritional beverages that provide electrolytes and carbohydrates. Research has also shown that many of these products have no beneficial effect. Equine sports nutrition should use the same sound scientific principles to provide information to horse owners and trainers.

References

Robertson, R. J. 1991. Introductory notes on validation and application of ergogenics. In: D.R. Lamb and M.H. Williams (Eds.) Perspectives in Exercise Science and Sports Medicine. Vol. 4, Ergogenics Enhancement of Performance in Exercise and Sport. pp. xvii-xxii. Brown and Benchmark Press, Carmel, IN.

Spriet, L.L. 1997. Ergogenic Aids: Recent advances and retreats. In: D.R. Lamb and M.H. Williams (Eds.) Perspectives in Exercise Science and Sports Medicine.Vol. 4, Ergogenics Enhancement of Performance in Exercise and Sport. pp. 185-238. Brown and Benchmark Press, Carmel, IN.

CAN FEED CAUSE A POSITIVE BLOOD TEST IN RACEHORSES? SOME RECENT INFORMATION ON THE EFFECT OF DIETARY SUPPLEMENTS ON PLASMA tCO_2 CONCENTRATION IN HORSES

KENNETH H. MCKEEVER
Rutgers - The State University of New Jersey, New Brunswick, NJ

An extensive amount of published scientific research has established that the measurement of plasma total carbon dioxide (tCO_2) concentration is a scientifically valid method for detecting the administration of alkalinizing agents to horses. However, questions exist as to whether various common management and nonmanagement factors (e.g., electrolyte supplementation, ration formulation, environmental temperature, breed, etc.) inadvertently cause an elevation in plasma tCO_2 concentration. This paper will review some of the recent research conducted at Rutgers and elsewhere on the effects of various feeding practices, in particular, electrolyte and feed supplements on plasma tCO_2 concentrations. Information gained will be useful to trainers and veterinarians who wish to avoid having their animals inadvertently exceed established threshold limits.

Milkshakes and Their Detection

In recent years, sodium bicarbonate and other alkalinizing agents have been administered to horses with the goal of buffering the decrease in pH or acidosis that occurs with high-intensity exercise. This practice, commonly referred to as "milkshaking," has become more sophisticated and the administration of "other alkalinizing agents" is perceived as a threat to the integrity of the sport of racing (Rose and Lloyd, 1992; Irvine, 1992; Lloyd and Rose, 1992; Hinchcliff et al., 1993) and a potential threat to the health and welfare (Roelofson, 1992; Frey et al., 1995; Rivas et al., 1996) of the equine athlete. Therefore, racing agencies throughout the world have supported research to develop methods to detect the administration of alkalinizing agents (Irvine, 1992; Lloyd and Rose, 1992; Slocumbe et al., 1995; Auer, 1993; Lorimer, 1998).

Extensive published scientific data has established the validity of the use of plasma total carbon dioxide concentration (tCO_2) by itself to determine if a horse has been given an alkalinizing agent (Auer, 1993; Lloyd and Rose, 1993; Slocumbe et al., 1995; Frey et al., 1999; Greene et al., 1999; Kauffman et al., 1999). Put simply, Lloyd and coworkers explain that plasma tCO_2 concentration is a measure of bicarbonate together with dissolved carbon dioxide (Lloyd et al., 1992). Lloyd further states that the actual bicarbonate concentration is about 95% of tCO_2 value.

This strong statistical relationship between bicarbonate concentrations and plasma tCO_2 concentration is a fact that is detailed in basic physiology and biochemistry textbooks (Tenney, 1970; Martin, 1981; Guyton, 1981) and has been accepted as valid in several other papers that detail the validity of using plasma tCO_2 concentrations to detect the administration of alkalinizing agents.

The aforementioned scientific data, published in internationally recognized scientific journals and proceedings, has made the use of tCO_2 alone an accepted method in racing jurisdictions both in the United States (Maryland, New Jersey, Illinois, New York, etc.) and throughout the world (Australia, New Zealand, Hong Kong, etc.). This testing is performed either before or after a race; however, in many jurisdictions, prerace sampling has fallen out of favor, since it was found that the timing of administration of an alkalinizing agent allowed some horses to circumvent the test. Postrace testing can be affected by intense exercise, which causes an acidosis and a decrease in plasma tCO_2 concentration. However, the work of Frey et al. (1995) demonstrated that plasma tCO_2 concentrations return to prerace levels within one hour of the race. Therefore, regulations have established a postrace threshold on samples taken a minimum of one hour after the cessation of exercise. In several states, including New Jersey, postrace testing is used to identify horses that may have been administered a substance that alters plasma tCO_2 concentration. Another effective paradigm used in some states is to have all horses report to a secured paddock area several hours before major races. In this format prerace testing has been shown to be effective as racing officials can monitor the horses and any overages can be handled as scratches.

The threshold limits used in New Jersey were established after a study of more than 250 horses. Lorimer and coworkers (1998) demonstrated that the mean plasma tCO_2 concentration measured in New Jersey Standardbred horses on an off day, when they were not likely to have been given an alkalinizing agent, was ~30 mMol/L. The highest reading of tCO_2 was 34 mMol/L, a value well below the threshold established in New Jersey. Several other studies of hundreds of horses (Rose and Lloyd, 1992; Lloyd and Rose, 1992, Auer et al., 1993) conducted around the world have consistently demonstrated that, in nonmilkshaked populations, the mean plasma tCO_2 concentration averages ~30 mMol/L with very little variation around that mean. This makes sense physiologically as blood pH and acid:base status is regulated. For optimum cellular function, a horse's body will "fight" to maintain acid:base homeostais around a set point with narrow variation. Based on measured population data, many racing jurisdictions (e.g., Maryland, Illinois, New Jersey, etc.) have used concentrations that are 4 standard deviations from the norm to establish a threshold of 37 mMol/L (39 mMol/L for horses on Lasix) and to ensure against false positives.

In New Jersey and other jurisdictions, regulations have been established in consultation with horse owners and trainers that allow the horse owner to place a horse into quarantine, where plasma tCO_2 concentration can be measured under controlled conditions. Almost all horses placed into quarantine exhibit plasma

tCO_2 concentrations near to the mean of the normal population; thus, elevated plasma tCO_2 concentrations previously measured postrace are usually due to either the deliberate or inadvertent administration of an alkalinizing agent. It is the latter circumstance that was of concern in recent research conducted at Rutgers and elsewhere.

Are There Naturally High Plasma tCO_2 Concentrations?

One defense that trainers, horse owners, and veterinarians have used has been that their animal has a naturally high plasma tCO_2 concentration (Vine, 1998). To this end, several papers have looked at common conditions affecting plasma tCO_2 concentration. Slocumbe and coworkers (1995) demonstrated that there is only a very minor, statistically significant, variation across time. More importantly, their data demonstrated that those "cyclical" variations were physiologically insignificant, and even the difference between the highest and lowest points in the day would not push a normal horse near to the established threshold. Slocumbe et al. (1995) further demonstrated that alterations in breathing only cause minor alterations in plasma tCO_2 concentrations. Irvine (1992) and Slocumbe et al. (1995) demonstrated that excitement does not affect plasma tCO_2 concentration. Irvine further demonstrated that there was no effect of sex or age on bicarbonate status. Slocumbe et al. (1995) demonstrated that transportation did not affect plasma tCO_2 concentration. Several studies, including that of Frey et al. (1995), have demonstrated that blood pH and bicarbonate concentrations return to prerace or pre-warm-up levels by one hour postexercise. Those studies are the basis for collecting postrace/postexercise samples at least one hour after exercise. Finally, it is well established that Lasix alters plasma tCO_2 concentration. That is why most states allow a higher plasma tCO_2 for horses on Lasix.

Effect of Dietary Manipulation

Another area of concern to horse owners is whether their feed can cause an inadvertently high plasma tCO_2. Part of the rationale for these concerns has been based on a report suggesting that horses in Australia appeared to have higher plasma bicarbonate concentrations when compared to North American horses. The Australian data suggests that pasture-fed horses and horses fed diets with coarse roughage may have slightly higher plasma bicarbonate concentrations compared to horses fed higher quality forage (Kauffman, et al., 1999). Upon closer examination, however, the difference between pasture feeding and formulated feeds was minimal. Furthermore, an examination of data from several studies from Australia and New Zealand demonstrates that the normal mean value for plasma tCO_2 concentrations in racehorses in those countries was ~30 mMol/L.

Several other studies have examined manipulation of the protein, fat, and starch concentration of rations given to horses. Graham-Thiers et al. (1999) reported on the effects of high versus low protein diet on differences in plasma bicarbonate concentrations. While there were differences in HCO_{3-} and acid:base status during exercise, there were no differences due to treatment before or at 30 minutes after exercise. This suggests that manipulating protein concentrations in the ration should not affect prerace or postrace markers of bicarbonate status. Taylor et al. (1995) examined the effects of dietary fat on acid-base variables before and during exercise, before and after training. They reported that there were no effects of feeding increased dietary fat on venous pH or plasma bicarbonate concentrations. Interestingly, data are mixed as far as the effects of carbohydrates/starch. Work by Ralston et al. (1993) reported a decrease in blood pH due to starch intake with dietary cation-anion difference (DCAD) held constant. Mueller et al. (1999), however, found that blood HCO_{3-} concentration was greater in horses that consumed diets containing a high DCAD compared to horses that had consumed diets with a low DCAD. They also found that starch intake or source had no significant effect on blood HCO_{3-} concentration. One should thus take care when using a ration formulation that alters the DCAD. Depending upon the ingredients, that manipulation does appear to affect blood pH and blood HCO_{3-} concentrations and could push a horse's plasma tCO_2 concentration upwards. Nevertheless, when one looks at the values presented in published studies, the variation due to DCAD manipulation can only account for a small portion of an increase in plasma tCO_2 concentration. With reference to the effect of diet on plasma tCO_2 concentrations, the studies mentioned above are limited as the researchers have only looked at acid:base status in general terms and have not focused on the effects of feeds on plasma tCO_2 concentration. Furthermore, they have not examined changes in postexercise plasma tCO_2 concentrations as measured in most racing jurisdictions. However, one recent report by Kauffman et al. (1999) has examined the effects of various common dietary regimens on plasma tCO_2 concentrations.

In that study, Kaufman et al. (1999) tested the effect of five different rations on plasma tCO_2 concentrations. One ration treatment consisted of pasture, and another consisted of a pellet formulated with a coarse forage and grain combination similar to that used in Australia. The other three diets were pelleted with varying alfalfa and grain combinations representing 100%, 60%, and 40% alfalfa. Mean plasma tCO_2 concentrations ranged from 25.6 mMol/L to 29.1 mMol/L. The authors found that for the most part these dietary manipulations caused a very minimal change or no change in plasma tCO_2 concentration. They also demonstrated that, while pasture horses had slightly higher plasma tCO_2 concentrations, the difference was minor. The authors did report a transient effect when changing from one diet to another. Thus, one should take care when introducing a new feed. One should also note that the diets used in the study above were carefully formulated to exclude ingredients that could have an alkalinizing effect. Some ration formulations can have bicarbonates and other ingredients that can alter DCAD and/or have an alkalinizing effect that can have the potential to alter plasma tCO_2 concentrations. Horse owners and trainers should check their feed label to make sure that their ration does not contain ingredients such as bicarbonate or other alkalinizing agents that could be a problem.

Recent Rutgers Equine Science Center Studies

Effect of Electrolyte Supplements. It has become extremely popular for horse owners/trainers to give their animals a variety of electrolyte supplements to replace salts lost in the sweat. In theory, the simplest products on the market may actually have an acidifying effect and should not be a worry. However, many of the newer electrolyte supplements have a long list of ingredients, and some of these ingredients may have an alkalinizing effect. Researchers at Rutgers have recently conducted a series of studies to test the hypothesis that several common electrolyte supplements (Lyte-Now, Stress-Dex, Summer Games, Electroplex, Enduramax, Acculytes, Perform n' Win) would alter preexercise and postexercise plasma tCO_2 concentration in normal healthy horses. Horses were tested before and after a simulated race test performed on a high-speed treadmill. It was found that the electrolyte supplements did not alter plasma total carbon dioxide concentrations in unfit Standardbred horses. However, one should caution that the products mentioned above are just a few of the many products on the market. Some electrolyte supplements do contain ingredients (such as sodium bicarbonate) with an alkalinizing effect. Thus, an owner or trainer should check the label before giving electrolytes to his horse or wait to supplement until after the postrace testing has been performed.

Dietary Supplements. As mentioned above, diet manipulations have been hypothesized to have the potential to affect acid:base status in the horse. Inadvertent elevation of tCO_2 through dietary changes can thus be a potential problem for racehorse trainers/owners. Another study was performed at Rutgers to test the hypothesis that dietary supplements used in horses in New Jersey (Omelene 200™, Strategy™, Drive™) would alter plasma tCO_2 concentrations before and after exercise. That research demonstrated that none of the diets (Omelene 200™, Strategy™, Drive™) examined had an effect on plasma tCO_2 concentrations measured before and after a simulated race test.

Exercise Training. Plasma tCO_2 concentrations measured in unfit horses in the two Rutgers studies were slightly higher than those reported for fit racehorses (Lorimer, 1998). We speculated that the repeated challenge of exercise training and racing may chronically lower plasma tCO_2 concentrations in the fit horse. To test that hypothesis, a third study was conducted to compare the plasma tCO_2 concentrations measured in unfit horses with eighteen horses that were being moderately trained as part of another experiment. Each group underwent similar housing, feeding, and watering protocols. Moderately trained horses had a significantly lower plasma tCO_2 concentration compared to the untrained horses, and the mean (31.4 mMol/L) for the trained horses was similar to previously reported data (Lorimer, 1998) for fit racehorses sampled on an off day when they were unlikely to have been given an alkalinizing agent or milkshake. These results are similar to data reported by Irvine (1992).

Quarantine-Induced Detraining. Another area of concern in New Jersey has been the effect of the limited amount of exercise performed by horses during quarantine. Some horse owners have suggested that the limited exercise and stall rest associated with quarantine may have an effect on plasma tCO_2 concentration. Data indicated that two days of detraining does not affect plasma tCO_2 concentration.

Conclusions

Data demonstrate that normal healthy horses defend blood pH, blood bicarbonate concentration, and plasma tCO_2 concentration. Studies to date have documented minimal changes due to normal diet or electrolyte supplementation; however, alterations in DCAD or addition of alkalinizing agents to a ration may influence plasma tCO_2 concentration. Trainers and owners are cautioned to examine the label of ingredients for any product they may give their horses.

References

Auer, D.E., K.V. Skelton, S. Tay, and F.C. Baldock. 1993. Detection of bicarbonate administration (milkshake) in Standardbred horses. Austr. Vet. J. 70:336-340.

Frey, L.P., K.H Kline, J.H. Foreman, A.H. Brady, and S.R. Cooper. 1995. Effects of warming-up, racing and sodium bicarbonate in Standardbred horses. Equine Vet. J. Suppl. 18:310-313.

Frey, L., K. Kline, J. Foreman, J.T. Lyman, and P. Butadom. 1999. Effects of alternate alkalinizing compounds on blood plasma acid-base balance in exercising horses. In: Proc. 16th Equine Nutr. and Physiol. Soc. Symp., pp. 161-162.

Graham-Thiers, P.M, D.S. Kronfeld, and K.A. Kline. 1999. Dietary protein influences acid-base responses to repeated sprints. Equine Vet. J. Suppl. 30:463-467.

Greene, A., K. Kline, and J. Foreman. 1999. Comparison of three blood gas machines for determination of plasma tCO_2 in horses administered sodium bicarbonate. In: Proc. 16th Equine Nutr. and Physiol. Soc. Symp., p. 380.

Guyton A.C. 1981. Transport of oxygen and carbon dioxide in the blood and body fluids. A.C. Guyton (Ed.) In: Textbook of Medical Physiology (6th Ed.). pp. 512-515. Saunders, Philadelphia.

Hinchcliff, K.W., K.H. McKeever, et al. 1993. Effects of oral sodium loading on acid:base response to exercise in horses. In: Proc. 13th Equine Nutr. and Physiol. Soc. Symp., pp. 121-123.

Irvine, C.H.G. 1992. Control of administration of sodium bicarbonate and other alkalis: The New Zealand experience. In: Proc. 9th Internat. Conf. Racing Analysts and Veterinarians, pp.139-143.

Kauffman, K.F., K.H. Kline, J.H. Foreman, and J.T. Lyman. 1999. Effects of diet on plasma tCO_2 in horses. In: Proc.16th Equine Nutri. and Physiol. Soc. Symp., pp. 363-364.

Lloyd, D.R., and R. J. Rose. 1995. Effects of sodium bicarbonate on acid-base status and exercise capacity. Equine Vet. J. Suppl. 18:323-325.

Lloyd, D.R., and R. J. Rose. 1995. Effects of sodium bicarbonate on acid-base status and exercise capacity. Equine Vet. J. Suppl. 18:323-325.

Lloyd, D., P. Reilly, and R. Rose. 1992. The detection and performance effects of sodium bicarbonate administration in the racehorse. In: Proc. 9th Internat. Conf. Racing Analysts and Veterinarians, pp. 131-138.

Lloyd, D.R., and R. J. Rose. 1992. Issues relating to use of products that can produce metabolic alkalosis prior to racing. Austr. Equine Vet. 10:27-28.

Lloyd, D.R., and R.J. Rose. 1996. The effects of several alkalinising agents on acid-base balance in horses. In: Proc. 11th Internat. Conf. Racing Analysts and Veterinarians, pp. 104-110.

Lorimer, P. 1998. Report of the NJ State Police Racing Commission Drug Detection Laboratory.

Martin, D.W. 1981. The chemistry of respiration. In: D.W. Martin, P.A. Mayes, and V.W. Rodwell (Eds.) Harper's Review of Biochemistry (18th Ed).pp. 516-526., Lange Inc., Los Altos, CA.

Mueller, R.K., D.R. Topliff, D.W. Freeman, C. MacAllister, S.D. Carter, and S.R. Cooper. 1999. Effect of varying DCAD on the acid-base status of mature sedentary horses with varying starch source and level of intake. Animal Science Research Report, Oklahoma State University, pp. 189-193.

Ralston, S.A., C. Puzio, and D. Cuddeford. 1993. Dietary carbohydrate, acid/base status and urinary calcium and phosphorus excretion in horses. In: Proc.13th Equine Nutr. and Physiol. Soc. Symp., pp. 42-43.

Rivas, L.J., and K.W. Hinchcliff. 1996. Sodium bicarbonate and performance horses: Effects on blood and urine constituents and a review of beneficial and adverse effects. In: Proc. Amer. Assoc. Equine Pract.. 42:90-92..

Roelofson, R. 1992. Sucrose and bicarbonate overloading in Standardbred horses in Ontario. In: Proc. 9th Internat. Conf. Racing Analysts and Veterinarians. pp. 145-147.

Rose, R.J., and D.R. Lloyd. 1992. Sodium bicarbonate: More than just a milkshake? Equine Vet. J. 24:75-7.

Slocumbe, R., P. Huntington, et al. 1995. Plasma total CO_2 and electrolytes: Diurnal changes and effects of adrenaline, doxapram, rebreathing, and transport.

Equine Vet. J. Suppl. 18:331-336.

Tenney, S.M. 1970. Respiration in mammals. In: M.J. Swenson (Ed.) Dukes' Physiology of Domestic Animals (8th Ed.). pp. 316-317. Cornell University Press, Ithaca, NY.

Vine, J.H. 1998. Plasma total carbon dioxide concentrations in racehorses: challenges to test results. Proc. 12th Internat. Conf Racing Analysts and Veterinarians, Vancouver, Canada, pp. 32-36.

ORAL JOINT SUPPLEMENTS: PANACEA OR EXPENSIVE FAD?

STEPHEN DUREN
Kentucky Equine Research, Inc., Versailles, Kentucky

Introduction

Athletic competition often requires horses to run, jump, turn, start, and stop, placing an enormous strain on the skeletal system. As such, a performance horse may fail to reach its athletic potential or a seasoned athlete may not stay at the top of its sport because of lameness. Injuries and diseases of the joints are common causes of lameness. Because joint problems can be a limiting factor in career longevity of athletic horses, care and maintenance of joints is a major concern among horsemen.

Joint health is an evolving science. Researchers are investigating many novel equine joint therapies. A relatively new approach to joint health is the use of oral joint supplements. Advertisements for joint supplements are in almost every horse-related periodical, and tack store shelves are lined with concoctions designed to improve joint health. Despite their prevalence in the market, much confusion exists regarding these products. The following is a brief summary of the information available on joint supplements.

Joint Supplements as Nutraceuticals

Joint supplements are loosely classified as nutraceuticals. The term "nutraceutical" combines the word "nutrient" (a nourishing food or food component) with "pharmaceutical" (a medical drug). The word nutraceutical has been used to describe a broad list of products sold under the premise of being a dietary supplement (i.e., a food), but for the expressed intent of treatment or prevention of disease. In the case of joint supplements, they are sold as dietary supplements with a twist. The claims (usually made by manufacturers) of their ability to aid in equine joint health provides the twist. A potential difference between a feed and a nutraceutical is that a nutraceutical is unlikely to have an established nutritive value. Feeds are required to have nutritive value and are accountable, via labeling, for these values. Another difference between a feed (food) and a nutraceutical is that feed is "generally recognized as safe (GRAS)." Nutraceuticals may contain substances that are "natural" but may not be generally recognized as safe. The primary stumbling block in adding the "active" compounds found in joint supplements into horse feed is that these substances do not have a GRAS statement on file with feed regulatory agencies. Thus, inclusion of the joint supplement in the feed and listing its name on the feed tag are illegal due to the lack of established safety data.

The definition of nutraceutical includes the statements "for disease treatment and prevention" and "administered with the intent of improving the health and well-being of animals." When a dietary supplement, nutraceutical, or other feed is used for the treatment or prevention of disease, in essence it then becomes a drug. Drugs are subject to an approval process prior to marketing. To be approved, a drug must demonstrate safety and efficacy for its intended use. Drugs that are not properly approved are subject to regulatory action.

From this discussion, it seems joint supplements fall somewhere in between food and drug. They have many advantages over foods or drugs because they are not required to list ingredients and nutrient profiles as required by feeds, and in many cases are intended to treat or prevent disease without first undergoing proper drug approval. Determining if a product is a food, or is subject to regulation as a drug, is a function of the manufacturer's claims that establish intent.

The Goal of Joint Supplements

With vague label information, it is difficult to determine what the manufacturers of joint supplements intend as an exact function for their products. It is not difficult, however, to determine what is implied and expected by horse owners who buy the products. In most cases, joint supplements are fed to horses for one of two purposes. The first intended purpose is to heal the lame or to make chronically unsound horses sound. Unfortunately, horses can be lame for a number of reasons, and a single joint supplement could not possibly be successful in treating all causes of lameness. Even with other, more studied approaches to treating lameness, recovery is not expected in every case.

The second intended purpose consumers have for feeding oral joint supplements is to prevent joint problems from ever occurring. Unfortunately, many horse owners have seen the career of a talented horse cut short due to joint problems. These owners have since vowed to do "everything possible" to prevent the problem from occurring in other performance horses. Again, this expectation may be unrealistic due to the vast number of opportunities that athletic horses have to take a bad step and become injured. Do oral joint supplements work in horses? Some horse owners swear by them, while others do not see results. The unrealistic goals that both consumers and manufacturers have placed on joint supplements, horse to horse variability, and different underlying causes of lameness explain at least some of the differences of opinion regarding effectiveness of oral joint supplements. The key to understanding the efficacy of a joint supplement is to first comprehend the basics of joint anatomy and physiology. An understanding of the tissues involved in a joint and of normal joint function will provide rationale for many of the ingredients used in joint supplements.

The Equine Joint

A joint is the union of two bones, regardless of the location in the body. A joint allows controlled movement of bones relative to each other, thus allowing the skeleton to move. Joints found in the leg of a horse endure incredible pressure during movement. Normal horse movement begins with muscle contraction. Shortening of muscle fibers moves the bones via tendons that attach muscle to bone. Excellent descriptions of normal joint movement were written by Karen Briggs and published in The Horse (March, 1997 and November, 2000). The following is a summary of those descriptions taken with permission from The Horse.

In a healthy joint, the ends of the bones are coated with a thin layer of friction-reducing articular cartilage. They are also surrounded by a joint capsule with a tough outer layer (to connect the bones and protect the joint) and a permeable inner layer, or synovial membrane, which secretes synovial fluid and allows the passage of nutrients and other elements from the bloodstream. Synovial fluid, a slippery, viscous liquid that many researchers describe as being about the same consistency as egg whites, fills the joint capsule, nourishes the articular cartilage, and provides essential lubrication.

Synovial fluid is a nutrient-rich brew that contains proteins, enzymes, water, leukocytes, and a key ingredient, sodium hyaluronate, which is responsible for the fluid's elastoviscous qualities. Sodium hyaluronate (formerly known as hyaluronic acid) is a negatively-charged sugar chain, or glycosaminoglycan (GAG), which arranges itself in complicated coils, adapting to the pressure changes in the joint capsule as the horse moves. It assures the unhindered passage of metabolites to and from tissues throughout the joint, and also serves as a stabilizer and shock absorber for the structures that are undergoing continual, changing mechanical stresses.

Articular cartilage, the other main shock-absorbing component of a joint, is an efficient but flawed structure. Its structural framework is a web of collagen fibers, with cells called chondrocytes scattered along the matrix. Chondrocytes produce giant proteoglycan molecules that bind the GAGs. The GAGs in turn extract and loosely hold large amounts of positively-charged water molecules. When cartilage is damaged, there is a decrease in the number of GAGs; therefore, the cartilage holds less water.

Among the talents of cartilage, it conforms to the bone surfaces for a tight fit between weight-bearing bones; it spreads pressure evenly over a broad area; and it manages the water in its matrix, squeezing it out when the joint is under pressure, and drawing it back in when the joint is not under pressure. This in and out movement of the fluid transports nutrients throughout the cartilage. In a way, cartilage also acts like a sponge, conforming to loading demands by changing its shape and size, and regaining its original shape when the pressure is off. This "squeeze film lubrication" is the most important part of cartilage on cartilage lubrication. This cartilage lubrication is much like hydroplaning – there is a thin coat of water between surfaces acting to decrease the coefficient of friction.

But here is the downside. Cartilage is one of the body's most primitive structures. It has no blood or nerve supply of its own, so cartilage has little or no ability to heal or repair itself. Only in rare cases when the cartilage is torn directly off the bone can healing take place (because the resulting space allows capillaries to break through and patch up the holes with fibrocartilage). Even then, the repair work is substandard and will not stand up to repeated stresses. As a result, although cartilage performs admirably under normal conditions, it only takes a 5-10% overload of work stresses to begin deteriorating.

Joint Damage

Lameness can result from damage to any of the tissues associated with the joint. If ligaments, tendons, or muscles are disrupted due to injury, instability of the joint can result. This ultimately results in a change in the normal range of motion of a joint and lameness. Likewise, disease of the supporting bone can lead to collapse of the joint surface and painful lameness. Damage to the articular cartilage such as breakdown of collagen and loss of proteoglycan result in weakened cartilage. This weakened cartilage develops cracks and holes and loses its smooth articulating surface, resulting in lameness. Similarly, damage to the synovial membrane and changes in the makeup of the joint fluid result in alternations in normal joint viscosity and still another reason for lameness. So what is the underlying reason for joint damage? The answer is quite simple – inflammation.

Inflammation is normally a protective mechanism initiated by the body in response to injury. It is often localized to a particular area of the body and begins as a result of injury to or destruction of body tissue. It is the initial response in a series of events that lead to the attempted repair of the injured tissue. Inflammation causes blood vessels to dilate and allows fluid and cells to leak out. The cells that are released into tissues during inflammation are primarily white blood cells. In turn white blood cells release a variety of chemicals and enzymes into the inflamed area. The inflammation response in a joint is a process designed to break down and remove injured or foreign material. The process of breaking down and removing the foreign bodies from the area changes the chemical makeup of the fluid in the joint, introducing excess fluids and a high concentration of destructive enzymes and prostaglandins into a closed area (the joint capsule). This destroys the lubricating GAGs. The synovial fluid begins to lose viscosity. The chondrocytes eventually suffer from a compromised nutrient supply and cannot keep up with repairs. The cartilage develops damaged areas, opening the bone ends to direct trauma. The bone responds with a defense that only causes further destruction; it lays down new bone to strengthen the surface (sclerosis) and extends its margins in the form of bone spurs. If left unchecked, this inflammation, known as arthritis, will totally destroy the joint.

Treatment Strategies

Many options exist for treating joint disease in horses. The major treatment goals are to reduce inflammation, to improve joint fluid, and to improve cartilage. Treatments to accomplish these goals generally fall into two categories, physical therapies and medical therapies. Physical therapies include rest, bandaging, application of heat, application of cold, and mild, controlled exercise to maintain range of motion. Forty years ago, medical therapies to treat joint disease were limited to liniments, blisters, sweats, poultices, application of DMSO (dimethyl sulfoxide, an anti-inflammatory), NSAIDs (nonsteroidal anti-inflammatory drugs such as phenylbutazone), and corticosteroids injected directly into the joint.

Treatment options for horses with joint disease began to change about 30 years ago when scientists first attempted to replace some of the natural constituents of joint fluid and/or cartilage, with the hope that the body could use those building blocks to restore normal joint function. The first product used was hyaluronate. Hyaluronate is a proteoglycan and an important component of joint fluid and joint cartilage. Hyaluronate can be injected directly into the joint, and more recently, a new form of the drug can be injected systemically. Hyaluronate is thought to increase the viscosity of synovial fluid, inhibit some of the damaging enzymes, and promote the synthesis of more sodium hyaluronate. Polysulfated glycosaminoglycan (PGAG) is another powerful class of drugs used for the treatment of joint disease. Remember that GAGs are negatively-charged molecules that bind and hold water. The water helps the articular cartilage manage the pressure of weight bearing. These drugs have been shown to be anti-inflammatory and to increase the production of the proteoglycan component of cartilage. PGAGs can be injected intra-articularly or intramuscularly to achieve positive treatment results.

Oral Joint Supplements – Proposed Mode of Action

About 10 to 15 years ago, supplement manufacturers combined many of the materials found in healthy joints into an oral supplement. The thinking process was quite simple: put the building blocks for a sound joint in a bucket, feed it to the horse, and let him absorb and utilize the materials to repair joint tissues. With this logic, treatment options went from intimidating needles to a harmless scoop of powder or pellets. The manufacturers of joint supplements typically include a number of ingredients that may have beneficial results. The average joint supplement will contain nutrients, derivatives of nutrients, and herbs.

In order for a joint supplement to achieve its desired effect in a living horse, several things need to happen. First, the substance must get absorbed across the gut. Second, the substance must get to the joint following absorption. Finally, if the substance gets to the joint, the body must utilize it for repair functions. Two of the most common ingredients included in joint supplements are chondroitin sulfate and glucosamine.

With respect to chondroitin sulfate, absorption is debatable due to its large molecular weight (size). Chondroitin sulfate is typically obtained from bovine, whale, and shark cartilage. Several studies have characterized the intact absorption as low; however, more studies are under way that will use digestive data from horses. If chondroitin sulfate is absorbed and if chondroitin sulfate reaches the joint, what is the potential mode of action? As you may remember, articular cartilage consists of water, collagen, and proteoglycan. Chondroitin sulfate is the primary GAG that makes up the proteoglycans found in joint cartilage. It is known that joint injury and the ensuing inflammation cause a reduction in the amount of proteoglycan. Thus, chondroitin sulfate theoretically could help replace proteoglycan. Chondroitin sulfate has also been proposed to inhibit the action of some enzymes associated with cartilage breakdown and to have general anti-inflammatory properties. Data to support the proposed actions of chondroitin sulfate in in vitro studies have shown positive results. Definitive data to document the effect of chondroitin sulfate in living horses is not available at the present time. Data in other models (humans, rats, and dogs) does not automatically hold true for horses. So, the jury is still out with respect to chondroitin sulfate and its influence on joint health in horses.

Glucosamine is added to oral joint supplements either as hydrochloride or sulfate. As suspected, considerable debate exists as to the best form of glucosamine. Regardless of the exact chemical form, glucosamine is a significantly smaller molecule when compared to chondroitin sulfate. By most estimates, the absorption of glucosamine from the digestive tract does not seem to be a problem. However, specific horse absorption data have not been published in the scientific literature. If glucosamine is absorbed and if glucosamine reaches the joint, what is the potential mode of action? Glucosamine is a precursor to the disaccharide unit of glycosaminoglycan (GAG), which comprises the proteoglycan found in articular cartilage. In vitro data support the concept that glucosamine may stimulate synthesis of proteoglycan and collagen by chondrocytes. Experiments conducted in humans found glucosamine sulfate significantly more effective than placebo in improving pain and joint motion. Therefore, glucosamine may possess anti-inflammatory properties. Unfortunately, specific data in living horses are unavailable at the present time to definitively answer the questions surrounding the efficacy of glucosamine for joint health.

In addition to chondroitin sulfate and glucosamine, supplement manufacturers often include other ingredients necessary for synthesis of joint tissues. Included on the list of possible joint supplement additives are MSM (methylsulfonylmethane), copper, zinc, manganese, and vitamin C. MSM is a source of sulfur, a component that is necessary to strengthen collagen. The trace minerals copper, zinc, and manganese are each involved as cofactors for synthetic production of joint materials.

Finally, vitamin C is necessary for collagen formation. It is not known if these additives have any special benefit in oral joint supplements.

The bottom line regarding the efficacy of oral joint supplements is unclear. Many knowledgeable horsemen have used joint supplements on horses in their care with glowing success. Others have tried supplements and reported no detectable difference in their horses. Scientifically, many potentially promising benefits of oral supplements exist, but to date the efficacy of oral joint supplements in horses is unproven. Further, information on how much ingredient or which combination of ingredients is necessary to facilitate a joint response is totally absent. The unfortunate thing about the lack of definitive information is that many horse owners are considering themselves scientists and making their horses research subjects. The good news is that controlled research is being conducted to answer important questions surrounding oral joint supplements.

The Potential Problem with Joint Supplements

Do oral joint supplements actually contain the amount of active ingredient indicated on the label? This is a huge problem as published analytical reports conclude that 84% of human over-the-counter glucosamine/chondroitin products do not meet label claims. Another study on oral chondroprotective products intended for animals indicated that 70% of products did not meet label claim. With regulatory agencies overrun with new joint products, who is monitoring quality control of both raw ingredients and finished product? Further, who is policing labels and advertisements for implied drug claims? Are studies being done that will answer concerns regarding safety of joint products? These are all fair questions with few answers. Supplement manufacturers are beginning to appreciate the necessity of this information and have begun to organize themselves in an effort to answer consumer concerns.

THE DIAGNOSTIC POTENTIAL OF EQUINE HAIR: A COMPARATIVE REVIEW OF HAIR ANALYSIS FOR ASSESSING NUTRITIONAL STATUS, ENVIRONMENTAL POISONING, AND DRUG USE AND ABUSE

MARK DUNNETT
Royal Veterinary College, University of London, UK

Introduction

At first glance hair may appear to be perceived as a rather unprepossessing tissue; however, on closer scrutiny the truth is somewhat different. Early anatomical opinion considered the skin and hair as simply a passive barrier to fluid loss and mechanical injury. More recently, it has become apparent that the common integument of the skin and hair has to be regarded as a complex organ in which regulated molecular and cellular processes control essential physiological responses to environmental variables.

Hair has many functions, but most importantly it serves to help regulate body temperature and to provide a protective barrier against the horse's environment (Tregear, 1965). For example, there is a greater density of hair growth over those regions of the skin exposed to direct sunlight (Pilliner and Davies, 1996). Coat color is of some importance in thermal regulation, with light-colored coats being more effective in hot, sunny weather (Lyne and Short, 1965; Scott, 1988). Glossiness of coat hair is also important in reflecting solar radiation. Tropical breeds tend to have glossy coats that reflect solar radiation well (Hayman and Nay, 1961; Holmes, 1970). Equine skin carries several types of hair: temporary hair that comprises the majority of the coat; tactile hairs of the muzzle, ears, and eyes; and the permanent hair of the mane, tail, feathers, and eyelashes. These permanent hairs are anatomically located to provide protection in a number of ways. The mane helps to shed rainwater and to insulate the head and the major blood vessels to the brain (Pilliner and Davies, 1996), and the eyelashes protect against corneal impact injury. The various functions of hair are given in Table 1.

Table 1. Functions of hair (Stenn, 2001).

Decoration, social communication, and camouflage
Protection against trauma and insect penetration
Protection against electromagnetic radiation
Provide sensory assessment of the environment
Insulation against heat loss and gain
Mechanism of outward transport of social environmental signals (sebum and pheromones)

The Structure, Composition, and Growth of Hair

Structure of the hair shaft. The hair shaft is an end product of hair follicle growth and specialization and consists of three distinct structural components: a protective outer cuticle, an intermediately located cortex, and a central medulla (Harkey, 1993). A cross-sectional view of the hair shaft is shown in Figure 1. This illustrates the "tiled" structure of the overlapping cells of the outer cuticle that anchors the hair shaft to the follicle by interlocking with cells of the inner root sheath.

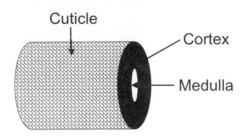

Figure 1. Cross section of the hair shaft.

The cortex constitutes the bulk of the hair shaft and comprises approximately 85% keratin, which is made up of matrix and fibrous proteins (Cone and Joseph, 1996). The protein fibers cross-link to form the structure of the hair and to provide its mechanical strength. The structural proteins of hair are interspaced with air gaps known as fusi. The cortex also contains melanin granules. Melanins (eumelanin and pheomelanin) are the pigments that give hair its color. The medulla is constructed of loosely packed, randomly orientated rectangular cells that shrivel when dehydrated, leaving a series of empty spaces (vacuoles) along the central axis of the hair shaft (Chatt and Katz, 1989). In general, the number of medulla cells, and thus the area of the medulla, increase with increasing hair fiber diameter. The fine hair of the equine coat contains predominantly cuticle and cortex cells, whereas the hair of the mane and tail contain a relatively large proportion of medulla cells (Talukdar et al., 1972; Harkey, 1993).

Chemical composition of the hair shaft. Hair is essentially a partially crystalline, cross-linked, and orientated polymeric protein structure. In addition to protein, the hair shaft comprises a number of different biochemical components including melanins, water, lipids, and inorganic minerals in variable amounts. Approximate proportions are given in Table 2.

Hair protein content derives primarily from the combination of three distinct structural keratins. These are designated as low-sulphur, high-sulphur, and high-tyrosine, high-glycine keratins. The sulphur content of hair is derived mainly from the proportion of sulphur-containing amino acids present, principally cysteine and to a lesser extent methionine. The lipid content of hair contains substances

Table 2. Approximate proportions of the various constituents of human hair

Constituent	Proportion (%)
Protein (keratins)	80-85
Water	<15
Lipids	1-9
Melanins	0.3-1.5
Inorganic minerals	0.25-0.95

such as free fatty acids and triglycerides. Melanins are polymeric substances produced from the oxidation of the amino acid tyrosine, through the action of the enzyme tyrosinase. In humans the melanin content of hair varies considerably between individuals and between races (Borges et al., 2001). The keratinized region of the hair shaft that extends beyond the epidermis of the skin (as the visible hair) is a dehydrated structure. The water content of the hair derives from atmospheric moisture and sweat and varies directly with the ambient relative humidity of the environment (Figure 2)(Robbins, 1979). Both trace elements and heavy metals such as lead, cadmium, and mercury can be found in hair. The concentrations of amino acid, lipids, and trace elements in hair are subject to variation due to factors such as genetics, diet, disease, environment, weathering, and cosmetic treatment.

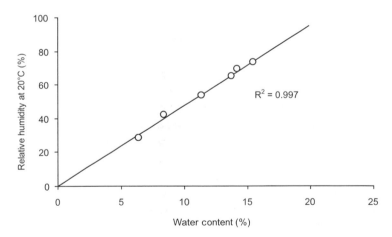

Figure 2. Relationship between hair water content and relative humidity.

Structure of the hair follicle. The hair follicle that produces the hair shaft is a miniature organ that contains muscular, vascular, and glandular components (Chatt and Katz, 1989). Follicles vary from site to site and generate hair shafts of varying shape, size, curl, and color depending on the anatomical location (Stenn and Paus,

2001). Unlike many species, including dogs and cats, that have compound hair follicles producing both primary and secondary hairs, the horse has simple follicles that generate only single hairs at any one time (Talukdar et al., 1972; Lloyd, 1993).

Simple follicles are associated with arrector pili muscles and both apocrine sweat and sebaceous glands. Contraction of the arrector muscle erects the hair shaft, influencing ventilation and heat loss from the skin, and is also associated with signaling in the fight-flight response to perceived danger. The sebaceous glands produce sebum, a lipid-based substance that coats the hair and skin to provide a protective barrier to repel water, to inhibit the growth of microorganisms (Lewis, 1995), and to prevent the penetration of toxic substances (Vale and Wagoner, 1997).

The follicle also comprises a dermal papilla, an inner and outer root sheath, and a bulge region (Figure 3). The dermal papilla directs the development of the follicular structure by supplying a permissive signal for continued growth of the hair. The hair bulb consists of proliferative epithelial cells that produce the inner and outer root sheaths and the hair matrix (Lloyd, 1993).

A further characteristic of the hair follicle as an organ is the presence of a range of enzyme systems that function to regulate the biochemical constitution of the tissue. The hair follicle contains a wide array of active enzyme systems including alcohol dehydrogenase, phosphorylase, NADPH reductase, glysosyltransferase, esterases, carboxylases, and succinic dehydrogenase (Jarrett, 1977; Potsch et al., 1997).

Hair growth cycle. The hair shaft develops via synthesis of matrix cells within the bulb. These cells move upwards and differentiate to form the various layers of the hair shaft and the surrounding root sheaths. When the hair shaft reaches the bulge area of the follicle, keratinization (hardening) occurs through protein cross-linking via formation of disulphide between adjacent cystine (amino acid) residues. The hair shaft then extrudes from the skin. The actual dynamics of hair growth is dependent on the rate of cell proliferation (Blume et al., 1991).

All mature hair follicles undergo a growth cycle comprising a period of active hair growth (anagen), a transitional period (catagen), a period of rest (telogen), and shedding (exogen) (Harkey, 1993; Lloyd, 1993; Stenn and Paus, 2001). The various stages of hair growth are shown in Figure 4, beginning with anagen in which the follicle is actively producing the hair shaft. During catagen active growth ceases and the follicle begins a shrinking process that ends in the telogen phase, where an inactive club hair is formed (Randall and Ebling, 1991).

At the end of the telogen phase, a new anogen phase begins. This is characterized by regeneration of the hair matrix from stem cells in the permanent part of the follicle, under the influence of the dermal papilla (Galbraith, 1998). A new hair shaft is then produced, the growth of which causes the previous club hair to be shed.

The duration of the hair growth cycle as a whole, and the duration of the individual phases within, varies between species, individuals, and anatomical sites. This cyclical activity is the mechanism by which animals change their pelage to meet the requirements of growth and seasonal climatic fluctuations (Randall and Ebling, 1991). It has also been proposed that the hair growth cycle protects against improper follicular formation and malignant degeneration (Stenn and Paus, 2001).

Hair Growth Rate in Horses: Non-Dietary Factors

The permanent hairs of the equine mane and tail undergo continual growth. Two studies involving small numbers of horses (four animals or less) over short periods of time suggest that the rate of growth of the mane is relatively constant (Whittem et al., 1998; Popot et al., 2000). In a much larger investigation involving 29 horses of different breeds, we found that mane and tail growth was essentially linear over a 12-month period (Figure 3). Although there was a degree of variability in the rates of hair growth in the mane and tail, when viewed on a month to month basis, no clear pattern was evident, and we were unable to correlate the fluctuations with climatic changes. The rate of growth varied between the mane and tail and within different regions of the mane (Figure 3). Rate of hair growth in the mane was lowest in the region near the withers and highest near the poll. The rates of growth of both the mane and tail were greater in native breeds of ponies than in Thoroughbreds, with crossbreds falling in between (Dunnett et al., 2002). We could find no clear effect of age or gender on hair growth rate in the mane or tail.

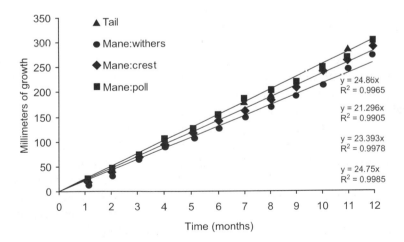

Figure 3. Cumulative mane and tail growth over time.

Effect of photoperiod. The seasonal growth and shedding of the pelage is something familiar to all owners of horses and domestic pets. Seasonal fluctuations in hair growth in the dog have been studied by Butler and Wright (1981) and Gunaratnam and Wilkinson (1983). This phenomenon is common to wild and domesticated mammalian species. For example, hair growth is minimal or absent in winter in cattle (Dowling and Nay, 1960) and cats (Baker, 1974; Ryder, 1976). Wool growth in sheep reaches a maximum during summer or early autumn and is minimal in midwinter (Coop, 1953). Even in humans hair is subject to small but significant seasonal variation with hair growth peaking in late summer and early autumn (Randall and Ebling, 1991; Courtois et al., 1996). Changes in photoperiod during spring, late summer, and early autumn influence hair growth through the eyes, hypothalamus, hypophysis, pineal gland, thyroid gland, adrenal gland, and gonads. Growth also has an intrinsic or inherent cyclic rhythm, and the timing of the cycle can be altered by systemic factors such as hormonal changes. Although many exogenous and endogenous factors can affect the rate of hair cycling, none alter the sequence.

Equine pelage, like that in most mammals, is affected by changes in photoperiod. Time of onset and rate of coat shedding is increased in fillies exposed to artificially extended photoperiods (Wesson and Ginther, 1982) and mares (Oxender et al., 1977; Kooistra and Ginther, 1975). A study of seasonal changes in pony colts (Fuller et al., 2001) found that metabolic and pelage responses to photoperiod change were not immediate but lagged behind abrupt day length transitions by 5 to 8 weeks. Reports of seasonal changes in equine pelage indicate that the greatest rate of growth occurs during the autumn (Popot et al., 2000). Possible photoperiodic changes in the permanent hair of the mane and tail have yet to be investigated. Our own work has indicated that there may be a tendency for both mane and tail hair growth to increase during autumn; however, this apparent increase could not be statistically proven.

Melatonin. The effect of melatonin on mammalian pelage change is well-known. Light receptors in the eye ultimately relay changes in daylight length to the pineal gland, which synthesizes melatonin. As daylight decreases, melatonin synthesis increases and vice versa (Bergfelt, 2000).

Androgens. The influence of androgenic steroids such as testosterone on hair growth in horses has apparently not been investigated. Red deer stags, however, produce androgen-dependent long mane hairs during the breeding season (Thornton et al., 2001). Changes in circulating androgen levels in humans have also been postulated to affect hair growth, although this has not been proven (Randall and Ebling, 1991; Messenger, 1993).

Prolactin. Prolactin has been shown to affect hair follicle cycling in many mammals. Seasonal increases in circulating prolactin levels have been shown to be statistically related to shedding of the winter coat in male ponies (Argo et al., 2001).

Furthermore, administration of recombinant porcine prolactin to seasonally anestrous mares induced pelage shedding within 14 days (Thompson et al., 1997).

Thyroxine. Hair growth also appears to be influenced by systemic thyroxine levels. Increased thyroxine levels have been shown to stimulate hair growth in both humans (Parker, 1981) and dogs (Gunaratnam, 1986). Thyroxine deficiency has also been shown to be a common feature in diffuse alopecia (Ebling, 1981). There have been no extensive studies to investigate the effect of thyroxine levels on hair growth in horses; however, coarser coat hair growth occurs in thyroidectomized mares (Lowe et al., 1987).

Effect of climatic variables. Through the effect on melatonin and prolactin production, day length clearly affects pelage growth in mammals including horses, although no direct effect on equine mane and tail growth has been demonstrated. The effects of other climatic variables such as temperature, intensity of solar radiation, and relative humidity have not been extensively studied. Cold-housed young (7-month-old) Standardbred horses produced 1.4 to 2 times more coat hair than warm-housed horses of the same age and breed (Cymbaluk, 1990).

Dietary Factors Affecting Hair Growth Rate and Quality: Amino Acids, Lipids, Essential Elements and Trace Minerals, Vitamins, and Selenium

Hair follicles are metabolically active tissues that require nutrients to support both structural and functional activities (Galbraith, 1998). As such, nutrition has a profound effect on both its quality and quantity. Poor nutrition may produce, and therefore be reflected by, a dull, dry, brittle, or thin hair coat. Pigmentary disturbances may also occur. Nutritional factors that influence hair growth are very complex and can be interrelated. Those most commonly associated with poor hair quality and hair loss have been summarized by Lewis (1995). They comprise dietary deficiencies of protein, phosphorus, iodine, zinc, and vitamins A and E, as well as dietary excesses of selenium, iodine, and vitamin A. Other possible nutritional imbalances that can affect hair growth include B-vitamin and vitamin C deficiencies, copper and cobalt deficiencies, and molybdenum toxicosis (Scott, 1988).

Protein and amino acids

Hair is predominantly a protein-based tissue with a high percentage of sulphur-containing amino acid residues. The amino acid composition of hair protein has been extensively studied in many species, including humans (Robbins, 1979) and horses (Samata, 1985; Samata and Matsuda,1988). The most abundant amino acids in equine hair are cystine, glutamic acid, serine, arginine, leucine, proline, and glycine. Samata and Matsuda (1988) observed differences in the amino acid content of equine hair between different breeds (Figure 4); however, no attempt was made to offer a possible explanation, and these apparent differences may have arisen due to methodological error or limited sample population. It was also reported that hair keratin amino acid content could be related to plasma amino acid levels, but no further details were offered (Samata and Matsuda 1988).

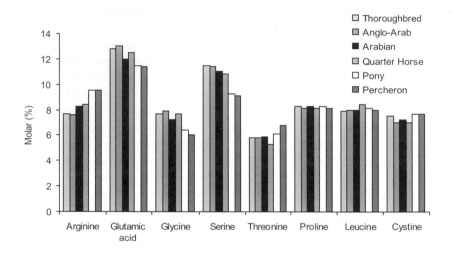

Figure 4. Differences in amino acid content in hair between equine breeds.

In mammals, normal hair growth and skin keratinization requires about 25% of an animal's daily protein requirement (Scott, 1988; Muller, 1989). Consequently, protein deficiency arising through starvation, low protein diet, or chronic catabolic disease results in hair production of abnormal texture and decreased length and diameter. In more extreme instances, diffuse thinning of the coat or alopecia can occur (Scott, 1988). Protein deficiency causes hair growth and shedding to be slowed (Lewis, 1995). The most important requirement for hair keratin synthesis is the sulphhydryl-containing amino acid cysteine, as it is ultimately oxidized to form the stable disulphide bonds that give keratin its structure, strength, and stability. Keratin is approximately 4% sulphur. Highest hair cysteine concentrations are found in the cuticle and cortex, and the lowest in the root sheaths (Rook and Dawber, 1982). Horses, like nonruminants, are unable to absorb inorganic sulphur and must meet their sulphur requirements through organic forms, such as the preformed sulphur-containing amino acids in plants: methionine, cysteine, and cystine (Lewis, 1995). Methionine can be converted to cysteine in the liver, and cystine is reduced to cysteine in the liver and blood. Despite the popularity of supplemental organic forms of sulphur, such as methylsulphonylmethane (MSM), there appear to be no reported specific sulphur deficiencies in the horse that could impair keratin synthesis. Whether sulphur supplementation (via sulphur-containing amino acids or MSM) and/or supplementation with other amino acids in horses with adequate dietary supplies can improve hair quality is uncertain. In other species, particularly sheep, increases in dietary sulphur content can, within certain limits, increase sulphur amino acid content in hair and can lead to increased hair growth rate and quality.

Lipids

The lipid content of hair is comprised of free fatty acids, monoglycerides, diglycerides, triglycerides, wax esters, hydrocarbons, and alcohols predominantly derived from surface deposition of sebum and apocrine secretions (Chatt and Katz, 1989). However, a proportion of hair lipid has been shown to form an integral part of the hair structure in humans. These integral hair lipids include cholesterol sulphate and ceramides (similar to those found in the keratinized portion of the epidermis), in addition to cholesterol, fatty alcohols, and free fatty acids. The predominant fatty acid, comprising 40% of the total fatty acids in the integral lipid faction, was identified as 18-methyl-eicosanoic acid (Wertz and Downing, 1988). Sebum and apocrine secretions normally coat the hair. These secretions of the sebaceous and apocrine glands are necessary to form a barrier to repel water and to protect against infection from microorganisms (Baxter and Trotter, 1969). Chronic illness may induce decreased production of sebum and apocrine secretions, resulting in dry lusterless hair. Such poor hair quality, in addition to hair thinning or alopecia, can also arise from essential fatty acid deficiency. Linoleic acid is an essential fatty acid needed for sebum production. Although essential fatty acid deficiencies are seen in dogs (Muller, 1989) and pigs (Scott, 1988), this condition does not appear to occur in horses (Lewis, 1995).

There has been a widely held belief that fat supplementation, particularly with oils rich in linoleic acid, will increase the quantity of sebum produced and thus lead to hair with a glossier appearance. Conclusive data to support this assumption have been lacking; however, Harris et al. (1998) observed significant improvements in coat, mane, and tail appearance (gloss and softness) following fat supplementation. There was also reportedly a significant increase in sebum and apocrine-secretion production. Recently, it has been demonstrated by administration of radio-labelled free fatty acids that dietary linoleic and linolenic acids are incorporated into guinea pig hair, presumably via sebum (Fu et al., 2001).

Carbohydrates

The main energy source for the hair follicle is glucose. During anagen the outer root sheath of the follicle is rich in glycogen, the storage form of glucose. This glycogen reserve disappears during catagen and is absent during the telogen phase (Jarrett, 1977; Rook and Dawber, 1982).

Essential elements and trace minerals

Few essential elements and trace minerals appear to have significant and clearly defined roles in relation to hair growth and quality. Those that do include iodine, zinc, and copper.

Iodine. This element is essential for the production of thyroxine. The effects of thyroxine on hair growth and quality have been discussed earlier. Iodine deficiency produces diffuse alopecia with premature telogenesis and hypoplastic hair follicle in all domestic species (Scott, 1988; Muller, 1989).

Zinc. Zinc is an essential element to many metalloenzymes and metabolic processes, including keratogenesis. It is also a cofactor for RNA and DNA polymerases and is involved in the synthesis of free fatty acids and vitamin A metabolism. Deficiency of zinc through low-zinc diets, high-calcium diets, phytates, or other chelators have been reported to cause alopecia in several species including dogs, goats, cattle, sheep, and pigs (Scott, 1988; Muller, 1989). There appear to be no reports of clinical zinc deficiency in horses, but experimentally induced zinc deficiency leads to hair loss (Harrington et al., 1973).

Copper. This element is essential in various enzyme systems including those involved in melanin synthesis, keratin synthesis, and disulphide bond linkage (Jarrett, 1977; Underwood, 1977). Copper deficiency results in fiber depigmentation and loss of hair tensile strength and elasticity leading to breakage. However, copper deficiency has not been observed in horses.

Molybdenum. Although not involved in keratogenesis and hair growth, excessive dietary levels of molybdenum can cause reduced hair growth and loss in hair quality. This is not a direct effect of molybdenum on hair but arises from interference with hepatic storage of copper and copper deficiency. However, there appear to be no reported cases of molybdenum toxicosis in horses.

Vitamins

Vitamins are essential to the promotion and regulation of a multitude of vital physiological and metabolic processes common to many organ systems in the horse.

Consequently, any disruption to the dietary supply or in vivo synthesis of vitamins has the potential to affect hair growth to a greater or lesser degree. In practice vitamin deficiencies are rare causes of disturbed hair growth in domestic mammals, including horses (Scott, 1988; Muller, 1989).

Vitamin A and β-carotene. Vitamin A is formed in the small intestine primarily from the enzyme-catalyzed cleavage of dietary ß-carotene. Vitamin A is required for healthy epithelial tissue formation through participation in glycoprotein synthesis that controls cell differentiation and gene expression. Correct cell differentiation is essential for the production of healthy inner and outer root sheath and hair matrix cells. Vitamin A deficiency can occur in foals and foaling mares. This results in rough, dry, dull, brittle, and long coat hair in both foals and mares (Donoghue et al., 1981; Evans et al., 1977). Similar coat hair defects are also observed in vitamin A toxicosis (Donoghue et al., 1981). More recently, in vitro experiments have shown that a vitamin A analogue, 13-cis-retinoic acid, alters equine hair sheath-shaft interactions. It was further hypothesized that in vivo hair sheath growth may be mediated by the follicle at the level of the sebaceous gland or by the sebaceous gland itself through the action of a biochemical factor analogous with vitamin A (Williams et al., 1996). Interestingly, some ß-carotene not cleaved in the gastrointestinal tract is absorbed and transported, bound to HDL lipoproteins, to various tissues, including the skin and corpus luteum. There are reported to be a number of poorly understood intrinsic mechanisms that regulate hair growth (Scott, 1988), and it is therefore possible that ß-carotene in the skin may directly affect hair growth by some unknown mechanism. Alternatively, ß-carotene could influence hair growth indirectly through its involvement in progesterone secretion from the corpus luteum.

B-complex vitamins. Since many of the B vitamins are involved in regulation of energy metabolism and protein synthesis, their deficiencies can lead to decreased feed intake, inadequate protein supply, increased protein catabolism, reduced keratogenesis, and therefore impaired hair growth and shedding. Extreme biotin deficiencies induced experimentally in a number of species, but not horses, resulted in hyperkeratosis of the follicular epithelia, alopecia, and depigmentation of the hair (Grieve, 1963; Misir et al., 1986). Biotin-containing supplements are widely marketed for promoting growth of equine hoof horn, a keratin-containing tissue. There is some evidence to suggest that biotin administration improves hair growth in swine (Bryant et al., 1985) but there appears to be no similar scientific evidence pertaining to its administration in horses. Furthermore, there is currently no clinical evidence for biotin deficiency in horses.

Vitamin C. Ascorbic acid (vitamin C) is important for hair growth and stability through facilitating the formation of disulphide linkages in keratin, and a vitamin C-responsive alopecia in recognized in calves (Goldsmith, 1983; Scott, 1988). No similar condition has been reported in horses. Adequate supply of ascorbic acid is also necessary for synthesis of both steroid hormones and hydroxyproline. Steroids, such as the androgens, are suspected of having a regulatory role in hair follicle cycling. Hydroxyproline is a major constituent of collagen and therefore connective tissue. Normal collagen is essential for the structural integrity of inner and outer hair root sheaths.

Vitamin E. This vitamin, in conjunction with selenium, provides the natural antioxidant system that helps to maintain cell membrane stability. Vitamin E functions as a free radical scavenger that protects cells from damage arising from reactive oxygen species (radicals), a major source of which is lipid metabolism. A high fat diet can lead to relative vitamin E deficiency. Subsequent free radical production and resultant membrane damage can lead to loss of cellular integrity and hair loss.

Selenium

Selenium performs a number of roles pertaining to cellular function and is a necessary constituent of the diet. However, chronic toxicity occurs when dietary levels exceed 5 mg/kg, and acute toxicity evolves when levels reach 25-50 mg/ kg. Toxic selenosis occurs occasionally in horses (Crinion and O'Connor, 1978; McLaughlin and Cullen, 1986; Dewes and Lowe, 1987; Witte et al., 1993). In this condition it is assumed that selenium substitutes for sulphur in sulphur-containing amino acids forming selenomethionine, selenocysteine, and selenocystine. Incorporation of absorbed seleno-amino acids during keratogenesis results in reduced capacity to form disulphide cross-links causing reduced structural integrity. Selenosis in horses generally occurs in areas of high soil selenium content and develops through chronic ingestion of selenium-concentrating plants and water of high selenium content. The condition results in progressive loss of hair from the mane, tail, and fetlocks and in extreme cases a generalized alopecia.

Hair Analysis: An Historical Perspective

Hair analysis was first applied in the middle of the 19th century. Casper (1857-1858) recorded its use to detect the presence of arsenic in hair from a suspected murder victim 11 years postmortem. The technique then appears to have been dormant for almost 100 years until in 1945 Flesch (1945) proposed that hair might be considered a metabolic end product and excretory organ, the trace element composition of which reflected the medium from which it was formed.

Early values for metal concentrations in hair were reported by Goldblum et al. (1953). A year later, Goldblum et al. (1954) described the detection of the first organic drug, phenobarbitone, in hair. Forshufvud et al. (1961) and Smith et al. (1962) used hair analysis to investigate suspicions that the Emperor Napoleon had been poisoned with arsenic. The results of the analysis indicated repeated exposure to arsenic. No firm conclusion as to the source of the arsenic could be drawn as it appears that pigments based on arsenic were used in wallpaper manufacture in the early 19th century.

The application of hair analysis to monitor exposure to heavy metals and nutritional trace elements continued through the 1960s and 1970s. The theory that hair could be used as a means to identify and track prior exposure to heavy metal toxins was explored and exploited with varying degrees of success in diverse situations. Hair analysis was used to trace the history and extent of exposure to mercury in cases of suspected poisoning in Iraq arising from consumption of bread produced from grain contaminated with mercurial fungicide. Other uses of the technique were to monitor occupational and lifestyle exposures to heavy metal toxins, such as mercury in dental technicians and lead from traffic exhaust emissions in school children.

The application of hair analysis for the detection of abuse of controlled drugs and to establish an individual's history of use was initiated by Baumgartner et al. (1979), who applied the technique to the detection of opiates in samples from drug addicts. Over the next decade, the application of the technique was expanded to encompass a range of drugs of abuse, including phencyclidine (Baumgartner et al., 1981), barbiturates (Smith and Pomposini, 1981), and cocaine (Valente et al., 1981). The subsequent 20 years has seen an exponential increase in the development, validation, and application of hair analysis to the detection of a wide range of abused and therapeutic drugs in human hair (Tagliaro et al., 1997; Nakahara, 1999; Gaillard and Pepin, 1999).

Hair Analysis to Assess Nutritional Status

Hair analysis for assessment of nutritional status (for essential elements and trace minerals) has been evaluated and employed for several decades. However, it is only within the last 10 to 20 years that increasing use of spectroscopic methods, making multi-element analysis possible, and improvements in analytical methodologies have provided a more reliable, rapid, and comparatively inexpensive diagnostic technique (Chyla and Zyrnicki, 2000). Hair is a potentially useful tissue for trace element analysis insofar as it is easily collected and transported, has high concentrations of trace elements, and may be representative of nutritional status over an extended time period. This last point may provide a benefit over plasma and urine samples, as transient fluctuations arising from recent dietary intake may be avoided.

Hair analysis has been used in the past in attempts to measure whole-body status of trace minerals such as calcium and phosphorus (Sippel et al., 1964; Wysocki and Klett, 1971); copper, molybdenum and iron (Cape and Hintz, 1982); and zinc, copper, and selenium (Wichert et al., 2002). However, the potential benefits of hair analysis can only be realized if measured hair concentrations are indicative of whole-body status and can accurately and consistently reflect nutritional imbalances. To date, there remain questions over the validity of hair analysis for the assessment of whole-body trace element status in horses (Hintz. 2000).

Monitoring Heavy Metal Exposure and Other Environmental Toxins

Hair analysis has been utilized extensively to investigate human exposure to a number of toxic heavy metals and other elements including lead, cadmium, mercury, and arsenic, and to track the history of such exposure. This topic has been reviewed extensively by Chatt and Katz (1989). The technique has been much less widely applied in animal toxicological studies, although it has been used to identify environmental exposure to heavy metals (Burger et al., 1994) and selenium (Clark et al., 1989; Edwards et al., 1989) in wildlife, and selenosis in domestic animals (Mihajlovic, 1992). Levine et al. (1976) reported that lead levels in blood and coat hair from a number of dead small and large animals that had been grazing pasture near a lead smelter were significantly elevated.

Environmental exposure of horses to a number of toxic elements has been investigated by hair analysis. Cadmium exposure of horses in central Europe in relation to their age, gender, breed, and location was examined by hair analysis. Cadmium was detectable in hair samples and was accumulated to a greater extent in geldings than mares (Anke et al., 1989). Hair analysis was used to monitor exposure of horses, sheep, and alpacas to a number of toxic heavy metals and other elements including cadmium, chromium, nickel, and bromine in vehicle emissions (Ward and Savage, 1994). Elevated lead and cadmium levels were found in horse hair and blood samples. Lead contents in blood and hair were significantly correlated (r = +0.69). Exposure of horses to toxic levels of selenium via forage ingestion has been investigated by hair analysis. Hair selenium concentrations in coat, mane, and tail hair samples ranged from 0.3–7.1 mg/kg. Hair selenium concentrations were strongly correlated with serum concentrations (r = 0.76–0.94) (Witte et al., 1993). Hair selenium concentrations are partially cumulative and reflect historical exposure to this element.

Dauberschmidt and Wennig (1998) used hair analysis to investigate pesticide exposure in humans. DDE and other polychlorinated biphenyls (PCB) were detected at concentrations of 0.5-4.9 pg/mg. As yet, assessment of the exposure of horses to environmental pesticide residues by hair analysis has not been attempted.

Another unevaluated potential application of hair analysis is in instances of plant-induced toxicosis in horses. Although plant poisoning in horses continues to be a problem in many countries throughout the world, its economic impact is unclear, as comparatively few poisonings are confirmed, and the actual extent of the problem is not clearly known. In the UK, however, approximately 500 horses each year die from hepatic disease resulting from the ingestion of common (or tansy) ragwort. The hepatotoxins in this plant are a group of substances known as pyrrolizidine alkaloids. In addition to causing primary hepatic failure, these substances are also carcinogenic and teratogenic (Lewis, 1995). These substances, in common with other alkaloids present in many other plants, should be chemically amenable to deposition in equine hair and therefore subsequent detection. We are currently developing analytical techniques to detect and identify alkaloid plant toxins in equine hair.

Hair Analysis and Drug Use: Residue Monitoring in Stock Production, Pre-Purchase Examinations, and Sports Anti-Doping Control

The use of hair analysis for the detection of drug administration in horses has only begun to be evaluated within the last 5 years. Horses can be subject to drug abuse in several instances. The growth-promoting potential of anabolic steroids such as testosterone, nandrolone, and stanozolol, and repartitioning agents such as clenbuterol (Ventipulmin), albuterol, and brombuterol, can be abused during bloodstock breeding to enhance muscular development of young horses. A multitude of performance-altering drugs including central nervous system stimulants and sedatives have been and continue to be misused during training and competition in equine sports such as racing and show jumping. Nonsteroidal anti-inflammatory analgesic drugs such as phenylbutazone (bute) and anti-inflammatory corticosteroids including dexamethasone are known to be used to mask lameness in horses during pre-purchase veterinary examinations. Furthermore, in the European Union many therapeutic drugs intended for use in equine veterinary medicine are no longer permitted to be used for treatment in horses intended for human consumption.

In 1997 we began a long-term investigation to study the incorporation of therapeutic and illicit drugs in equine mane and tail hair and to evaluate the potential for hair analysis for the retrospective detection of drug use and misuse in horses. We have shown that a number of antibiotics including sulphonamides, trimethoprim, metronidazole, and procaine benzylpenicillin can be detected in mane and tail hair samples up to two years after systemic administration (Dunnett and Lees, 2000; Dunnett et al., 2002). We have also detected a number a range of methylxanthine drugs and metabolites including caffeine and theobromine in mane and tail hair (Dunnett et al., 2002). Deposition of a number of other drugs in equine hair has recently been reported, including morphine (Beresford et al., 1998), diazepam, and clenbuterol (Popot et al., 2000). Cocaine, however, was not detected in mane hair following systemic administration (Whittem et al., 2000).

Thoroughbred racehorses can fail postrace drug tests for prohibited substances through ingestion of a number of potential feed contaminants. Some examples of prohibited substances that can occur in feedstuffs are shown in Table 3.

Table 3. Examples of prohibited substances that occur in feedstuffs.

Arsenic	Hyoscine
Atropine	Lupanine
Borneol	Menthol
Bufotenine	Morphine
Caffeine	Oryzanol
Camphor	Sparteine
Dimethylsulphoxide	Theobromine
Hordenine	

It is possible that the application of hair analysis provides additional analytical evidence to that normally achieved from blood or urine analysis. Analysis of hair, unlike that of urine and blood, may demonstrate that the presence of the drug in the horse's system arose from the chronic ingestion of contaminated feed rather than from an acute drug administration. The potential routes for the incorporation of drugs and other substances, including trace minerals, into hair is shown in Figure 5.

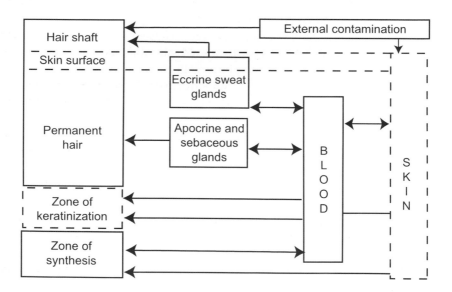

Figure 5. Potential routes of incorporation of drugs and other substances into hair (Henderson, 1993).

References

Anke, M., T. Kosla, and B. Groppel. 1989. The cadmium status of horses from central Europe depending on breed, sex, age and living area. Arch. Tierernahr. 39:657-683.

Argo, C.M., M.G.R. Collingsworth, and J.E. Cox. 2001. Seasonal changes in reproductive and pelage status during the initial quiescent and first active breeding seasons of the peripubertal pony colt. Anim. Sci. 72:55-64.

Baker, K.P. 1974. Hair growth and replacement in the cat. Br. Vet. J. 130:327-335.

Baumgartner, A.M., P.F. Jones, W.A. Baumgartner, and C.T. Black. 1979. Radioimmunoassay of hair for determining opiate-abuse histories. J. Nucl. Med. 20:748-752.

Baumgartner, A.M., P.F. Jones, and C.T. Black. 1981. Detection of phencyclidine in hair. J.Forensic Sci. 26:76-581.

Baxter, M., and D. Trotter. 1969. The effect of fatty materials extracted from keratins on the growth of fungi, with particular reference to the free fatty acid content. Sabouraudia 7:199-206.

Beresford, G.D., T.A. Gourdie.and E. Whittem. 1998. Analysis of morphine in equine hair samples by GC/MS. Proc. 13th Internat. Conf. of Racing Analysts and Veterinarians. Vancouver, BC, Canada.

Bergfelt, D.R. 2000. Anatomy and physiology of the mare. In: Equine Breeding Management and Artificial Insemination. p. 141-164. W B Saunders, London.

Blume, R.A., J. Ferracin, M. Verschoore, J.M. Czernielewski, and H. Schaefer. 1991. Physiology of the vellus hair follicle: Hair growth and sebum excretion. Br. J. Dermatol. 124:21-28.

Borges, C.R., J.C. Roberts, D.G. Wilkins, and D.E. Rollins. 2001. Relationship of melanin degradation to actual melanin content: Application to human hair. Anal Biochem. 290:116-125.

Bryant, K.L., E.T. Kornegay, and J.W. Knight. 1985. Supplemental biotin for swine III. J. Anim. Sci. 60:154-162.

Burger, J., M. Marquez, and M. Goechfeld. 1994. Heavy metals in the hair of opossum from Palo Verde, Costa Rica. Arch. Environ. Contam. Toxicol. 27:154-161.

Butler, W.F., and A.I. Wright. 1981. Hair growth in the greyhound. J. Small Anim. Pract. 22:655-661.

Cape, L., and H.F. Hintz. 1982. Influence of month, colour, age, corticosteroids and dietary molybdenum on mineral concentration of equine hair. Am. J. Vet. Res. 43:1132-1136.

Casper, J.L. 1857-1858. Praktisches handbuch der gerichtlichen medizin, (2 vol.). A. Hirschwald, Berlin.Chatt, A., and S.A. Katz. 1989. Hair Analysis:

Applications in the Biomedical and Environmental Sciences. VCH Publications, New York.

Chyla, M.A., and W. Zyrnicki. 2000. Determination of metal concentrations in animal hair by the ICP method. Comparison of various washing procedures. Biol. Trace Element Res. 75:187-194.

Clark, D.R., P.A. Ogasawana, G.J. Smith, and H.M. Ohlendorf. 1989. Selenium accumulation by raccoons exposed to irrigation drain water at Kesterson National Wildlife Refuge, California, 1986. Arch. Environ. Contam. Toxicol. 18:789-794.

Cone, E.J., and R.E. Joseph. 1996. The potential of bias in hair testing for drugs of abuse. In: Drug Testing in Hair. p. 69-93. CRC Press, London.

Coop, I.E. 1953. Wool growth as affected by nutrition and climate factors. J. Agric. Sci. 43:456-463.

Courtois, M., G. Loussouarn, S. Horseau, and J.F Grollier. 1996. Periodicity in the growth and shedding of hair. Br. J. Dermatol. 134:47-54.

Crinion, R.A.P., and J.P. O'Connor. 1978. Selenium intoxication in horses. Irish Vet. J. 30:81-86.

Cymbaluk, N.F. 1990. Cold housing effects on growth and nutrient demand of young horses. J. Anim. Sci. 68:3152-3162.

Dauberschmidt, C., and R. Wennig. 1998. Organochlorine pollutants in human hair. J. Anal. Toxicol. 22:610-611.

Dewes, H.F., and M.D. Lowe. 1987. Suspected selenium poisoning in a horse. N. Z. Vet. J. 35:53-54.

Donoghue, S., D.S. Kronfeld, and S.J. Berkowitz. 1981. Vitamin A nutrition of the equine. J. Nutr. 111:365-374.

Dowling, D.F., and T. Nay. 1960. Cyclic changes in the follicles and hair coat in cattle. Aust. J. Ag. Res. 11:1064-1071.

Dunnett, M., E. Houghton, and P. Lees. 2002. Deposition of etamiphylline and other methylxanthines in equine mane hair following oral administration. Proc. 14th Internat. Conf. of Racing Analysts and Veterinarians. R & W Publications, Orlando, Florida.

Dunnett, M., and P. Lees. 2000. Hair analysis as a novel investigative tool for the detection of historical drug use/misuse in the horse. Proc. 8th Internat. Congr. of the European Assoc. of Veterinary Pharmacologists and Toxicologists, Jerusalem, Israel.

Ebling, F.J. 1981. Hormonal control of hair growth. In: C.E.O. Orfanos, G.S. Montagna, and G.S. Stuttgen (Eds.) Hair Research. pp. 195-204. Springer-Verlag, Berlin.

Edwards, W.C., D.L. Whitenack, J.W. Alexander, and M.A. Solangi. 1989. Selenium toxicosis in three California sealions (*Zalophus californianus*). Vet. Hum. Toxicol. 31:568-570.

Evans, J.W., A. Borton, H.F. Hintz,.and D.L. Van Vleck. 1977. The Horse. W H Freeman and Co., New York.

Flesch, P. 1945. Physiology and Biochemistry of the Skin. S. Rothman (Ed.). pp. 601-661. University of Chicago Press, Chicago.

Forshufvud, S., H. Smith, and A. Wassen. 1961. Nature 192:103-105.

Fu, Z., N.M. Attar-Bashi, and A.J. Sinclair. 2001. 1-14C-linoleic acid distribution in various tissue lipids of guinea pigs following an oral dose. Lipids 36:255-260.

Fuller, Z., J.E. Cox, and C.M. Argo. 2001. Photoperiod entrainments of seasonal changes in the appetite, feeding behaviour, growth-rate and pelage of pony colts. Anim. Sci. 72:65-74.

Gaillard, Y., and G. Pepin. 1999. Testing hair for pharmaceuticals. J. Chromatogr. B. Biomed. Sci. Appl. 733:231-246.

Galbraith, H. 1998. Nutritional and hormonal regulation of hair follicle growth and development. Proc. Nutr. Soc. 57:195-205.

Goldblum, R.W., S. Berby, and A.B. Lerner. 1953. The metal content of skin, nails and hair. J. Invest. Dermatol. 20:13.

Goldblum, R.W., L.R. Goldbaum, and W.N. Piper. 1954. Barbiturate concentrations in the skin and hair of guinea pigs. J. Invest. Dermatol. 22:121-128.

Goldsmith, L.A. 1983. Biochemistry and Physiology of the Skin. Oxford University Press, Oxford.

Grieve, J.H. 1963. Effects of thyroid and biotin deficiences on canine demodicosis. Diss. Abstr. 24:1757.

Gunaratnam, P. 1986. Effects of thyroxine on hair growth in the dog. J. Small Anim. Pract. 27:17-29.

Gunaratnam, P., and G.T. Wilkinson. 1983. A study of normal hair growth in the dog. J. Small Anim. Pract. 24:445-453.

Harkey, M.R. 1993. Anatomy and physiology of hair. Forensic Sci. Int. 63:9-18.

Harrington, D.D., J. Walsh, and V. White. 1973. Clinical and pathological findings in horses fed zinc deficient diets. Proc. Equine Nutr. and Physiol. Soc. Symp., p. 51.

Harris, P.A., J.D. Pagan, K.G. Crandell, and N. Davidson. 1998. Effect of feeding thoroughbred horses a high unsaturated or saturated vegetable oil supplemented diet for 6 months following a 10 month fat acclimation. Proc. 5th Internat. Conf. on Equine Exercise Physiol., Utsunomiya, Japan.

Hayman, R.H., and T. Nay. 1961. Observation on hair loss and shedding in cattle. Aust. J. Agric. Res. 12:513-527.

Hintz, H.F. 2000. Hair analysis as an indicator of nutritional status. J. Equine Vet. Sci. 21:199.

Holmes, C.W. 1970. Effects of air temperature on body temperatures and sensible heat loss of Fresian and Jersey calves at 12 and 76 days of age. Anim. Prod. 12:493-501.

Jarrett, A. 1977. The Hair Follicle. Academic Press, London.

Kooistra, L.H., and O.J. Ginther. 1975. Effect of photoperiod on reproductive activity and hair in mares. Am. J. Vet. Res. 36:1413-1419.

Levine, R.J., R.M. Moore, G.D. Maclaren, W.F. Barthel, and P.J. Landrigan. 1976. Occupational lead poisoning, animal deaths, and environmental contamination at a scrap smelter. Am. J. Public Health 66:548-552.

Lewis, L.D. 1995. Equine Clinical Nutrition: Feeding and Care. Williams and Wilkins, London.

Lloyd, D.H. 1993. Structure, function and microflora of the skin. Manual of Small Animal Dermatology. P. Harvey, R.G. Harvey, and I.S. Mason (Eds.). pp. 10-22. British Small Animal Veterinary Association, Cheltenham, UK..

Lowe, J.E., R.H. Foot, B.H. Baldwin, R.B. Hillman, and F.A. Kallfelz. 1987. Reproductive patterns in cyclic and pregnant thyroidectomized mares. J. Reprod. Fertil. Suppl. 35:281-288.

Lyne, A.G., and B.F. Short. 1965. Biology of the Skin and Hair Growth. Angus and Robertson, Sydney. McLaughlin, J.G., and J. Cullen. 1986. Clinical cases of chronic selenosis in horses. Irish Vet. J. 40:136-138.

Messenger, A.G. 1993. The control of hair growth: An overview. J. Invest. Dermatol. 101:4S-8S.

Mihajlovic, M. 1992. Selenium toxicty in domestic animals. Glas. Srp. Akad. Nauka. Med. 42:131-144.

Misir, R., R. Blair, and C.E. Doige. 1986. Development of a system for clinical evaluation of the biotin status of sows. Can. Vet. J. 27:6-12.

Muller, G.H. 1989. Small Animal Dermatology. W B Saunders Company, Philadelphia. Nakahara, Y. 1999. Hair analysis for abused and therapeutic drugs. J. Chromatogr. B. Biomed. Sci. Appl. 733:161-180.

Oxender, W.D., P.A. Noden, .and H.D. Hafs. 1977. Estrus, ovulation, and serum progesterone, estradiol, and LH concentrations in mares after an increased photoperiod during winter. Am. J. Vet. Res. 38:203-207.

Parker, F. 1981. Skin and hormones. In: Textbook of Endocrinology. R. H. Williams (Ed.). pp. 1080-1098.W B Saunders, Philadelphia.

Pilliner, S., and Z. Davies. 1996. Equine Science, Health and Performance. Blackwell Science, London.

Popot, M.A., S. Boyer, P. Maciejewski, P. Garcia, L. Dehennin, and Y. Bonnaire. 2000. Approaches to the detection of drugs in horse hair. Proc. 13th Internat. Conf. of Racing Analysts and Veterinarians, Cambridge, UK.

Potsch, L., G. Skopp, and M.R. Moeller. 1997. Biochemical approach on the conservation of drug molecules during hair fibre formation. Forensic Sci. Int. 84:25-35.

Randall, V.A., and F.J.G. Ebling. 1991. Seasonal changes in human hair growth. Br. J. Dermatol. 124:146-151.

Robbins, C.R. 1979. Chemical and Physical Behaviour of Human Hair. Van Nostrand Reinhold Co., New York.

Rook, A., R. Dawber. 1982. Diseases of the Hair and Scalp. Blackwell Scientific Publications, Oxford.

Ryder, M.L. 1976. Seasonal changes in the coat of the cat. Res. Vet. Sci. 21:280-283.

Samata, T. 1985. A biochemical study of keratin. I. Amino acid compositions of body hair and hoof of Equidae. J. Fac. General Educ. Azabu. Univ. 18:17-34.

Samata, T., and M. Matsuda. 1988. Studies on the amino acid compositions of the equine body hair and the hoof. Jpn. J. Vet. Sci. 50:333-340.

Scott, D.W. 1988. Large Animal Dermatology. W B Saunders, Philadelphia.

Sippel, W.L., J. Flowers, J. O'Farrell, W. Thomas, and J. Powers. 1964. Nutrition consultation in horses by aid of feed, blood and hair analysis. Proc. Amer. Assoc.Equine Pract. 10:139-152

Smith, F.P., and M.S. Pomposini, M.S. 1981. Detection of phenobarbital in bloodstains, semen, seminal stains, saliva, saliva stains, perspiration stains and hair. J. Forensic Sci. 26:582-586

Smith, H., S. Forshufvud, and A. Wassen. 1962. Nature 194:725-726.
Stenn, K.S., and R. Paus. 2001. Controls of hair follicle cycling. Physiol. Rev. 81:449-494.

Tagliaro, F., F.P. Smith, Z.D. Battisti, G. Manetto, and M. Marigo. 1997. Hair analysis, novel tool in forensic and biomedical sciences: New chromatographic and electrophoretic/electrokinetic analytical strategies. J. Chromatogr. B. 689:261-271.

Talukdar, A.H., M.L. Calhoun, and A.W. Stinson. 1972. Microscopic anatomy of the skin of the horse. Am. J. Vet. Res. 33:2365-2390.

Thompson, D.L., R. Hoffman, and C.L. DePew. 1997. Prolactin administration to seasonally anoestrous mares: Reproductive, metabolic and hair-shedding responses. J. Anim. Sci. 75:1092-1099.

Thornton, M.J., N.A. Hibberts, T. Street, B.R. Brinklow, A.S.I. Loundon, and A.V. Randall. 2001. Androgen receptors are only present in mesechyme-derived dermal papilla cells of red deer (*Cervus elaphus*) neck follicles when raised androgens induce a mane in the breeding season. J. Endocrinol. 168:401-408.

Tregear, R.T. 1965. Hair density, wind speed and heat loss in mammals. J. Appl. Physiol. 20:796-801.

Underwood, E.J. 1977. Trace Elements in Human and Animal Nutrition. Academic Press, New York.

Vale, M.M., and D.M. Wagoner. 1997. The Veterinary Encyclopedia for Horsemen. Equine Research Inc., Texas.

Valente, D., M. Cassini, M. Pigliapochi, and G. Vanzetti. 1981. Hair as the sample in assessing morphine and cocaine addiction. Clin. Chem. 27:1952-1953.

Ward, N.I., and J.M. Savage. 1994. Elemental status of grazing animals located adjacent to the London Orbital (M25) motorway. Sci. Total Environ. 146:185-189.

Wertz, P.W., and D.T. Downing. 1988. Integral lipids of human hair. Lipids 23:878-881.

Wesson, J.A., and O.J. Ginther. 1982. Influence of photoperiod on puberty in the female pony. J. Reprod. Fertil. Suppl. 32:269-274.

Whittem, T., C. Davis, G.D. Beresford, and T. Gourdie. 1998. Detection of morphine in mane hair of horses. Aust. Vet. J. 76:426-427.

Whittem, T., J. Foreman, and S. Wood. 2000. Disposition of cocaine in plasma and mane hair of horses after intravenous, buccal and rectal administration. Proc. 8th Internat. Congr. of the European Association of Veterinary Pharmacologists and Toxicologists, Jerusalem, Israel.

Wichert, B., T. Frank, and E. Kienzle. 2002. Zinc, copper and selenium status of horses in Bavaria. J. Nutr. 132:1776S-1777S.

Williams, D., P. Siock, and, K. Stenn. 1996. 13-cis-retinoic acid affects sheath-shaft interaction of equine hair follicles in vitro. J. Invest. Dermatol. 106:356-361.

Witte, S.T., L.A. Will, C.R. Olsen, J.A. Kinker, and P. Miller-Graber. 1993. Chronic selenosis in horses fed locally produced alfalfa hay. J. Am. Vet. Med. Assoc. 202:406-409.

Wysocki, A.A., and R. Klett. 1971. Hair as an indicator of the calcium and phosphorus status of ponies. J. Anim. Sci. 32:74-78.

FEEDING MANAGEMENT

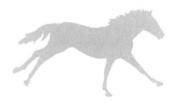

FEEDING MANAGEMENT OF HORSES UNDER STRESSFUL CONDITIONS

JOE D. PAGAN

Kentucky Equine Research, Inc., Versailles, KY

Most performance horses train and compete under a variety of stressful conditions that adversely affect health and performance. Feeding management is of critical importance to reduce many of these problems. Additionally, pre-competition feeding can significantly affect performance. Feeding management affects a number of different aspects of equine health and performance including gastrointestinal function, hydration, electrolyte status, and substrate selection during exercise. This paper will review these key areas of performance horse nutrition and give practical recommendations about how to feed horses under stressful conditions.

Digestive Function

Horses have evolved over millions of years as grazers, with specialized digestive tracts adapted to digest and utilize diets containing high levels of plant fiber. They are capable of processing large quantities of forage to meet their nutrient demands. In an attempt to maximize growth or productivity, horses are often fed diets which also contain high levels of grains and supplements. Unfortunately, this type of grain supplementation often overshadows the significant contribution that forages make in satisfying the horse's nutrient demands.

Horses are classified anatomically as nonruminant herbivores or hindgut fermenters. The large intestine of the horse holds about 80 to 90 liters (21 to 24 gallons) of liquid and houses billions of bacteria and protozoa that produce enzymes which ferment plant fiber. The by-products of microbial fermentation provide the horse with a source of energy and micronutrients. The equine digestive tract is designed in this fashion to allow the horse to ingest large quantities of forage in a continuous fashion. The small capacity of the upper part of the tract is not well suited for large single meals, a fact which is often ignored by horsemen. Large single meals of grain overwhelm the digestive capacity of the stomach and small intestine resulting in rapid fermentation of the grain carbohydrates by the microflora in the hindgut. This fermentation may result in a wide range of problems including colic and laminitis.

The fact that horses are hindgut fermenters has several implications for the person feeding the horse. First, since horses are designed to live on forages, any feeding program that neglects fiber will result in undesirable physical and mental consequences. Horses have a psychological need for the full feeling that fiber provides. Horses fed fiber-deficient diets will in extreme cases become chronic woodchewers. It is also important to maintain a constant food source for the beneficial bacteria in the hindgut. Not only does their fermentation of the fiber provide a great deal of energy for the horse, but their presence prevents the proliferation of other, potentially pathogenic bacteria. Horses, like man, need a certain amount of bulk to sustain normal digestive function. Horses have an immense digestive system designed to process a large volume of feed at all times. Deprived of that bulk, the many loops of the bowel are more likely to kink or twist, and serious colic can result.

The optimal quantity of forage intake varies by discipline. Endurance horses benefit from high forage intakes during both training and competition. Research conducted in Germany (Meyer et al., 1987) has underscored the importance of fiber in maintaining gut health. Their experiments have shown that a diet high in fiber resulted in an increased water intake. Further, animals supplemented with a simple hay and salt diet had 73% more water in their digestive tracts after exercise and approximately 33% more available electrolytes than animals on a low-fiber diet. The additional water and electrolytes in the digestive tract of the animals fed high-fiber diets is probably due to the high water-holding capacity of plant fiber. More importantly, the water and electrolyte pool created by a high-fiber diet can be used to combat dehydration and electrolyte imbalances which derail so many performance horses.

In Thoroughbred racehorses, excess gut fill during competition may be detrimental because additional energy must be expended to carry the extra weight of the ingesta. Therefore, a feeding strategy must be followed that tapers forage intake before a race. KER conducted a study to determine the effects of restricted hay intake on the metabolic responses of horses to high-intensity exercise (Rice et al., 2001). We hypothesized that, compared to ad libitum hay intake, a regimen of restricted hay feeding starting three days before a standardized exercise test would decrease body weight and reduce energy expenditure during running.

Four conditioned Thoroughbred horses were studied in a 2 x 2 crossover design. Initially, the length of time required for adaptation to ad libitum (AD LIB) intake of grass hay was determined. Thereafter, the metabolic responses to sprint exercise (SPR) were examined in two dietary periods, each five days in duration: 1) AD LIB, where horses had free-choice access to hay; and 2) Restricted (RES), where hay intake was restricted (~1% of body weight) for three days before the exercise test. Feed and water were removed four hours before the exercise test.

After measurement of body weight, horses completed a warm-up followed by 2 min at 115% of maximum oxygen uptake, then a 10-min walking recovery (REC).

During the three days before SPR, hay intake in AD LIB averaged (± SE)10.1 ± 0.9 kg, whereas intake during RES was 4.3 ± 0.2 kg. Pre-exercise bodyweight was significantly lower in RES (528 ± 5 kg) than in AD LIB (539 ± 4 kg)(Figure 1). During SPR, total mass-specific VO_2 was higher (P=0.02) in RES (243 ± 8 ml/kg/2 min) than in AD LIB (233 ± 10 ml/kg/2 min). Conversely, accumulated oxygen deficit was higher (P<0.01) in AD LIB (89.4 ± 2.2 ml O_2/kg) than in RES (82.4 ± 1.7 ml O_2/kg). Peak plasma lactate was also higher in AD LIB (22.2 ± 1.2 mM) than in RES (19.1 ± 2.1 mM), and VO_2 during recovery was 10% higher (P=0.12) in AD LIB.

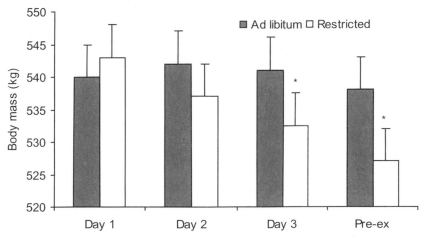

Figure 1. Body weight in the AD LIB and RES hay intake groups for the three-day period preceding the exercise test. Pre-ex = Body weight measured five min before the exercise test. *Significant (P<0.05) difference Ad libitum vs. Restricted.

The main findings of this study were:1) compared to ad libitum hay feeding, three days of restricted (1% of body weight) hay intake was associated with an approximately 2% decrease in body weight, and 2) the reduction in body weight associated with restricted hay feeding resulted in an increase in the mass-specific rate of oxygen consumption during sprint exercise, with a corresponding decrease in anaerobic energy expenditure. The anaerobic contribution to energy expenditure during exercise was lower in RES than in AD LIB as evidenced by lower values for accumulated oxygen deficit (Figure 2) and peak plasma lactate concentrations.

Currently, it is recommended that performance horses receive hay at a minimum of 1% of body weight per day to satisfy requirements for long-stem fiber and to minimize digestive upsets. In this context, relative to the restriction protocol used in this study, more severe or long-term restrictions of hay intake are not recommended. Nonetheless, on the basis of our results, further studies that examine the relationship between fiber intake, body weight, and exercise metabolism and performance are warranted.

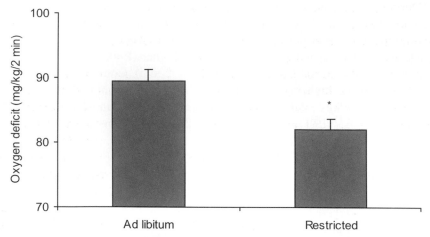

Figure 2. Accumulated oxygen deficit during 2 min of exercise at 115% of maximal oxygen uptake in the AD LIB and RES treatments. *P<0.05 RES vs AD LIB.

Gastric Ulcers

Performance horses are generally kept in confinement during training without access to grazing. This combined with large quantities of grain intake leads to a number of gastrointestinal problems such as gastric ulcers and colic. Many studies since the mid-1980s have documented that gastric ulcers are commonplace in racehorses. An early postmortem study in Hong Kong (Hammond et al., 1986) of 195 Thoroughbred racehorses showed that 80% of the horses in active training had ulcers. The incidence of ulcers in horses retired from racing for one month or longer was 52%. Murray et al. (1989) examined the stomachs of 187 horses ranging in age from one to 24 years. Eighty-seven horses had clinical problems including recurrent colic, poor body condition, or chronic diarrhea. One hundred horses had no clinical signs of gastrointestinal problems. Ninety-two percent of the horses with clinical problems had gastric ulcers. Surprisingly, 52% of the horses displaying no clinical signs also had lesions. Racehorses in training had a higher incidence of ulcers (89%) than non-racers (59%).

More recently, two studies evaluated the incidence of gastric ulcers in California racehorses. In one postmortem study of 169 horses, 88% of Thoroughbred horses in training had ulcers (Johnson et al., 1994). A gastroendoscopic study of 202 Thoroughbred horses in training showed that 81% had ulcers (Vatistas et al., 1994). Each of these studies produced remarkably similar results. Eighty to ninety percent of racehorses in training have gastric ulcers. Most of these lesions occur in the region of the stomach above the margo plicatus, with very few lesions in the glandular portion. The upper half of the stomach consists of squamous epithelial cells that are very similar to the tissue found in the esophagus. Ulcers in this part of the stomach are more similar to esophagitis (heartburn) in humans than the ulcers that occur in the glandular region of the human stomach. It has also been determined that equine gastric ulcers are not caused by *Helicobactor pylori* bacteria, which are a common cause of ulcers in humans.

Dr. M.J. Murray of the Marion du Pont Scott Equine Medical Center in Leesburg,Virginia has proposed that the major cause of gastric ulcers in horses is prolonged exposure of the squamous mucosa to gastric acid. Unlike the glandular portion of the stomach, this tissue does not have a mucous layer and does not secrete bicarbonate onto its luminal surface. The only protection that this portion of the stomach has from gastric acid and pepsin comes from saliva production. If adequate saliva is not produced to buffer the gastric acid and coat the squamous epithelium, gastric irritation occurs and lesions may develop.

The high incidence of ulcers observed in performance horses is a man-made problem resulting from the way that we feed and manage these horses, since ulcers are extremely rare in horses maintained solely on pasture. Horses evolved as wandering grazers with digestive tracts designed for continual consumption of forage. Meals of grain or extended periods of fasting lead to excess gastric acid output without adequate saliva production.

Horses secrete acid continually whether they are fed or not. The pH of gastric fluid in horses withheld from feed for several hours has consistently been measured to be 2.0 or less (Murray, 1992). Horses that received free-choice timothy hay for 24 hours had mean gastric pHs that were significantly higher than fasted horses (3.1 in fed versus 1.5 in fasted horses)(Murray and Schusser, 1989). Higher pHs in hay-fed horses should be expected since forage consumption stimulates saliva production. Meyer et al. (1985) measured the amount of saliva produced when horses ate either hay, pasture, or a grain feed. When fed hay and fresh grass, the horse produced 400-480 grams of saliva per 100 g of dry matter consumed. When a grain-based feed was offered, the horses produced only about half (206 g/100 g dry matter) as much saliva.

Most horses in training are confined for most of the day and fed large grain meals. Often, racehorses are fasted for an extended period before exercise, allowing gastric acid to accumulate in the stomach. Intense exercise further increases the production of gastric acid so that the squamous mucosa of the stomach gets thoroughly bathed in acid during work.

Treating ulcers involves either inhibiting gastric acid secretion or neutralizing the acid produced. There are three classes of drugs that can be used to inhibit gastric acid secretion:

1) Histamine type-2 antagonists (H2 antagonists). H2 antagonists act by competing with histamine for histamine type-2 receptor sites on the parietal cell, and therefore blocking histamine-stimulated gastric acid secretion. The two most popular H2 antagonists used in horses are cimetidine

(Tagamet) and ranitidine (Zantac).

2)   H+/K+ ATPase inhibitors. Direct inhibition of the proton pump can be achieved by substituted benzimidazoles. The only proton pump inhibitor licensed in the United States and Europe is omeprazole.

3)   Prostaglandin analogues.

An alternative to suppression of acid production is to neutralize stomach acid and protect the squamous mucosa from exposure to acid. The natural buffering mechanism in the horse is from saliva production and indeed the most effective way to treat ulcers is simply to turn the animal out on pasture. In situations where this is not possible, administration of antacids may be a useful adjunct to acid suppression therapy in horses.

Time of Feeding Before Competition

One of the most frequently asked questions regarding feeding the performance horse is when to feed before a competition. Three experiments were conducted by Kentucky Equine Research in conjunction with the Waltham Centre for Equine Nutrition and Care to evaluate if feeding hay with and without grain affects glycemic response and hematological responses in Thoroughbred horses at rest and during a simulated competition exercise test (CET) on a high-speed treadmill (Pagan and Harris, 1999). The first experiment evaluated how feeding forage along with grain influences plasma variables and water intake. The second experiment was conducted to determine whether these changes affect exercise performance. The third experiment was performed to determine how forage alone affects exercise response.

Feeding hay either before or with grain significantly reduced the glycemic response of the grain meal. Insulin production post feeding was also reduced. In addition, when hay was fed, total plasma protein (TP) became significantly elevated within one hour. Interestingly, feeding only grain resulted in essentially no change in TP, even though the level of grain intake was the same that elicited a large change when hay alone was fed. Water intake was significantly influenced by time of hay feeding. Following hay feeding, water intake was greatly increased. The increase in water intake also corresponded to increased TP, suggesting that decreased plasma volume may have triggered a thirst response. Feeding grain before exercise with or without hay reduced free fatty acid availability and increased glucose uptake into the working muscle (Figure 3). This would not be beneficial for horses competing in the speed and endurance phase of a three-day event.

Feeding only forage before exercise had a much smaller effect on glycemic and insulin response to exercise than a grain meal. Additionally, feeding forage did not affect FFA availability. In horses fed a pre-exercise meal of hay, TP was elevated before and during exercise, and heart rate was elevated during the gallop in the horses receiving ad libitum hay the night before exercise. Both of these responses in the hay-fed horses were probably due to increased gut fill and a movement of water from the plasma into the gut. Horses that grazed in paddocks the night before exercise did not suffer from reduced plasma volume or elevated heart rates during exercise. This is probably because water was able to equilibrate between the plasma volume and gut so there was no reduction in plasma volume before exercise.

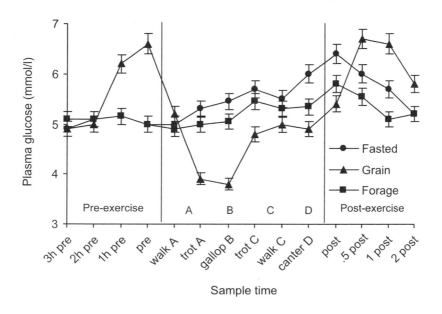

Figure 3. Plasma glucose before, during, and after competition exercise test (CET).

The results of these experiments indicate that feeding hay along with grain will result in a decrease of plasma volume and increase in body weight which may be detrimental to performance. Feeding grain either with or without hay two hours before exercise will reduce FFA availability and increase glucose uptake by the working muscle. This is probably not desirable during prolonged exercise. Feeding only forage before competition does not appear to interfere with FFA availability and has no adverse effects other than possibly reducing plasma volume and increasing body weight. If forage is fed in small amounts or if time in a grass paddock is limited, then these effects will probably be minimal. Since completely withholding forage may lead to stomach ulcers, the slight risk of reduced plasma volume and increased gut fill is more than outweighed by the potential benefit to the horse's long-term health and well-being.

Electrolyte Supplementation

Electrolytes are a critical component of a performance horse's nutritional program since they play an important role in maintaining osmotic pressure, fluid balance, and nerve and muscle activity. During exercise, sodium (Na^+), potassium (K^+), and chloride (Cl) are lost in large quantities through sweating. Loss of these electrolytes causes fatigue and muscle weakness and decreases the thirst response to dehydration. It is vitally important that performance horses begin competition with optimal levels of fluids and electrolytes in their bodies and that these important nutrients are replaced throughout prolonged exercise.

Sweat Losses

It is important to have some idea of the magnitude of electrolyte loss a horse incurs during exercise before a feeding program can be developed to replace these losses. Because most electrolyte losses in the horse occur through sweating, one method of calculating electrolyte requirements can be based on different amounts of sweat loss. Table 1 contains the levels of Na^+, Cl, and K^+ required per day by a horse at rest and after exercising hard enough to lose 5, 10, 20, or 40 liters of sweat.

Table 1. Total daily electrolyte requirements (grams/day) as a function of sweat loss.

		Sweat loss (liters/day)			
Electrolyte	*Rest*	*5 liters*	*10 liters*	*20 liters*	*40 liters*
Sodium (Na+)	15-20	33	50	85	155
Chloride (Cl)	27-33	55	83	139	251
Potassium (K+)	40-50	46	52	64	88

The amount of sweat loss will depend on a number of factors such as duration and intensity of exercise, temperature, and humidity. In general, horses exercising at low intensity (12-18 km/hr) will lose between 5 and 10 liters of sweat per hour. During higher intensity exercise (30-35 km/hr), sweat loss levels reach as high as 15 liters per hour. At the 1996 Olympic Games in Atlanta, horses lost an average of 18.4 kg of body weight during the speed and endurance phase of the three-day event, which translates to a sweat loss of around 15 liters.

Electrolyte Requirements During Endurance Training

Daily electrolyte requirements can be estimated by calculating the total amount of mileage logged weekly by the horse, taking into account the environmental conditions under which the training occurs (Table 2). For example, if an endurance horse were logging 50 km of work per week in a cool environment (20-25°C), it would only require about 60-120 grams (2-4 ounces) of a well-formulated electrolyte supplement to meet its daily electrolyte requirements. The lower range of supplementation would be adequate if the horse were also receiving adequate forage and a grain mix that contained supplemental salt, as well as access to a salt block. Horses at rest will normally consume around 50 grams of salt per day from a salt lick.

Table 2. Total daily electrolyte requirements (grams/day) as a function of training intensity and environment.

| Electrolyte | *Weekly mileage and training environment* | | | | | |
	50 km/wk (cool[1])	50 km/wk (hot[2])	75 km/wk (cool)	75 km/wk (hot)	100 km/wk (cool)	100 km/wk (hot)
Sodium (Na+)	24	32	27	40	32	48
Chloride (Cl)	40	54	47	67	54	80
Potassium (K+)	43	46	44	49	46	51
Daily electrolyte	60-120 g	90-150 g	75-130 g	120-170 g	90-150 g	140-200 g
supplementation[3]	2-4 oz	3-5 oz	2.5-4.5 oz	4-6 oz	3-5 oz	5-7 oz

[1] 20-25° C
[2] 33-35° C
[3] Based on the composition of KER Summer Games Electrolytes. The amount of daily electrolyte supplementation will depend on the amount of electrolyte already in the ration and whether the horse has access to a salt block.

As training mileage and environmental temperature increase, so does the requirement for electrolyte supplementation. Horses that are training heavily (100 km/week) in a hotter environment (33-35°C) may need 140-200 grams (5-7 ounces) of supplemental electrolytes daily.

The recommendations given above are based on supplementing electrolytes at the same rate daily even though the amount of exercise performed each day will vary. This is probably a reasonable approach to supplementation except for days when the training distance is especially long. For those days, additional supplementation may be warranted. As a rule of thumb, 60 grams (2 ounces) of electrolyte supplementation are required for each hour of exercise in moderate climates. This rate of supplementation will double in hot environments when sweat loss is extensive. A long training ride of 60 km (~4 hours) in moderate temperatures would therefore produce enough sweat loss to require 240 grams (8 ounces) of electrolyte supplementation. This level of supplementation would need to be partially provided during the ride (60 grams at 20 and 40 km) using an oral electrolyte paste with the remainder of the electrolyte administered after the ride.

If the horse will not consume this quantity of electrolyte (120 grams or 4 ounces) in a single meal, 60 grams can be administered as a paste at the end of the ride. When administering oral electrolyte pastes, it is absolutely essential that the horse have access to drinking water. If the horse refuses to drink, do not administer an electrolyte paste.

Supplementation During Endurance Competition

There is a great deal of controversy about how to administer electrolytes during competition. Competitors have used a number of different strategies successfully, and the recommendations given here are not necessarily the only way to achieve success.

During competition, sweat losses can be very large. Using the sweating rates described earlier, an endurance horse will lose between 45 and 60 liters of sweat during a 160-km ride. This represents electrolyte losses of 460-690 grams. Additionally, 9-14 grams of calcium and 5-8 grams of magnesium will be lost through sweating. It is debatable whether all of these losses can or need to be completely replaced during the competition. Research has shown that endurance horses participating in 80-160 km events often have a fluid deficit of 20 to 40 liters despite having access to water and electrolytes during the ride. Canadian researchers have shown, however, that endurance horses with less pronounced fluid and electrolyte alterations during a competitive ride were more successful than those with greater changes (Lindinger and Ecker, 1995). Therefore, it is absolutely essential that a large proportion of the electrolytes and water lost in sweat be replaced during the ride.

Pre-ride electrolyte loading. The endurance horse must start the competition with adequate stores of both water and electrolytes. This can be accomplished in two ways. First, the endurance horse should be on a high level of forage (hay or pasture) intake before a ride. When a horse is fed liberal quantities of forage, it can store extra water and electrolytes in its large intestine. These stores can be called on to replace sweat losses early in the ride. Second, extra electrolytes can be administered the night before and the morning of the ride. The horse's system is finely tuned to balance the amount of electrolytes and water that it stores in its body at rest, so excessive pre-ride electrolyte supplementation should be avoided. Moderate supplementation (60 grams the night before and 60 grams the morning of competition) will insure that the horse has adequate electrolytes within its body and will provide additional electrolyte stores within the gastrointestinal tract.

Electrolyte supplementation during competition. Electrolytes should be supplemented throughout competition. The type of electrolyte supplement used during competition is slightly different than that which is used during training.This electrolyte should provide additional calcium and magnesium along with sodium, potassium, and chloride. If calcium and magnesium losses are not replaced by mobilization of skeletal stores or by supplementation, metabolic disturbances such as thumps may occur. Electrolytes should be administered to horses at each vet check and at water stops along the trail. The best way to administer electrolytes is in the form of a paste. Pastes are commercially available, or they can be made up fresh at the vet check by diluting an electrolyte powder in applesauce, water, or liquid antacid. A reasonable dose of electrolyte powder (or equivalent) is 60 grams at each vet check. Thirty- to 60-gram doses of electrolyte can be administered on the trail. It is worth reemphasizing that the horse must have access to drinking water when receiving concentrated electrolyte pastes. These pastes are hypertonic (a greater concentration of electrolytes) compared to blood and will effectively draw fluid out of the horse into the gut if they are not diluted by drinking water. Administering large doses of electrolytes without adequate water intake will result in serious problems including colic, dehydration, and possibly death.

How well will this electrolyte supplementation program replace losses from sweating? Endura-Max powder and Endura-Max Plus paste are calcium- and magnesium-containing electrolytes formulated specifically for endurance competition. Supplementation with 300 grams of Endura-Max powder (60 grams at five vet checks) along with five tubes of Endura-Max Plus paste on the trail will provide 336 grams of sodium, potassium, and chloride, the quantity of electrolytes lost in 33 liters of sweat. If the horse consumed enough water to complement this level of electrolyte intake, then it would finish the ride with a fluid deficit of between 12-27 liters. While this level of fluid deficiency is as good or better than what has been reported in the literature, why not try to replace all of the electrolytes lost during the ride? The answer lies in the horse's ability to absorb and retain large quantities of electrolytes in a short period of time. Sodium is actively transported across the intestinal wall by an energy-requiring process. The maximal rate of sodium transport is not known. Practical experience has shown that the levels of supplementation described above can be safely administered. Higher levels may be possible, but the risk of complications related to malabsorption will certainly increase.

Post-ride supplementation. Administering 120-240 grams (4-8 ounces) of electrolyte over the 24-hour post-ride period can eliminate most of the post-ride electrolyte deficit. A portion of this can be given as a paste shortly after the conclusion of the ride followed by top-dressing supplementation of electrolyte on the next two or three meals.

Fat Adaptation Spares Glucose Utilization

Fatigue during prolonged submaximal exercise may result from depletion of intramuscular or hepatic glycogen stores (Derman and Noakes, 1994; Snow et al., 1981). Previous research has demonstrated that the inclusion of fat in the equine diet will affect substrate selection and utilization during exercise (Potter et al.,

1992, Kronfeld et al., 1994). Field trials with endurance horses have suggested that fat adaptation will protect against drops in blood glucose (Hintz, 1982; Slade et al., 1975) and treadmill studies have demonstrated muscle glycogen sparing effects in horses fed fat-supplemented diets (Griewe et al., 1989; Pagan et al., 1987). The degree to which fat adaptation will affect substrate utilization has not been previously quantified. Therefore, KER conducted a study to determine the effects of a fat-supplemented diet on carbohydrate and fat oxidation in conditioned horses during low-intensity exercise (Pagan et al., 2002). We hypothesized that short-term feeding (<10 weeks) of a fat-supplemented diet would result in adaptations that decrease carbohydrate oxidation and increase the utilization of fat for energy during exercise. This increase in fat utilization would be reflected by decreases in glucose turnover (glucose R_a and R_d) and respiratory exchange ratio during exercise.

Five mature Arabians were studied. The study was conducted as a crossover design with two dietary periods, each of 10 weeks duration: a) a control (CON) diet, and b) a fat-supplemented (FAT) diet. The total amount of digestible energy (DE) supplied by the fat in the CON and FAT diets was calculated to be 7% and 29%, respectively. During each period, the horses completed exercise tests before the start of the period (Week 0) and after 5 and 10 weeks on the diet consisting of 90 minutes of running (treadmill at 3° incline) at a speed calculated to elicit 35% VO_2max. Oxygen consumption (VO_2), carbon dioxide production (VCO_2), and respiratory exchange ratio (RER) were measured at 5-minute intervals. For determination of glucose kinetics, a stable isotope ([6-6-d_2] glucose) technique was used.

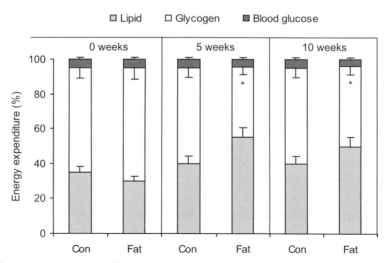

Figure 4. Relative contributions of energy from different substrate sources for three periods during 90 minutes of exercise at 36 ± 1% of maximum oxygen uptake. Values are means ± SE for five horses. *Significantly different from CON, P < 0.05.

Compared to a control diet, consumption of a fat-supplemented diet (~29% of DE from fat) was associated with an altered metabolic response to low-intensity exercise (Figure 4) as evidenced by:

1. A more than 30% reduction in the production (glucose R_a) and utilization (glucose R_d) of glucose after 5 and 10 weeks of fat feeding;

2. A decrease in respiratory exchange ratio after 5 and 10 weeks of fat feeding;

3. A decrease in the estimated rate of whole-body carbohydrate, attributable to decreases in muscle glycogen and plasma glucose utilization; and

4. An increase in the whole-body rate of lipid oxidation during exercise.

These metabolic adaptations which were evident after five weeks of fat supplementation would be advantageous during prolonged exercise, wherein the reduced reliance on carbohydrate for energy would preserve this more limited energy resource and delay the onset of fatigue associated with carbohydrate depletion. Further studies are warranted to investigate the mechanisms underlying this response to fat feeding.

References

Derman, K.D., and T.D. Noakes. 1994. Comparative aspects of exercise physiology. In: D.R. Hodgson and R.J. Rose (Eds.) The Athletic Horse: Principles and Practice of Equine Sports Medicine. W.B.Saunders Company, Philadelphia. pp. 13-25.

Griewe, K.M., T.N. Meacham, and J.P. Fontenot. 1989. Effect of added dietary fat on exercising horses. In: Proc. 11th Equine Nutr. Physiol. Symp. pp. 101-106.

Hammond, C.J., D.K. Mason, and K.L. Watkins. 1986. Gastric ulceration in mature Thoroughbred horses. Equine Vet. J. 18:284-287.

Hintz, H.F. 1982. Nutritional requirements of the exercising horse – A review. In: D.H. Snow, S.G.B. Persson and R.J. Rose (Eds.) Equine Exercise Physiology. Granta Editions, Cambridge, UK. pp. 275-290.

Johnson, W., G.P. Carlson, N. Vatistas, J.R. Snyder, K. Lloyd, and J. Koobs. 1994. Investigation of the number and location of gastric ulcerations in horses in race training submitted to the California racehorse postmortem program. In: Proc. Amer. Assn. Equine Pract. Conv.

Kronfeld, D.S., P.L. Ferrante, and D. Grandjean. 1994. Optimal nutrition for athletic performance, with emphasis on fat adaptation in dogs and horses. J. Nutr. 124:2745S-2753S.

Lindinger, M.I., and G.L. Ecker. 1995. Ion and water losses from body fluids during a 163 km endurance ride. Equine Vet. J., Suppl. 18:314-322.

Meyer, H., M. Coenen, and C. Gurer. 1985. Investigations of saliva production and chewing in horses fed various feeds. In: Proc. Equine Nutr. Physiol. Symp., pp. 38-41.

Meyer, H., H. Perez, Y. Gomda, and M. Heilmann, 1987. Postprandial renal and fecal water and electrolyte excretion in horses in relation to kind of feedstuffs, amount of sodium ingested and exercise. In: Proc. Equine Nutr. Physiol. Symp. p. 67.

Murray, M.J. 1992. Aetiopathogenesis and treatment of peptic ulcer in the horse: a comparative review. Equine Vet J. Suppl. 13:63-74.

Murray, M.J., C. Grodinsky, C.W. Anderson, P.F. Radue, and G.R. Schmidt. 1989. Gastric ulcers in horses: A comparison of endoscopic findings in horses with and without clinical signs. Equine Vet J. Suppl. 7:68-72.

Murray M.J., and G. Schusser. 1989. Application of gastric pH-metry in horses: Measurement of 24 hour gastric pH in horses fed, fasted, and treated with ranitidine. J. Vet. Intern. Med. 6:133.

Pagan, J.D., B. Essen-Gustavsson, A. Lindholm, and J. Thornton. 1987. The effect of dietary energy source on exercise performance in Standardbred horses. In: J.R. Gillespie and N.E. Robinson (Eds.) Equine Exercise Physiology 2. ICEEP Publications, Davis, California. pp. 686-700.

Pagan, J.D., R.J. Geor, P.A. Harris, K. Hoekstra, S. Gardner, C. Hudson, and A. Prince. 2002. Effects of fat adaptation on glucose kinetics and substrate oxidation during low-intensity exercise. Equine Vet. J., Suppl. 34:33-38.

Pagan, J.D., and P.A. Harris. 1999. The effects of timing and amount of forage and grain on exercise response in Thoroughbred horses. Equine Vet. J, Suppl 30:451-457.

Potter, G.D., S.L. Hughes, T.R. Julen, and D.L. Swinney. 1992. A review of research on digestion and utilization of fat by the equine. Pferdeheilkunde, 119-123.

Rice, O., R. Geor, P. Harris, K. Hoekstra, S. Gardner, and J. Pagan. 2001. Effects of restricted hay intake on body weight and metabolic responses to high-intensity exercise in Thoroughbred horses. In: Proc. 17th Equine Nutr. Physiol. Symp., pp. 273-279.

Slade, L.M., L.D. Lewis, C.R. Quinn, and M.L. Chandler. 1975. Nutritional adaptation of horses for endurance performance. In: Proc. 17th Equine Nutr. Physiol. Symp.

Snow, D.H., P. Baxter, and R.J. Rose. 1981. Muscle fiber composition and glycogen depletion in horses competing in an endurance ride. Vet Rec. 108:374.

Vatistas, N.J., J.R. Snyder, G. Carlson, B. Johnson, R.M. Arthur, M. Thurmond, and K.C.K. Lloyd. 1994. Epidemiological study of gastric ulceration in the Thoroughbred racehorse: 202 horses, 1992-1993. In: Proc. Amer. Assn. Equine Pract. Conv., p. 125-126.

AN OUNCE OF PREVENTION:
FEEDING MANAGEMENT TO MINIMIZE COLIC

KRIS PURCELL
Carson Valley Large Animal, Gardnerville, Nevada

The threat of colic lurks in the subconscious of all present-day equine caretakers. Even the hobbyist makes calculated decisions to avoid this dreaded condition – cooling the horse thoroughly before allowing it to drink, gradually switching from one feed to another, and periodic dosing with proven deworming agents. By definition, colic means any abdominal pain. However, the term has evolved to define a condition rather than a clinical sign.

In recent decades, great advances have been made in understanding the etiology and pathogenesis of abdominal disease in horses, including those factors directly related to feeding management. Accompanying these advances have been noteworthy strides in the prevention and treatment of colic.

The Equine Digestive Tract

Horses are classified as hindgut fermenters, meaning bacteria aid in the digestion of feedstuffs in the latter part of the gastrointestinal tract (the cecum and large intestine). The gastrointestinal system of a horse measures, on average, 100 feet long and holds approximately 48 gallons of water and ingesta. The gastrointestinal tract begins with the stomach, which holds approximately 2-4.5 gallons of fluid or food. Acid production and enzyme secretion are the primary functions of this organ.

Food is passed from the stomach to the small intestine, which consists of the duodenum, jejunum, and ileum. The duodenum is the site of bile and pancreatic enzyme secretion, fluids which help digest fats, proteins, and carbohydrates. The jejunum is the site of absorption of amino acids, mono- and diglycerides, fatty acids, glucose, vitamins, minerals, electrolytes, and a small amount of water. The jejunum is suspended by a sheet of mesentery, which is anchored via a stalk to the dorsal roof of the abdomen. This allows the jejunum to be mobile, but this mobility can lead to torsion, or twisting on itself, which can be a cause of colic. The ileum is the last section of the small intestine. It is short and has a muscular wall. The ileum acts as a one-way valve for ingesta to pass into the cecum.

The large intestine begins with the cecum. This is actually a fermentation vat where roughage undergoes microbial digestion. The cecum is 3.5 feet long and holds 7 to 8 gallons of fluid and up to 15 gallons of ingesta. B vitamins and volatile fatty acids are also produced here as a result of microbial fermentation. The ingesta leaves the cecum and passes to the large colon, which is approximately 11 feet long with an 18-gallon capacity. The large colon accounts for 40% of the total capacity of the equine gut. Water and volatile fatty acids are absorbed here. The fermentation process produces gas, which can be a cause of colic if it is allowed to build up within the large intestine. Pain is caused by gastrointestinal tract wall distention, displacement of the large colon, or torsion caused by the gas distention. Increased gas production can be caused by an increase in carbohydrate load, bowel obstruction, or altered motility of the bowel.

The small colon is approximately ten feet long. This segment of the gastrointestinal tract does not have any absorptive functions. This is where the ingesta is formed into fecal balls. The terminal section of the gastrointestinal tract is the rectum, which is approximately one foot long.

The incidence of colic per section of gastrointestinal tract is as follows: stomach 12%, small intestine 33%, cecum 6%, large colon 49%, small colon 7%, and rectum <1%.

Types of Colic

Many factors may cause the pain associated with colic. The most common are:

1. Spasms caused by contractions of the bowel wall.

2. Distention from a buildup of gas, fluid, or ingesta that causes expansion of the bowel.

3. Traction, a result of pulling on the bowel.

4. Ischemia (decreased blood flow) of the gastrointestinal tract because of dehydration, blockage of a blood vessel by a clot, or compression of a blood vessel.

5. Inflammation caused by stress, parasites, nonsteroidal anti-inflammatory drugs, sand, infectious colitis, or ingested toxins.

In a study that reviewed colic cases examined by veterinarians on the farm, 46% were spasmodic or gas colics, 29% were large colon impactions, 6% were strangulating obstructions, 8% were the result of enteritis, and 11% were from undiagnosed causes.

Colic risk factors can be divided into intrinsic factors and management practices, including environmental control. The intrinsic factors play a small role in the overall risk of colic. There does not appear to be any breed or gender predilection for colic. Mares may show more signs of colic late in pregnancy due to fetal movement. One study showed the incidence of colic is greatest among horses 2 to 10 years old. Further examination of this group revealed colic was related more to the stressful occupations (racing, three-day eventing, etc.) of the horses in this age group rather than age.

Management appears to play the greatest role in decreasing the risk of colic. Pasture turnout with a fresh water source appears to carry the lowest colic risk because horses are able to continually ingest small amounts of food throughout the day. Inclusion of concentrates in the diet tends to increase the likelihood of colic, and the risk escalates as the amount of concentrates fed increases. Feeding horses up to 5.5 pounds of concentrates slightly increased the risk of colic compared to feeding only roughage. Feeding 5.5 to 11 pounds of concentrate was five times more likely to cause colic than feeding only roughage. Horses eating more than 11 pounds of concentrate were six times more likely to colic.

Processed feeds are more easily digested than whole grains. Large amounts of pelleted feed or grain cannot be digested efficiently by the small intestine. The concentrate is passed into the cecum and large intestine where it is fermented by microbial flora, causing gas production and increasing acidity within the bowel. Fermentation causes water to be transferred from the bloodstream into the bowel lumen, which causes mild, transient dehydration. This dehydration persists for approximately eight hours after eating a high carbohydrate meal. Feeding a large amount of grain daily in multiple meals does not appear to decrease the risk of colic because the large intestine has very little time to restore its normal balance before the next feeding.

The horse's gastrointestinal system is designed to process roughage diets. Fresh grass in early spring is considered a readily digestible carbohydrate. Therefore, there may be an increased risk of spasmodic colic in horses grazing pasture if they have not previously been kept on pasture.

High-quality hay is important in decreasing the risk of colic. Abruptly changing from a high-quality hay to a poorer quality hay may predispose the horse to impaction due to decreased digestibility.

Alfalfa has been associated with enterolith formation. The problem with alfalfa may lie in its high protein content rather than its mineral content. A by-product of protein digestion is ammonium ion production. In an alkaline environment, such as that possible in the colon, these ions can form a complex with available magnesium and phosphorus. Over time these complexes may enlarge and become "stones." These stones can become so large they may block narrow portions of the large intestine, such as the pelvic flexure or the transverse colon. Enteroliths are found in horses in any part of the country but seem to be more predominant in the western United States, presumably because alfalfa is the primary source of roughage.

Parasites

Internal parasites were a significant cause of colic prior to the development of anthelmintics effective against the larval stages of strongyles. Today, this type of colic is rare if the horse is dewormed with ivermectin or ivermectin-type products. After large strongyle (bloodworm) larvae are ingested, they penetrate the bowel lining and migrate along the blood vessels. Many tend to lodge within the cranial mesenteric artery, the primary vessel that supplies blood to the gastrointestinal tract. Blockage of this vessel can cause damage to the bowel by decreasing its blood supply.

Small strongyle (cyathostome) larvae are ingested and then burrow into the lining of the large intestine, where they may remain dormant for up to two years. In this hypobiotic state, they are resistant to most anthelmintics and may cause weight loss, poor coat condition, delayed growth, colic, and/or diarrhea. It is suspected that warming environmental temperatures may stimulate the emergence of these larvae. Only three products have been shown to be effective in decreasing the number of cyathostome larvae. Strongid C is a daily dewormer that kills the larvae before they reach the hypobiotic state. Moxidectin (Quest) is in the same family as ivermectin. A double dose of fenbendazole (Panacur Power Pack) can be given for five days to penetrate cyathostome larvae in their hypobiotic state. Worming with a double dose of fenbendazole is recommended in the fall for cooler climates and in July for the southwestern and south-central states. For the deep South, it is recommended in May and November due to year-round grazing.

Summary

The strategy for preventing colic is multifactorial. The following management principles can help reduce the risk of colic in horses.

1. *Match the horse's normal diet.* Feed a high-quality roughage diet with very few soluble carbohydrates. The bulk of the diet should be roughage (hay or pasture), which should average 1-2% of the body weight per day. If grain must be fed to meet energy requirements, at least 50% of the total diet should be roughage. Fat may be added to the diet to increase the caloric density of the grain without causing the digestive problems associated with overfeeding carbohydrates. Horses can eat two cups of corn oil per day with no digestive upset. Fat can be added in the form of corn oil, vegetable oil, or rice bran.

2. *Mimic the horse's natural feeding schedule.* Allowing free choice hay to horses kept in stalls or paddocks will mimic the horse's grazing behavior. Overweight horses should be fed 1% of their body weight, and this can be divided into two or three feedings. Horses are creatures of habit, so feeding at approximately the same times every day will help decrease the risk of colic. Feeding grain without access to roughage between the feedings has been shown to increase the concentration of gastric acid and bile, which can cause severe gastric or duodenal ulceration within 14 hours of fasting.

Feeding small amounts of grain throughout the day will help decrease the carbohydrate load on the large intestine as long as the grain is kept to three pounds or less per meal.

3. *Afford the horse daily or near-daily exercise.* Colic risk is lower for horses on pasture. If full pasture turnout is not an option, the horse should be turned out daily for as long as possible. If no turnout is available, the horse should be ridden, walked, or otherwise exercised daily.

4. *Make diet alterations gradually.* Make dietary changes over a period of one to two weeks. Concentrate can be increased by ½ pound per day. When changing hay, mix the old hay with the new to allow the gastrointestinal tract to adapt. If the horse is to be confined to a stall due to an injury, decreasing the grain will help prevent colic.

5. *Provide good-quality feedstuffs.* All feeds offered to horses and ponies should be the highest quality. Avoid feeding any concentrate that is spoiled or contaminated. Horses will not often eat feed that is spoiled, but all suspected rancid feed should be discarded even if horses will consume it. Do not assume that feed is free of contamination simply because horses will eat it. The remains of rodents or other animals (mice, snakes, etc.) should deem any feed unsuitable for consumption.

   Hay should be leafy and soft with fine stems. Grass and legume hays harvested before maturity are more readily digested by horses and ponies and are therefore less likely to cause colic. Some owners are under the erroneous assumption that obese or laminitic horses should be given mediocre or poor-quality hay because overfeeding has been destructive to their well-being in the past. Instead, such horses should be fed the best quality grass hay possible doled in judicious portions.

   Alfalfa hay should be thoroughly inspected for blister beetles. As few as two or three beetles can induce colic or colitis in an otherwise healthy horse. Purchasing alfalfa hay from a reputable dealer is one way to avoid blister beetle poisoning, but because beetles usually swarm and infestation is hit-and-miss, inspection of every bale is worthwhile.

6. *Use only feeds formulated for horses.* Cattle, pig, and chicken feeds are not suited for consumption by horses. The nutritional requirements of horses are completely different than those for other species. A far more important reason for avoiding feeds formulated for other species exists. Certain additives in these feeds are poisonous to horses. For example, monensin, a common ingredient in cattle and poultry feeds, is highly toxic to horses and may predispose a horse to colic, general weakness, and death.

7. *Allow free access to fresh water.* Horses should have clean water available to them at all times. The only exception to this hard-and-fast rule is the

restriction of water immediately following intense exercise that has resulted in elevated body temperature and increased respiration rate. However, a horse can be offered two or three sips periodically during the cooling out period to help lower core body temperature. Particular attention should be paid to water consumption in the winter. Some horses drink less as water temperatures fall to near freezing. If this is the case, warm water should be offered to the horse at least twice a day during periods of persistent cold temperatures. Allowing the horse the opportunity to drink during transport and long-term exercise may also prevent an episode of colic.

8.   *Put the horse on a regular deworming program.* The cost of deworming is minimal, especially when compared to the benefits. Consult a veterinarian when devising a deworming program as this individual is most likely aware of the primary parasitic threats in the region. Regular deworming may also save on out-of-pocket feed expenses because the feed will be utilized for sustaining the body processes of the horse and not the life cycles of internal parasites.

9.   *Schedule regular dental care.* Annual dental examinations will ensure that feed is chewed properly and maximal nutrients are delivered to the gastrointestinal tract for absorption. Dental abnormalities can severely hamper the mechanical breakdown of grains, particularly unprocessed cereal grains such as whole oats. If teeth are left unchecked, sharp points may develop on the molars, and these may cause extreme discomfort to the horse. Some horses may eventually refuse to eat due to the pain caused by dental abnormalities.

10.   *Manage the environment.* Keep the horse's environment free of debris. Ingested foreign materials such as rubber or baling twine can cause colic by blocking the digestive tract. Minerals and other material may surround an object and form a stone that can lead to blockage. Although most horses will not eat toxic plants if other food is available, owners should monitor the pasture and hay bales for suspect plants.

Colic has plagued horses for centuries, even prior to domestication. Unfortunately, eliminating colic completely from the inventory of equine health concerns is unrealistic despite continued research efforts of scientists worldwide. However, reducing the occurrence of colic is possible when sound management practices are followed punctiliously.

BAG O' BONES: MANAGING THE UNDERWEIGHT HORSE

KATHLEEN CRANDELL
Kentucky Equine Research, Inc., Versailles, Kentucky

Nothing is more frustrating than trying to get weight on a horse and seeing no results. Although putting weight on a horse may be accomplished simply by feeding more calories, the problem often requires a more thorough probe into what is causing static weight. The probable causes and changes in diet or management that will give the skinny horse every opportunity to gain weight are outlined here. The first part will discuss factors that may keep a horse from gaining weight or may cause a horse to lose weight. The second part will review methods of increasing calories in the diet to achieve weight gain.

Reasons for Weight Loss

Insufficient caloric intake is the primary cause of failure to maintain sufficient body condition in horses. A variety of reasons may account for caloric deficiency. Some are easy to pinpoint and simple to address, such as parasite loads or teeth problems. Others are impossible to diagnose without euthanizing the horse and performing a necropsy. Physical problems of the digestive tract account for many of these problems, but there may be psychological and environmental reasons as well.

PARASITES

Internal parasites can be a major contributing factor to weight loss or inability to put on weight, although severe cases of parasitism are not as common as in years past because of improved dewormers and deworming programs. The ravages of internal parasites can be disastrous for several reasons. First, parasites may compete directly for the nutrients inside the digestive tract. They may also cause damage to the intestinal lining, making it difficult to absorb nutrients. Damage to the intestinal lining can diminish production of enzymes needed to prepare food particles for absorption. Competition for protein by parasites can affect absorption of nutrients because some are dependent on protein to transport them through the intestinal lining. The damage can also cause swelling of the intestinal lining which can draw electrolytes, sugars, and amino acids (building blocks of protein) back into the intestines to be eliminated with the manure. In older horses, wasting of muscle tissue may be a result of years of parasitic damage to the intestines, making it difficult for protein and other nutrients to be absorbed in adequate quantities. Therefore, the animal becomes protein deficient and starts to break down its own muscle tissue to supply protein for essential body processes. For this reason, diets formulated for senior horses typically have higher protein. An effective deworming program should keep parasites from being a reason for weight loss. Examination of fecal samples by a veterinarian will reveal the efficacy of a deworming program. Deworming strategies should be discussed with a veterinarian who is familiar with regional parasite populations.

TEETH

If a horse is not maintaining weight, the first thing that should be checked is the condition of teeth. Proper dentition is essential to a horse because of the nature of its diet. Horses evolved eating coarse roughage and plant materials that require thorough grinding by the molars to break down the particle size of the food. Enzymes and microbes of the gastrointestinal tract readily digest feedstuffs that have been crushed into minute particles. Problems with dentition can have deleterious effects on the body condition of a horse.

Perhaps the most common dental problem is irritation or laceration of the cheek, tongue, or gums by sharp edges or points of the teeth. Normal wear and tear induced by chewing can reshape the edges of the teeth, sometimes making them sharp enough to cut into the parts of the mouth they contact. This makes chewing painful. A horse with points will often reduce the quantity of feed consumed or will eat more slowly than normal. Pain caused by points can be alleviated by floating the teeth, a procedure in which a dental rasp is used to smooth sharp edges.

A dental problem particular to young horses is the presence of caps that will not dislodge appropriately. By the time a horse achieves maturity, it will have had two sets of teeth. Immature horses possess deciduous or milk teeth that are gradually replaced by permanent teeth. As permanent teeth erupt and grow, milk teeth are generally ousted. In some instances, a portion of a milk tooth, a cap, may remain. Caps can make chewing difficult and should be removed if discovered. Young horses that roll feed in their mouths and spill feed from their mouths should have their teeth inspected for the presence of caps.

Infections in gums or teeth, cracked or broken teeth, and poor mouth conformation (severe parrot mouth or undershot jaw) can also cause reduced feed intake. In aged horses, loss of molars is a primary concern when discerning a cause for weight loss. As time takes its toll on the horse, dentition can become wavy and teeth may start to fall out. When a horse does not properly grind his food because of molar loss or misalignment, the food enters the digestive tract in particles too large for proper breakdown by digestive enzymes in the small intestine and microbes in the large intestine and cecum. If this is the case, feed is of little energetic benefit to the horse and weight loss will result. Receding incisors, another problem common in aged horses, may cause difficulty in tearing grass when grazing. Inadequate intake of forage will result. Aged horses that have spent a lifetime cribbing may be doubly prone to receding incisors. For these reasons many commercial senior feeds are designed to provide a complete diet, including forage, in small particle size. These feeds can be softened with water and made into gruel so they do not require any chewing to be of benefit to the horse.

Careful observation of the eating habits of a horse will likely reveal a dentition problem. Slow eating, reluctance to drink cold water, tilting the head while chewing, wallowing food around in the mouth before swallowing, balling up food in the mouth, and dropping food may indicate a tooth problem. However, some horses may not exhibit abnormalities in food intake or mastication but may still be losing weight from a chronic tooth ailment. Most equine veterinarians are knowledgeable in proper dental care and can perform a thorough examination of the mouth. In areas of the country with exceptionally large horse populations, an equine dentist may be available to diagnose and alleviate dental quandaries. If the problems are permanent (as in tooth loss), adjustments of the diet should be made to address the problem.

DIGESTIVE TRACT PROBLEMS

Any physiological problem that keeps food from getting to the intestines for absorption can cause weight problems. If swallowing is painful or difficult, the horse will not want to eat. Things that may cause problems with swallowing could be nerve damage from equine protozoal myelitis (EPM), obstructions from abscesses or strangles, and muscle weakness caused by hyperkalemic periodic paralysis (HYPP) or botulism. Partial esophageal obstruction can occur from abnormal growths, scar tissue from an episode of choking, or a foreign object lodged in the throat. Esophageal obstruction narrows the passageway for food, making it difficult for the horse to swallow. Horses that have chronic choke may have an esophageal obstruction that instigates the problem. The only way to effectively diagnose esophageal narrowing is by endoscopic exam or x-ray. If there is no way to clear the obstruction, dietary adjustments should be made so that the type of food offered is easily swallowed.

Gastric ulcers can cause reduced appetite in horses because of a painful or uncomfortable stomach. The end result is a horse who is not able to consume enough calories to maintain weight. The incidence of ulcers in horses is surprisingly high. Surveys done on performance horses have found ulcers in about 80% of racehorses in training and as many as 50% in other types of performance horses. Horses that live on pasture most of the day rarely develop ulcers. Gastric ulcers develop in the horse when the acidity of the stomach is too high. The main precipitants for gastric ulcers in horses are a high grain and low forage diet, meal feeding instead of continuous forage availability, overtraining, and other stresses of a performance schedule. Signs associated with gastric ulcers are irritability, picky eater, chronic colic, diarrhea, and inability to gain weight. Some horses have all of the signs, some have only one, and some do not exhibit any, yet have the problem. Medications have been developed to help heal gastric ulcers, and antacids are currently being marketed to prevent gastric acid accumulation in the stomach. Antacids can also be used to prevent ulcers from occurring or recurring.

Problems that can occur in the small intestine, large intestine, and cecum may influence the nutrient absorption. Chronic diarrhea can contribute directly to weight loss because nutrients move too quickly through the digestive tract, thereby escaping absorption. There are many causes of diarrhea in the horse. Countless bacteria reside in the equine digestive tract, and a delicate balance exists between bacterial types. If the balance of the different types shifts, the ecosystem in the hindgut can disintegrate. Dysfunction of the bacteria may result in the inability of digesta to be broken down into small enough particles for absorption. Inadequately digested feed often results in diarrhea. Viruses can also disrupt the health of the bacterial population of the hindgut and cause detrimental effects. Viral and bacterial pathogens can induce damage and sloughing of the intestinal lining.

No magic potion is marketed which will return the bacterial population of the hindgut to a state of normalcy, but there are a few products that may help. Probiotics are frequently used to help repopulate the gut with beneficial bacteria. One old-fashioned probiotic recipe called for a bucket of feces from a healthy horse mixed with water. The preparation was then given to the horse through a nasogastric tube. Today, there are neater, but not necessarily more effective, ways to rebalance the microbe population of the hindgut. Endurance enthusiasts have been known to feed yogurt with live cultures to their horses for the probiotic effect. Commercial probiotic pastes or liquids with *Lactobacillus* and/or *Streptococcus faecium* are available, as are bagged products with yeasts and probiotics designed as daily supplements. Probiotics are very useful when a horse has been stressed by trailering, change of home, deworming, or antibiotic treatment. When there is no apparent reason for a horse to have a problem putting on weight, sometimes just the addition of probiotics and yeast supplement to the diet will bring the horse around.

DISEASE

Chronic and acute disease can interfere with the horse's ability to maintain weight. Many diseases affect the body by disturbing protein use. Without proper amounts of protein, the body cannot rebuild damaged tissues, make transport proteins that carry other nutrients through the blood to target sites, make clotting factors for blood, and carry on a host of other physiological functions. When the body cannot get enough protein from the diet, it begins to break down the existing protein in the body to use for its most important functions. Muscle is the most abundant storehouse of protein in the body. Muscle wasting is an indicator of protein deficiency, either from dietary inadequacy or disease interfering with protein utilization.

Chronic liver disease may result in weight loss due to the decreased ability to handle protein and fat properly. Normally, dietary protein and fat make their way to the liver after being absorbed from the intestines into the blood or lymphatic system. The liver acts as the master coordinator for nutrients, directing amino acids and fatty acids to fulfill assignments elsewhere in the body. When the liver is not functioning properly, many other systems in the body are affected with the end result of weight loss. Liver function can be assessed with a simple blood chemistry analysis.

Malfunctioning kidneys may also cause weight loss. Acute or chronic kidney disease can result in protein loss in the urine. Horses with kidney problems will usually drink excessive amounts of water and urinate frequently. Kidney function can also be assessed with a simple blood chemistry.

Certain problems occurring in the body will result in an abnormal increase in the distribution of energy usually necessary for normal body processes. Abscesses within the body cavity will rob large amounts of energy from the horse, resulting in chronic weight loss. Cancer has the same effect on metabolism. Horses with chronic obstructive pulmonary disease (COPD) burn more calories than horses with normal breathing patterns because of the physical effort required to breathe. Pituitary adenoma (Cushing's syndrome) also can place metabolism in high gear, burning the body's energy stores excessively. Common ailments such as a heart murmur can cause problems because of the disruption of blood flow that carries nutrients throughout the body.

ENVIRONMENT

Horses are like humans in the sense that environment may affect appetite. An uncomfortable or unhappy horse may prefer to indulge in a stable vice such as cribbing, weaving, or stall walking, thereby wasting valuable calories. The result is detrimental to the horse's ability to maintain weight. The ideal solution is to find out what the horse does not like about the environment. This is often challenging to find or, if found, impossible to change. The next best approach is to increase the caloric density of the diet.

Herd dynamics may account for poor condition and is frequently the cause in pasture or lot environments. Horses low in the pecking order will be granted only limited access to feed by horses higher in the social hierarchy. Timid horses will waste away rather than fight for a chance at the food if it is hoarded by the more dominant horses in a group. In group feeding situations, generous space should separate piles of hay. If grain is group fed, the grain buckets or feeders should also be spaced accordingly. Providing one or two extra servings of hay or grain to the group may be beneficial because less dominant horses will have more options from which to choose should they be intimidated by another horse.

Chronic pain is often overlooked as a cause of weight loss in horses. The body's response to pain is the release of adrenaline (epinephrine), which puts the body in a state of catabolism. Catabolism causes the breakdown of body energy stores that ultimately results in chronic weight loss. The discomfort can also dampen the appetite of the horse.

Numerous causes can account for a horse's inability to maintain weight aside from not consuming sufficient calories. Quick and easy solutions cure some problems, but for other problems there may be no solution but to deal with the animal as it is.

Putting Weight on the Horse

Sometimes, getting a thin horse to gain weight is simply a matter of increasing the caloric density of the diet. Other times, the diet may need to be higher in calories because of a medical, psychological, or environmental problem. Various strategies for increasing calories in the equine diet can be adapted to meet the needs of the horse.

HARD KEEPERS

The metabolic rate determines whether a horse is an easy or hard keeper, and the variation between horses can be extreme. Metabolism is the speed at which the body burns fuels for energy in order to maintain normal body functions. A slow metabolism is one that can function on little input of fuel energy. Conversely, a fast metabolism is one that needs a higher caloric intake in order to function properly. In general, members of certain breeds have faster metabolisms and need more food to maintain body condition than members of other breeds. For example, Thoroughbreds usually eat more per pound of body weight than draft horses. There is also variety within a breed. For instance, some Thoroughbreds are easy keepers while others require intense management to maintain body weight. Temperament often goes hand in hand with metabolic rate. A nervous horse may require more calories than a calm-tempered one to maintain the same body condition. A tense horse may spend more time stall walking or weaving while the calm horse conserves energy stores.

A thin horse requires energy in the diet to ensure proper functioning of body processes and to build fat stores. Energy is a general term, yet many horsemen associate the word energy with mental energy. In this article, energy refers to the potential of a feed to fuel body functions and exercise. Weight gain in the horse can be attributed to protein or fat deposition. When a horse does not have enough calories or protein in the diet, the body will break down its own muscle tissue and deplete much of the adipose tissue or fat. This results in emaciation with poor muscle definition and protruding bones. When the diet has excessive calories, the body will build muscle and adipose stores. The simple solution to low weight is to increase the caloric content of the diet while ensuring adequate protein content. The three nutrients that can supply energy to increase the caloric content of the diet in the horse are fiber, starch, and fat. Each nutrient is utilized for energy in a slightly different way in the body, which, depending on the horse, can be advantageous or not.

FIBER

Of the three major energy sources for the horse, fiber is the most important, most underestimated, and the safest. Fiber is the major component of grass and hay. Some horses can maintain their weight on fiber sources alone. For the hard keeper, however, fiber alone will not maintain weight, but there are fiber-feeding strategies that can increase the ability of the horse to derive energy from fiber.

The fiber portion of a plant consists primarily of cellulose, hemicellulose, and lignin. Residing in the intestinal tract of the horse (cecum and colon) are billions of microbes that break down the fiber into a physiological usable form, volatile fatty acids. These volatile fatty acids pass into the bloodstream of the horse where they can be transported to sites that need energy or tucked away as energy stores in the form of adipose tissue or muscle glycogen. Most of the cellulose and hemicellulose (digestible fiber) is easily digested by intestinal microbes. The lignin is not digestible (indigestible fiber). Therefore, as lignin content of a feed increases, digestibility decreases. As digestibility plummets, less energy is available to the horse. Lignin is the carbohydrate that gives the most structural support to a plant; rigid-stalked vegetation will contain more lignin than limp-stalked plants. For instance, there is little lignin in the soft leaves of the alfalfa plant, but a much higher content of lignin is present in the rigid stem. If there are more leaves and fewer stems, or if the stems have not matured to become stiff and inflexible, the digestible fiber portion of the hay will be higher. A young plant harvested prior to maturity will have a lower lignin content than a plant allowed to mature before cutting. Fresh spring grass is much higher in digestible fiber than parched summer grass. A horse can derive more energy from a high-quality, early harvested hay (whether grass or legume) than a mature hay. Pasture is also a source of fiber. The digestibility of pasture is usually higher than hay, because the curing process of haymaking results in digestible fiber losses.

When comparing the energy content of alfalfa and grass hays, alfalfa hay can provide a horse with more energy than grass hay of similar quality. On the other hand, a low-quality alfalfa hay which is composed of more stem than leaf is not a rich source of energy. More energy could be provided with a grass hay that has very little stem and an abundance of visible green grass blades. Maximizing forage quality should be the first dietary adjustment when trying to achieve weight gain.

When quality fiber in the form of pasture or hay is not available, or if the horse does not readily eat hay, there are alternative fiber sources that may add energy to the diet. The most common are beet pulp, soy hulls, wheat bran, and alfalfa pellets or cubes. Beet pulp is about 80% digestible fiber (as compared to 50% for the average hay). Soy hulls are a by-product of soybean production. Soy hulls are the skin of the bean (not the husk or pod) that is knocked off before oil is extracted from the bean. Commonly used in commercial horse feeds, soy hulls are slightly lower in digestibility than beet pulp. If a commercially designed horse feed has soy hulls listed as one of the primary ingredients, it will be a good source of highly digestible fiber.

Wheat bran is commonly thought of as a fiber source, but it actually has about the same amount of fiber as oats. Wheat bran is a rich energy source because it is abundant in digestible fiber and starch. Wheat bran contains a large quantity of phosphorus, which can potentially disrupt the calcium and phosphorus ratio in the diet. On the flip side, wheat bran complements a diet high in alfalfa hay, which is usually rich in calcium.

When good-quality forage is unavailable or if hay intake is minimal or difficult for a horse, the diet of the horse can be supplemented with alfalfa pellets or cubes. Both products are made with alfalfa that has been harvested when digestible fiber is at its peak. Thus, alfalfa pellets and cubes provide energy to the horse. Alfalfa hay is often combined with timothy hay or whole corn plants to create cubes lower in protein and calcium content than pure alfalfa cubes. A word of caution when feeding pellets: some hay should still be fed if possible because of the important laxative effect of long fiber in the diet.

Supplements are available that may help with fiber digestion if the horse has a problem with the balance of microbes in the cecum or colon. Yeast has been researched and found to improve fiber digestibility. Some commercial feeds come with yeast already added, and yeast products can be top-dressed. Probiotics are also thought to help improve fiber digestibility. Because the microbial population in the hindgut can shift out of balance, researchers believe the addition of more bacteria in the form of a probiotic restores bacterial stability, thereby improving digestion of forage. Some commercial products are available that combine yeast and a probiotic for maximal regeneration and efficiency of the microbial population.

STARCH

When a horse cannot maintain weight on hay or grass alone, the addition of starch in the form of grains has been the most traditional method of increasing the energy density of the diet. Obtaining energy from starch is actually more efficient because it is a simple enzymatic process. The end result is having to feed fewer pounds of grain than hay to supply the equivalent amount of energy to the horse. Grains are an excellent source of starch for the horse, but they can be hazardous to the digestive tract.

The starch molecules found in grains are complex polysaccharides which, when attacked by the enzyme amylase in the small intestine, can be broken down to very simple sugars which are easily absorbed into the bloodstream. From there, the sugars in the blood are distributed to where they may be needed by the body for energy or they may be stored as muscle glycogen or adipose tissue for future use.

The limiting factor to starch digestion in the horse is the production of amylase in the intestinal tract. Amylase production has been found to be quite variable among horses. Without sufficient amylase in the intestinal tract, much of the starch in the diet passes through to the large intestine where it is fermented. This is undesirable for two reasons. The amount of energy produced from starch by fermentation is less than the amount produced by enzymatic activity, and excessive fermentation of starch drops the pH of the hindgut which will decrease the efficiency of the bacteria which digest fiber and produce energy.

To further complicate the situation, not all starch molecules are created equal. Studies have shown that the oat starch molecule is small and easily digested by amylase. On the other hand, the starch molecules of corn and barley are large and not easily digested. Heating corn or barley changes the nature of the starch molecule and makes it more easily digested by amylase. Therefore, it is better to feed steam rolled or cooked barley and steam flaked or super flaked corn than their untreated counterparts. The process of pelleting involves heat that results in improved enzymatic digestion of corn; extruding improves it even more. When deciding on a commercial mix for the horse, look for one that uses grains that have been processed to allow for optimal digestion in the small intestine of the horse.

While grain is a concentrated source of energy for the horse, there are some inherent dangers with feeding excessive amounts. When desperately trying to get a difficult horse to gain weight, it is often tempting to keep increasing the amount of grain being fed. Unfortunately, there is a point of no return when a horse gets too much grain in its digestive tract and the delicate balance of the microbial population is thrown off kilter. At this point, many horses also lose their appetite for forage and the situation worsens. No matter how much grain you feed, the horse will probably lose more weight. The minimal amount of forage a horse requires is 1% of its body weight. Therefore, a 1000-pound horse needs a minimum of 10 pounds of hay per day in order to maintain a reasonable balance of the microbial population. The rest of the diet should be designed around the minimal forage requirement.

The danger of feeding too much starch occurs because certain horses have a sensitivity to starch overload, perhaps precipitated by low amylase production. The cascade of problems begins with too much grain passing from the small intestine to the cecum and colon. Starch in the grain is fermented by bacteria inhabiting the cecum and colon. The by-product of starch fermentation is lactic acid, a substance that alters the pH of the hindgut to be more acidic. The acidic environment kills the bacteria. As the bacteria die they produce endotoxins that can cause colic. The endotoxins that pass into the bloodstream cause blood vessels to constrict. This decreases blood flow to the sensitive laminae in the hoof, which can induce laminitis. Horses that suffer from starch sensitivity should not be given high-grain diets.

As with forage digestion, supplements designed to aid in starch digestion or utilization have been developed. Although there has not been definitive research performed on the benefit of adding enzymes to the diet, the theory is well founded. If amylase is the limiting factor in small intestinal grain digestion, adding amylase to the feed may reduce the amount of grain channeling into the cecum and colon. Although there are a few feeds and supplements containing enzymes on the market, their efficacy is still questionable. Enzymes are proteins that are sensitive to acidic environments. Such environments denature the enzymes thereby making them inactive. All feed passes through the acidic stomach before reaching the small intestine; so how much enzyme will actually reach the intestine intact and not be denatured? More research is necessary to establish the efficacy of feeding supplemental enzymes.

Supplemental chromium may improve the metabolism of starch. The action of chromium does not have as much to do with aiding digestion as it does with the way the body handles the rise in blood glucose resulting from starch digestion and the consequential rise in insulin. Chromium yeast has been effective in reducing the incidence of chronic founder in some ponies and the incidence of chronic tying up in some horses with intolerance to high-grain diets.

FAT

Almost all performance horses have some type of fat added to their diet, whether it is a slug of corn oil, a scoop of rice bran, a handful of linseed, or a commercial high fat feed. Traditionally, fat was added to give the coat a healthy shine. However, recent research has brought to light an even better reason for feeding fat – it is an excellent energy source. Added dietary fat has proven to be an invaluable tool for packing weight on a hard keeper. Feeding fat is advantageous for several reasons. It is more concentrated, energy from fat does not make a horse flighty as energy from grain can do, and horses on high-fat diets exhibit more endurance.

Differences among fat sources make some more useful than others under different circumstances. There are major differences between vegetable fats (oils) and animal fats. The primary disadvantage of feeding animal fats is palatability; oils are much more appealing to the horse, although many commercial animal fats have flavorings added to improve the taste. Corn oil typically has remained the star in palatability studies, but most oils are palatable when offered without corn oil as a choice. The second obstacle is digestibility. Animal fat is only about 75% digestible while oil is closer to 95%. With small intakes of animal fat the digestibility difference is insignificant, but when higher levels are fed, that portion of indigestible fat can start to play havoc with the balance of microbes in the hindgut. Loose, runny feces are a sign that improper fat digestion is occurring.

A third obstacle involves the long-term maintenance of horses on animal fat. Horses may tire of the flavor and go off of an animal fat product before refusing a vegetable oil.

Other common sources of fat include rice bran, linseed, sunflower seeds, full-fat soybeans, and coconut meal (copra meal). Rice bran is an excellent product for improving body condition of thin horses because it is a good combination of rice oil and highly digestible fiber. Rice bran can be added to the regular grain to increase the caloric density of the ration. Linseed, sunflower seeds, and other seeds provide fat in the diet. However, a notable problem does arise when feeding vast amounts of seeds. As quantities of seeds fed increases, consumption will frequently slow, sometimes to the point of total refusal. Roasted soybeans are also great in small quantities but will increase the protein percentage of the diet too much if fed in larger amounts.

A high-fat diet is an invaluable tool for achieving weight gain in a skinny horse as long as the gastrointestinal tract of the horse will tolerate the fat. Normally horses have no problem digesting fat as long as it is introduced gradually into the diet. The greatest advantage of using fat as an energy source is that it helps to avoid excessive intakes of grain. Dietary fat works best when fed in conjunction with grain and/or highly digestible fiber sources like beet pulp (not neglecting good-quality hay or pasture). Many new feeds are appearing on the market that incorporate high fat levels (>6%) with high-fiber ingredients like beet pulp or soy hulls.

Conclusion

Some horses are metabolically inclined to be hard keepers while others have medical, psychological, or environmental reasons for having difficulty in maintaining weight. Increasing the caloric intake of a horse is not problematic if careful attention is paid to the feedstuffs offered to the horse. Manipulation of the amount and variety of energy sources will often achieve ideal body condition for the hard keeper.

HIDDEN KILLERS: MOLDS AND MYCOTOXINS

MIKE MURPHY
Department of Veterinary Diagnostic Medicine, University of Minnesota, St. Paul, Minnesota

Mold Diseases

Many diseases in horses have been associated with the presence of molds. These diseases involve guttural pouches, lungs, eyes, skin, the reproductive system, and the body as a whole.

GUTTURAL POUCHES

Molds have been isolated from infected guttural pouches in horses worldwide. Such associations have been made in India (Pal, 1996), Korea (Ha Tae Yong et al., 1995), France (Guillot et al., 1996), Japan (Takatori et al., 1984; Yoshihara et al., 1994), Italy (Gresti et al., 1993), and the United States.

The most common molds isolated from equine guttural pouches are *Aspergillus*, *Penicillium*, and *Candida* (Grabner, 1987). Perhaps the most important report for this group is a case where a liquid pellet feed binder was found to be the source of infection for a horse with guttural pouch disease. *Aspergillus* sp. was cultured from the guttural pouch, the mixed feed, and the liquid pellet binder (McLaughlin and O'Brien, 1986).

Early reports did not identify the particular species of *Aspergillus*. Several secondary problems were identified early on, including erosion of the internal carotid artery, cranial nerve damage (Hilbert et al., 1981), and blindness (Hatziolos et al., 1975). Later studies reported the species of *Aspergillus* responsible for disease.

Aspergillus nidulans is the *Aspergillus* species most frequently isolated from equine guttural pouches. The association between *Aspergillus nidulans* and guttural pouch mycosis was first recognized in the early 1970s (Johnson et al., 1973; Johnson and Attleberger, 1973). Soon thereafter an association between *Aspergillus nidulans* guttural pouch mycosis and nosebleeds was made (Lingard et al., 1974). Coughing, nasal discharge, and loss of 100 kg in 16 days occurred in a horse with *Aspergillus nidulans* guttural pouch mycosis (Krogh and Lundegaard, 1986). *Aspergillus nidulans* guttural pouch mycosis has been recognized in India (Pal,

139

1996), Korea (Ha TaeYong et al., 1995), France (Guillot et al., 1996), and Japan (Takatori et al., 1984; Kanemitsu et al., 1995). *Aspergillus nidulans* has recently been renamed *Emericella nidulans*. Horses have bled to death after erosion of the carotid artery due to *Emericella nidulans* infection of the guttural pouch (Guillot et al., 1997; Matsuda et al., 1999). *Emericella nidulans* and *Aspergillus fumigatus* were isolated from the guttural pouches of four Thoroughbreds using endoscopy. Three of the horses were killed because of their poor prognosis (Anzai et al., 2000).

Two other species of *Aspergillus* are commonly isolated from equine guttural pouches. *Aspergillus fumigatus* from a guttural pouch infection has caused an atlanto-occipital joint infection (Dixon and Rowlands, 1981) and nasal discharge (Greet, 1981). Guttural pouch mycosis has also been caused by *Aspergillus ochraceus* (Gresti et al., 1993).

A *Penicillium* sp. mold was isolated from the guttural pouch of a horse with a fistula that developed from a guttural pouch mycosis (Jacobs and Fretz, 1982).

LUNGS

Aspergillus has also been associated with lung lesions in horses. Both acute and chronic forms of the disease have been identified (Sudaric et al., 1979). An association between GI disease and pulmonary aspergillosis has been suspected. Invasive pulmonary aspergillosis was identified in 19 horses; 16 of them also had entercolitis (Slocombe and Slauson, 1988). Endocarditis and pulmonary aspergillosis developed in an 8-year-old Quarter Horse after surgery (Pace et al., 1994). Three Thoroughbreds died after a five-day illness of apathy, fever, lacrimation, and dyspnea after being transferred to a new stable. They died with thrombosis, hemorrhage, and tissue necrosis. A diagnosis of pneumonia caused by *Aspergillus niger* was made (*Rhizopus stonifer* was also isolated) (Carrasco et al., 1997). The sudden death of two horses was attributed to the rapid and acute development of pulmonary aspergillosis. One horse developed it after surgery, the other while being treated for equine protozoal myelitis (Johnson et al., 1999).

EYES

A variety of molds has been isolated from the eyes of horses with keratitis (Hamilton et al., 1994). *Alternaria, Aspergillus, Actinomyces, Candida, Fusarium, Penicillium*, and *Mucor* have been isolated from 11 cases of keratomycoses in Pennsylvania (Beech et al., 1983). Additionally, *Rhizopus* (Scherzer et al., 1998), *Cephalosporium*, and *Phycomyces* have been isolated. *Aspergillus* is the most prevalent (Moore et al., 1983). Of 31 keratomycosis cases in Texas, 11 were *Aspergillus* and four were *Penicillium* (Coad et al., 1985).

Aspergillus and *Fusarium* are most commonly isolated. Of 39 horses treated for ulcerative keratomycosis, *Aspergillus* was isolated from 13 and *Fusarium* from 10 (Andrew et al., 1998). *Aspergillus* and *Fusarium* sp. were also reported in a second study (Kern et al., 1983). *Aspergillus flavus* (Grahn et al., 1993; Collins et al., 1994), *Aspergillus fumigatus* (Aho et al., 1991), and *Aspergillus oryzae* (Marolt et al., 1984) are the most commonly reported *Aspergillus* species. *Fusarium* has been isolated in a number of cases also (Mitchell and Attleburger, 1973; Hodgson and Jacobs, 1982). Of six cases with keratomycosis, *Aspergillus* was isolated from three, *Fusarium* from two, and *Cladosporium* from one (Peiffer, 1979).

REPRODUCTIVE SYSTEM

Molds have also been reported to cause abortions as well as uterine and placental infections. Fungi were cultured from nine of 100 aborted horses in India. *Candida tropicalis* was in three, *Aspergillus fumigatus* in three, *Candida albicans* in two, and *Cryptococcus laurentii* in one (Monga et al., 1983). Of 2000 pregnancies followed in India, 175 abortions occurred. Six were caused by fungi. The fungi involved were *Mucor* (three), *Aspergillus* (two), and *Microsporum* (one) (Garg and Manchanda, 1986). *Aspergillus fumigatus* has been diagnosed as the cause of abortion in two Thoroughbred mares (Plagemann et al., 1992).

Aspergillus fumigatus and *Candida albicans* were isolated from mares with uterine infections (Blue, 1983). Fungi isolated from the uteri of mares with endometritis are *Actinomyces, Aspergillus, Candida, Coccidiodes, Hansenula, Monosporium, Mucor, Nocardia, Paecilomyces,* and *Trichosporon* (Pugh et al., 1986). Of 27 mares with chronic infertility problems, *Alternaria* sp., *Aspergillus flavus, A. fumigatus, A. niger, Mortierella wolfi,* and *Mucor* sp. were isolated from cervical, vaginal, or clitoral fossa swabs (Verma and Gupta, 1983). Of 200 cases of infective placentitis, 37 were caused by *Aspergillus fumigatus* and 14 by *Absidia* sp. (Whitwell and Powell, 1988).

SKIN

Of 1090 horses examined, most had *Trichophyton equinum* skin disease, but *Aspergillus* infection was common (Takatori et al., 1981).

SEPTICEMIA

An 18-year-old Morgan had a 10-day history of watery diarrhea, depression, and dysphagia. It died four days after being referred to a veterinary teaching hospital. *Aspergillus niger* was identified as the cause of vasculitis and brain infarction (Tunev et al., 1999). *Mucor* and *Rhizopus* were associated with a horse that developed myocarditis and nephritis after surgery (Peet et al., 1981).

IMMUNOSUPPRESSION

Horses have developed systemic mold infections after corticosteroid treatment or natural immunosuppression. Fatal pulmonary infections with *Aspergillus flavus* and *A. niger* developed after corticosteroid immunosuppression (Weiler et al., 1994) or colic treatment (Smith et al., 1981). A horse with myelomonocytic leukemia developed pulmonary aspergillosis after phenylbutazone and corticosteroid therapy (Blue et al., 1987) or without such therapy (Buechner-Maxwell et al., 1994). A chronic bronchopulmonary *Aspergillus* infection was diagnosed in a 30-year-old Saddlebred with Cushing's syndrome (Carrasco et al., 1996).

Mold Allergies

Chronic obstructive pulmonary disease (COPD) is also referred to as "heaves," "broken wind," or "pulmonary emphysema." The syndrome was first reported in the early 1970s. Eight horses were reported as having an allergic pneumonitis that was clinically and pathologically similar to farmer's lung in humans (Paul et al., 1972). The pathology has been described as peribronchitis, perivasculitis, and interstitial pneumonitis with foci and nodules of macrophages containing refractile particles of inorganic dust in alveoli (Chen et al., 1989). Considerable work has gone into determining the factors that predispose horses to the disease.

Molds were one of the predisposing factors initially considered. Using the method available at the time, exposure of horses to *Penicillium*, *Alternaria*, *Epicoccum*, and *Cladosporium* molds was found to have little relationship to the existence of the disease (Halliwell et al., 1979). Poor ventilation of the stable did seem to increase the chance of a horse becoming affected with COPD. However, gender, body weight, and season of onset of coughing did not seem to influence occurrence of the disease (McPherson et al., 1979b). After ruling out several factors, an immune component was investigated.

The possibility of COPD as a hypersensitivity disease has been considered (McPherson et al., 1979a; McGorum et al., 1993) and gained acceptance. Currently, evidence indicates that COPD is a delayed hypersensitivity response to inhaled antigens, particularly molds. It involves increased histamine, thromboxane, and 15-hydroxyeicosatetraenoic acid in bronchoalveolar lavage fluid (BALF), and decreased prostaglandin E$_2$ in airway mucosa (Robinson et al., 1996).

Despite these advances, the diagnosis of COPD was elusive, largely because investigators focused on skin reactions and serum antibody titers. Although horses with COPD had strong skin reactions after intradermal injections of mold extracts, there was no correlation between fungal contamination and the incidence of COPD. *Aspergillus*, *Alternaria*, and *Hormodendron* extracts were tested (Eyre et al., 1972). Of 237 horses tested, 100 of which had COPD, no relationship between COPD and type I skin reactions was seen. Although many horses gave a type III reaction to *Micropolyspora faeni* (Eriksen and Olson, 1990), more recent studies of dermal and pulmonary reactivities to *M. faeni*, *A. fumigatus*, and *T. vulgaris* indicate that intradermal testing is of limited value in investigating COPD (McGorum, 1993b).

Studies focusing on serum antibody titers have been equally disappointing. Circulating precipitins to *Micropolyspora faeni* and *Aspergillus fumigatus* were not restricted to horses with COPD, but did occur more frequently in horses with COPD (Lawson et al., 1979). In 119 serum samples, antibodies against *M. faeni* were demonstrated in 11, and among these, COPD was only confirmed in four (Eriksen et al., 1986). Serological tests are of little value in the diagnosis of COPD (Madelin et al., 1991). In eight horses tested with 67 extracts from different allergens, significant difference was evident between horses with COPD and healthy horses in only 3% of the possible extracts (Evans et al., 1992). Higher titers of anti-*Micropolyspora faeni*, anti-*Aspergillus fumigatus,* and anti-hay mold precipitins were observed in the serum samples of horses positive for equine influenza antibodies (Chabchoub et al., 1994). Fortunately, BALF has been investigated.

Recently, use of BALF has shed light on the diagnosis of COPD. *Micropolyspora faeni* and *Aspergillus fumigatus* were identified as common causes of respiratory hypersensitivity in horses affected with COPD (McPherson et al., 1979a). An ELISA was used to measure specific antibodies to *Micropolyspora faeni* and to *Aspergillus fumigatus* in the serum and BALF of normal horses, horses with COPD, and horses with other respiratory diseases. Elevated antibody results were not detected in the sera of any horses, but IgE and IgA antibodies to both allergens were significantly elevated in BALF of COPD horses (Halliwell et al., 1993). Horses with COPD have significantly higher levels of BALF IgE and IgG to *A. fumigatus* antigens but no significant differences in serum (Schmallenbach et al., 1998).

Treatment has been developed. Sodium cromoglycate (80 mg) prevented exacerbation of the respiratory disease for four to five days after exposure to *Micropolyspora faeni* (Murphy et al., 1979).

Mycotoxins (Forage)

FESCUE

Fescue toxicosis in horses has been recognized for decades. Nevertheless, the mechanism of action and successful management practices are only now being reported. The prevalence of exposure, clinical signs, management, and treatment reports are briefly summarized.

Despite decades of knowledge of the potential for toxicosis from endophyte-infested fescue, many horses remain exposed. Of 207 equine owners and veterinarians responding to a recent survey, fescue was the predominant forage on 50% of pastures and was present on 70%. Almost 50% of the broodmares in the survey were exposed to endophyte-infected fescue, and 43% had signs of toxicosis requiring treatment or management to reduce the problem (Anas et al., 1998).

The clinical signs of fescue toxicosis are well known. Pregnant mares develop agalactia, stillbirth, and thickened and retained placentas (Bennett-Wimbush and Loch, 1998). In addition, mares have dystocias (McCann et al., 1992), increased gestation length, increased foal and mare mortality, weak and dysmature foals, and increased sweating during warm weather (Cross et al., 1995). The prevalence of clinical signs is not the same in each case. For example, in one study approximately 26% of 1010 mares on fescue pasture had fescue toxicosis, 53% had agalactia, 38% had prolonged pregnancy, 18% had abortions, and 9% had thickened placentas (Garrett et al., 1980).

Mares are not the only horses affected. Average daily gain for yearlings is lower on fescue with high infection rates versus low infection rates (Aiken et al., 1993). Fiber digestibility of endophyte-positive hay is lower than that for endophyte-negative hay (McCann et al., 1992).

The mechanism for these signs long eluded researchers but may now have been discovered. Decreased perfusion of peripheral tissues (Adney et al., 1993) and impaired endometrial cup function mechanisms were investigated (Brendemuehl et al., 1996). Reduced serum prolactin and progesterone and increased serum estradiol 17 beta levels have been observed (Cross et al., 1995). At this point, it appears that ergovaline in tall fescue infested with *Neotyphodium coenophialum* explains the clinical signs and laboratory results previously reported (McClusky et al., 1999).

Fescue toxicosis may be dealt with by managment or treatment. A rotational grazing technique allows use of fescue for growing horses. Even though endophyte-infected tall fescue hay may be less digestible in horses than uninfected hay (Redmond et al., 1991), young growing horses being exercised can efficiently use the endophyte-infected fescue on a short-term basis (Pendergraft et al., 1993). Similar techniques can be used in mares.

If mares are removed from fescue late in gestation, most signs of toxicosis can be eliminated or reduced. Withdrawal from infected fescue before parturition results in a rise in serum prolactin levels, allowing milk production (Redmond et al., 1991). Mares moved to endophyte-free pasture at 305 to 310 days of gestation delivered live foals and lactated normally. Supplementation of energy requirements to these mares while grazing endophyte-infected fescue was of little or no benefit (Earle et al., 1990).

Effective treatments after signs develop are also being developed. Selenium treatment is not effective (Monroe et al., 1988). Fluphanazine has been considered (Bennett-Wimbush and Loch, 1997), and domperidone looks promising. Daily oral doses of 1.1 mg/kg body weight domperidone prevented symptoms of fescue toxicosis in late gestation mares on endophyte-infested fescue forage (Cross et al., 1999). A single injection of a long-acting dopamine receptor antagonist may be beneficial in reducing the effects of fescue toxicosis in pregnant mares grazing endophyte-infected tall fescue pastures (Bennett-Wimbush and Loch, 1998).

RYEGRASS

Ataxia, tremors, and paralysis were observed in a group of horses and then several weeks later in a second group ingesting the same hay. The horses were ingesting ryegrass hay containing 5 to 6 mg lolitrem B/kg (Van Oldruitenborgh-Oosterbaan et al., 1999). A stallion ingesting 1.5 and 2.5 mg lolitrem B/kg also experienced ryegrass staggers. Trembling, hyperexcitability, and abdominal muscular spasms developed suddenly in ponies fed exclusively ryegrass seed cleanings shown to contain 5.3 mg lolitrem B/kg (Munday et al., 1985; Hintz, 1990).

SWEET CLOVER

Spontaneous nosebleeds developed in a 6-year-old Percheron mare fed weathered sweet clover (McDonald, 1980).

RED CLOVER

Excessive salivation and increased water consumption were observed in horses eating red clover or lucerne infested with *Rhizoctonia leguminicola*. Slaframine was associated with the parasympathetic signs (Socket et al., 1982). The slaframine breaks down with time. It fell from 100 mg/kg to 7 mg/kg after ten months of storage (Hagler and Behlow, 1981).

ALSIKE CLOVER

Photosensitization and biliary fibrosis may occur in horses ingesting alsike clover (*Trifolium hybridum*) (Nation, 1989). Chronic or nervous clinical signs and liver disease, including biliary fibrosis and epithelial proliferation, may occur (Nation, 1991). Icterus and photosensitization are followed by nervous signs in almost 80% of cases (Zientara, 1993). Icterus of the sclera, oral and vulvar membranes and dermatitis of the muzzle and vulva, as well as increased serum liver enzymes have recently been reported in horses ingesting alsike clover (Colon et al., 1996).

Mycotoxins (Grains)

FUMONISIN

Fumonisins are new mycotoxins that are of great significance to horse owners. Like aflatoxin, they are suspected of being carcinogenic, so feed entering interstate commerce will be subject to regulation based on its fumonisin content. FDA's guidance document issued June 6, 2000 indicates that corn or corn by-products intended for horses may contain five ppm fumonisin B_1, plus B_2, plus B_3, but comprise no more than 20% of the diet.

Fumonisins are produced by *Fusarium moniliforme*, which causes "stalk rot" in corn. Fumonisin toxicosis in horses has primarily been caused by corn screenings or corn-containing feed. Fumonisin causes equine leukoencephalomalacia (ELEM), liver necrosis, and occasionally death in horses. Quite a number of field and experimental reports have substantiated this.

Although "moldy corn poisoning" of horses has been recognized for decades, fumonisin was not identified as the causative agent until 1988. Investigators in South Africa were the first to make the connection (Marasas et al., 1988; Kellerman et al., 1990; Thiel et al., 1991; Sydenham et al., 1992; Sydenham et al., 1993). Since then, fumonisin toxicosis in horses has been recognized in Italy (Carmelli et al., 1993), Australia (Shanks et al., 1995), Hungary (Fazekas and Bajmicy, 1996; Fazekas et al., 1997), Mexico (Rosiles et al., 1996), France (Guerre et al., 1997), Turkey (Akar and Sarii, 1998), and the United States. The reports from North America are summarized.

In the United States, several cases of fumonisin toxicosis were diagnosed in 1989 and 1990. No clinical cases occurred in horses ingesting feed with less than eight ppm fumonisins (Wilson et al., 1990; Ross et al., 1991a,b). In 1991 and 1992, fumonisin B_1 and B_2 were detected at concentrations higher than 10 ppm in 16% of 291 Indiana corn samples tested (Binkerd et al., 1993), so studies of the dose to produce toxicity were initiated.

A pony fed a diet of 22 ppm fumonisin for 55 days suddenly died (Wilson et al., 1991; Wilson et al., 1992; Ross et al., 1993). *Fusarium moniliforme* was isolated from each feed sample of 125 horses affected with ELEM (Wilson et al., 1990a,b,c). One hundred donkeys died in Mexico with ELEM after ingesting feed containing 0.67 to 13.3 mg fumonisin B_1 (Rosiles et al., 1998), and four Thoroughbreds developed ELEM after ingesting corn containing 46 to 53 µg/g fumonisin B_1 (Mallmann et al., 1999).

Fusarium moniliforme produces fumonisin B_1, B_2, and B_3. Early studies focused on fumonisin B_1, but it now appears that fumonisin B_2 can also contribute to toxicosis (Ross et al., 1994). Fumonisin B_2 at 75 ppm (0.75 mg/kg body weight daily) caused hepatotoxicity and ELEM in ponies. Fumonisin B_2 is more effective than fumonisin B_3 in causing toxicity (Riley et al., 1997). The fumonisins appear to cause ELEM by interfering with myelin synthesis.

Both fumonisin B_1 and B_2 disrupt sphingolipid metabolism (Riley et al., 1997). So, the ratio of sphinganine to sphingosine may be elevated in horses exposed to fumonisin B_1 or B_2 (Goel et al., 1996). This testing of serum or liver is being used to diagnose exposure to fumonisin. Aflatoxin is the other mycotoxin that is a suspected carcinogen.

AFLATOXIN

Aflatoxin is primarily produced by *Aspergillus* molds and occasionally by *Penicillium* molds. Grain in interstate commerce is currently regulated based on its aflatoxin concentration because it is a suspected carcinogen. The major concerns to horse owners though are liver disease, death, and abortion.

Signs of aflatoxicosis in nonpregnant horses include mild fever, anorexia, depression, incoordination, and marked swelling of the supraorbital fossae (Poomvises et al., 1982; Asquith et al., 1983). Signs of inappetence, depression, tremors, and prostration have also been reported (Cysewski et al., 1982). Liver disease develops in horses receiving more than 0.075 mg/kg aflatoxin B_1 (Cysewski et al., 1982), but liver enzymes return to normal within 10 days of removing the source (Aller et al., 1981).

Equine deaths have been reported in field and experimental cases. Three horses had severe hepatic necrosis and died after ingesting corn containing aflatoxin B_1, B_2 and M_1 at 114, 10 and 6 ppb, respectively (Vesonder et al., 1991).

All ponies given 4 mg/kg aflatoxin B_1 died and half given 2 mg/kg died (Bortell et al., 1983). Death occurred at 12 to 16 days in horses dosed with 0.3 mg/kg aflatoxin B_1, at 25 to 32 days if dosed with 0.15 mg/kg, and at 36 to 39 days if dosed with 0.075 mg/kg (Cysewski et al., 1982). Mortality rates of 25% are reported in field cases (Poomvises et al., 1982).

Abortion is not reported in most species ingesting aflatoxin unless the dam is quite ill. However, a report of 17 of 63 mares aborting 6- to 9-month-old feti after ingesting feed containing 250 ppb aflatoxin B_1 exists (Xie et al., 1991).

ERGOT

Symptoms of ergot toxicosis developed in several horses fed Bermuda grass hay (Lindley, 1978). *Achnatherum inebrians* (drunken horse grass) in China contained ergonovine and lysergic acid amide at 2500 and 400 mg/kg, respectively (Miles et al., 1996).

DEOXYNIVALENOL

Reduced general condition was noted in horses fed for six to eight weeks on oat samples containing 20 ppm deoxynivalenol and 2 ppm zearalenone (Bauer and Gedek, 1980).

Table 1. Molds, mycoses and allergies in horses.

Mold	System	Mold	System
Absidia	Reproductive	Candida tropicalis	Reproductive
Actinomyces	Eyes	Cephalosporium	Eyes
Actinomyces	Reproductive	Cladosporium	Eyes
Alternaria	Eyes	Coccidiodes	Reproductive
Alternaria	Reproductive	Cryptococcus laurentii	Reproductive
Aspergillus	Eyes	Emericella nidulans	Guttural pouch disease
Aspergillus	Guttural pouch disease	Fusarium	Eyes
Aspergillus	Lungs	Hansenula	Reproductive
Aspergillus	Reproductive	Micropolyspora faeni	COPD
Aspergillus	Skin	Microsporum	Reproductive
Aspergillus flavus	Eyes	Monosporium	Reproductive
Aspergillus flavus	Reproductive	Mortierella wolfi	Reproductive
Aspergillus flavus	Septicemia	Mucor	Eyes
Aspergillus fumigatus	COPD	Mucor	Reproductive
Aspergillus fumigatus	Eyes	Mucor	Septicemia
Aspergillus fumigatus	Guttural pouch disease	Nocardia	Reproductive
Aspergillus fumigatus	Reproductive	Paecilomyces	Reproductive
Aspergillus nidulans	Guttural pouch disease	Penicillium	Eyes
Aspergillus niger	Lungs	Penicillium	Guttural pouch disease
Aspergillus niger	Reproductive	Phycomyces	Eyes
Aspergillus niger	Septicemia	Rhizopus	Septicemia
Aspergillus ochraceus	Guttural pouch disease	Rhizopus stonifer	Eyes
Aspergillus oryzae	Eyes	Rhizopus stonifer	Lungs
Candida	Eyes	Trichophyton equinum	Skin
Candida	Guttural pouch disease	Trichosporon	Reproductive
Candida	Reproductive		
Candida albicans	Reproductive		

Table 2. Molds and mycotoxins in horse feeds.

Mold	Source	Mycotoxin
Acremonium coenophialum	Fescue	Ergovaline
Aspergillus	Grain	Aflatoxin
Claviceps purpura	Small grains	Ergot
Fusarium	Grain	Oxynivalenol
Fusarium moniliforme	Grain	Fumonisin
Neotyphodium coenophialum	Fescue	Ergovaline
Penicillium	Grain	Aflatoxin
Rhizoctonia leguminicola	Legumes	Slaframine

References

Abdel-Hamid AM. Detection of aflatoxins in Egyptian feedstuffs. Annals Ag Sci, Moshtohor. 1985, 23: 2, 649-657.

Abney LK; Oliver JW; Reinemeyer CR. Vasoconstrictive effects of tall fescue alkaloids on equine vasculature. J Eq Vet Sci. 1993, 13: 6, 334-340.

Aho R; Tala N; Kivalo M. Mycotic keratitis in a horse caused by *Aspergillus fumigatus*. The first reported case in Finland. Acta Vet Scandinavica. 1991, 32: 3, 373-376.

Aiken GE; Bransby DI; McCall CA. Growth of yearling horses compared to steers on high- and low-endophyte infected tall fescue. J Eq Vet Sci. 1993, 13: 1, 26-28.

Akar F; Sarii M. A new mycotoxin group: fumonisins. Veteriner Kontrol ve Arastirma Enstitusu Mudurlugu Dergisi. 1998, 23: 37, 145-153.

Allen VG. Fescue problems. Eq Vet Data. 1983, 4: 1, 8-9.

Aller WW Jr.; Edds GT; Asquith RL. Effects of aflatoxins in young ponies. Am J Vet Res. 1981, 42: 12, 2162-2164.

Anas K; Cross DL; Poling R; Redmond LM; Campbell CE. A survey concerning the equine fescue toxicosis malady. J Eq Vet Sci. 1998, 18: 10, 631-637.

Andrew SE; Brooks DE; Smith PJ; Gelatt KN; Chmielewski NT; Whittaker CJG. Equine ulcerative keratomycosis: visual outcome and ocular survival in 39 cases (1987-1996). Eq Vet J. 1998, 30: 2, 109-116.

Angusbhakorn S; Poomuises P; Romruen K; Newberne PM. Aflatoxicosis in horses. J Am Vet Med *Assoc*. 1981, 178: 3, 274-278.

Animal Health 1975. Report of the Chief Veterinary Officer. 1977.

Anzai T; Takatori K; Shimozawa K; Manglai D. Fungal and bacterial isolation from inflamed guttural pouches. Drug susceptibility of the isolates. J Japan Vet Med Assoc. 2000, 53: 2, 63-66.

Archer M. Further studies on palatability of grasses to horses. *J Br Grassland*

Soc. 1978, 33: 4, 239-243.

Asmundsson T; Gunnarsson E; Johannesson T. "Haysickness" in Icelandic horses: precipitin tests and other studies. Eq Vet J. 1983, 15: 3, 229-232.

Archer M. The species preferences of grazing horses. J British-Grassland-Society. 1973, 28: 3, 123-128.

Asquith RL; Smith JE (ed.); Henderson RS (ed.). Mycotoxicoses in horses. Mycotoxins and animal foods. 1991, 679-688.

Asquith RL; Edds GT. Investigations in equine aflatoxicosis. Proc Am Assoc Eq Pract. 1980 publ. 1981, No. 26, 193-200.

Asquith RL; Diener UL (ed.); Asquith RL (ed.); Dickens JW (ed.). Biological effects of aflatoxins: horses. Aflatoxin and *Aspergillus flavus* in corn. 1983, 62-66.

Attleberger MH; Chick EW (ed.); Balows A (ed.); Furcolow L (ed.). Opportunistic fungus infections in large animals seen at autopsy. Opportunistic fungal infections. Proceedings of the Second International Conference. 1975, 293-299.

Bacon CW; Bennett RM; Hinton DM; Voss KA. Scanning electron microscopy of *Fusarium moniliforme* within asymptomatic corn kernels and kernels associated with equine leukoencephalomalacia. Plant Disease. 1992, 76: 2, 144-148.

Bauer J; Binder S. Fumonisins in feedstuffs: their occurrence and the relevance of a new group of *Fusarium* toxins. Tierarztliche-Umschau. 1993, 48: 11, 718-720, 727.

Bauer J; Gedek B. *Fusarium* toxins as a cause of feed refusal and fertility disorders in the horse. Tierarztliche-Umschau. 1980, 35: 9, 600-603.

Beech J; Sweeney CR; IrbyN. Keratomycoses in 11 horses. Eq Vet J. 1983, Suppl. 2, 39-44.

Bennett-Wimbush K; Loch WE. A preliminary study of the efficacy of fluphenazine as a treatment for fescue toxicosis in gravid pony mares. J Eq Vet Sci. 1998, 18: 3, 169-174.

Bennett-Wimbush K; Loch WE. The efficacy of fluphenazine as a treatment for fescue toxicosis in gravid pony mares. Proceedings of the Fifteenth Equine Nutrition and Physiology Symposium, Fort Worth, Texas, USA, 28-31 May, 1997. 1997, 281-282.

Binkerd KA; Scott DH; Everson RJ; Sullivan JM; Robinson FR. Fumonisin contamination of the 1991 Indiana corn crop and its effect on horses. J Vet Diagnostic Investigation. 1993, 5: 4, 653-655.

Bistner SI; Riis RC. Clinical aspects of mycotic keratitis in the horse. Cornell Vet. 1979, 69: 4, 364-374.

Blomme E; Piero FD; La Perle KMD; Wilkins PA. Aspergillosis in horses: a review. Eq Vet Ed. 1998, 10: 2, 86-93.

Blood DC; Henderson JA; Radostits OM. Diseases caused by fungi. Veterinary Medicine. A textbook of the diseases of cattle, sheep, pigs and horses.

1979, 5th edition, 718-727. Bailliere Tindall.; London; UK.

Blue J; Perdrizet J; Brown E. Pulmonary aspergillosis in a horse with myelomonocytic leukemia. J Am Vet Med Assoc. 1987, 190: 12, 1562-1564.

Blue MG. Mycotic invasion of the mare's uterus. Vet Rec. 1983, 113: 6, 131-132.

Bortell R; Asquith RL; Edds GT; Simpson CF; Aller WW. Acute experimentally induced aflatoxicosis in the weanling pony. Am J Vet Res. 1983, 44: 11, 2110-2114.

Brendemuehl JP; Carson RL; Wenzel JGW; Boosinger TR; Shelby RA. Effects of grazing endophyte-infected tall fescue on eCG and progestogen concentrations from gestation day 21 to 300 in the mare. Theriogenology. 1996, 46: 1, 85-96.

Bridges CH; Wyllie TD(ed.); Morehouse LG (ed.). Mycotoxicoses in horses. Mycotoxin fungi, mycotoxins, mycotoxicoses. Volume 2. 1978, 173-181.

Brown ACL. Animal health 1974. Report of the Chief Veterinary Officer. 1975.

Buechner-Maxwell V; Zhang-Chong H; Robertson J; Jain NC; Antczak DF; Feldman BF; Murray MJ. Intravascular leukostasis and systemic aspergillosis in a horse with subleukemic acute myelomonocytic leukemia. J Vet Internal Med. 1994, 8: 4, 258-263.

Bushee EL; Edwards DR; Moore PA. Quality of runoff from plots treated with municipal sludge and horse bedding. Transactions of the ASAE. 1998, 41: 4, 1035-1041.

Caramelli M; Dondo A; Cortellazzi GC; Visconti A; Minervini F; Doko MB; Guarda F. Leukoencephalomalacia in the equine caused by fumonisins: first report in Italy. Ippologia. 1993, 4: 4, 49-56.

Carrasco L; Tarradas MC; Gomez-Villamandos JC; Luque I; Arenas A; Mendez A. Equine pulmonary mycosis due to *Aspergillus niger* and *Rhizopus stolonifer*. J Comparative Pathology. 1997, 117: 3, 191-199.

Carrasco L; Mendez A; Jensen HE. Chronic bronchopulmonary aspergillosis in a horse with Cushing's syndrome. Mycoses. 1996, 39: 11-12, 443-447.

Carvajal M; Barcenas E; Sanchez R; Mendoza S; Gomez H; Cardenas E. *Fusarium* related to leukoencephalomalacia and brain edema of horses. Proceedings Japanese Assoc Mycotoxicology. 1988, Supplement No. 1, 133-134.

Chabchoub A; Ghram A; Louzir H; Boussetta M; Jomaa I; Aouina T. Investigation of anti-equine influenza antibodies in the sera of horses with chronic pulmonary disease. Revue-de-Medecine-Veterinaire. 1994, 145: 5, 343-348.

Chabchoub A; Louzir H; Aouina T; Grham A. Detection by ELISA of anti-*Micropolyspora faeni*, anti-*Aspergillus fumigatus* and anti-hay mould antibodies in the serum of horses with chronic pulmonary disease in north eastern Tunisia. Pratique Veterinaire Eq. 1994, 26: 3, 175-180.

Chen HT; Zhu XQ; Ni JB; WangWH; Jia N. Pathological study on heaves in horses in Gansu province. Acta Veterinaria et Zootechnica Sinica. 1989,

20: 1, 55-59. Coad CT; Robinson NM; Wilhelmus KR. Antifungal sensitivity testing for equine keratomycosis. Am J Vet Research. 1985, 46: 3, 676-678.

Codazza D; Maffeo G; Giongo P; Gavazzi L; Proverbio E. Changes in some blood chemistry values of young trotters fed cereals contaminated with aflatoxin B1. Clinica Veterinaria. 1980, 103: 9-10, 577-584.

Collins MB; Ethell MT; Hodgson DR. Management of mycotic keratitis in a horse using a conjunctival pedicle graft. Australian Vet J. 1994, 71: 9, 298-299.

Colon JL; Jackson CA; Del Piero F. Hepatic dysfunction and photodermatitis secondary to alsike clover poisoning. Compendium Continuing Ed Practicing Vet. 1996, 18: 9, 1022-1026.

Consalvi PJ. Enilconazole: a new compound for the external treatment of dermatomycoses in dog, horses and cattle. Pratique Medicale Chirurgicale Animal Compagnie. 1983, 18: 1, 61-64.

Cross DL; Redmond LM; Strickland JR. Equine fescue toxicosis: signs and solutions. J An Sci. 1995, 73: 3, 899-908.

Cross DL; Anas K; Bridges WC; Chappell JH. Clinical effects of domperidone on fescue toxicosis in pregnant mares. Proceedings of the 45th Annual Convention of the American Association of Equine Practitioners, Albuquerque, New Mexico, 5-8 December 1999. 1999, 203-206.

Cysewski SJ; Pier AC; Baetz AL; Cheville NF. Experimental equine aflatoxicosis. Toxicol Appl Pharm. 1982, 65: 3, 354-365.

Davis EW; Legendre AM. Successful treatment of guttural pouch mycosis with itraconazole and topical enilconazole in a horse. J Vet Internal Med. 1994, 8: 4, 304-305.

Dirscherl P; Grabner A; Buschmann H. Responsiveness of basophil granulocytes of horses suffering from chronic obstructive pulmonary disease to various allergens. Vet Immunol Immunopath. 1993, 38: 3-4, 217-227.

Dixon PM; Rowlands AC. Atlanto-occipital joint infection associated with guttural pouch mycosis in a horse. Eq Vet J. 1981, 13: 4, 260-262.

Dovgich NA. Dermatomycoses of animals and man caused by *Alternaria alternata* (Fr.) Keissler. Mikrobiologicheskii-Zhurnal. 1981, 43: 3, 382-383.

Earle WE; Cross DL; Hudson LW; Redmond LM; Kennedy SW. Effect of energy supplementation on gravid mares grazing endophyte-infected fescue. J Eq Vet Sci. 1990, 10: 2, 126-127, 129-130.

Edwards DR; Moore PA Jr.; Workman SR; Bushee EL. Runoff of metals from alum-treated horse manure and municipal sludge. J Am Water-Resources-Associa-tion. 1999, 35: 1, 155-165.

El Dessouki S. Aflatoxins in cosmetics containing substrates for aflatoxin-producing fungi. Food Chem Toxicology. 1992, 30: 11, 993-994.

Eriksen L; Olsen SN. Skin tests in horses. Use in the diagnosis of respiratory allergies. Dansk-Veterinaertidsskrift. 1990, 73: 10, 538-544.

Eriksen L; Deegen E (ed.); Beadle RE. Studies on *Micropolyspora faeni* and chronic obstructive pulmonary disease (COPD). Lung function and respiratory diseases in the horse. International Symposium in Hannover, Germany, June 27-29, 1985. 1986, 32-34.

Eriksson NE; Holmen A. Skin prick tests with standardized extracts of inhalant allergens in 7099 adult patients with asthma or rhinitis: cross-sensitizations and relationships to age, sex, month of birth and year of testing. J Investigational Allergology Clin Immunol. 1996, 6: 1, 36-46.

Erturk E; Alibasoglu M. Fungus diseases of domestic animals in Ankara. Veteriner Fakultesi Dergisi. 1974, 21: 3-4, 224-242.

Evans TJ; Youngquist RS; Loch WE; Cross DL. A comparison of the relative efficacies of domperidone and reserpine in treating equine "fescue toxicosis". Proceedings of the 45th Annual Convention of the American Association of Equine Practitioners, Albuquerque, New Mexico, 5-8 December 1999. 1999, 207-209.

Evans AG; Paradis MR; O' Callaghan M. Intradermal testing of horses with chronic obstructive pulmonary disease and recurrent urticaria. Am J Vet Res. 1992, 53: 2, 203-208.

Eyre P. Equine pulmonary emphysema: a bronchopulmonary mould allergy. Veterinary-Record. 1972, 91: No.6, 134-140.

Falk-Ronne J; Gravesen S; Larsen L; Svenningsen J. Microorganisms in the air of a horse stable. Concentrations of *Aspergillus fumigatus* and actinomycetes with the use of straw and shredded newspaper as bedding material. Dansk-Veterinaertidsskrift. 1984, 67: 21, 1079-1083.

Fazekas B; Bajmocy E; Glavits R; Fenyvesi A. Fumonisin mycotoxicoses in Hungary. Leukoencephalomalacia in horses, fattening pulmonary oedema in pigs. Magyar-Allatorvosok-Lapja. 1997, 119: 3, 137-142.

Fazekas B; Bajmicy E. Occurrence of equine leukoencephalomalacia caused by fumonisin-B1 mycotoxin in Hungary. Magyar-Allatorvosok-Lapja. 1996, 51: 8, 484-487.

Ficken MD; Cummings TS; Wages DP. Cerebral encephalomalacia in commercial turkeys. Av Diseases. 1993, 37: 3, 917-922.

Firth EC; Pearce SG; Grace ND; Fennessy PF. Health care of the pregnant mare: evidence for copper supplementation. Ippologia. 1999, 10: 2, 49-52.

Flore JA; Hansen E; Johnson J; Wisse J; Whalon M; Bird G; Jones A; Schenk AME (ed.); Webster AD (ed.); Wertheim SJ. Low input production of peach (*Prunus persica* cv. 'Newhaven'). Proceedings of the Second International Symposium on Integrated Fruit Production, held at Veldhoven, Netherlands, 24-28 August 1992. Acta-Horticulturae. 1993, No. 347, 65-74.

Freeman DE; Ross MW; Donawick WJ; Hamir AN. Occlusion of the external carotid and maxillary arteries in the horse to prevent hemorrhage from guttural pouch mycosis. Vet Surgery. 1989, 18: 1, 39-47.

Gabal MA; Awad YL; Morcos MB; Barakat AM; Malik G. Fusariotoxicoses of farm animals and mycotoxic leucoencephalomalacia of the equine associated with the finding of trichothecenes in feedstuffs. Vet Hum Toxicol. 1986, 28: 3, 207-212.

Garg DN; Manchanda VP; Chandiramani NK. Etiology of postnatal foal mortality. Indian J Comparative Microbiology, Immunology Infectious Diseases. 1985, 6: 1, 29-35.

Garg DN; Manchanda VP. Prevalence and aetiology of equine abortion. Indian J An Sci. 1986, 56: 7, 730-735.

Garrett LW; Heimann ED; Pfander WH; Wilson LL. Reproductive problems of pregnant mares grazing fescue pastures. J An Sci. 1980, 51: Suppl. 1, 237.

Gedek B; Bauer J; Ueno Y (ed.). Trichothecene problems in the Federal Republic of Germany. Trichothecenes. Chemical, biological toxicological-aspects. 1983, 301-307.

Gehlen H; Stadler P; Zentek J; Deegen E. Ulcerative stomatitis in a horse. Tierarztliche Praxis. Ausgabe-G,-Grosstiere-Nutztiere. 1999, 27: 5, 256-257,285-287.

Geisel O. Aspergillosis in animals, a brief review. Tierarztliche-Umschau. 1982, 37: 6, 403-404, 406-7.

Gerber H; Hockenjos P; Lazary S; Kings M; De Weck A. Histamine release from equine leucocytes provoked by fungal allergens. Deutsche-Tierarztliche-Wochenschrift. 1982, 89: 7, 267-270.

Goel S; Schumacher J; Lenz SD; Kemppainen BW. Effects of *Fusarium moniliforme* isolates on tissue and serum sphingolipid concentrations in horses. Vet Hum Toxicol. 1996, 38: 4, 265-270.

Gonzalez C-HE; Ruiz M-A. Phycomycotic granuloma in horses: aetiology and pathogenesis. Revista Instituto Colombiano Agropecuario. 1975, publ. 1976, 10: 2, 175-185.

Grabner A. Diagnosis and treatment of guttural pouch mycoses in the horse. Tierarztliche Praxis. 1987, Suppl. 2, 10-14.

Grahn B; Wolfer J; Keller C; Wilcock B. Equine keratomycosis: clinical and laboratory findings in 23 cases. Progress Vet Comparative Ophthalmology. 1993, 3: 1, 2-7.

Green P; Rose HR. Suspected gangrenous ergotism in a wild roe deer (Capreolus capreolous). Deer, J Br Deer Soc. 1995, 9: 8, 512-513.

Green EM; Loch WE; Messer NT; Blake-Caddel L. Maternal and fetal effects of endophyte fungus-infected fescue. Proceedings of the Thirty-Seventh Annual Convention of the American Association of Equine Practitioners, San Francisco, California, December 1-4, 1991. 1992, 29-44.

Green SL; Spencer CP; Wells M; Sausville D. Radiographic diagnosis. Vet Radiology. 1989, 30:4, 181-3.

Green EM; Loch WE; Messer NT; Blake-Caddel L. Maternal and fetal effects of endophyte fungus-infected fescue. Proceedings of the Thirty-Seventh Annual

Convention of the American Association of Equine Practitioners, San Francisco, California, December 1-4, 1991. 1992, 29-44.

Greet TRC. Nasal aspergillosis in three horses. Vet Rec. 1981, 109: 22, 487-489.

Gresti A De; Barone P; Perniola N. A case of guttural pouch mycosis caused by *Aspergillus ochraceus*: diagnosis and therapy. Ippologia. 1993, 4: 3, 81-86.

Guerre P; Bailly JD; Le Bars J; Raymond I; Burgat V. Fumonisin poisoning in horses. 23rd day of equine research, Institut du Cheval, Paris, France, 26 February 1997. 1997, 43-52.

Guillot J; Collobert C; Gueho E; Mialot M; Lagarde E. *Emericella nidulans* as an agent of guttural pouch mycosis in a horse. J Med Vet Mycology. 1997, 35: 6, 433-435.

Guillot J; Ribot X; Cadore JL; Bornert G. Aspergillosis in the guttural pouch of horses. Bulletin Mensuel Societe Veterinaire Pratique France. 1996, 80: 4, 141-162.

Ha TY; Cho CJ; Bak-UB; Kim SJ. Two cases of guttural pouch mycosis in racehorses caused by *Aspergillus nidulans*. Korean J Vet Clin Med. 1995, 12: 1, 65-72.

Hacking A; Harrison J; Jarvis B; Skinner FA (ed.); Carr JG (ed.). Microbiology in agriculture, fisheries and food. Society for Applied Bacteriology Symposium Series. 1976.

Hagler WM; Behlow RF. Salivary syndrome in horses: identification of slaframine in red clover hay. Appl Environmental Microbiology. 1981, 42: 6, 1067-1073.

Halliwell REW; Fleischman JB; Mackay-Smith M; Beech J; Gunson DE. The role of allergy in chronic pulmonary disease of horses. J Am Vet Med Assoc. 1979, 174: 3, 277-281.

Halliwell REW; McGorum BC; Irving P; Dixon PM. Local and systemic antibody production in horses affected with chronic obstructive pulmonary disease. Vet Immunol Immunopath. 1993, 38: 3-4, 201-215.

Hamilton HL; McLaughlin SA; Whitley EM; Gilger BC; Whitley RD. Histological findings in corneal stromal abscesses of 11 horses: correlation with cultures and cytology. Eq Vet J. 1994, 26: 6, 448-453.

Harbers LH; McNally LK; Smith WH. Digestibility of three grass hays by the horse and scanning electron microscopy of undigested leaf remnants. J An Sci. 1981, 53: 6, 1671-1677.

Hatziolos BC; Sass B; Albert TF; Stevenson MC. Blindness in a horse probably caused by gutturomycosis. Zentralblatt-fur-Veterinarmedizin. 1975, 22B: 5, 362-371.

Hatziolos BC; Sass B; Albert TF; Stevenson MC. Ocular changes in a horse with gutturomycosis. J Am Vet Med Assoc. 1975, 167: No.1, 51-54.

Hilbert BJ; Huxtable CR; Brighton AJ. Erosion of the internal carotid artery and cranial nerve damage caused by guttural pouch mycosis in a horse. Australian Vet J. 1981, 57: 7, 346-347.

Hintz HF. Tall fescue pasture for horses. Eq Practice. 1987, 9: 2, 5-6.

Hintz HF. Ergotism. Eq Practice. 1988, 10: 5, 6-7.

Hintz HF. Molds, mycotoxins, and mycotoxicosis. Vet Clinics No Am, Eq Practice. 1990, 6: 2, 419-431.

Hirooka EY; Viotti NMA; Marochi MA; Ishii K; Veno Y. Equine leukoencephalomalacia in North Parana. Revista de Microbiologia. 1990, 21: 3, 223-227.

Hodgson DR; Jacobs KA. Two cases of fusarium keratomycosis in the horse. Vet Rec 1982, 110: 22, 520-522.

Hunt WF. Research on foal growth under various pasture conditions. Proceedings of the Annual Seminar of the Equine Branch of the NZVA, Hamilton, May 1997. Pub Vet Cont Ed, Massey University. 1997, No. 174, 27-35.

Ikede BO (ed.). Tropical Veterinarian, volume 1, number 1 (August 1983). 1983, 60pp.; ISSN 0253-4851.

Jackson SG; Pagan JD; Dyke TM. Nutrition and productivity: Practical problems related to nutrition. Equine neurology and nutrition. Proceedings of Eighteenth Bain-Fallon Memorial Lectures, Stamford Grand Hotel, Glenelg, South Australia, Australia 22nd-26th July 1996. 1996, 131-148.

Jacobs KA; Fretz PB. Fistula between the guttural pouches and the dorsal pharyngeal recess as a sequela to guttural pouch mycosis in the horse. Canadian Vet J. 1982, 23: 4, 117-118.

Jarnagin JL; Thoen CO. Isolation of *Dermatophilus congolensis* and certain mycotic agents from animal tissues: a laboratory summary. Am J Vet Res. 1977, 38: 11, 1909-1911.

Johnson JH; Attleberger M. A case of guttural pouch mycosis caused by *Aspergillus nidulans*. Vet Med Sm An Clinician. 1973, 68: No.7, 771-774.

Johnson JH; Merriam JG; Attleburger M. A case of guttural pouch mycosis caused by *Aspergillus nidulans*. Vet Med Sm An Clinician. 1973, 68: 7, 771-774.

Johnson PJ; Moore LA; Mrad DR; Turk JR; Wilson DA. Sudden death of two horses associated with pulmonary aspergillosis. Vet Rec. 1999, 145: 1, 16-20.

Kamphues J. Risks through poor hygiene quality in feeds for horses. Nutrition and nutritional related disorders in the foal. Proceedings of the 2nd European conference on horse nutrition, Celle, Germany, 16-17 May 1996. Pferdeheilkunde. 1996, 12: 3, 326-332.

Kanemitsu H; Goryo M; Okada K. Two cases of equine mycotic epistaxis. J Japan Vet Med Assoc. 1995, 48: 8, 547-550.

Kellerman TS; Marasas WFO; Thiel PG; Gelderblom WCA; Cawood M; Coetzer JAW. Leukoencephalomalacia in two horses induced by oral dosing of fumonisin B_1. Onderstepoort J Vet Res. 1990, 57: 4, 269-275.

Keratomycosis in the horse. Eq Practice. 1979, 1: 5, 32-37.

Kern TJ; Brooks DE; White MM. Equine keratomycosis: current concepts of diagnosis and therapy. Eq Vet J. 1983, Suppl. 2, 33-38.

Khan ZU; Misra VC; Randhawa HS. Precipitating antibodies against *Micropolyspora faeni* in equines in north western India. Antonie van Leeuwenhoek. 1985, 51: 3, 313-319.

Khmelevskii BN; Pilipets ZI; Malinovskaya LS; Kostin VV; Komarnitskaya NP; Ivanov VG. Prophylaxis of mycotoxicoses in animals. 1985, p. 271.

Khmelevskii BN; Pilipets ZI; Malinovskaya LS; Kostin VV; Komarnitskaya NP; Ivanov VG. Prophylaxis of mycotoxicoses in animals. 1985. Agropromizdat; Moscow; USSR.

Krogh HV; Lundegaard HC. A case of guttural pouch mycosis in a horse. Nordisk Veterinaermedicin. 1986, 38: 2, 85-89.

Laurent D; Pellegrin F; Kohler F; Costa R; Thevenon J; Demersemen P; Guillaumel J; Platzer N. Is fumonisin B responsible for equine leucoencephalomalacia? Toxicon-Oxford. 1992, 30: 5-6, 530; Abstracts of plenary lectures, slide and poster presentations at the tenth World Congress on Animal, Plant and Microbial Toxins, Singapore, 3-8 November, 1991.

Laurent D; Pellegrin F; Kohler F; Costa R; Thevenon J; Lambert C; Huerre M. Fumonisin B$_1$ in equine leucoencephalomalacia pathogenesis. Microbiologie, Aliments, Nutrition. 1989, 7: 3, 285-291.

Lawson GHK; McPherson EA; Murphy JR; Nicholson JM; Wooding P; Breeze RG; Pirie HM. The presence of precipitating antibodies in the sera of horses with chronic obstructive pulmonary disease (COPD). Eq Vet J. 1979, 11: 3, 172-176.

Leslie JF; Doe FJ; Plattner RD; Shackelford DD; Jonz J. Fumonisin B$_1$ production and vegetative compatibility of strains from *Gibberella fujikuroi* mating population 'A' (*Fusarium moniliforme*). Mycopathologia. 1992, 117: 1-2, 37-45.

Ley WB. Management of the foaling mare: prefoaling considerations. Vet Med. 1994, 89: 6, 559-569.

Lhafi A. Poisoning of equids by *Stachybotrys atra* in Morocco. Bulletin Office International des Epizooties. 1991, 103: 12, 912-915; Fr version on pages 897-900.

Lim CW; Rim BM. The current status of fumonisin toxicosis in domestic animals. A review. Korean J Vet Res. 1995, 35: 2, 405-416.

Lindley WH. Ergot toxicosis. Modern Vet Practice. 1978, 59: 6, 463-464.

Lingard DR; Gosser HS; Monfort TN. Acute epistaxis associated with guttural pouch mycosis in two horses. J Am Vet Med Assoc. 1974, 164: 10, 1038-1040.

Loistl A. Intradermal allergen testing of horses with chronic obstructive bronchitis. 1996, p. 144.

Madelin TM; Clarke AF; Mair TS. Prevalence of serum precipitating antibodies in horses to fungal and thermophilic actinomycete antigens: effects of environmental challenge. Eq Vet J. 1991, 23: 4, 247-252.

Mallmann CA; Santurio JM; Dilkin P. Equine leukoencephalomalacia associated with ingestion of corn contaminated with fumonisin B$_1$. Revista-de-Microbiologia. 1999, 30: 3, 249-252.

Maragos CM. Capillary zone electrophoresis and HPLC for the analysis of fluorescein isothiocyanate-labeled fumonisin B$_1$. J Ag Food Chem. 1995, 43: 2, 390-394.

Marasas WFO; Wyllie TD (ed.); Morehouse LG (ed.). Lupinosis. [I] In cattle. [II] In horse. [III] In sheep. [IV] In swine. [V] In laboratory animals and dogs. Mycotoxic fungi, mycotoxins, mycotoxicoses. Volume 2. 1978, 161-163, 186187, 213-217, 275-277, 484-487.

Marasas WFO; Kellerman TS; Gelderblom WCA; Coetzer JAW; Thiel PG; Van Der Lugt JJ. Leukoencephalomalacia in a horse induced by fumonisin B$_1$ isolated from *Fusarium moniliforme*. Onderstepoort J Vet Res. 1988, 55: 4, 197-203.

Marolt J; Naglic T; Hajsig D. *Aspergillus oryzae* as the causal agent of keratomycosis in a horse. Tierarztliche-Praxis. 1984, 12: 4, 489-492.

Matsuda Y; Nakanishi Y; Mizuno Y. Occlusion of the internal carotid artery by means of microcoils for preventing epistaxis caused by guttural pouch mycosis in horses. J Vet Med Sci. 1999, 61: 3, 221-225.

McCann JS; Heusner GL; Amos HE; Thompson Jr DL. Growth rate, diet digestibility, and serum prolactin of yearling horses fed non-infected and infected tall fescue hay. J Eq Vet Sci. 1992, 12: 4, 240-243.

McCann JS. Ramifications of endophyte infected tall fescue in horse production systems. Proceedings 1990, Georgia Nutrition Conference for the Feed Industry, Atlanta Airport Hilton, Atlanta, Georgia, November 13-15. 1990, 84-91.

McCluskey B; Traub-Dargatz J; Garber L; Ross F. Survey of endophyte infection and its associated toxin in pastures grazed by horses. Proceedings of the 45th Annual Convention of the American Association of Equine Practitioners, Albuquerque, New Mexico, 5 8 December-1999. 1999, No., 213-216.

McDonald GK. Moldy sweetclover poisoning in a horse. Canadian-Veterinary-Journal. 1980, 21: 9, 250-251.

McGorum BC; Dixon PM; Halliwell REW. Responses of horses affected with chronic obstructive pulmonary disease to inhalation challenges with mould antigens. Eq Vet J. 1993, 25: 4, 261-267.

McGorum B. Differential diagnosis of chronic coughing in the horse. Vet Rec Editorial Espanol. 1994, 7: 2, 88-90, 92-93; first published in En in In Practice (1994) 16 (3) 55-60.

McGorum BC; Dixon PM; Halliwell REW. Evaluation of intradermal mould antigen testing in the diagnosis of equine chronic obstructive pulmonary disease. Eq Vet J. 1993, 25: 4, 273-275.

McKenzie RA; Mallett K (ed.); Grgurinovic C. Mycoses and macrofungal poisonings of domestic and native animals. Fungi of Australia. Volume 1B. Introduction fungi in the environment. 1996, 213-223.

McLaughlin SA; Brightman AH; Helper LC; Manning JP; Tomes JE. Pathogenic bacteria and fungi associated with extraocular disease in the horse. J Am Vet Med Assoc. 1983, 182: 3, 241-242.

McLaughlin BG; O' Brien JL. Guttural pouch mycosis and mycotic encephalitis in a horse. Canadian Vet J. 1986, 27: 3, 109-111.

McNally LK; Harbers LH; Smith WH. Nutritive value of three Kansas hays for the mature horse. Transactions of the Kansas Academy of Science. 1980, 83: 1, 36-43.

McPherson EA; Lawson GHK; Murphy JR; Nicholson JM; Breeze RG; Pirie HM. Chronic obstructive pulmonary disease (COPD) in horses: aetiological studies: responses to intradermal and inhalation antigenic challenge. Eq Vet J. 1979, 11: 3, 159-166.

McPherson EA; Lawson GHK; Murphy JR; Nicholson JM; Breeze RG; Pirie HM. Chronic obstructive pulmonary disease (COPD): factors influencing the occurrence. Eq Vet J. 1979, 11: 3, 167-171.

McPherson EA; Lawson GHK; Murphy JR; Nicholson JM; Breeze RG; Pirie HM. Chronic obstructive pulmonary disease (COPD) in horses: aetiological studies: responses to intradermal and inhalation antigenic challenge. Eq Vet J. 1979, 11: 3, 159-166.

Meacham VB; Meacham TN; Fontenot JP. Seasonal differences in apparent digestibility of fescue pasture by horses. Animal Science Research Report, Virginia Agricultural Experiment Station. undated, No. 5, 131-133.

Menchaca ES; Moras EV; Pelliza R; Barboni de Stella AM. Infectious diseases of Thoroughbreds. II. Infertility in mares due to *Candida albicans*, *Aspergillus fumigatus* and *Rhizopus equi*. Revista Militar Veterinaria. 1981, 27: 127-128, 117-118, 120-121.

Menchaca ES; Moras EV; Barboni de Stella AM; Palacios-Bacque H. Infectious diseases of Thoroughbreds. I. Genital infections causing infertility. Revista Militar Veterinaria. 1981, 27: 127-128, 109-112, 114-115.

Meyer H; Heckotter E; Merkt M; Bernoth EM; Kienzle E; Kamphues J. Current problems in veterinary advice on feeding. 6. Adverse effects of feeds in horses. Deutsche Tierarztliche Wochenschrift. 1986, 93: 10, 486-490.

Miles CO; Lane GA; Di Menna ME; Garthwaite I; Piper EL; Ball OJP; Latch GCM; Allen JM; Hunt MB; Bush LP; Fletcher I; Harris PS; Min-FK. High levels of ergonovine and lysergic acid amide in toxic *Achnatherum inebrians* accompany infection by an *Acremonium*-like endophytic fungus. J Ag Food Chem. 1996, 44: 5, 1285-1290.

Mirocha CJ; Abbas HK; Vesonder RF. Absence of trichothecenes in toxigenic isolates of *Fusarium moniliforme*. Applied Environmental Microbiology. 1990, 56: 2, 520-525.

Mitchell JS; Attleburger MH. Fusarium keratomycosis in the horse. Vet Med Sm An Clinician. 1973, 68: 1, 1257-1260.

Monga DP; Tiwari SC; Prasad S. Mycotic abortions in equines. Mykosen. 1983, 26: 12, 612-614.

Monroe JL; Cross DL; Hudson LW; Hendricks DM; Kennedy SW; Bridges Jr. WC. Effect of selenium and endophyte-contaminated fescue on performance and reproduction in mares. J Eq Vet Sci. 1988, 8: 2, 148-153.

Moore CP; Fales WH; Whittington P; Bauer L. Bacterial and fungal isolates from Equidae with ulcerative keratitis. J Am Vet Med Association. 1983, 182: 6, 600-603.

Morgan SE. Feeds, forages, and toxic plants. Eq Practice. 1996, 18: 1, 8-12.

Munday BL; Monkhouse IM; Gallagher RT. Intoxication of horses by lolitrem B in ryegrass seed cleanings. Australian Vet J. 1985, 62: 6, 207.

Murphy JR; McPherson EA; Lawson GHK. The effects of sodium cromoglycate on antigen inhalation challenge in two horses affected with chronic obstructive pulmonary disease (COPD). Vet Immunol Immunopath. 1979, 1: 1, 89-95.

Nation PN. Hepatic disease in Alberta horses: a retrospective study of "alsike clover poisoning" (1973-1988). Canadian Vet J. 1991, 32: 10, 602-607.

Nation PN. Alsike clover poisoning: a review. Canadian Vet J. 1989, 30: 5, 410-415.

Nelson GH; Christensen CM; Keyl AC; Ribelin WE; Garner GB; Connell CN; Mortimer PH; Di Menna ME; White EP; Marasas WFO; Kellerman TS; Kurmanov IA; Smalley EB; Scheel LD; Cysewski SJ; Mantle PG; Hintikka EL; Bridges CH; Armbrecht BH; Mortimer PH; Krogh P; Kurtz HJ; Mirocha CJ; Austwick PKC; Peckham JC; Joffe AZ; Carlton WW; Szczech GM; Sinnhuber RO; Wales JH; Wyllie TD (ed.); Morehouse LG (ed.). Mycotoxic fungi, mycotoxins, mycotoxicoses. An encyclopedic handbook. Volume 2. Mycotoxicoses of domestic and laboratory animals, poultry, and aquatic invertebrates and vertebrates. 1978.

Norred WP; Bacon CW; Porter JK; Voss KA. Inhibition of protein synthesis in rat primary hepatocytes by extracts of *Fusarium* moniliforme-contaminated corn. Food Chem Toxicol. 1990, 28: 2, 89-94.

Norred WP; Wang E; Yoo H; Riley RT; Merrill Jr. AH. In vitro toxicology of fumonisins and the mechanistic implications. Mycopathologia. 1992, 117: 1-2, 73-78.

Olesen J (ed.). Review of research and investigations in the agricultural economic associations 1971. Olesen, J. (Compiler)): Crop production work in the agricultural associations 1971.: Planteavlsarbejdet i landboforeningerne 1971. 1972, 1001-1154.

Ostergaard H. Photosensitization in horses. Alsike clover can cause photosensitization. Dansk Veterinaertidsskrift. 1992, 75: 2, 49.

Pace LW; Wirth NR; Foss RR; Fales WH. Endocarditis and pulmonary aspergillosis in a horse. J Vet Diagnostic Investigation. 1994, 6: 4, 504-506.

Pal M. Guttural pouch mycosis in a horse: the first reported case in India. Revista Iberoamericana Micologia. 1996, 13: 2, 31-32.

Palti J. Toxigenic fusaria, their distribution and significance as causes of disease in animal and man. 1978, 110pp.; Acta Phytomedica No.6.

Palyusik M. Mycotoxicoses. Wiener-Tierarztliche-Monatsschrift. 1977, 64: 8-9; 10, 211-220; 259-266.

Palyusik M. Equine leukoencephalomalacia (ELEM) - a disease caused by Fumonisin B₁ toxin. Review article. Magyar Allatorvosok Lapja. 1993, 48: 4, 206-207.

Park DL; Rua Jr. SM; Mirocha CJ; Abd-Alla EAM; Weng CY. Mutagenic potentials of fumonisin contaminated corn following ammonia decontamination procedure. Mycopathologia. 1992, 117: 1-2, 105-108.

Patten VH; Rebhun WC; Shin SJ; McDonough PL. Rapid laboratory diagnosis of mycotic keratitis in the horse. American Association of Veterinary Laboratory Diagnosticians: Abstracts 33rd Annual Meeting, Denver, Colorado, October 79, 1990. 1990, 15.

Pauli B; Gerber H; Schatzmann U. 'Farmer's lung' in the horse. Pathologia et Microbiologia. 1972, 38: No.3, 200-214.

Pearce SG; Grace ND; Firth EC; Wichtel JJ; Holle SA; Fennessy PF. Effect of copper supplementation on the copper status of pasture-fed young Thoroughbreds. Eq Vet J. 1998, 30: 3, 204-210.

Pearce SG; Grace ND; Wichtel JJ; Firth EC; Fennessy PF. Effect of copper supplementation on copper status of pregnant mares and foals. Eq Vet J. 1998, 30: 3, 200-203.

Peet RL; McDermott J; Williams JM; Maclean AA. Fungal myocarditis and nephritis in a horse. Australian Vet J. 1981, 57: 9, 439-440.

Pendergraft J; Arns MJ; Brazle FK. Tall fescue utilization by exercised yearling horses. J Eq Vet Sci. 1993, 13: 10, 548-552.

Pereira J; Do Valle LAC. Hosts of *Phomopsis phaseoli f.* sp. *meridionalis*, causal agent of soybean stem canker. Fitopatologia-Brasileira. 1997, 22: 4, 553-554.

Pereira AM; Tamarisho K; Macruz R; Salvadori MC. Aflatoxins in the feed of racehorses at the Sao Paulo Jockey Club. Atualidades Agroveterinarias. 1978, 6: 34, 6-8.

Pier AC; Newberne PM; Munro IC; Scott PM; Moodie CA; Willes RF; Wilson BJ; Harbison RD; Nelson GH; Christensen CM; Mirocha CJ; Smalley EB; Burfening PJ; Cysewski SJ; Wilson BJ; Maronpot RR; Hildebrandt PK; Carlton WW; Tuite J; Caldwell R; Richard JL; Lillehoj EB; Wessel JR; Stoloff L; Crump MH; Anon. Mycotoxicoses of domestic animals. J Am Vet Med Assoc. 1973, 163: 11, 1259-1302.

Placinta CM; D' Mello JPF; Macdonald AMC. A review of worldwide contamination of cereal grains and animal feed with Fusarium mycotoxins. An Feed Sci Technology. 1999, 78: 1-2, 21-37.

Plagemann O; Weber A; Singer H. *Aspergillus fumigatus* as the cause of abortion in two Thoroughbred mares. Tierarztliche-Umschau. 1992, 47: 12, 881-882.

Plattner RD; Ross PF; Reagor J; Stedelin J; Rice LG. Analysis of corn and cultured corn for fumonisin B$_1$ by HPLC and GC/MS by four laboratories. J Vet Diagnostic Investigation. 1991, 3: 4, 357-358.

Poomvises P; Gesmankit P; Inpanbutr N; Angsuphakorn S; Tawasin A; Bourke JM (ed.); Ashelford PJ (ed.). Equine aflatoxicosis. [Abstract]. Fourth International Conference, Control of the use of drugs in racehorses, Melbourne, May 1981. Proceedings of the scientific sessions. 1982, 95-96.

Porter JK; Voss KA; Bacon CW; Norred WP. Effects of *Fusarium moniliforme* and corn associated with equine leukoencephalomalacia on rat neurotransmitters and metabolites. Proceedings Society Experimental Biology Medicine. 1990, 194: 3, 265-269.

Pugh DG; Bowen JM; Kloppe LH; Simpson RB. Fungal endometritis in mares. Compendium Continuing Education Practicing Veterinarian. 1986, 8: 4, S173S177, S180-S181.

Pugh DG; Schumacher J. Management of the broodmare. Proceedings of the 36th Annual Convention of the American Association of Equine Practitioners Lexington, Kentucky, December 2-5 1990. 1991, 61-78.

Putman MR; Bransby DI; Schumacher J; Boosinger TR; Bush L; Shelby RA; Vaughan JT; Ball D; Brendemuehl JP. Effects of the fungal endophyte *Acremonium coenophialum* in fescue on pregnant mares and foal viability. Am J Vet Res. 1991, 52: 12, 2071-2074.

Rade C; Koch W; Leibold W; Kamphues J; Kienzle E (ed.); Tennant B. Antibodies against moulds and mites in sera of young horses experimentally exposed to those agents via oral and inhalative challenge. Proceedings of the Conference of the European Society of Veterinary and Comparative Nutrition, Munich, Germany, 19-21 March 1997. Journal of Animal Physiology and Animal Nutrition. 1998, 80: 2-5, 239-245.

Ragheb RR; Maysa H; Shaker KH; Rawia KH; Ebrahim. Mycotoxicosis as a field problem in equine. Egyptian J Comp Path Clin Pathology. 1995, 8: 2, 39-57.

Ramachandran S. Equine respiratory disease: 2. Mycotic and helminthic causes. Centaur-Mylapore. 1995, 11: 4, 69-79.

Rawlinson RJ; Jones RT. Guttural pouch mycosis in two horses. Australian Vet J. 1978, 54: 3, 135-138.

Reddy DN; Nusrath M. Aflatoxin contamination in pulses from tribal areas of Medak district, Andhra Pradesh. Current Science, India. 1983, 52: 21, 1024.

Redmond LM; Cross DL; Strickland JR; Kennedy SW. Efficacy of domperidone and sulpiride as treatments for fescue toxicosis in horses. Am J Vet Res. 1994, 55: 5, 722-729.

Redmond LM; Cross DL; Jenkins TC; Kennedy SW. The effect of *Acremonium coenophialum* on intake and digestibility of tall fescue hay in horses. J Eq Vet Sci. 1991, 11: 4, 215-219.

Redmond LM; Cross DL; Gimenez T; Hudson LW; Earle WF; Kennedy SW. The effect of phenothiazine and withdrawal time on gravid mares grazing endophyte-infected tall fescue. J Eq Vet Sci. 1991, 11: 1, 17-22.

Redmond LM; Cross DL; Gimenez T; Hudson LW; Earle WF; Kennedy SW. The effect of phenothiazine and withdrawal time on gravid mares grazing endophyte-infected tall fescue. J Eq Vet Sci. 1991, 11: 1, 17-22.

Regius-Mocsenyi A. Zinc, manganese, copper, molybdenum, nickel and cadmium status of the cattle, sheep and horse. 5th paper: nickel status. Allattenyesztes-es-Takarmanyozas. 1991, 40: 2, 151-162.

Rice LG; Ross PF. Methods for detection and quantitation of fumonisins in corn, cereal products and animal excreta. J Food Protection. 1994, 57: 6, 536-540.

Riet-Correa F; Meirelles MA; Soares JM; Machado JJ; Zambrano AF. Leukoencephalomalacia in horses fed mouldy maize (*Fusarium moniliforme* mycotoxin). Pesquisa-Veterinaria-Brasileira. 1982, 2: 1, 27-30.

Riley RT; Wang E; Merrill Jr. AH. Liquid chromatographic determination of sphinganine and sphingosine: use of the free sphinganine-to-sphingosine ratio as a biomarker for consumption of fumonisins. J AOAC International. 1994, 77: 2, 533-540.

Riley RT; Showker JL; Owens DL; Ross PF. Disruption of sphingolipid metabolism and induction of equine leukoencephalomalacia by *Fusarium proliferatum* culture material containing fumonisin B_2 or B_3. Environmental Toxicology and Pharmacology. 1997, 3: 3, 221-228.

Roberge R; Ladenheim S; Mahood CFP; Lesser RW; Roberts RR; Slovis CM; Molavi A; Blumberg EA; Shepherd SM; Whye Jr. DPW; Werman HA; Kelen GD; Schillinger D (ed.); Harwood-Nuss A (ed.). Infections in Emergency Medicine. Vol. 1. 1989, Churchill Livingstone; New York; USA.

Robertson-Smith RG; Jeffcott LB; Friend SCE; Badcoe LM. An unusual incidence of neurological disease affecting horses during a drought. Australian Vet J. 1985, 62: 1, 6-12.

Robinson NE; Derksen FJ; Olszewski MA; Buechner-Madxwell VA. The pathogenesis of chronic obstructive pulmonary disease of horses. Br Vet J. 1996, 152: 3, 283-306.

Rohrbach BW; Green EM; Oliver JW; Schneider JF. Aggregate risk study of exposure to endophyte-infected (*Acremonium coenophialum*) tall fescue as a risk factor for laminitis in horses. Am J Vet Res. 1995, 56: 1, 22-26.

Rosiles MR; Garcia TM; Ross FP. Physico-chemical confirmation of fumonisin B_1 in maize and in feed for horses which had died of leukoencephalomalacia. Veterinaria-Mexico. 1996, 27: 1, 111-113.

Rosiles MR; Bautista J; Fuentes VO; Ross F. An outbreak of equine leukoencephalomalacia at Oaxaca, Mexico, associated with fumonisin B_1. J Vet Med. Series A. 1998, 45: 5, 299-302.

Ross PF; Rice LG; Osweiler GD; Nelson PE; Richard JL; Wilson TM. A review and update of animal toxicoses associated with fumonisin-contaminated feeds and production of fumonisins by *Fusarium* isolates. Mycopathologia. 1992, 117: 12, 109-114.

Ross PF; Ledet AE; Owens DL; Rice LG; Nelson HA; Osweiler GD; Wilson TM. Experimental equine leukoencephalomalacia, toxic hepatosis, and encephalopathy caused by corn naturally contaminated with fumonisins. J Vet Diag Investigation. 1993, 5: 1, 69-74.

Ross PF; Rice LG; Reagor JC; Osweiler GD; Wilson TM; Nelson HA; Owens DL; Plattner RD; Harlin KA; Richard JL; Colvin BM; Banton MI. Fumonisin B_1 concentrations in feeds from 45 confirmed equine leukoencephalomalacia cases. J Vet Diagnostic Investigation. 1991a, 3: 3, 238-241.

Ross PF; Nelson PE; Richard JL; Osweiler GD; Rice LG; Plattner RD; Wilson TM. Production of fumonisins by *Fusarium moniliforme* and *Fusarium proliferatum* isolates associated with equine leukoencephalomalacia and a pulmonary edema syndrome in swine. Applied Environmental Microbiology. 1990, 56: 10, 3225-3226.

Ross PF; Rice LG; Plattner RD; Osweiler GD; Wilson TM; Owens DL; Nelson HA; Richard JL. Concentrations of fumonisin B_1 in feeds associated with animal health problems. Mypathologia. 1991b, 114: 3, 129-135.

Ross PF. What are we going to do with this dead horse? J AOAC International. 1994, 77: 2, 491-494.

Ross PF; Nelson PE; Owens DL; Rice LG; Nelson HA; Wilson TM. Fumonisin B_2 in cultured *Fusarium proliferatum*, 6104, causes equine leukoencephalomalacia. J Vet Diagnostic Investigation. 1994, 6: 2, 263-265.

Ross PF; Rice LG; Wilson TM; Osweiler GD; Nelson HA; Plattner RD; Reagor JC; Harlin KA; Colvin BM; Banton MI. Fumonisin B_1 concentrations in feeds from 40 confirmed equine leukoencephalomalacia cases. American Association of Veterinary Laboratory Diagnosticians: Abstracts 33rd Annual Meeting, Denver, Colorado, October 7-9, 1990. 1990, 60.

Scherzer S; Nell B; Suchy A. Five cases of keratomycosis in the horse in Austria. Wiener Tierarztliche Monatsschrift. 1998, 85: 5, 154-162.

Schmallenbach KH; Rahman I; Sasse HHL; Dixon PM; Halliwell REW; McGorum BC; Crameri R; Miller HRP. Studies on pulmonary and systemic *Aspergillus fumigatus*-specific IgE and IgG antibodies in horses affected with chronic obstructive pulmonary disease (COPD). Vet Immunol Immunopath. 1998, 66: 3-4, 245-256.

Schumacher J; Mullen J; Shelby R; Lenz S; Ruffin DC; Kemppainen BW. An investigation of the role of *Fusarium moniliforme* in duodenitis/proximal jejunitis of horses. Vet Hum Toxicol. 1995, 37: 1, 39-45.

Schurg WA; Pulse RE; Holtan DW; Oldfield JE. Use of various quantities and forms of ryegrass straw in horse diets. J An Sci. 1978, 47: 6, 1287-1291.

Seahorn TL; Beadle RE. Summer pasture-associated obstructive pulmonary disease. Eq Practice. 1994, 16: 7, 39-41.

Shanks G; Tabak P; Begg AP; Bryden WL. An outbreak of acute leukoencephalomalacia associated with fumonisin intoxication in three horses. Australian Eq Vet. 1995, 13: 2, 17-18.

Slocombe RF; Slauson DO. Invasive pulmonary aspergillosis of horses: an association with acute enteritis. Vet Pathology. 1988, 25: 4, 277-281.

Smith DA; Maxie MG; Wilcock BP. Disseminated mycosis: a danger with systemic corticosteroid therapy. Canadian Vet J. 1981, 22: 9, 276.

Sockett DC; Baker JC; Stowe CM. Slaframine (*Rhizoctonia leguminicola*) intoxication in horses. J Am Vet Med Association. 1982, 181: 6, 606.

Stef Anon B; Volpelli LA; Bovolenta S; Pinosa M. Estimation of fescue hay intake in horses using the n-alkanes method. Zootecnica e Nutrizione Animale. 1999, 25: 6, 243-248.

Steiss JE; Brendemuehl JP; Wright JC; Storrs DP. Nerve conduction velocities and brain stem auditory evoked responses in normal neonatal foals, compared to foals exposed to endophyte-infected fescue in utero. Progress Vet Neurology. 1991, 2: 4, 252-260.

Step DL. Equine leukoencephalomalacia. Eq Practice. 1993, 15: 10, 24-30.

Sudaric F; Marzan B; Ozegovic L. Pathological changes in acute and chronic *Aspergillus* pneumonia of horses. Veterinaria, Yugoslavia. 1979, 28: 3, 383-396.

Swerczek TW; Kirkbride CA (ed.). Perinatal mortality in foals caused by fescue grass toxicosis. Laboratory diagnosis livestock abortion. 1990, Ed. 3, 214-216.

Sydenham EW; Shephard GS; Thiel PG. Liquid chromatographic determination of fumonisins B_1, B_2, and B_3 in foods and feeds. J AOAC International. 1992, 75: 2, 313-318.

Sydenham EW; Shephard GS; Thiel PG; Marasas WFO; Rheeder JP; Peralta-Sanhueza CE; Gonzalez HHL; Resnik SL. Fumonisins in Argentinian field-trial corn. J Ag Food Chem. 1993, 41: 6, 891-895.

Szigeti G; Erdos A; Krause B. Feeding of fusariotoxin (T_2 toxin) contaminated maize as a predisposing factor in pyosepticaemia of horses. Magyar-Allatorvosok-Lapja. 1977, 32: 4, 243-245.

Takatori K (et al.). Fungal flora of equine skin with or without dermatophytosis. J Japan Vet Med Assoc. 1981, 34: 12, 580-584.

Takatori K; Kamada M; Fukunaga Y; Kumanomido T; Hirasawa K; Nigishi M; Takada K; Oikawa M. *Emericella nidulans* isolated from horses with guttural pouch mycosis in Japan. Bulletin Eq Res Institute. 1984, No.21, 81-87.

Takatori K; Ichijo S; Konishi T; Tanaka I. Occurrence of equine dermatophytosis in Hokkaido. Japanese J Vet Sci. 1981, 43: 3, 307-313.

Taylor MC; Loch WE. Toxicity in pregnant pony mares grazing Kentucky-31 [fescue] pastures. J An Sci. 1983, 57: Suppl.1, 311.

Thiel PG; Marasas WFO; Sydenham EW; Shephard GS; Gelderblom WCA. The implications of naturally occurring levels of fumonisins in corn for human and animal health. Mycopathologia. 1992, 117: 1-2, 3-9.

Thiel PG; Shephard GS; Sydenham EW; Marasas WFO; Nelson PE; Wilson TM. Levels of fumonisins B_1 and B_2 in feeds associated with confirmed cases of equine leukoencephalomalacia. J Ag Food Chemistry. 1991, 39: 1, 109-111.

Thomson JR; McPherson EA; Lawson GHK; Wooding P; Brown R. A study of the possible role of chymotrypsin in the aetiology of equine chronic obstructive pulmonary disease (COPD). Vet Immunol Immunopath. 1983, 4: 3, 387-395.

Tietjen U. Occurrence, clinical course and treatment of diseases from mycotoxins in horses and poultry since 1981. 1989.

Traub JL; Potter KA; Bayly WM; Reed SM. Alsike clover poisoning [in a horse]. Modern Vet Practice. 1982, 63: 4, 307-309.

Tunev SS; Ehrhart EJ; Jensen HE; Foreman JH; Richter RA; Messick JB. Necrotizing mycotic vasculitis with cerebral infarction caused by *Aspergillus niger* in a horse with acute typhlocolitis. Vet Pathol. 1999, 36: 4, 347-351.

Uboh CE; Rudy JA; Railing FA; Enright JM; Shoemaker JM; Kahler MC; Shellenberger JM; Kemecsei Z; Das DN; Soma LR; Leonard JM. Postmortem tissue samples: an alternative to urine and blood for drug analysis in racehorses. J Analytical Toxicology. 1995, 19: 5, 307-315.

Uhlinger C. Leukoencephalomalacia. Veterinary Clinics of North America, Equine Practice. 1997, 13: 1, 13-20.

Uppal PK; Yadav MP. Equine respiratory diseases and their diagnosis. Centaur. 1987, 4: 2, 67-72.

Valdez H; Peyton LC. Idiopathic thrombocytopenia associated with hematoma of the maxillary sinus. J Eq Med Surg. 1978, 2: 9, 379-383.

Van Essen GJ; Blom M; Gremmels-Gehrmann JF. Ryegrass staggers in horses. Tijdschrift voor Diergeneeskunde. 1995, 120: 24, 710-711.

Van Nieuwstadt RA; Kalsbeek HC. Guttural pouch mycosis in a horse: local treatment with enilconazole administered through a permanent cannula. Tijdschrift voor Diergeneeskunde. 1994, 119: 1, 3-5.

Van Oldruitenborgh-Oosterbaan MMS; Schipper FCM; Goehring LS; Gremmels JF. Pleasure horses with neurological signs: EHV1 infection or mycotoxin intoxication? Tijdschrift-voor-Diergeneeskunde. 1999, 124: 22, 679-681.

Varner DD; Blanchard TL; Brinsko SP. Estrogens, oxytocin and ergot alkaloids - uses in reproductive management of mares. Proceedings Annual Convention American Association Equine Practitioners. 1989, 34: 219-241.

Verma R; Gupta BR. Isolation of monomorphic fungi from reproductive tract of mares. Indian J Comparative Microbiology, Immunology Infectious

Diseases. 1983, 4: 3, 169-170.

Vesonder R; Haliburton J; Stubblefield R; Gilmore W; Peterson S. *Aspergillus flavus* and aflatoxins B$_1$, B$_2$, and M$_1$ in corn associated with equine death. Archives Environmental Contamination Toxicology. 1991, 20: 1, 151-153.

Vesonder R; Haliburton J; Golinski P. Toxicity of field samples and *Fusarium moniliforme* from feed associated with equine-leucoencephalomalacia. Archives Environmental Contamination Toxicology. 1989, 18: 3, 439-442.

Villahoz MD; Moras EV; Barboni AM; Scharf V; Mechaca ES; De Guglielmone R. Reproductive problems in pregnant mares grazing fescue pasture in Argentina. Proceedings 10th International Congress on Animal Reproduction Artificial Insemination, Urbana Champaign, 10-14 June 1984. 1984, II: 100.

Vissiennon T; Hennig T; Bergmann A; Wernery U (ed.); Wade JF (ed.); Mumford JA (ed.); Kaaden OR. Mycoallergens in stable bedding: their incidence and importance to respiratory diseases. Equine infectious diseases VIII: Proceedings of the Eighth International Conference, Dubai, 23rd-26th March 1998. 1999, 71-75.

Wagner PC; Miller RA; Gallina AM; Grant BD. Mycotic encephalitis associated with a guttural pouch mycosis. J Eq Med Surgery. 1978, 2: 7-8, 355-359.

Weiler H; Staib F; Keller H; Stacker W. Guttural pouch mycosis in horses. A contribution to its pathology and aetiology. Pferdeheilkunde. 1991, 7: 3, 179-181, 183-187.

Weiler H; Zapf F; Hummel PH. Invasive pneumomycosis in a horse. Contribution to the pathological picture and serological diagnosis. Pferdeheilkunde. 1994, 10: 3, 177-184.

Whitwell KE; Powell DG. Infective placentitis in the mare. Equine infectious diseases V. Proceedings of the fifth International Conference, Lexington, Kentucky, USA, October 7-10, 1987. 1988, 172-180.

Wichtel JJ; Whitacre MD; Yates DJ; Van Camp SD. Comparison of the effects of PGF2alpha and bromocryptine in pregnant beagle bitches. Theriogenology. 1990, 33: 4, 829-836.

Wilson TM; Ross PF; Nelson PE. Fumonisin mycotoxins and equine leukoencephalomalacia. J Am Vet Med Assoc. 1991, 198: 7, 1104-1105.

Wilson TM; Ross PF; Rice LG; Osweiler GD; Nelson HA; Owens DL; Plattner RD; Reggiardo C; Noon TH; Pickrell JW. Fumonisin B$_1$ levels associated with an epizootic of equine leukoencephalomalacia. J Vet Diagnostic Inestigation. 1990a, 2: 3, 213-216.

Wilson TM; Ross PF; Owens DL; Rice LG; Green SA; Jenkins SJ; Nelson HA. Experimental reproduction of ELEM. A study to determine the minimum toxic dose in ponies. Mycopathologia. 1992, 117: 1-2, 115-120.

Wilson TM; Ledet AE; Owens DL; Rice LG; Nelson HA; Ostweiller GD; Ross PF. Experimental liver disease in ponies associated with the ingestion of a corn-based ration naturally contaminated with fumonisin B_1. American Association of Veterinary Laboratory Diagnosticians: Abstracts 33rd Annual Meeting, Denver, Colorado, October 7-9, 1990. 1990b, 61.

Wilson TM; Nelson PE; Marasas WFO; Thiel PG; Shephard GS; Sydenham EW; Nelson HA; Ross PF. A mycological evaluation and in vivo toxicity evaluation of feed from 41 farms with equine leukoencephalomalacia. J Vet Diagnostic-Investigation. 1990c, 2: 4, 352-354.

Wisniewska-Dmytrow H; Kozak A; Zmudzki J. Fumonisins - biochemical and biological characteristics. Medycyna-Weterynaryjna. 1996, 52: 3, 159-162.

Worthington WE; Chick EW (ed.); Balows A (ed.); Furcolow ML (ed.). Opportunistic fungus infections of horses. Opportunistic fungal infections. Proceedings of the Second International Conference. 1975, 287-292.

Xie YF; Wang ZX; Qin S; Li ZS; Liu XY; Liu BF; Wang QA; Zhao ZX; Song ZZ. Abortion in horses caused by aflatoxins. Acta Vet Zootechnica-Sinica. 1991, 22: 2, 145-149.

Yoshihara T; Katayama Y; Kuwano A; Nakajima H (ed.); Plowright W. The pathological observations of guttural pouch mycosis of horses. Equine infectious diseases VII: Proceedings of the Seventh International Conference, Tokyo, Japan 8th11th June 1994. 1994, 357-358.

Zientara S. Hepatic encephalopathy in mares in western France. Bulletin des GTV. 1993, No. 3, 77-84.

FEEDING FAT TO MANAGE MUSCLE DISORDERS

STEPHANIE VALBERG AND ERICA MCKENZIE
University of Minnesota, St. Paul, Minnesota

Excerpted from: McKenzie, E.M., S.J. Valberg, and J. Pagan. Nutritional
management of exertional rhabdomyolysis. In: E. Robinson (Ed.) Current Therapy
in Equine Medicine 5.

Exertional rhabdomyolysis has been recognized in horses for more than 100 years
as a syndrome of muscle pain and cramping associated with exercise. In the last
ten to twelve years, research advances have provided greater insight into this
syndrome. Of greatest importance is the realization that exertional rhabdomyolysis
comprises several myopathies that, despite similarities in clinical presentation,
differ considerably in regards to pathogenesis (cellular events, reactions, and other
pathologic mechanisms occurring in the development of disease).

Tying-up is a common disorder in Thoroughbred racehorses. During the 1995
racing season, 1000 Thoroughbreds at Canterbury Park were evaluated. Five percent
of the horses exhibited signs of tying-up during the season. Of the two- and three-
year-old horses that presented with tying-up, 15% could not be raced at all that
season. Interestingly, if the horses that experienced tying-up could race, there was
no difference between their performances and those of matched control horses.

Exertional rhabdomyolysis continues to be a performance-limiting or career-
ending disorder for many equine athletes. Advances in the management of horses
with exertional rhabdomyolysis, particularly in the way they are fed, have
significantly reduced the impact of the disorder.

Clinical Signs of Rhabdomyolysis and Differential Diagnoses

Clinical signs of exertional rhabdomyolysis usually occur shortly after the beginning
of exercise. The most common sign is firm and painful muscles over the lumbar
(loin) and sacral (croup) regions of the topline, including the large gluteal muscles.
Excessive sweating, tachypnea (quick, shallow breathing), tachycardia (rapid
heartbeat), and muscle fasciculations are also noticed. In extreme cases, horses
may be reluctant or refuse to move and may produce discolored urine due to the
release of myoglobin from damaged muscle tissue. Episodes of ER vary from
subclinical to severe in which massive muscle necrosis and renal failure from
myoglobinuria occurs.

In order for exertional rhabdomyolysis to be confirmed, serum creatine kinase
(CK) and aspartate transaminase (AST) activity must be elevated during periods
of muscle stiffness. When muscle cells are damaged, CK and AST are released

into the bloodstream within hours. AST activity may be heightened in asymptomatic horses with chronic exertional rhabdomyolysis. If CK and AST values are not above normal, differential diagnoses should be considered for horses that are reluctant to move, recumbent, or producing off-colored urine. Such diagnoses include lameness, colic, laminitis, pleuropneumonia, tetanus, aorto-iliac thrombosis, intravascular hemolysis, bilirubinuria, or neurological disease. Causes of non-exercise-associated myopathies include infectious and immune-mediated myopathies (influenza, *Clostridium* sp., *Streptococcus* sp., *Sarcocystis* sp.); nutritional myodegeneration; traumatic or compressive myopathy; idiopathic pasture myopathy; and toxic muscle damage from the ingestion of monensin, white snake root, or vitamin D-stimulating plants.

Etiology and Pathophysiology of Exertional Rhabdomyolysis

Exertional rhabdomyolysis can be subdivided into one of two distinct forms–sporadic and chronic. Horses that experience a single episode or infrequent episodes of muscle necrosis with exercise are categorized as having sporadic exertional rhabdomyolysis, whereas horses that have repeated episodes of exertional rhabdomyolysis accompanied by increased muscle enzyme activity, even with mild exertion, are classified as having chronic exertional rhabdomyolysis.

Sporadic Exertional Rhabdomyolysis

Sporadic exertional rhabdomyolysis occurs most commonly in horses that are exercised in excess of their level of conditioning. This happens frequently when a training program is accelerated too abruptly, particularly after an idle period of a few days, weeks, or months. Endurance competitions held on hot, humid days may elicit sporadic exertional rhabdomyolysis in susceptible horses because of high body temperatures, loss of fluid and electrolytes in sweat, and depletion of muscle energy stores. These metabolic imbalances can lead to muscle dysfunction and damage. In some instances, horses seem more prone to exertional rhabdomyolysis following respiratory infections. Therefore, horses should not be exercised if they have a fever, cough, nasal discharge, or other signs of respiratory compromise.

Chronic Exertional Rhabdomyolysis

Chronic exertional rhabdomyolysis arises frequently from heritable myopathies such as polysaccharide storage myopathy (PSSM) or recurrent exertional rhabdomyolysis (RER). Other causes of chronic exertional rhabdomyolysis are probable; however, their etiopathologies remain unknown.

Polysaccharide storage myopathy affects primarily Quarter Horses and horses with Quarter Horse bloodlines such as Paints and Appaloosas. In addition, warmbloods and Morgans have been diagnosed with this disorder. PSSM is a glycogen storage disorder characterized by the accumulation of glycogen and abnormal polysaccharide complexes in 1-40% of skeletal muscle fibers. Muscle glycogen concentrations in affected horses are 1.5 to 4 times greater than in normal horses. Horses with PSSM typically have calm dispositions and are in good body condition. A change in exercise routine often triggers an episode of rhabdomyolysis. This change need not be profound; something as subtle and seemingly harmless as unaccustomed stall confinement may provoke an episode. Signs of PSSM include sweating, stretching out as if posturing to urinate, muscle fasciculations, and rolling or pawing following exercise. Severe cases may display stiffness and hesitance to move within minutes of starting exercise, and extreme cases may result in the horse being unable to stand and in discomfort even when lying down. Serum creatine kinase (CK) activity may be persistently elevated despite an extended period of rest.

A similar glycogen storage disorder has been reported in draft breeds. This syndrome is referred to as equine polysaccharide storage myopathy (EPSM). While similarities exist between PSSM and EPSM, draft horses with EPSM often exhibit signs not indicative of PSSM, including normal serum creatine kinase, difficulty backing and holding up limbs, a shivers-like gait, and loss of muscle mass. Some drafts afflicted with EPSM also show recumbency and weakness with only slight increases in serum CK and AST, and this combination of signs is not seen in horses with PSSM.

Recurrent exertional rhabdomyolysis commonly afflicts Thoroughbreds and likely Standardbreds and Arabians. In Thoroughbreds, RER has been identified as a heritable defect in intracellular calcium regulation leading to excessive muscular contraction and necrosis with exercise. In one investigation of heritability, a farm had 18 horses tie-up repeatedly over three years. Fourteen of the broodmares on this farm were bred to a particular stallion; all of the offspring experienced tying-up. When the same mares were bred to another stallion, only two of the offspring tied-up. On a different farm, one mare prone to tying-up produced six offspring with the disorder. At this juncture, a genetic connection is almost certain.

The most severely affected horses are nervous young (two-year-old) fillies in race training at tracks. The sex predilection for females, however, is not obvious in older horses with RER. Episodes of RER occur most often when horses are restrained during exercise, and incidences of RER may become more frequent as level of fitness increases. Clinical expression of RER is often stress-induced, and horses with RER are typically described as having nervous or very nervous temperaments. Older horses with RER may have muscle stiffness and soreness but only show overt evidence of tying-up after steeplechase or cross-country phases of a three-day event.

Diagnostic Approach to Chronic Exertional Rhabdomyolysis

A thorough and systematic diagnostic approach is recommended to help accurately establish and address possible causative factors for chronic exertional rhabdomyolysis. Muscle enzyme activity levels following light exercise (15 minutes of trotting on a longe line) may provide evidence for a diagnosis of subclinical rhabdomyolysis. In addition, horses experiencing intermittent episodes of rhabdomyolysis may also show abnormal elevations in CK after the same exercise test. The amount of exercise a horse tolerates without developing rhabdomyolysis can be used as a starting point for returning a horse to training.

Muscle biopsies are helpful in distinguishing PSSM from RER and in identifying other disorders that contribute to clinical signs of muscle stiffness. Biopsies taken on site are from the middle gluteal muscle using a modified Bergstrom biopsy needle and frozen immediately. Biopsies shipped by referring veterinarians are of the semimembranosus/tendinosis muscles performed by an open surgical technique. An experimental approach to identifying RER is to perform contracture tests on small intact pieces of muscle taken from between the ribs. The technique measures how the muscle responds to electrical stimulation (simulation of exercise) and to chemicals that are known to create cramps in human diseases similar to tying-up. Muscle from Thoroughbreds that tied-up reacted very differently compared to muscle from Thoroughbreds without the disorder in that it was much more sensitive to contractions induced by halothane, caffeine, and potassium. The contracture reaction indicated a possible problem with the way calcium is regulated inside the muscle cell.

Nutritional Management

Diet manipulation is becoming the method of choice in controlling exertional rhabdomyolysis, particularly in equine athletes that are closely monitored for pharmacological substances. A well-designed exercise program and a nutritionally balanced diet with appropriate caloric intake and adequate vitamins and minerals are the core elements of treating exertional rhabdomyolysis.

Vitamin E and selenium. Adequate amounts of vitamin E and selenium prevent the detrimental interaction of peroxides with lipid membranes of the muscle cell. Most horses with chronic rhabdomyolysis have adequate or more than adequate blood concentrations of vitamin E and selenium, and further supplementation has not been found to have protective effects on muscle integrity in exercising horses. Many feeds, particularly those designed for horses with rhabdomyolysis, provide adequate selenium supplementation and caution should be taken not to provide excessive selenium in the diet. Likewise, sufficient vitamin E is provided in most diets by green grasses, well-cured hay, and rice bran.

Electrolytes and minerals. Horses performing in hot weather often develop electrolyte imbalances. Free-choice access to loose salt or a salt block should be provided to these horses, or alternatively, one to four ounces of salt can be added to the feed daily. Extreme climatic conditions may necessitate the use of commercial electrolyte mixtures containing a 2:1:4 ratio of sodium:potassium:chloride. Fresh water should be available to horses at all times, especially if they are being supplemented with electrolytes.

Dietary imbalances of electrolytes, particularly deficiencies of sodium, potassium, and calcium, have been implicated in exertional rhabdomyolysis. Correction of imbalances may be crucial in the management of some exertional rhabdomyolysis cases.

Chromium. Supplementation with oral chromium (5 mg/day) has been reported to calm horses and improve their responses to exercise (e.g., lower peak concentrations of insulin, cortisol, and lactic acid). Chromium may assist glucose and glycogen metabolism, possibly by potentiating the action of insulin. The purported calming effect of chromium may be beneficial in horses with recurrent exertional rhabdomyolysis because it appears that stress is a critical precipitator of this disorder. Because PSSM horses display abnormal sensitivity to insulin, however, chromium supplementation may be counterproductive in these animals.

Effect of Modulation of Dietary Fat and Starch

Although PSSM and RER possess distinct etiologies, increasing dietary fat supplementation and decreasing dietary starch have resulted in beneficial effects to horses with both disorders. PSSM horses have enhanced insulin sensitivity, and reducing dietary starch as much as possible (by eliminating all grain) decreases the inevitable rise in glucose and insulin that occurs after consumption of concentrate feeds. With PSSM horses, even a slight amount of fat supplementation of a low to moderate caloric intake provides a favorable effect. In addition to diet alterations, improvement in clinical signs of muscle stiffness requires the addition of incrementally increasing amounts of daily exercise over one month.

While fat supplementation also helps horses with recurrent exertional rhabdomyolysis, the mechanism for this is not clearly understood. Unlike horses with PSSM, fat supplementation is only beneficial to RER horses when total dietary caloric intake is high. The beneficial effects of fat supplementation in RER horses may be due to the exclusion of dietary starch rather than specific protective effects of high dietary fat. Given the close relationship between nervousness and tying-up in horses with RER, assuaging anxiety and excitability by reducing dietary starch and increasing dietary fat may decrease predisposition to RER by making these horses calmer prior to exercise.

Fat Sources

Animal- and vegetable-based fats are the major sources of fat available for equine consumption. Examples of vegetable oils used for supplementation include corn, soy, peanut, coconut, safflower, linseed, flaxseed, and canola. Corn and soy oils are the most palatable. Vegetable oils are highly digestible (90-100%) and energy dense. While it can be messy to dole out, unpalatable to some horses, prone to rancidity in warm weather, and difficult to feed in large amounts, oil is an effective way to boost daily energy intake and may be the most economical way of providing fat to horses that do not require large amounts of supplementation. Horses receiving large amounts of oil may need vitamin E supplementation.

Animal fat varies in digestibility (75-90%). Because animal fat is more saturated, it tends to be solid at room temperature and would need to be melted before being top-dressed on feed. Most horses find animal-based fats less palatable than vegetable-based fats.

Rice bran contains about 20% fat as well as a considerable amount of vitamin E. Products containing rice bran are readily accepted by most horses. Commercial rice bran products are usually in powder or pellet form and are considerably more stable than animal fat and vegetable oils. Many rice bran-based products are balanced for calcium and phosphorus or are concurrently fed with a mineral supplement to offset the naturally high phosphorus content.

Controlled and field studies have shown that feeding 1.1 to 5 pounds of rice bran or rice bran-based products (Re-Leve by Hallway Feeds, Lexington, KY) to both PSSM and RER horses has resulted in significant improvement in disease.

Recommended Diets for Horses with PSSM and RER

Feeding recommendations for horses with chronic exertional rhabdomyolysis are displayed in Tables 1, 2, and 3. As with any horse, feeding forage at a rate of 1.5-2% of body weight is a fundamental part of the diet. The amount of fat supplied to horses with PSSM and RER is controversial. Part of this debate may be due to the fact that the diseases are often not distinguished. If PSSM horses are exercised regularly, many respond to low-calorie, low-starch diets that are only lightly supplemented with fat. Conversely, RER horses seem to benefit from fat supplementation only when they require high caloric intakes. Therefore, not all horses with exertional rhabdomyolysis require diets in which 25% of daily caloric intake is supplied by fat. In fact, such a diet is not always appropriate, is difficult to achieve in the face of high caloric requirements, and may result in problems with weight gain and unpalatable diets. Once caloric needs are assessed, a diet should be designed with an appropriate amount of fat and starch.

In Quarter Horse-related breeds, PSSM can usually be managed with grass hay or mixed hay and a fat supplement that is balanced for vitamins and minerals.

Starch should be decreased to less than 10% of daily digestible energy (DE) intake by eliminating grain and molasses. Rice bran can be gradually introduced into the diet as powder or as a pelleted feed. Some horses that will not eat powder will consume pelleted forms of rice bran (Equi-Jewel, Kentucky Performance Products, Versailles, KY). It is important for owners to understand that if horses eat the rice bran at a slower rate than sweet feed this can be beneficial as it reduces rapid absorption of starch. Depending on the caloric requirements of the horse, 1-5 pounds of rice bran can be fed but must be combined with a reduction in dietary starch to less than 10% of DE. An alternative source of fat is corn oil added to alfalfa pellets. An upper limit of 600 ml of oil per day is recommended, and additional vitamin E should be added to the diet. It is not possible to achieve the high caloric requirements for intense exercise using oil supplementation of alfalfa pellets, sweet feed, or rice bran without exceeding recommended maximum amounts of these products. To achieve the appropriate caloric intake for PSSM horses performing intense exercise, high-fat, low-starch pelleted feeds designed for PSSM horses in intense exercise are recommended (Table 1). Supplying fat at 6-10% by weight (or 15-20% of DE) of the entire ration to PSSM Quarter Horses (unless a higher energy intake is required for exercise) is likely quite sufficient for managing PSSM and further benefit from more fat has not been demonstrated in controlled trials. Note, however, that none of these diets will result in clinical improvement of muscle stiffness and exercise tolerance without gradually increasing the amount of daily exercise and maximizing access to turn-out.

Table 1. Feeding recommendations for an average-sized horse (500 kg) with chronic exertional rhabdomyolysis at varying levels of exertion.

	Maintenance	Light exercise	Moderate exercise	Intense exercise
Digestible Energy (Mcal/day)	16.4	20.5	24.6	32.8
% DE as NSC, PSSM horses	<10%	<10%	<10%	<10%
% DE as NSC, RER horses	20%	<20%	<20%	<20%
% DE as fat, PSSM horses	20%	20%	15%-20%	15%-20%
% DE as fat, RER horses	15%	15%	15%-20%	20-25%
Forage (% bwt)	1.5- 2.0 %	1.5- 2.0 %	1.5- 2.0 %	1.5- 2.0 %
Protein (grams/day)	697	767	836	906
Calcium (g)	30	33	36	39
Phosphorus (g)	20	22	24	26
Sodium (g)	22.5	33.5	33.8	41.3
Chloride (g)	33.8	50.3	50.6	62
Potassium (g)	52.5	78.3	78.8	96.4
Selenium (mg)	1.88	2.2	2.81	3.13
Vitamin E (IU)	375	700	900	1000

Daily requirements derived from multiple research studies (% NSC and % fat) and Kentucky Equine Research recommendations. From: McKenzie, E.M., S.J. Valberg, and J. Pagan. Nutritional management of exertional rhabdomyolysis. In: E. Robinson (Ed.) Current Therapy in Equine Medicine 5.

Thoroughbred horses with frequent episodes of rhabdomyolysis are usually being fed 5-15 pounds of sweet feed per day. The incidence of subclinical rhabdomyolysis is low in Thoroughbreds being fed a moderate caloric intake whether it is in the form of sweet feed or rice bran. However, when calories are increased by the addition of more sweet feed, the incidence of subclinical and clinical rhabdomyolysis is much greater. One way to lower serum CK after exercise when a high caloric intake is required is to feed a low-starch, high-fat ration. For RER horses, the recommendation is to feed no greater than 20% of daily DE as nonstructural carbohydrate and to supply 20-25% of daily DE from fat. The diet should contain no more than five pounds of sweet feed, 600 ml of vegetable oil, and five pounds of rice bran per day. For horses undergoing intense exercise, the combination of sweet feed and oil or sweet feed and rice bran does not achieve an adequate DE without feeding amounts of cereal grains that have been shown to elicit rhabdomyolysis in susceptible horses.

A specialized diet, Re-Leve, has been designed for intensely exercised horses with chronic exertional rhabdomyolysis. Re-Leve contains 13% fat by weight (rice bran and corn oil) or 20% DE as fat and only 9% DE as starch. This type of high-energy diet for RER horses might be provided through a combination of other commercially available grains, several fat supplements, and highly fermentable fiber sources (soy hulls, beet pulp). Other commercially available concentrates contain moderate amounts of fat (6-10%) and have lower NSC values (17–30% by weight). However, they cannot be fed in the quantities necessary to achieve the calories required to sustain intense exercise in RER horses without exceeding recommended NSC limits for these horses. They should therefore be combined with a fat supplement.

Expectations of fat supplementation. The time required for improvement in signs of exertional rhabdomyolysis is controversial. It has been suggested that a minimum of four months of supplementation is required and that relapses are associated primarily with disruption of supplementation. However, in the author's experience clinical improvement with PSSM is more dependent on the amount of daily exercise and turn-out than on the length or amount of dietary fat supplementation. For example, when serum CK was monitored daily post-exercise, levels were almost within the normal range after four weeks of daily exercise, without fat supplementation. In addition, when PSSM horses were turned out 24 hours a day on grass, post-exercise serum CK was normal compared to high activities during the same exercise test with stall-kept horses on a hay diet. Thus, it seems that consistent fat supplementation without implementing a structured daily exercise regime in PSSM horses is highly likely to result in failure, and confinement while consuming high levels of fat is likely to lead to obesity.

Surprisingly, recent studies in RER horses show that significant reductions or normalization of post-exercise serum CK activity occurs within a week of commencing a diet providing 20% DE as fat and 9% DE as starch. This low serum CK activity compared to the high CK activity observed in the same horses on an isocaloric diet where 40% DE was starch was not the result of any measurable change in muscle glycogen or metabolism during exercise. Potentially, the rapid response to decreasing starch and increasing fat was due to neurohormonal changes that resulted in a calmer demeanor, lower pre-exercise heart rates, and a decreased incidence of stress-induced rhabdomyolysis. Avoiding prolonged stall rest in fit Thoroughbreds with RER is also important since post-exercise CK activity is higher following two days of rest compared to values taken later in the week when performing consecutive days of the same amount of submaximal exercise. It is quite possible that exercise exerts beneficial effects on horses with chronic exertional rhabdomyolysis that are separate from the impact of reduction in dietary starch and/or fat supplementation. Failure to implement an appropriate exercise routine will likely lead to failure to control rhabdomyolysis.

Additional management strategies for chronic exertional rhabdomyolysis. Daily exercise appears to be crucial for successful dietary control of PSSM. It is recommended that turn-out and some exercise be started as soon as stiffness abates following an episode of rhabdomyolysis in PSSM horses, rather than waiting for muscle enzyme activity to normalize. Serum CK activity frequently remains increased in PSSM animals that are stall rested. Severely affected horses may only be able to manage a few minutes of exercise a day, but with gradually increasing intervals of walk and two minutes of trot (but no more than two-minute intervals) per day, many of these horses are capable of eventually accomplishing intense daily exercise without clinical rhabdomyolysis. Stall confinement should be kept to a maximum of 12 hours per day, and pasture turn-out is ideal.

RER horses are often very fit when they develop rhabdomyolysis and require only a few days off before commencing a reduced amount of training. Stall confinement should be kept to less than 24 hours if possible. Since RER appears to be a stress-related disorder, management strategies to reduce stress and excitability in these horses are important. These include turn-out, exercising or feeding these horses before other horses, providing compatible equine company, and the judicious use of low-dose tranquilizers during training. Anecdotal reports of increased nervousness have been received when selenium is supplemented at higher than the recommended levels. Feeds designed for RER should be evaluated for their selenium concentrations and should not be supplemented in addition if adequate levels are provided in the feed.

All supplemental feeds should be reduced in amount on days when energy requirements are not as high, particularly if the horse is at risk of weight gain. Other management strategies may help to decrease the intensity of the postprandial glycemic response, and include feeding small meals, providing at least 1.5-2.0% body weight per day in forage, and feeding a forage source either two hours before or concurrently with any grain. Avoiding high-starch supplements such as molasses is also important.

Table 2. Potential rations for a 500-kg horse with recurrent exertional rhabdomyolysis.

	Light exercise	*Moderate exercise*	*Intense exercise*
FORAGE	7-9 kg quality grass hay or pasture	7-9 kg quality grass hay or pasture	7-9 kg quality grass hay or 20:80 mix alfalfa/grass
PLUS:			
DIET 1:*	1.5 kg sweet feed + 1 kg rice bran	2 kg sweet feed + 1 kg rice bran	2.1 kg sweet feed + 1.4 kg of rice bran + 1.4 kg beet pulp**
OR: DIET 2:	1.5 kg of Re-Leve	3 kg of Re-Leve	5 kg of Re-Leve
OR: DIET 3:*	1 kg of sweet feed + 200 ml oil	2 kg of sweet feed + 500 ml oil	Combination cannot achieve required DE intake

*Vitamin and mineral supplement required for nonfortified feeds. The mineral recommended for the specific rice bran product should be provided (not necessary for Re-Leve).
**Soak beet pulp before feeding.
Addition of 50-100 g of salt per day to all rations is recommended based on level of exertion.
From: McKenzie, E.M., S.J. Valberg, and J. Pagan. Nutritional management of exertional rhabdomyolysis. In: E. Robinson (Ed.) Current Therapy in Equine Medicine 5.

Table 3. Potential rations for a 500-kg horse with polysaccharide storage myopathy.

	Light exercise	*Moderate exercise*	*Intense exercise*
FORAGE	7-9 kg quality grass hay or pasture	7-9 kg quality grass hay or pasture	7-9 kg quality grass hay or 20:80 mix alfalfa/grass
PLUS:			
DIET 1*	1.5 kg rice bran	2.25 kg rice bran	Cannot achieve required DE intake with rice bran alone
DIET 2	1.5 kg Re-Leve	2.5 kg Re-Leve	5 kg of Re-Leve
DIET 3*	1.8 kg alfalfa pellets + 475 ml oil	Combination cannot achieve required DE intake	Combination cannot achieve required DE intake

*Vitamin and mineral supplement required for nonfortified feeds. The mineral recommended for the specific rice bran product should be provided (not necessary for Re-Leve). Addition of 50-100 g of salt per day to all rations is recommended based on level of exertion. From: McKenzie, E.M., S.J. Valberg, and J. Pagan. Nutritional management of exertional rhabdomyolysis. In: E. Robinson (Ed.) Current Therapy in Equine Medicine 5.

Supplemental Reading

Beech, J. 1994. Treating and preventing chronic intermittent rhabdomyolysis. Vet. Med. 458-461.

De La Corte, F.D., Valberg, S.J., MacLeay, J.M., et al. 1999. The effect of feeding a fat supplement to horses with polysaccharide storage myopathy. J. World Equine Health 4:12-19.

Pagan, J.D. Carbohydrates in equine nutrition. 1997. In: Proc. 7th Equine Nutr. Conf. Feed Manufacturers. Kentucky Equine Research Inc., Lexington, KY, p. 45-50.

Valberg, S.J. 1996. Muscular causes of exercise intolerance in horses. Vet. Clin. North Am. Equine Pract.12:495-515.

Valberg, S.J., MacLeay, J.M., and Mickelson, J.R. 1997. Exertional rhabdomyolysis and polysaccharide storage myopathy in horses. Comp. Cont. Educ. Pract. Vet. 19:1077-1086.

Valberg, S.J., Mickelson, J.R., Gallant, E.M., et al. 1998. Exertional rhabdomyolysis in Quarter Horses and Thoroughbreds: One syndrome, multiple etiologies. Equine Exercise Physiology 5. Equine Vet. J. Suppl. 30: 533-538

Valentine, B.A., Van Saun, R.J., Thompson, K.N., et al. 2001. Role of dietary carbohydrate and fat in horses with equine polysaccharide storage myopathy. J. Am. Vet. Med. Assn.219:1537-1544

TRENDS IN FEEDING THE AMERICAN ENDURANCE HORSE

KATHLEEN CRANDELL
Kentucky Equine Research, Inc., Versailles, KY

Endurance riding is one of the fastest growing equestrian sports in the United States. Its popularity stems from the incredible bond that develops between a horse and rider after taking care of each other for so many hours on the trail. Because of this bond, endurance riders tend to be particular about wanting everything to be just right for their horses. Endurance riders, in general, are the most educated and open-minded about nutrition of their horses. Nutrition plays such an important role in the success of an endurance horse that endurance riders have to make proper nutrition a priority in their management.

Why does nutrition make or break an endurance horse? The type of work that is asked of the endurance horse, low-intensity and long-duration exercise, is dependent upon body stores of fuel in the form of glycogen and fat. Composition of the diet influences the type of fuels horses store. Manipulating the amounts of fiber, fat, and starch in the diet can influence which of the fuels is then utilized for energy. A balanced diet with adequate fiber, fat, and starch, as well as proper fortification of vitamins and minerals, will go a long way in determining whether an endurance horse can finish a race.

The United States Equestrian Team (USET) has a program for training endurance riders that have aspirations of competing internationally. The USET offers yearly clinics in which lessons are given on all aspects of the sport, such as riding, training, farriery, saddle fit, sport psychology, health issues, rider fitness, and horse nutrition. KER has provided a nutritionist to counsel each rider on his or her horse's nutritional program during these clinics over the past two years. The following is a summary of the data acquired from 37 riders participating in clinics in the East Coast, Central, and West Coast regions of the United States in 2001. Although the numbers may be small, the data appear to be closely representative of endurance horses in general.

The Horses

While any horse may have the ability to do endurance-type work, it appears that horses of Arabian descent excel in speed and endurance. Of the horses participating in the nutritional evaluation, 89% were of Arabian breeding, with 65% being purebred and 24% being crossbred. Arabians are generally not large horses, and the average weight of this group was 460 kg. The average age of the horses was 9.4 years, with a range of 4 to 21 years. Endurance horses are not permitted to enter any race of 50 miles or more until they are at least 5 years of age. With proper management, horses with good conformation and strong bone can compete into their late teens and early twenties.

Forage

There are many reasons why endurance horses do well in the United States. Most of these endurance horses have the advantage of being allowed to stay out on pasture as much as 24 hours per day. In this group of horses, at least 80% have 24-hour turnout. Not only is 24-hour turnout closer to the natural way in which horses evolved, but it also keeps bones stronger, muscles toned, and joints lubricated. Endurance horses that are kept in stalls are more likely to have muscle disorders and joint problems. Many regions of the country have quality pasture grasses so that the majority of the nutrition is coming from quality forage. Because Arabians are easy keepers by nature, quality pasture allows horses to maintain weight on little more than grass until they begin heavy work.

Regardless of pasture quality, horses will have to be supplemented with dry forage such as hay during some parts of the year. Over the years endurance riders have been advised to avoid pure alfalfa if at all possible because of the high protein and calcium content. In most regions of the country, grass hay is available and is the preferred forage for the endurance horse. Grass hay was being fed to 87% of the horses in the study. Only 22% received some alfalfa on a regular basis alone or in addition to grass hay. Alternative fiber sources like beet pulp are popular among endurance riders, and 60% of these riders fed beet pulp daily. This is in addition to the horses that were also getting beet pulp in their commercial concentrates. Beet pulp is rapidly becoming a common addition to the diets of endurance horses because of its high caloric and fiber content and its ability to hold large amounts of water.

Ideally, the endurance horse should get as many calories as possible from forage to avoid the complications of high-starch diets and muscle disorders. Forage in the hindgut also helps to delay the onset of dehydration during periods when the horse is working and not eating. The fiber holds water in reservoir. The average forage content of the diets for this group of horses was 78%, which is much higher in comparison to other types of sports horses.

Grain and Concentrates

Commercial concentrates are designed to take the guesswork out of balancing forage deficiencies of energy, protein, vitamins, and minerals. Still, some horse owners believe in keeping the feeding program simple by feeding straight grains. In this group, 32% fed some type of straight grain alone or with a commercial concentrate. The average intake of grain was 1.44 kg per day. Of those that fed straight grains, 67% fed grain plus a commercial concentrate; of the remaining 33%, three-fourths added some type of vitamin and mineral supplement, and only one-fourth fed grain alone. Commercial concentrates were by far the preferred method for addressing inadequacies of the forage with 89% feeding at least one type of commercial concentrate. The average intake of commercial concentrates was 2.27 kg per day. Most commercial concentrates are designed to be fed at a minimum feeding rate of 2.27 kg per day, which is exactly what the average intake was for this group of horses. When feeding lower than the recommended amount, the feed cannot provide the desired amounts of vitamins and minerals, and some sort of vitamin and mineral supplement is necessary.

Dietary Fat

Because these horses were on the low end of the grain or concentrate supplementation spectrum, they required additional calories from other sources. Feeding added fat to endurance horses has become very popular for various reasons. Research on feeding fat has demonstrated a glycogen sparing effect of high-fat diets. High-fat diets appear to influence fuel selection towards using triglycerides for energy during work, and the body store of triglycerides is by far the largest. Adding fat to the diet also increases the caloric density so that less high-starch feed is needed. Fat gives the horse physical energy without increasing mental energy, like high-starch diets. At least 54% of the horses were receiving additional fat in the form of oil or rice bran. Rice bran was being fed to 27% of the horses and other fat sources to 41%, with 14% getting both rice bran and oil. The fat source of choice was corn oil, but others included dry fat, coco soya, and flax. High-fat commercial concentrates (>6% fat) are also popular with endurance riders, with 51% of the riders feeding some type. Interestingly, 92% of the East Coast riders were feeding a high-fat concentrate, while only 32% of the Central and West Coast riders were. This may be attributed to high-quality, high-fat feeds being more readily accessible in the Eastern regions of the country. Even with all the fat supplementation, the average fat percentage of the total diet was still only 2.3%, ranging from as low as 1.4% to as high as 6.9%.

Calories and Protein

The amount of calories provided by the diet averaged around 24.1 Mcal digestible energy per day. The exact calculation of caloric intake is difficult to measure in those endurance horses that have ad libitum access to hay and/or pasture. The overall protein content of the diet averaged 10.2%, ranging from 6.2 to 15.7%, depending greatly on the type of forage offered. The commercial concentrates used had protein concentration ranging from 10 to 14%, with the majority of the riders preferring the 10% feeds.

Supplements

Balancing the diet is very important. One of the most important supplements for the endurance horse is salt because of the large amounts of salt lost in sweat. Surprisingly, only 35% of the riders offered horses free-choice access to salt. Again, regional differences were very distinctive because 75% of the East Coast riders offered salt, and only 16% in the West Coast and Central regions did. The higher humidity of the East Coast may be one reason for the difference; horses ridden on the East Coast may have a higher requirement. Only 5% of the riders feed a daily electrolyte, while all of them give electrolytes at a competition.

Use of other supplements varied; 35% fed an additional vitamin and mineral supplement to top off the commercial concentrate or grain. Selenium and vitamin E are of major concern for the endurance horse because of their importance in supporting muscle tissue. Only 19% fed a vitamin E and selenium supplement, but again regions were very distinctive. None of the horses in the West Coast or Central regions were being supplemented with vitamin E or selenium, while 67% of the horses on the East Coast were receiving it. The soils and consequentially the forages are very deficient in the East Coast and the Northwest. Only 16% of the riders were feeding some type of hoof supplement. Arabians have been bred to have strong hooves, and the limited use of hoof supplements attests to the hardiness of their feet.

The trend in feeding the modern-day endurance horse leans toward a higher forage, higher fat, and lower starch diet. Riders appear to be astute in balancing inadequacies of forage with grain concentrates and supplements. Their willingness to put the horse first and do whatever is necessary to supply all of the nutrients needed was very evident in the evaluation of the individual feeding programs.

SPORT HORSE NUTRITION—AN AUSTRALIAN PERSPECTIVE

ELIZABETH OWENS
Ridley AgriProducts, Brisbane, Australia

Introduction

To perform at Olympic-caliber competitions, horses must consistently maintain a level of athletic performance that strains their muscular, skeletal, and digestive systems. As the consulting nutritionist to the Australian Equestrian Team, I am primarily concerned with the nutritional challenges of our equine athletes. Much of the equine nutritional research and product development effort is directed at the racing industry, and while this information is useful, it is worth remembering that an elite performance horse is much different than a Thoroughbred racehorse. Moreover, each Olympic discipline attracts horses of different types, workloads, training programs, and feeding practices.

An extensive evaluation of feeding and work practices of members of Australia's equestrian team was conducted over a two-year period. The daily workloads, actual body weights, feed intakes, and feed analyses were ascertained for 22 elite horses, consisting of eventers, show jumpers, and dressage horses. Horses were evaluated for five consecutive days. All of the horses studied were stabled at night with limited or no access to pasture during the day.

The ultimate goal of this study was to ensure that the performances of Australia's equine athletes, both within and outside Australia, was not limited by suboptimal nutrition. To attain this goal, it was important to quantify the variation in standard nutritional parameters for each discipline and to understand the "hot buttons" for riders in the different disciplines.

This paper summarizes some of the outcomes from that feeding evaluation and provides some insight into current feeding practices of sport horses in Australia.

Daily Feed Intake

During the study, each horse was weighed at the same time each day using portable Tru-test scales, and every ingredient in each meal was weighed over a five-day period. Rejected feed was recorded and samples retained for analysis. Table 1 summarizes the average body weight and DM (dry matter) feed intake for all horses in each of the disciplines. In this evaluation, the eventing horses consumed an average of between 1.48 and 2.45% of body weight. The dressage horses consumed between 1.04 and 1.79% of body weight and the show jumpers between 1.09 and 2.55%. Recommendations by the NRC (1989) suggest daily feed intakes for working horses to be between 2 and 3% of body weight.

Table 1. Average daily intake of DM as a percentage of body weight (BWT) by discipline.

Discipline	Body weight	% of BWT as DM intake
Show jumpers	487.0	1.98
	493.3	1.17
	506.8	1.09
	514.8	2.08
	542.5	2.55
Dressage horses	533.2	1.36
	570.4	1.69
	608.0	1.79
	646.0	1.48
	657.6	1.04
	759.2	1.20
Eventers	483.4	2.12
	498.4	1.91
	502.8	2.05
	517.6	1.91
	529.2	2.45
	539.2	1.75
	546.8	1.48
	558.4	1.76
	582.0	1.76
	587.6	2.02
	615.6	1.63

In a study of 25 Thoroughbred and Standardbred racing stables in 1993, Southwood et al. found that the feed intake of the Thoroughbreds and Standardbreds studied was similar to NRC published requirements. In this study, the horse's body weight was estimated using the formula from Carroll and Huntington (1988), and the feed intake was recorded for only a single day. The results shown in Table 1 show less consistent agreement with NRC recommendations for feed intake and highlight the individuality of horses in their feed consumption and the importance of considering existing patterns of feed intake when recommending a diet change.

Results from this evaluation suggest that dressage horses in full work might be expected to consume between 1 and 2% of body weight, while eventers and show jumpers may consume between 1 and 2.75% of body weight. These results illustrate how important it is for each horse to be fed as an individual and why it is sometimes necessary to be critical of feed manufacturers' recommendations for feed allowances. Such feed intake allowances are frequently based on surveys done with racehorses, and direct application of the allowances to performance horses could result in unwanted weight gain and/or other undesirable side effects, such as colic, heat bumps, and behavioral modifications.

Body Weight

Variation in body weight of horses in the three disciplines is summarized in Figures 1, 2, and 3. Predictably, the dressage horses were the largest with average body weights between 533 and 759 kg. Four out of five of these horses were full or part warmblood, and as a group recorded the least variable body weights over the five-day evaluation period. This reflects the consistent pattern and intensity of work employed with these horses.

The eventers (all Thoroughbreds) had a standard deviation for body weight change over the five-day study period of between 1.673 and 10.64 kg. A change of 22 kg was recorded for one horse between a day of gallop work and a day of flat work when the horse was accidentally denied access to water.

The greatest daily change in body weight was reflected in the show jumpers that were either Thoroughbreds or Thoroughbred/warmblood crosses. This may be explained by two factors. Firstly, one group of horses had recently returned from a short layoff, so some of the variation could be explained through adaptation to higher energy diets following a week of fiber-based rations. Secondly, both groups of horses studied were fed hay by volume from variable-quality hay, which contributed to fluctuations in daily intakes of fiber by weight.

Generally, riders are not aware of the actual weights of their horses, nor the normal range for variation of those body weights in response to work intensity, climate, or feed changes. The three eventing horses that were fed four times daily and were most closely supervised by their riders showed the lowest daily variation in body weight of all the eventers and show jumpers.

Feed Ingredients and Analyses

There was a heavy reliance on roughage sources to provide macro- and microminerals. All horses were fed chaff with their concentrate meals. Both white and green chaffs were used. White chaff was either oaten or wheaten hay steam cut to 1 cm, and green chaff was lucerne steam cut to between 1 and 3 cm. Lucerne and grass hays were also fed in hay nets at night and/or on the ground during the day in the yards. The majority of horses received the appropriate amount of roughage in their diet (between 40 and 50%), but there was considerable daily variation as a result of the hay being fed by volume rather than by weight.

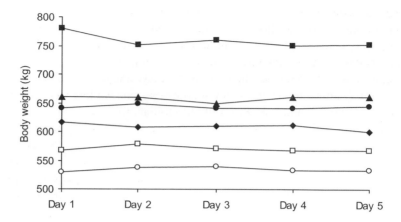

Figure 1. Daily body weight variation of dressage horses.

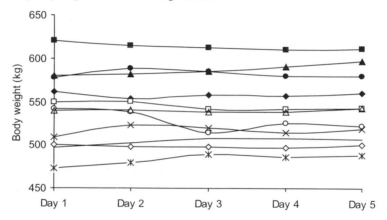

Figure 2. Daily body weight variation of eventers.

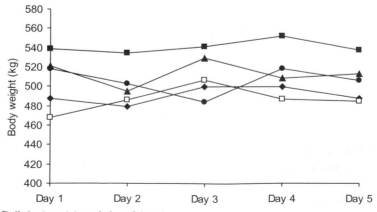

Figure 3. Daily body weight variation of show jumpers.

Lucerne is a source of calcium, but analysis of lucerne hays and chaffs used by participants in this evaluation showed that the calcium level varied from 0.67 to 1.75%. The iron content in one sample was 65 ppm, which is considerably less than the stated level of 225 ppm in the NRC. These results suggest that riders naively believe that the roughage will provide an adequate source of all major minerals for their horses. There is a need for an accurate and reproducible method for determining the digestible energy (DE) composition of feeds, both raw materials and compound feeds. Using the DHIA Laboratory in Ithaca, New York and the prediction equation of Pagan (1986), it was found that the estimated DE for a commercial extruded feed was only 12.86 MJ/kg versus a label claim of 16.9 MJ/ kg. This is a source of inaccuracy and misinformation for riders, veterinarians, and nutritionists trying to formulate balanced and appropriate rations for sport horses.

The majority of the dressage and eventing horses were fed home-mixed diets (grain-based) without inclusion of any fortification pellet or sweet feed. Three eventing horses were fed a fortified sweet feed, and the balance of the horses (show jumpers, eventers, and one dressage horse) received a pellet in conjunction with other diet components.

Some riders were feeding seaweed meal or liquid sea minerals in the belief that these products provided an adequate source of essential minerals for a working horse.

Dietary Deficiencies

Raw materials were analyzed by the laboratory at the University of New England and the DHIA Laboratory, and DE was estimated using the equation from Pagan (1986). Declared nutrient levels were used for proprietary feeds and supplements. Data from the NRC (1989) were used for the balance of nutrient data for each of the ingredients to produce an estimate of nutrient intake for each day of the evaluation. This information was then compared against predicted requirements gathered from Kentucky Equine Research's MicroSteed program and the NRC (1989) for mature horses in work. The requirements used were aimed at optimizing performance rather than preventing deficiency and are therefore higher than published data that addresses minimum requirements. Of the 22 horses studied, only one eventer and three dressage horses received no additional vitamin/trace mineral supplementation from either supplements or fortified feeds. Overall, 17 of the 22 horses were receiving suboptimal levels of vitamin E, less than 1000 IU/ day. Nine horses received intakes far below those recommended for sodium, and four were deficient in minor vitamins. All horses appeared to receive adequate calcium, phosphorus, magnesium, potassium, iron, and cobalt.

Feeding Practices and Management

FEEDING FREQUENCY

Of the horses studied, 15 were fed twice a day, three were fed three times a day, and four were fed four times a day. Under free-range conditions, a horse will graze between 50 and 70% of the time, ensuring a continuous intake of small amounts of grass. Restriction to twice-daily feeding increases the likelihood of colic, possibly affecting gastrointestinal tract distention, motility, and blood flow. There is a concurrent alteration in metabolic rate, circulation and concentration of cortisol, and concentrations of electrolytes.

To prevent digestion dysfunction (excessive gas production, colic, laminitis, and impaired fiber digestion) resulting from starch overload, grain intake in horses fed two or three times daily should be limited to 0.5 kg of grain per 100 kg of body weight. Most riders were aware of these potential problems but were unable or unwilling to modify current feeding management practices to cater to the idiosyncrasies of their horses' digestive systems. Three of the eventers consumed a grain portion well in excess of this recommended maximum, thus increasing the risk of colic in these animals.

By contrast, four of the eventers were subjected to increased feeding frequency and more personal supervision of their feeding management, resulting in these horses having the lowest variation in digestible energy intake and body weight.

FEEDING PRACTICES

In Australia, it is not common practice to wet hay. In this study, none of the participants soaked hay and usually only the night feed was dampened with molasses water. Two eventers were fed a wet feed once a week. It was into this feed only that the vitamin/mineral supplements were added. All feeds were mixed by volume, but one rider did weigh the horses' rations on a weekly basis and adjusted the volume-mix charts accordingly.

Most members of the elite equestrian squads in Australia are professional riders who are required to work a team of horses each day and combine teaching and training to supplement their incomes. This necessitates the employment of staff to supervise the daily management of their horses. As a result, the riders forfeit the intimate knowledge of their horses' feeding to their staff.

During this study, I discovered instances where riders were ignorant of their horses' level of feed intake and/or rejection and were unaware that certain ingredients were being excluded from the diet, due either to lack of availability or grooms who simply forgot to include that ingredient. Feeds prepared for one horse were mistakenly fed to another, and in a case already described, a horse was accidentally denied access to water because of staff negligence. These instances should not be viewed as the norm, but indicate that the nutritional adequacy of some Australian sport horses is compromised because riders do not believe that nutrition is worthy of their personal interest or attention.

NUTRITIONAL UNDERSTANDING

While some of the participants had a clear grasp of the principles of basic equine nutrition, several were confused about feeding and viewed nutrition as a low priority in the performance of their horses.

One rider who had been consistently advised against feeding large amounts of pollard (wheat bran) continued to do so because he had not detected any negative impact from this practice. By comparison, another rider adhered to the very best feeding practices and had previously utilized the services of a nutritionist to evaluate the nutritional adequacy of his feeding program.

The fact that the participants allowed the evaluation to be carried out at their stables demonstrated that they are willing to learn about nutrition. Without exception, the riders were interested in the outcome of the evaluation and the suggested diets that were provided.

Hot Buttons

It can be very dangerous to make generalizations about the feed preferences that riders in different disciplines have for their equine partners. For instance, it is commonly assumed that, because the majority of dressage competitors are female and that the horses are large warmbloods, a "non-heating" diet is preferred since the riders could not control such a big animal otherwise. While this may be the case for many hobbyists, riders at an elite level need a horse that is extremely fit. Long-term soundness, prevention of muscle soreness, and endurance to produce a top-level performance over three days of competition are the major goals.

Show jumpers do relatively little work compared to dressage horses or eventers–both in training and during competition–so feeding strategies need to be aimed at high energy for short duration work, body weight control, and soundness of legs and head.

All top-level horses spend months each year traveling and competing under stressful conditions. Highly palatable feeds that the horse will consistently clean up are of primary concern. Soundness and prevention of muscle damage is crucial. As the value of the animal increases, veterinary intervention to oversee such conditions may take precedence over nutritional solutions.

Lack of knowledge leads to the use of unproven herbal, homeopathic, medicinal, or other dubious alternatives for the treatment of performance-limiting conditions such as muscle soreness, mental tenseness, lameness, low feed intake, or respiratory disorders. Riders are often reluctant to share these "cures" with professionals charged with supervising the health of their horses. It should also be remembered that it is not always the rider who does the feeding; rather, the groom or head girl is frequently the individual overseeing the animals' daily feeding and management routines.

Ingrained, inappropriate feeding practices persist even among elite competitors. Quite often the lack of a problem is the greatest hindrance to improving feeding practices and nutrition of sport horses.

Conclusion

Australia continues to dominate international three-day events, having won three consecutive team gold medals in Olympic competition. At the Sydney Olympics, Australia also demonstrated improving competitiveness in dressage and show jumping. Sport horses are an important part of the Australian equine industry and meeting their nutritional requirements with a cost-effective diet that recognizes the limitations of ingrained feeding practices is a challenge.

In order to formulate a balanced ration for sporting horses today, we are faced with the dilemma of deciding what to measure, against which standards, and using what resources? Consistent, reproducible laboratory tests for DE determination of feedstuffs and finished feeds must be established in Australia and implemented by the major feed manufacturing companies. NRC figures, last published in 1989, do not take into sufficient consideration variations in workloads, feeding practices, or breed differences and address minimal, rather than optimal, nutritional requirements for performance. Actual body weights and weights of individual feed ingredients are a minimal requirement in any nutritional evaluation. Riders rarely take the time to measure these parameters themselves and in some cases cannot be relied upon to give an accurate record of a horse's feed status. Professionals who cater to riders of eventing horses need to be aware of the differences in both requirements and feeding practices of elite sport horses versus Thoroughbreds and/or Standardbreds.

References

Carroll, C. L., and P. J. Huntington. 1988. Body condition scoring and weight estimation of horses. Equine Vet. J. 20:40-45.

NRC. Nutrient Requirements of Horses (5th Ed.) National Academy Press, Washington, D.C., 1989.

Pagan, J. D., and H. F. Hintz. 1986. Equine Energetics. I. Relationship between body weight and energy requirements in horses. II. Energy expenditure in horses during submaximal exercise. J Anim Sci 63:815-830.

Southwood, L. L., D. L. Evans, W. L. Bryden, and R. J. Rose. 1993. Nutrient intake of horses in Thoroughbred and Standardbred stables. Aust Vet J 70:164-168.

NUTRITIONAL MANAGEMENT OF MARES—THE FOUNDATION OF A STRONG SKELETON

PETER J. HUNTINGTON[1], ELIZABETH OWENS[2], KATHLEEN CRANDELL[3], AND JOE PAGAN[3]

[1]Kentucky Equine Research Australasia, Brighton, Victoria, Australia
[2]Ridley AgriProducts PL, Wacol, Queensland, Australia
[3]Kentucky Equine Research, Versailles, Kentucky, USA

Introduction

The impact of a broodmare feeding program can be substantial on the skeletal development of the foal and the equine athlete. Among domestic animals, horses have the shortest period between parturition and rebreeding, and ideally the mare will be both lactating and pregnant simultaneously. Most horsemen have an appreciation for the obvious things that feeding affects such as fertility, milk production by mares, and the health of their foals. In recent years the importance of good nutrition during pregnancy has become more apparent. The goal of a feeding program for mares is to complement other facets of management so that total efficiency of the broodmare band is not compromised by nutrition and wastage of foals is minimized. One of the major causes of wastage is skeletal disease, and one of the most important periods for sound growth is the time prior to weaning when the foal is still nursing the mare. Studies of the incidence of osteochondritis dissecans (OCD) have shown that the disorder is very dynamic during the early months of life and that the highest recorded incidence occurs at 5 months of age. Many foals are still not weaned at this age and are reliant on nutrition from mare's milk, pasture and other forages, and concentrates from the mare's feed bin or creep feeder. Unfortunately, the pressures of the breeding season mean that many foals get more scrutiny and individual attention at or after weaning; by then, however, it may be too late.

Mares should be divided into four classes when considering their nutritional needs: (1) the maiden mare; (2) the barren and early pregnant non-lactating mare; (3) the mare in the last third of pregnancy; and (4) the lactating mare (and possibly pregnant as well).

Each of these classes of mares needs the same nutrients in the diet, but at different levels of intake, as nutrient requirements are based on the physiological state. In addition, foals within a breed vary in their metabolism and growth rate so they need to be fed differently. The contrast between the nutrient needs and feeding practices required by Thoroughbred mares and warmblood mares is striking. This paper will cover the important nutrient needs of different classes of mares and the feeding practices required in different management situations to achieve optimal nutrition for skeletal development.

193

Nutrient Needs of Mares

ENERGY AND PROTEIN

The requirements for energy and protein during pregnancy do not increase substantially until the last trimester of pregnancy, when 75% of the fetal growth occurs (Table 1). There are very few studies to verify energy and protein requirements for mares, and more work is needed to clarify differences in requirements between breeds. In other species, maternal malnutrition has been shown to lead to long-term changes in metabolic processes in the offspring. Could the performance potential of an equine athlete be influenced by intrauterine growth retardation that results from maternal malnutrition, disease, or reduced supply of nutrients to the fetus arising from placental or umbilical abnormalities? This topic has been covered in an excellent review article by Rossdale and Ousey (2002).

Table 1. KER nutrient requirements of the 500-kg light horse broodmare[1].

Nutrient	Early pregnancy	Late pregnancy	% change	Early lactation	% change	Late lactation
DE (MJ)	68	89	29	118	33	102
Protein (g)	697	938	35	1414	51	1217
Lysine (g)	24	33	38	50	52	43
Calcium (g)	30	47	57	61	30	47
Phosphorus (g)	20	31	55	41	32	31
Magnesium (g)	10	12	20	15	25	12
Zinc (mg)	337	450	34	600	33	500
Copper (mg)	112	150	34	150	0	125
Manganese (mg)	337	450	34	600	33	500
Selenium (mg)	1.9	2.2	16	3	36	2.5
Iodine (mg)	1.5	1.75	17	2.25	29	1.9
Vitamin A (IU)	37500	43750	17	75000	71	62500
Vitamin E (IU)	375	700	87	750	7	625

[1]Light horses include Thoroughbreds, Standardbreds, Arabians, Quarter Horses, and similar breeds. Many mares are heavier than 500 kg, but this weight is used for comparison purposes.

Kentucky Equine Research (KER) has developed estimated nutrient requirements for warmbloods that take into account differences in metabolism and growth rate between light horses and warmbloods (Table 2). This table shows that warmblood mares need less energy and protein and more minerals than light horse mares of the same weight.

Table 2. Comparison of nutrient requirements of 500-kg Thoroughbred (TB) and 700-kg warmblood (WB) mares during late pregnancy and early lactation.

	TB Late pregnancy	WB Late pregnancy	% difference	TB Early lactation	WB Early lactation	% Difference
Weight (kg)	575	800	40	500	700	40
DE (MJ)	89	97	9	118	112	-5
Protein (g)	938	1152	23	1414	1506	7
Lysine (g)	33	40	21	50	53	6
Calcium (g)	47	66	40	61	85	39
Phosphorus (g)	31	44	42	41	57	39
Magnesium (g)	12	17	42	15	21	40
Zinc (g)	450	630	40	600	840	40
Copper (mg)	150	210	40	150	210	40
Manganese (mg)	450	630	40	600	840	40
Selenium (mg)	2.2	3.1	41	2	4.2	40
Iodine (mg)	1.75	2.45	40	2.25	3.15	40
Vitamin A (IU)	43750	61250	40	75000	105000	40
Vitamin E (IU)	700	980	40	750	1050	40

It is thought that during energy or protein deprivation pregnant and lactating mares will draw upon stored reserves to maintain intrauterine growth of a fetus and milk production. During pregnancy, fetal growth is very slow during the early months. By the end of the seventh month of pregnancy, the fetus has only deposited 10% of the protein it will contain at birth. In the last four months of pregnancy, the fetus will deposit about 8 kg of protein as it grows to a birth weight of 50 kg (protein deposited and birth weight will vary depending on breed). During the last month of pregnancy alone, the fetus will deposit over 2.5 kg of protein into its body. Mares produce large quantities of milk and this dramatically increases demands for protein and energy. Milk production is estimated at between 3 and 4% of body weight during the first 2 months of lactation, and this declines to 2% of body weight after 5 months. Milk is 20-25% protein on a dry matter basis.

Gill et al. (1985) restricted mares to 70% of protein needs during pregnancy and lactation and found that birth weights were not affected, but growth rate of the foal to 90 days was reduced in the restricted group compared to mares fed normal diets during both pregnancy and lactation or those restricted during pregnancy but not lactation. These diets were not isocaloric. This effect of protein deprivation on the growth rate of foals was presumed to have occurred via an effect on milk production. The quality of protein supplied to the lactating mare may influence milk production and growth rate. Glade and Luba (1990) added soybean meal to the diet of Thoroughbred mares being fed a high-protein concentrate 2 weeks prior to and 7 weeks after foaling. The addition of 500 g of soybean meal prior to foaling and 750 g after foaling was matched by a reduction in concentrate intake so that the DE intake remained the same in both groups. The crude protein content of milk was significantly increased in the first 5 weeks of lactation, and the foals of soybean-supplemented mares grew 10% taller in the first 7 weeks of life. The control group of mares in this study were fed a 16% (as fed) crude protein concentrate and were supplied with crude protein and lysine in excess of National Research Council (NRC) requirements both before and after foaling. However, several studies have also shown that variations in protein and amino acid intake had no impact on the composition of mare's milk.

The impact of protein and energy restriction may depend upon the reserves the mare has to draw on. Pagan et al. (1984) found that there was no difference in the growth rate of pony foals on mares that were fed either 70% or 130% of their energy and protein requirements. Mares either lost or gained weight, but foal growth rate did not change. However, when mares were in poor body condition (a body condition score of 2) and had fewer reserves to draw on for the energy and protein required for milk production, growth rate of the foal was reduced. The same group of researchers found that feeding excess energy to pony mares led to reduced fat and protein content in the milk, which might reduce growth rate. Doreau and Boulet (1987) found that thin mares had lower milk production than fat mares.

Adding 5% fat to the diet of lactating mares led to an increase in milk energy production (Davison et al., 1991). Hoffman et al. (1996) found that mares fed a high-fat, high-fiber concentrate prior to and after foaling had higher levels of linoleic acid in their milk than mares fed a high-starch, high-sugar concentrate. This increased linoleic acid content may protect foals against the development of gastric ulcers, and the mares fed the high-fat, high-fiber diet also had higher immunoglobulin levels in their colostrum, which may improve protection against disease. Doreau et al. (1992) found that increasing the proportion of concentrates in the diet of the lactating mare from 5% to 50% led to an increased milk yield and lactose content, but it was more dilute with a lower protein concentration. This change led mares on the high-grain diet to gain weight but did not affect the growth of the foals.

Prolactin is a hormone that is important in parturition and milk secretion in the mare. Recent work has shown that energy restriction and low body condition can reduce prolactin secretion, and this could be an important consideration in lactating mares. Dry mares kept in poor to moderate condition produced less prolactin than mares kept in fat condition (Gentry et al., 2002), and geldings kept on a high-for-age diet that only supplied 70% of energy needs produced lower prolactin levels following stimulation with thyroid releasing hormone (Powell et al., 2003).

MINERALS

The requirements of horses for calcium, phosphorus, and magnesium were reviewed by Hintz at the 2000 KER Nutrition Conference. They are important minerals in the diet of pregnant and lactating mares because they are needed to supply the rapid growth of bone in the fetus in late pregnancy and in the foal prior to weaning. By 6 months of age, the foal has reached 85% of its height and has 68% of its bone mineral content. Many foals would not be weaned by this time, and if the mare were not being given supplementary feed, all of these minerals would have been supplied by the placental circulation, milk, and grass.

Martin et al. (1996) measured changes in serum concentrations of calcium (Ca) and parathyroid hormones in mares fed diets containing calcium concentrations below (0.35%) and above (0.55%) the NRC requirement of 0.45%. They found less extreme variations of serum total calcium, ionized calcium, and parathyroid hormone in the mares that were fed 0.55% calcium than in mares fed 0.35% calcium. They suggested that the optimal concentration of dietary calcium for prepartum mares was closer to 0.55% than 0.35%. Glade (1993) estimated metacarpal breaking strength (MBS) by transmission ultrasound of mares during the last 12 weeks of gestation and for 40 weeks after foaling. MBS increased during the last 6-10 weeks of gestation in mares fed amounts of calcium similar to NRC recommendations, but mares fed 20% less calcium than NRC recommendations did not have an increase in MBS. Importantly, foals of the mares fed the lower level of calcium had thinner mid-cannon circumference and mechanically weaker bones at birth than foals of control mares and the differences persisted for 40 weeks. These indicate that the pregnant mare probably needs more calcium intake than the NRC recommendation, but the optimal level has not been established.

It was estimated that mare's milk contains about 1.2 g of Ca/kg of fluid milk during early lactation (first three months) and 0.8 g of Ca/kg of fluid milk during late lactation (Schryver et al., 1986; Grace, 1999), so lactating mares need nearly three times the calcium intake of dry mares. Wide variation in calcium intake by mares has been shown to have no effect on concentration in milk in a number of studies (Lewis, 1995). However, Lewis (1995) cited a study in which milk calcium concentration was 40% lower in mares receiving 33% of dietary calcium needs, but levels were not increased above normal values in mares getting 250% of their daily requirement. Glade (1993) reported that mares fed the NRC recommended levels of calcium gradually lost bone density during the first 12 weeks of lactation, but density started increasing at that time and was fully restored at 24 weeks postparturition. Mares fed 20% less calcium than recommended, however, had not recovered bone density at 40 weeks after parturition even though the foals were weaned at 20 weeks.

Numerous studies have examined the impact of low dietary cation-anion balance (DCAB) on mineral excretion, and it has been found that low DCAB diets lead to increased calcium excretion (Baker et al., 1993). However, a number of studies on this topic have found that horses can compensate for increased calcium losses by increasing absorption, so that calcium balance is not affected. The most likely cause of a low DCAB diet is a high-grain, low-forage diet, and if this diet is not supplied with adequate supplementary calcium, deficiencies may occur. Another factor to consider is teeth. Correction of molar abnormalities in late pregnant mares was associated with significant increases in digestion and retention of calcium, phosphorus, and magnesium (Gatta et al., 2001).

Phosphorus (P) requirements also increase in late pregnancy and lactation in line with calcium. Donoghue et al. (1990) reported that phosphorus deficiencies were quite common in late pregnancy, while calcium deficiencies occurred in lactation. The phosphorus deposition in the fetus was estimated to be 9.4 g/day for a 500-kg mare during the last three months of gestation based on the body composition data from Dr. Helmut Meyer's laboratory (Drepper et al., 1992). Thus a 500-kg mare would require about 31g of P/day. The phosphorus content of liquid milk in early lactation was 0.75 g/kg and decreased to 0.50 g/kg during late lactation (NRC, 1989). This leads to a 30% increase in phosphorus needs in early lactation. Data from digestion studies at KER have shown that phosphorus digestibility is unaffected by calcium content, but calcium to phosphorus ratio was negatively correlated with fiber content in the diet (Pagan, 1998).

As with calcium and phosphorus, body composition data from the laboratory of Meyer (Drepper et al., 1982) were utilized to estimate magnesium (Mg) requirements of mares. Deposition of magnesium was calculated to be 0.3 mg/kg of body weight of the mare, and it was figured that a 500-kg late pregnant mare would need about 12 g of Mg/day. It was estimated that the magnesium concentration of milk averages 90 mg/kg during early lactation and a 500-kg mare would need about 15 g of magnesium during early lactation. It is possible that nutritionists should be concerned about the calcium to magnesium ratio in the diet of mares, as well as young horses, but there are no data to validate any suggested ratios. Data from digestion studies conducted at the KER laboratory have shown a positive correlation between calcium content and magnesium digestibility and a negative correlation with phosphorus content (Pagan, 1998).

Silicon is a mineral that does not receive much attention. It has an important role in bone calcification and is present in high concentrations in active growth areas of bone. Work at Texas A&M University on supplementation of sodium zeolite A (a source of silicon) to weanlings and yearlings showed that plasma silicon and radiographic bone density were increased (Frey et al., 1992). Would the young growing horse benefit if silicon were fed to the mare during pregnancy or lactation?

TRACE MINERALS

Copper (Cu) is essential for proper synthesis and maintenance of elastic connective tissue and detoxification of superoxide. Copper has received a great deal of attention since the last publication of the NRC because of its suggested role in the pathogenesis of developmental orthopedic disease (DOD). The 1989 NRC estimated that all classes of horses require 10 mg Cu/kg of dry diet. This appears accurate for horses at maintenance but other work suggests that the requirements of copper for young growing horses and broodmares are considerably higher, especially in certain breeds.

New Zealand researchers (Pearce et al., 1998a) studied the effect of copper supplementation on the incidence of DOD in Thoroughbred foals. Pregnant Thoroughbred mares were divided into either copper-supplemented or control groups. Live foals born to each group of mares were also divided into copper-supplemented or control groups. The four treatment groups were: (1) mares supplemented with copper, but their foals were not supplemented; (2) both mares and foals were supplemented with copper; (3) mares were not supplemented, but their foals received supplementation; (4) neither mares nor foals received supplementation.

Supplemented mares received 0.5 mg Cu/kg body weight daily (~250 mg), while copper-supplemented foals received 0.2 mg Cu/kg body weight from 21-49 days of age and 0.5 mg Cu/kg body weight (~100 mg) from 50 days to 150 days. Mares were supplemented for the final 13 to 25 weeks of gestation, and all mares and foals received concurrent selenium and zinc supplementation. At 150 days of age, the foals were sacrificed, and an exhaustive postmortem examination was performed. The number of articular and physeal cartilage lesions was noted for each treatment group along with a physitis score that was determined from radiographs of the distal metatarsus.

Copper supplementation of mares was associated with a significant reduction in the radiographic physitis scores of the foals at 150 days of age. Foals from mares that received no supplementation had a mean physitis score of 6, while foals out of supplemented mares had a mean score of 3.7. A lower score indicates less physitis. When only foals (but not mares) were supplemented with copper, no significant effect on physitis scores was noted. There was a significantly lower incidence of articular cartilage lesions in foals from mares supplemented with copper. However, no significant effects on lesions occurred in foals supplemented with copper.

Two North American dose-response studies examining the effect of increased dietary copper intakes on bone and cartilage abnormalities (Knight et al., 1990; Hurtig et al., 1993) found that the incidence of DOD was decreased by increasing the copper content of the diet above NRC recommendations. In Knight's study, mares were fed 32 ppm compared to 13 ppm. Because both mares and their foals received copper supplementation, it is difficult to determine whether the effect resulted from supplementation of the mare or the foal. New Zealand research (Pearce et al., 1998a,b) would suggest that supplementation of the pregnant mare is more important than supplementation of the foal. Oral copper supplementation of mares in late gestation altered the copper balance in these horses and resulted in an increase in the foal's liver copper stores at birth. Increased liver copper stores of the neonate may be important for ensuring healthy development of the skeleton during the period of maximum postnatal growth. Van Weeren et al. (2003) examined the copper status of foals at birth and the incidence of radiographic signs of OCD in warmblood foals genetically prone to OCD. The foals were evaluated at 5 months and 11 months of age. Radiographic score was not related to liver copper concentration at birth, but foals with high liver copper levels had improvements in the severity of OCD changes in the stifle from 5 months to 11 months. Foals with low liver copper levels at birth had more severe signs of OCD at 11 months than 5 months, indicating that copper is perhaps less involved as a cause of OCD and more important in repair of lesions.

These studies certainly provide proof that copper supplementation of mares and their foals can play an important role in skeletal development. Copper is not, however, the only factor involved in the pathogenesis of DOD, and it has been questioned whether the lesions produced by copper deficiency are the same as those most often seen in the field (Pagan, 2000). Copper deficiencies may either be primary in origin because of a lack of copper intake or induced (secondary) due to interactions with other substances in the ration. Zinc (Zn) and molybdenum (Mo) have often been implicated as minerals that can interfere with copper absorption in horses, but several studies have suggested that neither zinc nor molybdenum (Pagan, 2000) affects copper utilization when fed at levels found in practical diets. Pagan (1998b) found significant negative correlations between true copper digestibility and the concentration of both crude protein and calcium in 30 different diets. These interactions may be particularly relevant when horses are fed predominantly legume forage or given several calcium supplements.

Zinc is present as a component of many enzymes and the biochemical role of zinc relates largely to the functions of these enzymes. Pagan (1998) evaluated interactions between zinc digestibility and a number of nutrients in 30 different diets. The only nutrient that was significantly correlated to zinc digestibility was magnesium. None of the trace minerals, including iron, affected zinc digestibility. There are no studies examining the intake of zinc in the diets of mares and bone development in their offspring.

Manganese deficiency has not been seen in horses. From research in other animals, manganese is known to be involved in several metabolic processes including cartilage formation. Unfortunately, little research on this mineral has been conducted with horses.

Lewis (1995) and other authors stated that because milk is a poor source of trace minerals for the foal, there is no correlation between the amount of copper, iron, and zinc in the mare's diet and levels in the milk. In contrast, iodine and selenium concentrations in milk are correlated with consumption by the mare. However, the source of the trace minerals may have an impact.

A chelated mineral is a type of organic complex that has a specific chemical structure. Minerals are usually chelated to an amino acid to improve uptake by the digestive system. Trace minerals in organic sources are believed to be more available (more easily absorbed from the digestive tract) than inorganic sources. Unfortunately, few experiments have compared organic and inorganic sources of minerals in horse feeds.

A study conducted at the University of Florida (Ott et al., 1994) examined the influence of inorganic or organic trace mineral supplementation of late pregnant mares on the trace mineral status and growth of their foals. Mares were fed from 56 days prior to foaling to weaning at 112 days of age. Trace mineral supplementation of mares had little effect on their serum concentrations, reproductive performance, or weight gains. Supplementation had no impact on foal growth, development, or bone mineral deposition, but foals nursing mares receiving organic copper, zinc, and iron had significantly higher plasma copper levels at 112 days of age and higher zinc levels at 14 days after foaling. It could not be determined if this difference resulted from higher mineral levels in milk or from the foals eating the mare's feed. The beneficial effect on trace mineral levels in the plasma of foals was only noted with chelated minerals; however, the diets were supplemented with relatively low amounts of copper, zinc, manganese, and iron.

Other studies have not shown superior absorption of organic minerals. Organic mineral sources are considerably more expensive than inorganic sources. More research will be necessary to determine whether including organic mineral sources in horse feeds provides enough benefit to justify the additional cost and which classes of horse benefit most significantly from organic supplementation.

Iodine (I) is an essential nutrient for reproduction and normal physiological function in the horse. Thyroxine (T_4) contains iodine and this hormone, along with triiodothyronine (T_3), has powerful effects on the overall health of the horse. These hormones influence nearly every process in the body, from heat regulation and feed utilization to proper bone growth and maturation. Iodine deficiency may result in goiter as the thyroid becomes enlarged in an attempt to produce adequate levels of thyroxine. Goiter often occurs in the foal at birth. Foal goiter may result from a deficiency in iodine in the mare's ration during pregnancy, or it may be caused by a goitrogenic substance. Symptoms of iodine deficiency may be stillbirth or a very weak foal that cannot stand and nurse. The foal may also have a rough hair coat, contracted tendons, angular limb deformities, or other abnormal bone development. There can be dramatic seasonal variation in the iodine intake for grazing animals with low intakes recorded during spring when many mares are in the final stages of pregnancy (Caple, 1991).

While iodine deficiency is the primary cause of goiter in foals, excessive levels of iodine may also cause this condition. The maximal tolerable dietary concentration of iodine has been estimated to be 5 mg/kg (ppm) of dry matter (NRC, 1989), equivalent to 50 mg I/day for a horse consuming 10 kg of dry matter daily. The horses most sensitive to high iodine levels are foals from mares who are supplemented with high levels of iodine. Iodine is concentrated across the placenta and in milk so that the fetus and nursing foal receive much higher concentrations than are present in the mare's ration. Therefore, goiter may be present in newborn foals while sparing the mother. A dietary intake of 83 mg I/day is the lowest level reported to have caused goiter in a horse more mature than a suckling foal (Drew et al., 1975).

Baker and Lindsey (1968) reported that foals with goiter were born on three farms that were feeding mares high levels of iodine. The incidence of goiter was proportional to the level of iodine fed and was 3% on one farm feeding 48-55 mg I/day, 10% on a farm feeding 36-69 mg I/day, and 50% on another farm feeding 288-432 mg I/day. A nearby farm, which did not have any affected foals, fed iodine at a rate of 6.3-7 mg I/day. Drew et al. (1975) reported that on one stud farm in England four foals were born with greatly enlarged thyroids and leg weaknesses. One mare also had an enlarged thyroid. Feed analysis showed that the mares had received 83 mg I/day from a proprietary feed during pregnancy.

The year before the mares received a supplement which supplied about 12 mg I/day, and there was no problem with goiter on the farm.

It appears from these reports that around 50 mg of dietary iodine is required in the daily rations of mares to produce any incidence of goiters in their foals. Toxic dietary iodine concentrations may result from adding excessive supplemental iodine, such as from ethylenediamindihydroiodide (EDDI), to concentrates or from using feedstuffs high in iodine. A common feedstuff that may contain excess iodine is kelp (*Laminariales*), a specific family of seaweeds that may contain as much as 1,850 ppm iodine (NRC, 1989). Unfortunately, people have a tendency to classify all seaweeds as kelp. There are numerous other specific seaweeds that contain considerably less iodine than kelp (Pagan, 2000). The iodine content of seaweed meal and kelp products should be examined prior to feeding to pregnant mares and intake must be carefully controlled.

Selenium (Se) plays an important role in the maintenance of membrane integrity, growth, reproduction, and immune response. A deficiency of selenium in foals may produce white muscle disease, a myopathy which results in weakness, impaired locomotion, difficulty in suckling and swallowing, respiratory distress, and impaired cardiac function (Dill and Rebhun, 1985). Although nutritionists tend to think of selenium as an antioxidant with major roles in immune function and muscle, Hintz (1999) proposed a link between selenium and skeletal disorders. "Kaschin-Beck disease (a chondrodystrophy in men in China) is associated with selenium deficiency. It has also been suggested that the mold Fusarium might also be involved. A toxin extracted from *Fusarium tricenatum* can cause a decrease in collagen microfibroids in chicken embryo chondrocytes. The addition of selenium prevented the decrease (Reilly, 1996). It has been suggested that selenium might help prevent Kaschin-Beck disease by its effect on *Fusarium* in the food (Reilly, 1996). Tibial chondroplasia in growing chicks can be caused by *Fusarium*. Tibial chondroplasia in chicks is similar to osteochondrosis in foals. Would there be a benefit from increasing selenium intake if foals or mares were consuming moldy feed?"

VITAMINS

Vitamin A is best known for its role in vision but also has functions in reproduction, differentiation of epithelial cells, embryogenesis, and growth. Vitamin A is found in abundant quantities in fresh green forages in the form of carotenes, which are converted to vitamin A by enzymes in the intestinal mucosa. Once forage is cut, there is rapid oxidation of carotenes (up to 85% within the first 24 hours and then about 7% per month during storage), which results in hay being practically devoid of carotenes after extended storage (McDowell, 1989). Horses on hay-only diets had depletion of vitamin A liver stores over a relatively short period of time (Fonnesbeck and Symons, 1967; Greiwe-Crandell et al., 1995).

Vitamin A has a distinct role in growth of the horse. Both deficiency and toxicity of vitamin A adversely affect growth, body weight, and rate of gain in young growing ponies (Donoghue et al., 1981). This retardation of growth may have reflected impaired cell proliferation and differentiation. Bone remodeling is modulated by vitamin A in the growing animal. Vitamin A's role in bone remodeling is in the proper functioning of osteoclasts, the bone cells responsible for resorption of bone. Without sufficient vitamin A, excessive deposition of periosteal bone occurs. Vitamin A deficiency causes bones to be shorter and thicker than normal (Fell and Mellanby, 1950). This is in part caused by the dysfunction of osteoclasts but also by a reduction in the degradation of glycosaminoglycans and the synthesis of proteoglycans also caused by deficiency (Dingle et al., 1972).

It is possible that some of the systemic effects of vitamin A on growth, as well as the poor growth usually associated with vitamin A deficiency, are related to its effects on growth hormone secretion. Vitamin A takes different functional forms once it is working in the body, one of which is retinoic acid, which has been found to affect growth hormone regulation (Sporn et al.,1994). Retinoic acid can synergize with either thyroid hormone or glucocorticoids to enhance the transcriptional activity of the growth hormone gene and subsequently of growth hormone secretion from cells (Bedo et al., 1989). Retinoic acid is also essential for embroyonic development during pregnancy.

For horses grazing sufficient quantities of green pastures, their vitamin A requirement can be met entirely by the carotenes in the forage (Greiwe-Crandell et al., 1997a). In northern states and countries, vitamin A supplementation is particularly important because of the short growing season of grasses. Depletion of vitamin A reserves in pregnant mares was found within two months of a diet of hay and vitamin A-free concentrate. Subsequent supplementation of vitamin A palmitate at two times the NRC recommended level was not adequate to completely replete stores of vitamin A in mares with no access to pasture (Greiwe-Crandell et al., 1997a). Mares with access to green pastures had adequate liver stores of vitamin A regardless of vitamin A supplementation. Additional vitamin A palmitate did not induce any excesses of vitamin A in liver or serum (Greiwe-Crandell et al., 1997a). Further investigation on ß-carotene found carotenes in grass readily available as a source of vitamin A, but synthetic ß-carotene was not readily absorbed. Use of synthetic ß-carotene as a sole source of vitamin A could not meet vitamin A requirements of horses and is not recommended (Greiwe-Crandell et al., 1997b). Vitamin A has been found to be of critical importance to the late pregnant mare. Studies by Greiwe-Crandell (unpublished) showed that if mares are maintained on hay alone with no green pasture and no vitamin A supplementation, the subsequent growth rates of their foals are significantly reduced up until 12 months of age compared to foals of mares with adequate vitamin A intake.

Vitamin D is known as the sunshine vitamin since it is made on the skin from 7-dehydrocholesterol by a reaction catalyzed by ultraviolet (UV) light. The function of vitamin D is maintenance of calcium homeostasis in the blood (McDowell, 1989). Circulating calcium is used for normal mineralization of bone as well as for a host of other body functions. Parathyroid hormone (PTH) and calcitonin function with vitamin D to control blood calcium and phosphorus concentrations. When blood calcium is low, the parathyroid is stimulated to release PTH. PTH travels to the kidney and stimulates conversion of 25-OH vitamin D to form the active vitamin (1,25 OH vitamin D). Active vitamin D then stimulates intestinal calcium uptake, stimulates bone mineral release, and stimulates resorption of calcium by the kidney, all in an effort to restore blood calcium levels (Linder, 1991). Calcitonin regulates high serum calcium by depressing gut absorption, halting bone demineralization, and slowing resorption in the kidney.

Since vitamin D is readily synthesized and absorbed from the skin, is it necessary to supplement vitamin D in the diet? In modern horse production systems, show horses are often kept out of the sunlight to prevent dulling of the hair coat. For horses not exposed to sunlight or artificial light with an emission spectrum of 280-315 nm, the NRC (1989) has established a requirement for dietary vitamin D. Pregnant and lactating mares require 800 IU of vitamin D per kg of diet dry matter according to the NRC (1989). The actual vitamin D intake would likely be less than calculated since vitamin D is lost at a rate of 7.5% per month with hay storage (Lewis, 1995).

Vitamin D should not be given in an effort to treat developmental orthopedic disease (DOD) by increasing calcium and phosphorus absorption and bone mineralization. DOD has not been shown to be caused by vitamin D deficiency and supplementation with vitamin D will not make up for diets that are not properly fortified with calcium and phosphorus. Oversupplementation of vitamin D to horses is toxic and results in extensive mineralization of cardiovascular and other soft tissues (Harrington and Page, 1983). Care should be taken to remain well below the maximum tolerance level (2200 IU/kg diet) established by the NRC in 1989.

Vitamin K was the last fat-soluble vitamin to be discovered (McDowell, 1989). For many years, vitamin K has been known for its blood-clotting function. Recently, the carboxyglutamyl residues have been found in other proteins associated with a variety of tissues. Most notable is osteocalcin, a protein involved in bone metabolism. Osteocalcin is responsible for binding to hydroxyapatite and facilitating bone mineralization. Undercarboxylated osteocalcin does not bind hydroxyapatite with the same affinity as carboxylated osteocalcin (Knapen et al., 1989). If vitamin K is in short supply, one would expect to find irregularities in blood clotting along with undercarboxylated osteocalcin. However, it is suspected that osteocalcin is more sensitive to low vitamin K activity than are the blood-clotting proteins (Duren and Crandell, 1989). Therefore, it seems possible that bone tissue may be vitamin K deficient, while liver, and thus the blood-clotting mechanism, is vitamin K adequate. If vitamin K has a positive effect on net bone formation, it might be expected that vitamin K antagonists (coumarin) have an opposite effect. Pastoreau et al. (1993) reported that lambs treated with vitamin K antagonists (warfarin) had strongly decreased bone formation indicated by a 30% lower bone mass in three months compared to controls. A deficiency in vitamin K would be expected also to have negative consequences for bone health.

The NRC (1989) has not established requirements for vitamin K fortification of equine diets. Natural sources of vitamin K are phylloquinone, found in green leafy plants, and menaquinone, which is produced by bacteria in the digestive system. Both phylloquinone and menaquinone are converted to the active vitamin (hydroquinone) in the liver (Lewis, 1995). The NRC (1989) states that if the intake or intestinal synthesis of vitamin K is inadequate, horses will have an increased susceptibility to hemorrhage. With new functions of vitamin K being explored, the previous statement may no longer be true. With current research interest, look for nutrient requirements for vitamin K in horse diets in the near future. At the present time, the NRC (1989) indicates that oral intake of phylloquinone and menadione appears to be essentially innocuous in horses.

Feeding Practices

BODY CONDITION

One of the most important aspects of broodmare nutrition is keeping the mare out of negative energy balance and preventing significant loss of body condition. Mares have an optimum body condition and are probably most efficient when kept at or near that condition. Establishment of the ideal condition comes from a combination of visually appraising the mare's condition and recording her body weight over time. Mares can differ in shape and weight and be remarkably similar in condition. Mares in optimum condition should have adequate fat over the ribs, behind the shoulder, and over the topline. Ribs should be covered and not easily seen but should be readily palpated. Once the optimum condition is determined, it should be maintained as a minimal acceptable condition. There are times when maintaining this condition requires a lot of feed and other times when little feed is required.

A number of studies have demonstrated the link between body fat content, body condition scores, and fertility. Although reproductive efficiency will be enhanced if mares are kept in a body condition score range from 3 to 4.5, it has been suggested that obesity may lead to a reduced milk output (Kubiak et al., 1991). Mares should be managed to keep them in body condition scores of less than 4.5 to maintain milk production and prevent metabolic disorders such as laminitis. A body condition scoring system of 0 to 5 has been developed for use in Australia (Figure 1) (Huntington, 1991). The Texan 1-9 system is used in other countries.

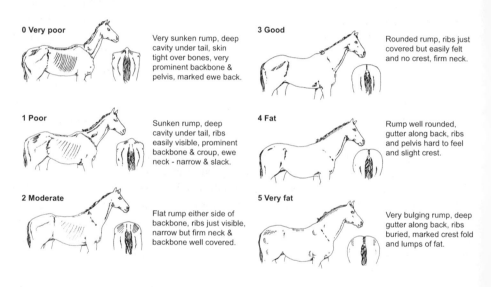

0 Very poor
Very sunken rump, deep cavity under tail, skin tight over bones, very prominent backbone & pelvis, marked ewe back.

1 Poor
Sunken rump, deep cavity under tail, ribs easily visible, prominent backbone & croup, ewe neck - narrow & slack.

2 Moderate
Flat rump either side of backbone, ribs just visible, narrow but firm neck & backbone well covered.

3 Good
Rounded rump, ribs just covered but easily felt and no crest, firm neck.

4 Fat
Rump well rounded, gutter along back, ribs and pelvis hard to feel and slight crest.

5 Very fat
Very bulging rump, deep gutter along back, ribs buried, marked crest fold and lumps of fat.

Figure 1. Body condition scoring system.

The effect of loss of body condition on reproductive performance is well documented. For this reason it is undesirable to send mares to stud too fat. The combination of a change of environment, pecking order, and feeding program may cause a mare to lose weight and reproductive efficiency. The only safe time to adjust a mare's body weight by diet is between weaning and the last 3 months of pregnancy.

There is anecdotal evidence that fat late pregnant mares have a greater incidence of delivering foals with angular limb deformities (ALD). In an Australian case report, a very high incidence of ALD was related to excessive energy intake in a group of thin mares, which led them to be obese at the time of foaling (Mason, 1981). It has been speculated that this relates to excessive internal fat in the mare leading to compression of movement of the foal in utero, but this seems an unlikely reason. Hormonal changes related to obesity such as insulin resistance may be more relevant explanations. Exercise is important for all horses and obese mares appear to move around paddocks less than mares that are not carrying an extra 100 kg of fat. This tends to perpetuate the obesity as energy consumption by exercise is reduced. Breeders should provide late pregnant mares with adequate opportunities for free-choice exercise. Hills are desirable as they increase the intensity of exercise but are not always available on horse farms. In some situations fat pregnant or barren mares would benefit from forced exercise on automatic walkers. While exercise is desirable, a study by Sparks (1999) showed that restriction of movement during pregnancy did not change the birth weights of foals when compared to mares allowed free exercise.

How much weight should a mare gain in pregnancy? Powell et al. (1989) showed that Quarter Horse mares gained 90 kg from day 65 to day 305 of pregnancy. Mares gained fat to day 205, were static during day 205 to 275, and lost weight in the last month of the study. In late pregnancy, the uterus and the growing foal consume 70% of the mare's blood glucose utilization (Rossdale and Ousey, 2002), and this is why some mares will lose weight in the last month before foaling. Very thin mares have been noted to reduce milk production and foal growth rate (Pagan et al., 1984; Gill et al., 1985; Doreau and Boulet, 1987), so keeping mares in good condition is desirable.

Although a few studs weigh their pregnant mares, it would appear to be desirable for mares to gain weight in late pregnancy. Studies conducted at Lindsay Park Stud (Baker, personal communication) have shown that early-foaling mares gained an average of 40 kg in the last 2 months while later foaling mares gained an average of 80 kg. The lower weight gain in the early-foaling mares was associated with changes in pasture quantity and quality and weather conditions during late winter compared with spring. It was also associated with lower birth weights, faster growth, and a higher incidence of valgus deformities of the knee. When management practices were changed to increase weight gain, this incidence of ALD in the foals born in August and early September was reduced. This change in management practices involved feeding greater amounts of a balanced concentrate feed so the mare would have received more energy, protein, and minerals. In contrast to these findings, Liu et al. (1984) have reviewed work from the United States and concluded that mares in good condition do not need to gain significant amounts of weight during late pregnancy in order to produce healthy foals.

FORAGES - PASTURE, HAY, AND CHAFF

Although the horse has evolved as a pasture-reared animal, the growth rate and reproductive efficiency of horses demanded by breeders means that many horses cannot be reared on pasture alone. However, it is desirable that the contribution to the diet of growing horses and mares made by pasture, chaff, and hay is maximized as horses are healthiest when fed a simple forage-based diet. Supplementation with concentrates or supplements is necessary to correct various nutrient deficiencies in forage.

To calculate accurately the contribution that forage makes to the horse's overall feeding program, forage intake as well as composition must be known. Weighing a dipper or using average figures can calculate chaff intake. Hay intake can be determined by simply recording the total weight of hay offered minus any hay wasted or refused. This does not take into account the differences in composition between hay that is eaten and hay that is wasted, but is accurate enough to do a good evaluation in the field.

The 1989 NRC gives estimates of forage and concentrate intakes based on the body weight of the animal and as a percentage of the total diet (Table 3). These figures can be used to establish reasonable concentrate and forage intakes for different classes of horses. Pasture intake is more difficult to estimate. Pasture intake will vary depending on the season, species, quality of pasture grazed, and the total amount of time that horses are allowed to graze. Another factor that has not been thoroughly studied is the effect that supplemental grain feeding has on pasture intake. Is pasture intake limited physically by the amount of time that a horse has to graze, or does the animal's total energy requirement dictate intake?

Table 3. Expected feed consumption by horses.

| | *% of body weight* | | *% of diet* | |
	Forage	*Concentrate*	*Forage*	*Concentrate*
Horse				
Maintenance/early pregnancy	1.5-2.0	0-0.5	100	0
Late pregnancy	1.0-1.5	0.5-1.0	70	30
Early lactation	1.0-2.0	1.0-2.0	50	50
Late lactation	1.0-2.0	0.5-1.5	65	35
Young horses				
Weanling	0.5-1.0	1.5-3.0	30	70
Yearling	1.0-1.5	1.0-2.0	40	60

Several studies have evaluated pasture intake (Table 4). Moffitt et al. (1987) estimated grazing forage dry matter intakes for ten 2-year-old horses during December, May, and August to be 9.6 kg, but younger horses have been shown to consume less pasture than mature mares. This may be one reason why maiden mares often struggle to maintain condition.

Table 4. Estimates of pasture dry matter intake by horses.

Class of horse	Pasture	Intake/hr (lb)	Duration (hrs)
Mature horse	Fescue	3.30	3
Mature horse	Alfalfa	3.63	3
2-year-old	Fescue	0.91	24
2-year-old	Orchard grass	0.85	24

Actual pasture intakes may be 4 to 7 times the dry matter intake as some green pastures can be only 15-25% dry matter.

In Australia, Martin et al. (1989) studied pasture intake of mares and found that late pregnant mares consumed pasture at the rate of 1.6% body weight (DM) while lactating mares ate 2.3% body weight (DM). Provision of 2 kg/d of a concentrate pellet resulted in reduced pasture intake. There is no doubt lactating mares can eat large amounts of pasture as mares of certain breeds can produce enough milk for rapid growth in their foals while on pasture alone. These mares are producing 3-4% of their body weight in milk and are probably consuming a similar quantity of pasture dry matter. Obviously the quality and quantity of pasture available have a significant bearing on the consumption level and the ability of the mare to produce enough milk on pasture alone.

Unlike horse breeders in New Zealand and the United States, many Australian breeders pay little attention to pasture analysis. The relevance of pasture analysis is to pinpoint nutrient deficiencies, which need to be determined so appropriate levels of mineral supplementation can be offered. Most pastures have higher calcium than phosphorus levels, a situation that matches the requirements of the horse. Of particular relevance to skeletal development is the low calcium and high phosphorus levels combined with very low availability of calcium in high-oxalate pastures such as kikuyu. Reversals of the normal calcium to phosphorus ratio can occur on a temporary basis in certain pasture types in late winter and early spring. The level of copper and zinc supplementation needed in late pregnancy can be determined best by pasture analysis at the relevant time of year.

THE BARREN AND EARLY PREGNANT NON-LACTATING MARE

Both of these classes of mares have the same nutrient requirements as the mature horse at maintenance (Table 1). The most common mistake made in feeding broodmares is overfeeding the early pregnant mare. About 80% of the growth of the foal in the pregnant mare occurs in the last 4 months of pregnancy. The goal for the early pregnant mares should be to maintain body condition. If good-quality pasture or hay is available, the normal mare should need no supplementary feed other than a trace-mineralized supplement and a salt block. Warmblood mares and other easy keepers do not need grain in most situations, as their efficient metabolism allows them to consume lower amounts of energy for maintenance (Table 2). Obviously, if pasture is limited or if hay is in short supply, pellets, grain, or sweet feed may be used to effectively meet the mare's energy needs. Another factor is weather; if winter rain and cold are factors, supplementary energy may be required. Intakes vary but should not exceed 3 kg concentrates for the average mare. Higher intakes may be needed if a gain in condition is desired and mares should be grouped accordingly. The mare should not put on too much weight in early pregnancy.

Many dry and early pregnant mares are fed a diet that does not contain any supplementary minerals or vitamins. While this diet will result in theoretical nutrient deficiencies, it does appear that mares, if they have access to some green pasture, can reproduce efficiently and have foals that develop normally under these conditions.

However, under dry conditions (summer or winter), the intake of vitamin A from pasture declines dramatically and added vitamin A from a feed or supplement may be needed. At this time it is likely that mares will be "hard fed" (fed a concentrate). Most, but not all, prepared feeds and supplements contain enough added vitamin A, and supplementary hay, provided it is fresh and has retained its vitamin A content, will also help add vitamin A to the diet.

THE MARE IN LATE PREGNANCY

As the mare enters the ninth month of pregnancy, her nutrient needs increase significantly because of the demands of rapidly increasing fetal growth. She needs more energy, protein, minerals, and vitamins than the early pregnant mare (Table 1). If the diet does not supply adequate nutrients for fetal growth then the mare can utilize her own reserves to an extent, but it would appear that these diets can also cause an increase in the incidence of developmental orthopedic disease. Some of these disorders may not present until after weaning, but the feeding of the mare in late pregnancy can have a major impact on the wastage rate and the development in young horses. One of the critical areas relates to trace mineral nutrition, as milk is a very poor source of trace minerals and the foal needs to store trace minerals in its liver to cope with the deprivation that occurs while it is on a milk-based diet.

Although the late pregnant mare is able to meet her energy needs from forage alone if she is grazing suitable pasture and hay, she is unable to meet her other nutrient requirements in this manner. If an abundant supply of good-quality pasture is available, one may feed a mare 1 kg of a 20-25% protein concentrate pellet that contains added minerals to meet the mare's nutrient needs. Clearly, this would apply more to the early foaling mare and breeds that hold condition well, as pasture availability may become marginal during the late autumn and throughout the winter.

A more common manner of meeting the late pregnant mare's nutrient needs is to provide her with 3-5 kg/d of a 13-15% protein feed such as that described in Table 5, so the mare is required to meet a smaller percentage of her nutrient needs with forage. If abundant grass, hay, or both are available, the mare fed in this manner will probably gain weight. The protein content of the pasture will determine the specific protein level required in the concentrate. A critical aspect of this phase of the nutritional management of the mare is to maintain body condition and perhaps even slightly increase fat stores.

Protein quality becomes an important issue in late pregnancy as birth weight can have a significant impact on the eventual body size or growth rate of the foal. The amino acid that is most likely to be deficient in the mare's diet is lysine. Lysine content in the protein of cereal grains and many other protein sources such as cottonseed meal and linseed meal is low. Lysine is plentiful in the protein from milk products and soybean meal. Therefore, it is important that the mare receives feeds that include plenty of lysine for proper fetal growth. In the last four months of pregnancy, the equine fetus will deposit about 8 kg of protein as it grows to an average birth weight of 55 kg. During the last month of pregnancy the fetus will deposit over 3 kg of protein into its body. If people are mixing their own feeds, then they should use soybean meal as the protein supplement of choice in late pregnancy or use a supplement pellet or a concentrate that has high lysine content (Table 5). The hay of choice for the late pregnant mare is obviously a legume, lucerne (alfalfa) or clover hay that has a high protein and lysine content.

The first foal of a mare is often smaller than subsequent foals. French research has identified that first foaling mares ate 10% less feed than multiparous mares, and the resulting foals were 10% lighter (Doreau et al., 1991). This difference in nutrient intake can be addressed by paying special attention to feeding of the late pregnant mare that is foaling for the first time. Older mares also benefit from the same individual attention.

Table 5. Key nutrient specifications of feeds for mares.

Nutrient feed intake	Balancer 1 kg	Mare feed 3 kg-7 kg
Protein (%)	20-25	13-15
Lysine (%)	1.5	0.7-0.75
DE (MJ/kg)	11	12.5
Calcium (%)	3.0	0.8
Phosphorus (%)	2.0	0.6
Magnesium (%)	1.0	0.25
Zinc (mg/kg)	400	120
Copper (mg/kg)	150	45

Selenium and iodine deficiencies in pasture can be regional in origin and can result in white muscle disease and hypothyroidism respectively in young foals. Both of these disorders are uncommon but in areas where selenium and iodine deficiency occurs, horse owners need to pay particular attention to the selenium and iodine content of a supplement or a feed.

THE LACTATING MARE

With the exception of the racehorse in heavy training, the lactating mare has the highest nutrient requirements of any class of horse. Although the mare has never been selected on the basis of her ability to produce milk, she actually does a very good job of it. Mares are thought to produce 3-4% and 2% of their body weight per day in early and late lactation, respectively. This milk production represents a significant daily secretion of nutrients by the mare. The amount of secreted energy, protein, vitamins, and minerals leads to an increased dietary requirement for these nutrients. In most parts of the world, it is doubtful that the Thoroughbred or Standardbred mare can do an acceptable job of raising a foal, conceiving, and maintaining a new pregnancy on pasture alone, so supplementary feeding will be needed. However, in countries like New Zealand, temperate climates and magnificent pastures mean that many mares do not require feeding to supply energy and protein needs for lactation. Other breeds such as warmbloods, Quarter Horses, and ponies do not need feeding unless pastures are very poor.

Unlike the late pregnant mare, energy intake is critical to the lactating mare. Therefore, a more appropriate feeding regime includes the use of a high-quality, energy-dense feed, such as the 13-15% protein feed previously discussed (Table 5). Assuming a minimal forage intake of 1.5% of body weight per day, practical ranges in feed intake are from 3.5-7 kg.

The extreme range seen in feed intakes of lactating mares points to the variability in the proportion of the mare's nutrient needs that is met by forage. As with other classes of mares, one should carefully monitor the condition of individuals. If mares are getting too thin, increase their feed. If they are getting fat, decrease it. Remember that many feeds designed for broodmares are formulated with Thoroughbred mares in mind. Feeding rates for other breeds (especially those breeds renowned for being able to survive on next to nothing) can be significantly lower than levels suggested for Thoroughbreds. In fact, some mares can survive on only pasture and a vitamin and mineral supplement, even when lactating, without any detriment to the foal or loss of condition.

Once again, lucerne hay or chaff or clover hay are the forages of choice for the lactating mare. Legume hay has a higher protein and energy content than grass hay. If grass hay or chaff is fed in large quantities, allowances need to be made in the formulation of a compatible concentrate. If the breeder is mixing his own feed, he needs to add some supplementary protein to the grains used. Oats will generally be the staple grain and supplementary protein can generally come from soybean meal, full-fat soybean meal, or lupins. Commercial balancers and concentrate that supply protein are also used. There is a practical limit to the intake of soybean meal per day and this is about 500 g. There are benefits to using pelleted concentrates or those that don't leave any fines in the feed bins. If mares are receiving more than 3 kg of concentrate feed per day, they should be fed twice a day. This also provides another opportunity for early detection of illness or disease in foals. Pellets are an economical alternative for feeding lactating mares, but only use pellets that are designed for mares.

One of the determining factors in the decision to creep feed foals revolves around the nutrient content of the mare's feed. If a suitable fortified feed is used, it may be preferable to provide enough feed so that the foal can eat with the mare. On the other hand, if pasture grasses are plentiful or if the supplement for the mare is just oats or unfortified grains, then a creep feed is more desirable. Foals and weanlings need more concentrated feeds than mares because they are growing rapidly and have restricted appetites.

Although the economics of feeding fat to lactating mares does not justify its widespread use, adding fat to the diet from oil, sunflower seeds, or rice bran can assist in maintaining a positive energy balance in the lactating mare. The fat content of prepared feeds is on the label or oil can be added to the feed. Remember that 2 cups of oil supplies about the same amount of energy as 1.2 kg of oats and could be a valuable aid in feeding the mare that is producing a large quantity of milk and losing weight.

Lactating mares require large amounts of quality protein. The lactating mare needs twice as much protein as the dry mare because a mare's milk is high in protein and contains 20-25% protein on a dry basis. Milk protein is high in lysine, and the mare requires high-quality protein in her diet to produce it. In fact, the quickest way to decrease milk production in a mare is to restrict her protein intake but this can cause a decrease in foal growth. Sometimes this strategy is useful with mares that milk too well and foals that are growing too fast; however, dietary restriction needs to be managed carefully in the mare that is being bred again that season. Mares that are in a negative energy balance will be less reproductively efficient, and while an improvement in the growth of the current foal may occur, conception may be hampered. It would be nice to find a method to reduce milk production without impacting reproduction.

Trace mineral fortification is not as important for lactating mares as for late pregnant mares because milk contains low levels of these nutrients. Research has shown that adding more to the lactating mare's diet does not increase the trace mineral content of the milk. Calcium and phosphorus are the minerals of prime concern at this stage. If the foal is sharing the mare's feed bin, however, appropriate trace mineral fortification would be valuable.

In summary, the critical aspect of feeding the broodmare is maintaining the mare in good condition by meeting her energy needs while ensuring that her protein, vitamin, and mineral intakes are appropriate for the stage in the reproductive cycle.

Most studs pay much more attention to feeding the young growing horse than the broodmare, yet an increased focus on the broodmare could increase fertility and produce better young horses.

References

Baker, H.J., and J.R. Lindsey. 1968. Equine goiter due to excess dietary iodine. J. Amer. Vet. Med. Assoc. 153:1618.

Baker, L.A., D.R. Topliff, R.G. Freeman, et al. 1993. Effect of dietary cation-anion balance on urinary mineral excretion in horses. In: Proc. Equine Nutr. Physiol. Soc. Symp. 13:44-49.

Bedo, G., P. Santisteban, and A. Aranda. 1989. Retinoic acid regulates growth hormone gene expression. Nature 339:231.

Bridges, C.H., and P.G. Moffitt. 1990. Influence of variable content of dietary zinc on copper metabolism of weanling foals. Amer. J. Vet. Res. 51:275-280.

Caple, I. 1991. Disorders of mineral nutrition in horses in Australia. In: Equine Nutr. Proc. 181 Post Grad. Comm. Vet. Sci. Sydney, 3-13.

Coger, L.S., H.F. Hintz, H.F. Schryver, and J.E. Lowe. 1987. The effect of high zinc intake on copper metabolism and bone development in growing horses. In: Proc. Equine Nutr. Physiol. Soc. Symp. 10:173-177.

Cymbaluk, N.F., H.F. Schryver, and H.F. Hintz. 1981. Influence of dietary molybdenum on copper metabolism in ponies. J. Nutr. 111:96-106.

Davidson K.E., G.D. Potter, L.W. Greene, et al. 1991. Lactation and reproductive performance of mares fed added dietary fat during late gestation and early lactation. J. Equine Vet. Sci. 11:111.

Dill, S.G., and W.C. Rebhun. 1985. White muscle disease in foals. Comp. Cont. Ed. 7:S627.

Dingle, J.T., H.B. Fell, and D.S. Goodman. 1972. The effect of retinol and retinal binding protein on embryonic skeletal tissue in organ culture. J. Cell Sci. 11:393.

Donoghue, S., T.N. Meacham, and D.S. Kronfeld. 1990. A conceptual approach to optimal nutrition of broodmares. Vet. Clinics North Amer. Equine Pract. 6:373-390.

Donoghue, S., D.S. Kronfeld, S.J. Berkowitz, and R.L. Copp. 1981. Vitamin A nutrition of the equine: Growth, serum biochemistry, and hematology. J. Nutr. 111:365.

Doreau, M., and S. Boulot. 1987. Milk yield and composition in mares either fat or thin at foaling. In: Proc. Equine Nutr. Physiol. Soc. Symp.

Doreau, M., S. Boulot, and W. Martin Rossett. 1991 Effect of parity and physiological state on intake, milk production, and blood parameters in lactating mares differing in body size. Anim. Prod. 53:111-118.

Drepper, K., J.O. Gutte, H. Meyer, and F.J. Schwarz. 1982. Energie und Nahrstoffbedard landwirtschaftylicher Nutztiere. Nr 2 Empfehlungen zur Energieund Nahrstoffversorgung der pferde. Frankfurt am main, Germany: DLG Verlag.

Drew, B., W.P. Barber, and D.G. Williams. 1975. The effect of excess iodine on pregnant mares and foals. Vet. Rec. 97:93.

Driscoll, J., H.F. Hintz, and H.F. Schryver. 1978. Goiter in foals caused by excess iodine. J. Amer. Vet. Med. Assoc. 173:858.

Fell, H.B., and E. Mellanby. 1950. Effect of hypervitaminosis on fetal mouse bone cultivated in vitro. Br. J. Med. 2:535.

Fonnesbeck, R.V., and L.D. Symons. 1967. Utilization of the carotene of hay by horses. J. Anim. Sci. 26:1030.

Food and Drug Administration. 1987. Food additives permitted in feed and drinking water of animals. Fed. Reg. 52 (Part 573, No. 65):10887.

Frape, D. 1998. Equine Nutrition and Feeding. (2nd Ed.). Blackwell Science Ltd., UK.

Frey, K.S., G.D. Potter, T.W. Odom, et al. 1991. Plasma silicon and radiographic bone density in weanling Quarter Horses fed sodium zeolite A. J. Equine Vet. Sci. 12:292-296.

Gatta, D., P. Krusic, S. Schramel, et al. 2001. Influence on corrected teeth on digestibility of macro-minerals and micro-minerals in pregnant mares. In: Proc. Equine Nutr. Physiol. Soc. Symp. 17:482-485.

Gentry, L.R., D.L. Thompson, G.T. Gentry, et al. 2002. The relationship between body condition, leptin, and reproductive and hormonal characteristics of mares during the seasonal anovulatory period. J. Anim. Sci. 80:2695-2703.

Gill R.J., G.P. Potter, J.L. Krieder, et al. 1985. Nitrogen status and postpartum LH levels of mares fed varying levels of protein. In: Proc. Equine Nutr. Physiol. Soc. Symp. 9:84-89.

Glade, M.J. 1993. Equine osteochondrosis in the 90's. J. Equine Vet. Sci. 13:14.

Glade, M.J., and N.K. Luba. 1990. Benefits to foals of feeding soybean meal to lactating mares J. Equine Vet. Sci., 10:422-428.

Grace, N.D., S.G. Pearce, E.C. Firth, and P.F. Fennessy. 1999. Concentrations of macromineral and micromineral elements in the milk of pasture-fed Thoroughbred mares. Aust. Vet. J. 77:177-180.

Greiwe-Crandell, K.M., D.S. Kronfeld, L.A. Gay, and D. Sklan. 1995. Seasonal vitamin A depletion in grazing horses is assessed better by the relative dose response test than by serum retinol concentration. J. Nutr. 125:2711.

Greiwe-Crandell, K.M., D.S. Kronfeld, L.A. Gay, D. Sklan, and P.A. Harris. 1997b. Daily beta-carotene supplementation of vitamin A depleted mares. In: Proc. Equine Nutr. Physiol. Soc. Symp. 15:378.

Greiwe-Crandell, K.M., D.S. Kronfeld, L.A. Gay, D. Sklan, W. Tiegs, and P.A. Harris. 1997a. Vitamin A repletion in Thoroughbred mares with retinyl palmitate or beta-carotene. J. Anim. Sci. 7:2684.

Griewe-Crandell, K.M., D.S. Kronfeld, G.A. Morrow, and W. Tiego. 1993. Vitamin A depletion in Thoroughbreds: A comparison of pasture and non-pasture feeding regimes. In: Proc. Equine Nutr. Physiol. Soc. Symp. 13:2.

Harrington, D.D., and E.H. Page. 1983. Acute vitamin D_3 toxicosis in horses: Case reports and experimental studies of the comparative toxicity of vitamins D_2 and D_3. J. Amer. Vet. Med. Assoc. 182:1358.

Hintz, H. 1999. The many phases of selenium. In: Proc. Kentucky Equine Research Nutrition Conference for Feed Manufacturers. 9:73-80.

Hintz, H. 2000. Macrominerals: Calcium, phosphorus and magnesium. In: Proc. Kentucky Equine Research Nutrition Conference for Feed Manufacturers. 10:121-131.

Hintz, H.F., R.L. Hintz, and L.D. van Vleck. 1989. Growth rate of Thoroughbreds: Effects of age of dam, year and month of birth, and sex of foal. J. Anim. Sci. 48:480-487.

Hoffman, R.M., D.S. Kronfield, L.A. Lawrence, W.L. Cooper, J.J. Danscario, and P.A. Harris. 1996. Dietary starch and sugar verses fat and fibre, growth and development of foals. Pferdeheilkunde. 12:312-316.

Huntington, P.J. 1991. Field estimation of body condition and weight. In: Equine Nutr. Proc. 181 Post Grad. Comm. Vet. Sci. 15-23.

Hurtig, M.B., S.L. Green, H. Dobson, Y. Mikuni-Takagaki, and J. Choi. 1993. Correlative study of defective cartilage and bone growth in foals fed a low-copper diet. Equine Vet. J. Suppl. 16:66-73.

Jackson, S.G., and J.D. Pagan. 1992. Equine nutrition: A practitioner's guide. In: Proc. Amer. Assoc. Equine Practnr. 37:409-432.

Knapen, M.H., J.K. Hamulyak, and C. Vermeer. 1989. The effect of vitamin K supplementation on circulating osteocalcin (bone Gla-protein) and urinary calcium excretion. Ann. Intern. Med. 111:1001.

Knight D.A, S.E. Weibroke, L.M. Schmall, et al. 1987. Copper supplementation and cartilage lesions in foals. In: Proc. Amer. Assoc. Equine Practnr. 33:191.

Knight, D.A, S.E Weisbrode, L.M Schmall, S.M Reed, A.A Gabel, L.R Bramlage, and W.I. Tyznik. 1990. The effects of copper supplementation on the prevalence of cartilage lesions in foals. Equine Vet. J. 22:426-432.

Kubiak, J.R., J.W. Evans, G.D. Potter, P.G. Harms, and W.L. Jenkins. 1991. Milk yield and composition in the multiparous mare fed to obesity. J. Equine Vet. Sci. 11:158.

Lewis, L.D. 1995. Equine Clinical Nutrition: Feeding and Care. Williams and Wilkins, Media, Pennsylvania.

Linder, M.C. 1991. Nutritional Biochemistry and Metabolism with Clinical Applications. Appleton and Lance. Norwalk, Connecticut.

Lui, P., C. Collyer, and H.F. Hintz. 1984. Body weights of mares in late gestation. Equine Pract. 16:13.

Martin, R.G., N.P. McMeniman, and K.F. Dowsett. 1989. Pasture intake of pregnant and lactating mares in South East Queensland. In: Proc. Equine Nutr. Physiol. Soc. Symp. 11:176-177.

Martin, K.L., R.M. Hoffman, and D.S. Kronfield. 1996. Calcium decreases and parathyroid hormone increases in the serum of periparturient mares. J. Anim. Sci. 74:834-839.

Mason, T.A. 1981. A high incidence of congenital angular limb deformities in a group of foals. Vet. Rec. 109:93.

McDowell, L.R. 1989. Vitamins In Animal Nutrition: Comparative Aspects to Human Nutrition. Academic Press, San Diego, California.

Moffit, D.L., T.N. Meacham, J.P. Fonternot, et al. 1987. Seasonal differences in apparent digestibilities of fescue and orchard grass/clover pastures. In: Proc. Equine Nutr. Physiol. Soc. Symp. 10:79-86.

NRC. 1980. Mineral tolerance of domestic animals. National Academy Press, Washington DC.

NRC. 1989. Nutrient Requirements of Horses (5th Ed.) National Academy Press, Washington DC.

Ott, E.A., and R.L. Asquith. 1987. The influence of trace mineral supplementation on growth and bone development of yearling horses. In: Proc. Equine Nutr. Physiol. Soc. Symp. 10:185-192.

Ott. E.A., and R.L. Asquith. 1994. Trace mineral supplementation of mares. J. Equine Vet. Sci. 14:93.

Pagan, J.D. 2000. Micromineral requirements in horses. In: Proc. Kentucky Equine Research Nutrition Conference for Feed Manufacturers. 9:107-119.

Pagan, J.D. 1998a. Nutrient digestibility in horses. In: J.D. Pagan (Ed.) Advances in Equine Nutrition. pp. 77-83. Nottingham University Press, United Kingdom.

Pagan, J.D. 1998b. Factors affecting mineral digestibility in horses. In: Proc. Kentucky Equine Research Nutrition Conference for Feed Manufacturers. 7:89-104.

Pagan, J.D., H.F. Hintz, and T.R. Rounsaville. 1984.The digestible energy requirements of lactating pony mares. J. Anim. Sci. 58:1382-1387.

Pastoureau, P., P. Vergnaud, P. Meunier, and P.D. Delmas. 1993. Osteopenia and bone remodeling abnormalities in warfarin-treated lambs. J. Bone Miner. Res. 8:1417

Pearce, S.G., E.C. Firth, N.D. Grace, and P.F. Fennessy. 1998a. Effect of copper supplementation on the evidence of developmental orthopedic disease in pasture-fed New Zealand Thoroughbreds. Equine Vet. J. 30:211-218.

Pearce, S.G., N.D. Grace, E.C. Firth, J.J. Wichtel, S.A. Holle, and P.F. Fennessy. 1998b. Effect of copper supplementation on the copper status of pasture-fed young Thoroughbreds. Equine Vet. J. 30:204-210.

Powell, D.M., L.M. Lawrence, and S. Hayes. 2003. Effect of dietary restriction and exercise on prolactin response to a thyrotropin releasing hormone challenge. Proc. Equine Nutr. Physiol. Soc. Symp. 18:271-272.

Powell, D.M., L.M. Lawrence, D.F. Parrett, et al. 1989. Body composition changes in brood-mares. In: Proc. Equine Nutr. Physiol. Soc. Symp. 11:91-94.

Reilly, C. 1996. Selenium in food and health. Blackie Academic, London.

Rossdale, P.D., and J.C. Ousey. 2002. Foetal programming for athletic performance in the horse: Potential effects of IUGR. Equine Vet. Ed. 4:127-142.

Schryver, H.F., O.T. Oftedal, J. Williams, et al. 1986. Lactation in the horse: The mineral composition of a mare's milk. J. Nutr. 116:2142-2147.

Sipple, W.L. 1969. A veterinarian's approach to stud farm nutrition. Equine Vet. J. 1:203.

Sparks, C.R., M.E. Topliff, D.W. Freeman, and J.E. Breazile. 1999. The influence of restricted movement on the physical fitness and well-being of pregnant mares. In: Proc. Equine Nutr. Physiol. Soc. Symp. 16:251-252.

Sporn, M.B., A.B. Roberts, and D.S. Goodman. 1994. The Retinoids: Biology, Chemistry, and Medicine (2nd Ed.) Raven Press, Ldt., New York.

Strickland, K.F., M. Woods, and J. Mason. 1987. Dietary molybdenum as a putative copper antagonist in the horse. Equine Vet. J. 19:50-54.

Thompson, K.N., J.P. Baker, and S.G. Jackson. 1988. The influence of supplemental feed on growth and bone development of nursing foals. J. Anim. Sci. 66:1692-1696.

van Weeren, P.R., J. Knapp, and E.C. Firth. 2003. Influence of liver copper status of mare and newborn foal on the development of osteochrondrotic lesions. Equine Vet. J. 35:67-71

Vermeer, C., B.L.M.G. Gijsbers, A.M. Craciun, M.C.L. Groenen-VanDooren, and M.H.J. Knapen. 1996. Effects of vitamin K on bone mass and bone metabolism. J. Nutr. 126:1187S.

Young, J.K., G.D. Potter, L.W. Green, S.P. Webb, J.W. Evans, and G.W. Webb. 1987. Copper balance in miniature horses fed varying amounts of zinc. In: Proc. Equine Nutr. Physiol. Soc. Symp. 10:153-157.

PERFORMANCE HORSES

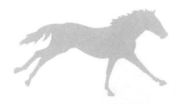

EFFECTS OF EXERCISE AND TRAINING ON SKELETAL DEVELOPMENT IN HORSES

LARRY A. LAWRENCE
Kentucky Equine Research, Versailles, Kentucky, USA

The main role of the equine skeleton is to provide structural support. Conformation determines the functional integrity and success of the gaits of athletic horses. The bones of the skeleton determine conformation or balance and structural correctness. The relationships of alignment, lengths, and angles of the bones of the skeleton have tremendous effects on the athletic ability and long-term soundness of horses. Bones must oppose muscular contraction to create movement and withstand the forces of the applied loads resulting from mass, gait, speed, and interactive forces with ground surfaces. Bone is also critical for protecting internal organs from injury. The skeletal system also includes tendons, ligaments, and cartilage. Each element of the musculoskeletal system must be functioning correctly in order for the horse to travel soundly. Acute malfunction of the skeletal system is most often associated with injury to the bones of the lower limb.

A horse galloping at race speed will place three times its body weight as force on the lower limb. There is a complicated support system for the skeleton; muscles, tendons, ligaments, cartilage, joint lubricants, and hoof structures help dissipate the forces of locomotion. But ultimately the strength of the bones of the legs must bear the loads created by exercise and training. Strength of bone is derived from a mineralized cartilaginous matrix. Strength is defined as the amount of force a bone can withstand per unit area.

When measuring breaking strength or the amount of force applied to a bone before failure, an important factor, the area moment of inertia, must also be calculated. The moment of inertia increases as the distance from the neutral axis (mechanical center) to the outermost point increases. Basically, as the bone gets bigger in diameter it gets stronger.

The bones of the skeleton are a dynamic tissue and are therefore responsive to forces placed upon them. Bone also responds physiologically to changes in calcium, phosphorus, and magnesium homeostasis and houses the bone marrow (site of red blood cell synthesis). The remodeling of bone in response to exercise is the result of signaling bone cells to remove bone via osteoclasts and then to build bone via osteoblasts.

The remodeling sequence includes (1) osteoclastic resorption; (2) preosteoblastic migration and differentiation into osteoblast; (3) osteoblastic matrix (osteoid) formation; and (4) mineralization (Mundy, 1999). Mature compact bone remodels in pockets known as bone-forming units. These pockets function independently and can be located throughout the skeleton. The remodeling of each pocket takes up to four months. The independent characteristics of bone remodeling suggest that the activation of the remodeling sequence can be controlled by local events in the bone microenvironment. The new bone is called the bone structural unit (BSU). Compact bone reacts more slowly to remodeling signals and is controlled by parathyroid hormone and 1, 25-dihydroxy vitamin D_3. Cortical bone comprises more than 80% of skeletal bone. Cancellous bone also remodels in response to local force stimuli, but because it is labile and subject to rapid turnover, it is also very responsive to mineral homeostasis, particularly changes in blood levels of calcium and phosphorus. Part of its responsiveness is related to its association with bone marrow, which has a high concentration of osteotropic cells (cytokines).

One theory of bone remodeling is that osteoclastic precursors recognize a change in the mechanical properties of bone, which signals a need for increased structural strength of new bone. While the exact signal for remodeling is unknown, the effective signal is strain. Strain is defined as the ratio of the change in length or dimension to the original dimension. Strains result from deformation of an object by a force. Force is mass times acceleration. Forces on bone can be applied in tension, compression, or shear. Shear forces result when there is bending or torsion and layers of material slide against each other. The minimum effective strain for modeling is reported to be 1500 to 3000 µε. The threshold for remodeling is thought to be much lower, between 100 and 300 µε. There also appears to be an optimum strain rate or number of strain cycles for maintenance of skeletal strength (Dalin and Jeffcott, 1994).

Exercise in Young Growing Horses

Initial mineralization of the cartilage models of the bones of foals takes place in the last three months of pregnancy and continues at an accelerated pace through the first year of life. The skeleton of the newborn foal contains only 17% of the adult bone mineral content. It consists mainly of cortical or compact bone and cancellous or trabecular bone. Figure 1 illustrates the degree of mineralization or the percentage of compact bone in relation to cancellous bone when compared to adults.

The two types of bone of most concern for growing horses are woven bone and lamellar bone. Woven bone is rapidly formed and characterized by loosely packed, large diameter collagen bundles. Woven and lamellar bone have osteocyes that are located within lacunae and interconnected via a network of fine canaliculi. Thicker collagen fiber bundles lie parallel to each other within the plane of each lamella (Figure 2). The orientation of collagen fibers can vary. Lamellar bone formation is a slow process, as lamellae are deposited along the long axis of the bone. In order for the bone growth to keep pace with the rapid growth in foals a combination of bone types are found. Fibrolamellar bone consists of circumferential layers of woven bone separated by radial struts (Riggs and Evans, 1990). Rather than concentric layers of lamellae forming around the entire bone, there are branches that radiate out from the center of the bone, similar to the branches on a tree. This allows the bone circumference to expand rapidly and lamellar bone is filled in at a slower rate.

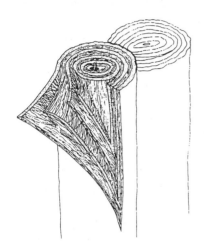

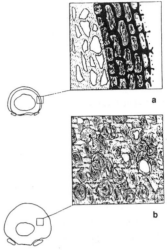

Figure 1. Degree of mineralization or percentage of compact bone in relation to cancellous bone when compared to adults.

Figure 2. Thicker collagen fiber bundles lie parallel to each other within the plane of each lamella.

Recent research supports the idea that bone morphology and mechanical and chemical properties can be affected by exercise or the lack of it from birth throughout the life of the horse. Barneveld and van Weeden (1999) reported significantly lower ($37 \pm 4\%$) bone density of the third tarsal bone of five-month-old foals that were housed in box stalls compared to pasture-raised and box-raised foals that were sprint-trained from one day of age. In a similar study from The Netherlands, the effects of exercise on the developing bones of newborn foals through weaning were examined. At weaning eight foals from a pasture group, a box stall group, and a box stall-sprint trained group were euthanized. The remaining 19 foals on the study were housed together in a large covered area with access to a paddock (van de Lest et al., 2003). The authors concluded that the bone mass (cross-sectional area and bone mineral density from subchondral bone at the femoropatellar joint) for the pastured horses and the sprint-trained horses was similar and significantly higher than the box-stalled group. However, the authors caution against the sprint training because of an inverse relationship between the bone morphogenic enzymes alkaline phosphatase and tartrate-resistant acid phosphatase and possible long-term effects. After six months of identical exercise, there were no differences between the groups.

Bell et al. (2001) kept 17 weanling Arabian horses either in stalls, on pasture 12 hours/day, or on pasture 24 hours/day for 56 days. Nutrient intakes were standardized via the use of ad libitum alfalfa hay in the stalled group. Radiographs were taken at 28-day intervals along with morphometric measurements. Radiographs were analyzed with photodensitometry. The partial-pasture turnout group and the full-pasture turnout group had increased bone mineral contents. Cannon bone circumference increased in both the pasture group and the partial pasture groups, but not in the stalled group.

Firth and coworkers (1999) subjected Dutch Warmblood foals to different exercise regimens. The foals were either box confined, box confined and sprint-trained daily, or kept at pasture until they were five months old. From six to 11 months, half of the horses were confined in a stall with daily turnout. Foals that were trained and turned out had greater bone density than confined foals. Foals with lower bone density had higher osteochondrosis scores and showed the most variability in growth rates during the first five months. At 11 months of age, there were no differences in bone density between groups. Raub et al. (1989) exercised a group of 10 Thoroughbred or Quarter Horse weanlings for 111 days and compared bone mineral content (BMC) estimated by photodensitometry to a group of 9 horses housed in stalls at night and turned out in pens during the day. The exercised group was trotted at a speed of 3.6 m/s starting at a distance of 0.4 km and gradually working up to 4.35 km/d. They were exercised five times each week. At the end of the 111-day period, the exercise group had 25% more estimated bone mineral content in the cannon bone than the non-exercise group.

Hoekstra et al. (1999) divided sixteen Arabian long yearlings that had been on pasture into two groups. One group was housed in box stalls while the second group was maintained on pasture. Radiographs were taken every 28 days for densitometry. Blood samples were taken every 14 days. After an 84-day pre-training period, six horses from each group were placed in a 56-day training period. Stalled horses had decreased BMC estimates at days 28, 56, and 140. Serum osteocalcin concentrations were lower at day 14 ($p < 0.05$) and urinary deoxypyridinaline (a bone resorption indicator) was greater at day 28. Nielsen et al. (1997) at Texas A&M University placed 53 eighteen-month-old Quarter Horses in race training. They were broken to ride and trained in a typical race-training program for 17 weeks. The horses then entered an 18-week racing period during which they were raced every other week for a total of nine races. Radiographs were taken of the left metacarpal on day 0, 62, 104, and 244. Decreases in radiographic bone aluminum equivalence (RBAE) of the lateral, medial, and dorsal cortices were observed from day 0 to day 62. After the initial decrease in estimated bone mineral, the RBAE increased by day 104 and day 244. The authors report that the introduction of speed work corresponded to the lowest RBAE readings.

Firth et al. (2000) summarized a series of studies examining the effects of training on two-year-old Thoroughbred fillies. They were treadmill trained at a gallop three times a week for 4.5 to 18 months. These trained fillies were compared with control fillies that were exercised only at a walk. In the trained horses, changes in bone mineralization were detected within three months. The changes consisted of thickened trabecular bone in the subchondral area, the cuboidal bones, and specific areas of the epiphysis of long bones. A companion study looked at the effects of exercising fillies on a training track compared to Thoroughbred fillies housed in stalls with turnout on dirt yards during the day. The training consisted of four weeks slow cantering, four weeks fast cantering, and then four weeks fast cantering with fast gallops included twice a week. Researchers reported increases in bone density of 36.8% in epiphysis of the metacarpal.

Sherman et al. (1995) measured the breaking strength, cross-sectional area, and area moments of inertia in the cannon bones of 24 Thoroughbreds in various stages of training from two to four years of age. Horses with the most training had greater cross-sectional areas and area moments of inertia. Greater cross-sectional areas and moments of inertia correlated with greater breaking load.

Thoroughbred Race Training

The strength and ability of the bone to resist a load or force placed upon it is dependent on the quality of the bone materially and on the size and shape of the bone. Davies and McCarthy (1994) reported that strains on the dorsal aspect of the third metacarpal increased linearly with speed and were higher in yearlings than mature racehorses. Nunamaker et al. (1990) reported that the third metacarpals of young Thoroughbreds have a fatigue life of 50,000 cycles when tested at strains recorded in young horses in training and more than a million at lower strains recorded in older horses. The authors state that clinically it is common to observe fatigue fractures occurring five months into training which should correspond to roughly the time it takes to complete 50,000 strides in typical training programs.

Davies (2001) further demonstrated differences between individual horses and between mature racehorses and naive Thoroughbreds that were significantly related to the geometry of the midshaft of the cannon bone. Horses with greater cross-sectional area and more bone deposited in the dorsal cortex had lower peak strains. The speed of ultrasound measurements is known to be faster in denser bones; however, Davies (2002) reported that ultrasound readings were faster in bones with higher strains. Davies (2002) stated that higher strains associated with stiffer and denser bones were not expected because faster ultrasound readings are associated with higher bone mineral contents. The author states that the remodeled bone deposited on the dorsal cortex of the third metacarpal is more porous than the original growth. The rapidly produced bone resulting from remodeling does not have the circumferential lamella organization of primary osteons; however, the increased strength associated with the changes in shape and increases in bone deposited in the areas of highest strain offsets any losses in strength associated with decreases in bone mineral in that area. Overall, the bone mineral content of the bone was not changed, but the distribution of the mineral was.

Remodeling is dependent on peak strain rates, though there is a maximum number of peak strain rates a bone can withstand. Peak strain rate can be altered with training but still may be limiting. Davies (2002) states that interaction between the size and shape of the bone and the quality of bone determines how much bone mass is needed to withstand racing speeds in an individual horse.

Boston and Nunamaker (2000) designed a survey study to determine the degree to which components of the training programs of two-year-old Thoroughbreds influenced their susceptibility to fatigue injury (bucked shins). They found that if more training effort was directed at short-distance breezing (15 m/s for 0.24 km/ week) and less to long-distance galloping (11 m/for 7.19 km/week) there was a significant reduction in the incidence of fatigue fracture. The exact type of exercise needed to develop young equine athletes for sustained sound performance will need to be established for all disciplines. Evidence suggests that early free exercise combined with training programs started in horses under three years of age will produce long-term effects, both positive and negative, depending on the ultimate performance and characteristics of breeds and individuals within breeds.

References

Barneveld, A., and P.R. van Weeren. 1999. Early changes in the distal intertarsal joint of Dutch Warmblood foals and the influence of exercise on bone density in the third tarsal bone. Equine Vet J Suppl 31:67.

Bell, R.A., B.D. Nielsen, K. Waite, D.S. Rosenstein, and M. Orth. 2001. Daily access to pasture turnout prevents loss of mineral in the third metacarpus of Arabian weanlings. J. Anim. Sci. 79:1142.

Boston, R. C., and D. M. Nunamaker. 2000. Gait and speed as exercise components of risk factors associated with onset of fatigue injury of the third metacarpal bone in two year old Thoroughbred racehorses. Amer. J. Vet. Res. 61:602.

Dalin, G., and J.B. Jeffcott. 1994. Biomechanics, gait and conformation. In: D.R. Hodgson and R.J. Rose (Eds.) The Athletic Horse. p. 27-48. W.B. Saunders Company, Sydney, AUS.

Davies, H.M.S., and R. N. McCarthy. 1994. Strain in the yearling equine metacarpus during locomotion. Equine Vet. J. Suppl. 17:25.

Davies, H.M.S. 2001. The relationship between surface strain and measurements of bone quality, quantity and shape. Equine Vet. J. Suppl. 33:16.

Davies, H.M.S. 2002. Dorsal metacarpal cortex ultrasound speed and bone size and shape. Equine Vet. J. Suppl. 34:337.

Firth, E.C., C.W. Rodgers, and A.E. Goodship. 2000. Bone mineral density changes in growing and training Thoroughbreds. In: Proc. Amer. Assoc. Equine Practnr. 46:295.

Firth, E.C., P.R. van Weeren, and D.U. Pfeiffer. 1999. Effect of age, exercise and growth rate on bone mineral density (BMD) in third carpal bone and distal radius of Dutch Warmblood foals with osteochondrosis. Equine Vet. J. Suppl. 31:74.

Hoekstra, K.E., B.D. Nielsen, M.W. Orth, D.S. Rosenstein, H.C. Schott, and J.E. Shelle. 1999. Comparison of bone mineral content and bone metabolism in stall- versus pasture-reared horses. Equine Vet. J. Suppl. 30:602.

Mundy, G.R. 1999. Bone Remodeling. In: Primer on Metabolic Bone Diseases and Disorders of Mineral Metabolism. (4th Ed.) p. 30-38. Lippincott Williams & Wilkins, Philadelphia.

Nielsen, B.D., G.D. Potter, E.L. Morris, T.W. Odom, D.M. Senor, J.A. Reynolds, W.B. Smith, and M.T. Martin. 1997. Changes in the third metacarpal bone and frequency of bone injures in young Quarter Horses during race training: Observations and theoretical considerations. J. Equine Vet. Sci. 17:541.

Nunamaker, D.M., C.M. Butterweck, and M.T. Provost. 1990. Fatigue fractures in Thoroughbred racehorses: Relationship with age, peak bone strain and training. J. Orthop. Res. 8:604.

Raub, R.H., S.G. Jackson, and J.P. Baker. 1989. The effect of exercise on bone growth and development in weanling horses. J. Anim. Sci. 67:2508.

Riggs, C.M., and G. P. Evans. 1990. The microstructural basis of the mechanical properties of equine bone. Equine Vet. Educ. 2:197.

Sherman, K.M., G.J. Miller, T.J. Wronski, P.T. Colahan, M. Brown, and W. Wilson. 1995. The effect of training on equine metacarpal bone breaking strength. Equine Vet. J. 27:135.

van de Lest, C.H., P.A. Brama, and P.R. van Weeren. 2003. The influence of exercise on bone morphogenic enzyme activity of immature equine subchondral bone. Biorheology 40(1-3):377-82.

FEEDING MORE AND GETTING LESS: EFFECTS OF HIGH GRAIN INTAKES ON DIGESTIVE CAPACITY AND GASTROINTESTINAL HEALTH OF PERFORMANCE HORSES

LAURIE M. LAWRENCE
University of Kentucky, Lexington, Kentucky

Exercise markedly affects nutrient requirements, especially the demand for energy. The daily digestible energy requirements for hardworking horses (racehorses, three-day event horses, endurance horses) are about double the requirements for a similar horse that is not in work. To meet the elevated energy demand, horse managers typically reduce hay intake and increase concentrate intake. According to reported surveys, racehorses weighing 450 to 550 kg frequently receive 3 to 6 kg of concentrate per day (Gallagher et al., 1988; Southwood et al., 1993) with anecdotal reports suggesting that some horses receive more than 8 kg of grain per day. At these rates of concentrate feeding, it is hard to imagine that horses could not be getting sufficient calories to maintain body weight. However, failure to maintain body condition is a common situation in intensely exercised horses. This paper will discuss some of the possible explanations for the apparent mismatch in calorie intake and energy balance in performance horses.

Energy Utilization

Not all of the energy consumed by horses is available for tissue use. In the United States, dietary energy recommendations for horses are based on digestible energy. Digestible energy (DE) is the difference in the gross energy of the feed consumed and the gross energy of feces (Figure 1). The amount of DE in a feed usually goes up as the amount of fiber goes down, so that a good-quality hay might contain 2 Mcal DE/kg dry matter (DM), while a cereal grain will contain 3.2 to 3.8 Mcal of DE/kg DM. Thus, it is a logical choice to replace hay with grain to increase energy intake. By replacing 5 kg of hay DM with 5 kg of grain DM, total DE intake can be increased 7 to 9 Mcal per day.

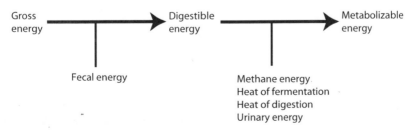

Figure 1. Schematic representation of energy partitioning.

As shown in Figure 1, DE can be further partitioned to metabolizable energy. Metabolizable energy (ME) accounts for losses due to methane, heat of fermentation, heat of digestion, and urinary energy. Because cereal grains are mostly digested in the small intestine, the losses due to fermentation (methane and heat) should be much smaller for grains than for hay. For ruminants, it can be estimated that approximately 25 to 35% of the DE contained in hemicellulose and cellulose is lost during fermentation. When starch is fermented the losses are lower (less methane is produced) but still significant. However, if starch bypasses rumen fermentation and is digested in the small intestine, the conversion of DE to ME is quite high, approximately 95%. Thus, the energetic differences between a diet of all hay and a diet containing hay and grain are magnified at the level of ME. Furthermore, there may be differences in the efficiency of utilization of the products of digestion between an all-hay diet and a diet containing hay and grain. Although the order of events is different for digestion in the horse, the relative losses associated with each type of digestion and the utilization of end products should be similar.

Figure 2 illustrates the potential differences in DE and ME from an all-hay diet and a mixed hay and grain diet. In the example shown here, about 75% of the DE consumed from an all-hay diet is available as ME, whereas almost 90% of the DE from a mixed diet is available as ME. Clearly, there is a theoretical advantage to feeding diets high in concentrate to performance horses with high energy requirements. But there are also potential disadvantages, and there is probably a point at which you can actually feed more, but get less. In Figure 2, it was assumed that all of the starch in the grain would be digested in the small intestine; however, this assumption is probably not valid in most horses.

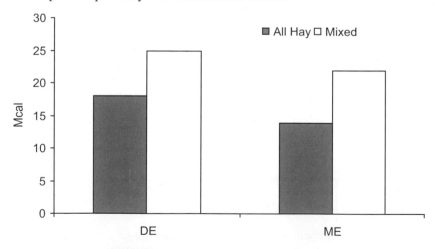

Figure 2. The amount of digestible energy (DE) and metabolizable energy (ME) available in diets containing either 10 kg of hay (All Hay) or 5 kg of hay and 5 kg of grain (Mixed). Note that the theoretical difference in ME between diets is greater than the difference in DE.

When Is More Really Less?

Several studies conducted in the last two decades suggest that the horse may have a limited ability to digest and absorb nonstructural carbohydrates (NSC), particularly starch, from the small intestine. When a small amount of oats was fed to horses, approximately 80% of the starch was digested and absorbed in the small intestine (Potter et al., 1992). When the amount of oats was increased, small intestinal starch digestibility decreased to 58%. Differences in small intestinal starch digestibility have also been reported among different types of grains (Kienzle et al., 1992; Radicke et al., 1991). Processing also appears to play a role in how well horses can digest starch in the small intestine (Potter et al., 1992). The amount of starch that can be tolerated will vary with type of grain and the type of processing; however, a few guidelines have been suggested. To minimize overflow to the large intestine, one researcher has suggested that the maximum amount of starch that should be fed at one meal is 3.50 to 4.0 g/kg BW (Potter et al., 1992). However, Cuddeford (1999) has suggested that other research supports a much lower value of 2.0 g/kg BW. If a concentrate feed contains 50% starch, the maximum amount of grain that could be fed without significant starch overflow to the large intestine is 4 g/kg BW or about 2 kg of grain/500 kg horse.

As more grain is fed, a greater percentage will flow to the large intestine and much of the energetic advantage of feeding grains will be lost. Harmon and McLeod (2000) have suggested that the energetic value of starch that is fermented is only about 75% of the value of starch that is digested in the small intestine.

Gastrointestinal Function

One of the consequences of high grain intakes in horses is the reduced amount of energy available from the grain when it bypasses digestion in the small intestine. Another consequence is the potential effect that excessive NSC flow to the large intestine could have on gastrointestinal function and health. At least one study in recent years has linked large concentrate meals to increased risk for gastrointestinal dysfunction. Tinker and coworkers (1997) examined some of the management factors related to colic incidence in horses. They reported an increased risk for colic when horses received more than 2.5 kg of grain per day, with a further increase in risk when grain intake exceeded 5 kg (Tinker et al., 1997). These amounts of grain are at or below expected intakes in racehorses but are within a range for which incomplete digestion of starch in the small intestine might be expected.

Why would high concentrate intakes increase the risk of colic? In a 1990 review, Clark concluded that large concentrate meals have the potential to alter gastrointestinal motility, stimulate large fluid shifts, and impact the gut microflora. Like the rumen, the equine large intestine is a complex ecosystem consisting of many different types of microbes. Mackie and Wilkens (1988) reported that horses consuming all-grass diets had glucolytic, amylolytic, proteolytic, cellulolytic, hemicellulolytic, and lactate-utilizing bacteria in the cecum and colon. It is generally accepted that the composition of the ruminant microbial population can be influenced by the type of substrate available as well as other factors such as pH. Using ponies, Kern et al. (1973) evaluated changes in the cecal microbial population to diets of all hay or 75% hay and 25% grain. Moore and Dehority (1993) characterized the microbial populations in ponies fed diets containing either a 90:10 or 60:40 hay:concentrate ratio. Kern et al. (1973) found that adding grain to the diet increased the total number of bacteria in the cecum. Moore and Dehority (1993) did not find a significant effect of diet on bacterial numbers in the cecum but did find increased microbial numbers in the colon. Neither study reported a marked effect of diet on the types of bacteria present, possibly because total feed intakes were moderate to low (1.5 to 2.0% of body weight). These results are in contrast to those obtained using a carbohydrate-overload model which found an increase in *Lactobacillus* and *Clostridium* spp. and a reduction in *Enterobacteriaceae* (Garner et al., 1978). These changes represent an increase in acid-producing bacteria and a decrease in acid-utilizing bacteria, particularly lactate utilizers, and would be expected to promote an acidic environment in the large intestine.

The effect of diet on large intestinal pH has been measured in several studies with horses. Figure 3 shows the effect of an all-hay meal or an all-concentrate meal on cecal pH in horses (Willard, 1975). A similar response was reported by Goodson et al. (1985). A reduction pH can have many potential effects on gastrointestinal function. Clark (1990) compared the effect of large concentrate meals in horses to the effects observed in cattle which include damage to the rumen epithelium and a reduction in rumen muscle tone.

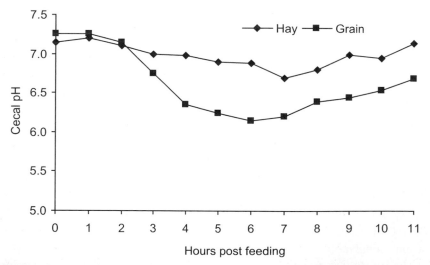

Figure 3. Changes in cecal pH following a meal of hay or a meal of grain (Willard, 1975).

Although the most marked effects of concentrate feeding are observed with the rapid, sudden consumption of large amounts of rapidly fermentable feeds, it is possible that a subacute acidosis may also occur in animals fed a high concentrate diet on a daily basis. In subacute ruminant acidosis, animals frequently exhibit inappetence, reduced weight gain, and reduced feed efficiency. Although subacute acidosis has not been widely recognized in horses, poor appetite is a condition reported in intensely exercised horses and horses receiving large amounts of grain (Ralston, 1992). Southwood et al. (1993) have reported that failure of horses to maintain feed intake is perceived as an important problem in racing stables. According to Owens (1993), the greatest potential to disturb the rumen environment occurs when animals are fed high concentrate diets at infrequent intervals (such as two times per day) and at high rates of feed intake. These characteristics would describe the feeding situation for many intensely exercised performance horses.

In addition to affecting gastrointestinal health, low large intestinal pH may affect digestive efficiency. In ruminants low pH can impair fiber digestion. Low pH may impair the attachment of microbes to cellulose and affect the ability of cellulolytic organisms to thrive, thus altering capacity for fiber digestion (Owens, 1993). In lactating dairy cows, 48 hour in situ neutral detergent fiber (NDF) digestibility was reduced from 51.3% to 36.9% for grass hay and from 49% to 37.2% for alfalfa hay (Krajcarski-Hunt et al., 2002). If a similar response occurred in horses, the effect on the amount of DE available from hay could be significant.

A few studies have examined the effect of forage:concentrate ratios on fiber digestibility in horses. Moore and Dehority (1993) did not find a difference in cellulose digestibility between an all-hay diet and a diet containing 60% hay and 40% concentrate fed to ponies at 1.5% of body weight. Hintz et al. (1971) compared nutrient disappearance from different segments of the gastrointestinal tract in ponies fed diets with varying forage:concentrate ratios. Diets were offered in isocaloric amounts so that the all-hay diet was fed at 2.1% of body weight and the 20% hay:80% concentrate diet was offered at 1.65% of body weight. Animals were slaughtered at 4 hours post-feeding and nutrient digestibilities determined using chromic oxide as a marker. In this study, increasing the amount of concentrate in the diet did not decrease fiber digestibility. However, in a study by Thompson (1982) where digestibility was measured using total fecal collections, fiber digestibility decreased with increasing concentrate intake. Cellulose and ADF digestibility were not decreased by changing the diet from all hay to 60% hay and 40% concentrate, but decreased digestibility of both components was noted when the concentrate portion of the diet was 60 or 80% of the total. Although feeding 80% of the total diet as concentrate may seem extreme, the horses in this study were consuming approximately 4.5 kg of grain per day (about 1% of BW), which is not unlike grain intakes reported for racehorses. Based on the results of these studies, it appears that diets containing large amounts of concentrate may depress the ability of horses to digest dietary fiber. It can be theorized that when large concentrate meals are fed, some NSC escapes small intestinal digestion and is fermented in the large intestine. Not only is the energetic value of the NSC lowered through fermentation, but the effects of fermentation (lowered pH) may depress fiber digestibility, thus producing a further negative effect on the energetic value of the diet.

Summary

Intensely exercised horses require high dietary energy intakes to maintain body weight. Typically these energy needs are met by increasing grain intake and reducing hay intake. When grain intakes are not excessive, this strategy works well because of the increased energy density of grain as well as the increased efficiency of energy use from glucose. However, as grain intakes exceed the capacity of the small intestine for starch digestion and absorption, a situation of diminishing returns is reached. These diminishing returns include a reduction in the amount of net energy derived from each unit of grain consumed and a potential decrease in fiber digestion. Observations in ruminants suggest that high concentrate intakes can produce a subacute acidosis that results in decreased feed intake as well as decreased feed efficiency. If a similar condition exists in horses, it could produce a situation where a horse is being fed more grain, but is still not maintaining body weight.

References

Clark, L. 1990. Feeding and digestive problems in horses. In: Veterinary Clinics of North America:Equine Practice 6(2):433.

Cuddeford, D. 1999. Starch digestion in the horse. In: Proc. 9th Equine Nutr. Conf. Feed Manufacturers. Kentucky Equine Research Inc., Lexington KY, p. 129.

Gallagher, K., J. Leech, and H. Stowe. 1988. Protein, energy and dry matter consumption by racing Thoroughbreds: A field study. J. Equine Vet. Sci. 12:43.

Garner H.E., J.N. Moore, and J.H. Johnson. 1978. Changes in the cecal microflora associated with the onset of laminitis. Equine Vet. J. 10:249.

Goodson, J., W.J. Tyznik, and J.H. Cline. 1985. Effects of an abrupt change from all hay to all concentrate on anaerobic bacterial numbers (grown on selective media), protozoal numbers, and pH of the cecum. In. Proc. Equine Nutr. Physiol. Symp., p. 52.

Harmon D., and K. McLeod. 2000. Glucose uptake and regulation by intestinal tissues: Implications and whole-body energetics. J. Anim. Sci. (E Supplement):E59.

Hintz, H.F., D.E. Hogue, E.F. Walker, J.E. Lowe, and H.F. Schryver. 1971. Apparent digestion in various segments of the digestive tract of ponies fed diets with varying roughage:grain ratios. J. Anim. Sci. 32:245.

Kern, D.L., L.L. Slyter, J.M. Weaver, E.C. Leffel, and G. Samuelson. 1973. Pony cecum vs steer rumen: The effect of oats and hay on the microbial ecosystem. J. Anim.Sci. 37:463.

Kienzle, E., S. Radicke, S. Wilke, E. Landes, and H. Meyer. 1992. Preileal starch digestion in relation to source and preparation of starch. Pferdeheilkunde (1st European Conference on Horse Nutrition): 103.

Krajcarski-Hunt, H., J.C. Plazier, J.P. Walton, R. Spratt, and B.W. McBride. 2002. Effect ofsubacute acidosis on in situ fiber digestion in lactating dairy cows. J. Dairy Sci. 85:570.

Mackie, R., and C. Wilkens. 1988. Enumeration of anaerobic bacterial microflora of the equine gastrointestinal tract. Appl. Env. Micro. 54:2155.

Moore, B.E., and B.A. Dehority. 1993. Effects of diet and hindgut defaunation on diet digestibility and microbial concentrations in the cecum and colon of the horse. J. Anim. Sci. 71:3350.

Owens, F.N. 1993. Ruminal fermentation. In: D.C. Church (Ed.) The Ruminant Animal.p. 145. Waveland Press, IL.

Potter, G.D., F.F. Arnold, D.D. Householder, D.H. Hansen, and K.M. Brown. 1992. Digestion of starch in the small or large intestine of the equine. Pferdeheilkunde (1st European Conference on Horse Nutrition): 107.

Radicke, S., E. Kienzle, and H. Meyer. 1991. Preileal apparent digestibility of oats and corn starch and consequences for cecal metabolism. In: Proc. Equine Nutr. Physiol. Symp., p. 43.

Ralston, S. 1992. Regulation of feed intake in the horse in relation to gastrointestinal disease. Pferdeheilkunde.(1st European Conference on Horse Nutrition):15.

Southwood, L.L., D.L. Evans, W.L. Bryden, and R.J. Rose. 1993. Nutrient intake of horses in Thoroughbred and Standardbred stables. Aust. Vet. J. 70:164.

Thompson, K. 1982. Apparent digestion coefficients and associative effects of varying hay-grain ratios fed to horses. M.S. Thesis, Univ. of Kentucky, Lexington.

Tinker, M.K., N.A. White, P. Lessard, C.D. Thatcher, K.D. Pelzer, B. Davis, and D.K. Carmel. 1997. Prospective study of equine colic risk factors. EquineVet. J. 29:454.

Willard, J. 1975. Feeding behavior in the equine fed concentrate versus roughage diets. Ph.D. Thesis. Univ. of Kentucky, Lexington.

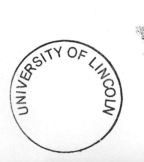

EXERCISE AND IMMUNE FUNCTION: NUTRITIONAL INFLUENCES

DAVID NIEMAN
Appalachian State University, Boone, North Carolina

Moderate Physical Activity and the Common Cold

Data from three randomized studies support the viewpoint that near-daily physical activity reduces the number of days with sickness (Nieman et al., 1990b, 1993, 1998c). In these studies, women in the exercise groups walked briskly 35-45 minutes, five days a week, for 12-15 weeks during the winter/spring or fall, while the control groups remained physically inactive. The results were in the same direction reported by fitness enthusiasts—walkers experienced about half the days with cold symptoms of the sedentary controls (Figure 1). A recent one-year epidemiological study of 547 adults demonstrated a 23% reduction in risk of upper respiratory tract infection (URTI) in those engaging in regular versus irregular moderate-to-vigorous physical activity (Matthews et al., 2000). In healthy elderly subjects, URTI symptomatology during a one-year period was inversely related to energy expended during moderate physical activity (Kostka et al., 2000).

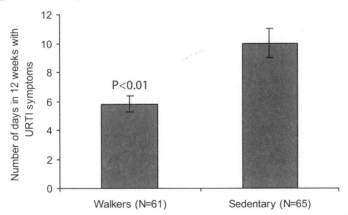

Figure 1. Near-daily brisk walking for 45 minutes per session is associated with significantly fewer days with URTI symptoms. This figure combines the results from two studies of 126 overweight women randomized to walking and non-walking groups. Data from Nieman et al., 1990b, 1998c. Mean ± SE.

Other research has shown that during moderate exercise, several positive changes occur in the immune system (Nehlsen-Cannarella et al., 1991; Nieman and Nehlsen-

Cannarella, 1994; Nieman et al., 1999, 2000a). Stress hormones, which can suppress immunity, and pro- and anti-inflammatory cytokines, indicative of intense metabolic activity, are not elevated during moderate exercise. Although the immune system returns to pre-exercise levels very quickly after the exercise session is over, each session represents a boost in immune surveillance that appears to reduce the risk of infection over the long term.

Although public health recommendations must be considered tentative, the data on the relationship between moderate exercise, enhanced immunity, and lowered risk of sickness are consistent with guidelines urging the general public to engage in near-daily brisk walking.

Is the Endurance Athlete at Risk for Respiratory Infection and Immune Suppression?

A common perception among elite endurance athletes and coaches is that overtraining lowers resistance to URTI such as the common cold and sore throats (Nieman, 2000b). In a 1996 survey conducted by the Gatorade Sports Science Institute, 89% of 2,700 high school and college coaches and athletic trainers checked "yes" to the question, "Do you believe overtraining can compromise the immune system and make athletes sick?" (Personal communication, 1997, Gatorade Sports Science Institute, Barrington, IL).

The results of epidemiological studies generally support the belief that URTI risk is elevated during periods of heavy training and in the 1-2 week period following participation in competitive endurance races (Nieman et al., 1990a). A high percentage of self-reported illnesses occur when elite athletes exceed individually identifiable training thresholds, mostly related to the strain of training (Foster, 1998). The majority of endurance athletes, however, do not report URTI after competitive race events. For example, only one in seven marathon runners reported an episode of URTI during the week following the March 1987 Los Angeles Marathon, compared to two in 100 who did not compete (Nieman et al., 1990a). URTI rates in marathon runners are even lower during the summer than winter/spring. In a study of 170 experienced marathon runners, only 3% reported an URTI during the week after a July marathon race event (Unpublished data, author, 1993). When athletes train hard, but avoid overreaching and overtraining, URTI risk is typically unaltered. For example, during a 2.5 month period (winter/spring) in which elite female rowers trained 2-3 hours daily (rowing drills, resistance training), incidence of URTI did not vary significantly from that of nonathletic controls (Nieman et al., 2000b).

Together, these data indicate that there is a relationship between exercise workload and infection (Figure 2). Most endurance athletes should experience low-to-normal URTI risk during periods of regular training, with URTI risk rising during periods of overreaching/overtraining and competition.

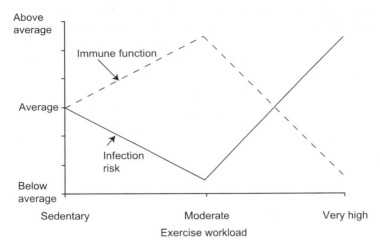

Figure 2. Infection risk and immune function are related to the exercise workload.

Is immune function in athletes modified in parallel with infection risk (Figure 2)? Two lines of investigation have provided insights both supporting and challenging this assumption (Nieman, 2000a):

•   Do the immune systems of endurance athletes and nonathletes function differently when in a state of rest?

•   Does heavy exertion lead to temporary but clinically significant changes in immunity (i.e., the "open window" theory)?

RESTING IMMUNE FUNCTION IN ATHLETES AND NONATHLETES

The immune system is remarkably adaptive in its defense capabilities. It is able to generate an enormous variety of cells and molecules capable of recognizing and eliminating a limitless variety of foreign invaders (Mackinnon, 1999). Attempts thus far to compare resting immune function in athletes and nonathletes have failed to provide evidence that athletic endeavor is linked to clinically important changes in immunity, despite compelling epidemiological data (Nieman et al., 1993, 1995, 2000b; Tvede et al., 1991). Of all immune measures, only NK cell activity has emerged as a somewhat consistent indicator differentiating the immune systems of athletes and nonathletes. NK cells are highly active cells that combat certain types of viruses and cancer cells. In a study comparing elite female rowers and controls, NK cell activity measured 1.6-fold higher in the rowers (Nieman et al., 2000b). Elevated NK cell activity has also been reported in runners and cyclists (Nieman et al., 1995; Tvede et al., 1991).

Neutrophils are important components of the innate immune system, aiding in the phagocytosis of many bacterial and viral pathogens, and the release of immunomodulatory cytokines. Neutrophils are considered to be the body's most effective phagocyte and are critical in the early control of invading infectious agents. Neutrophil function has been reported to be suppressed in athletes, but this has not been a consistent finding and may depend on the severity of training (Mackinnon, 1999).

Attempts thus far to link variances in both neutrophil function and NK cell activity with risk of infection have failed. Salivary IgA concentration warrants further research as a practical and inexpensive marker of potential infection risk in athletes. The secretory immune system of the mucosal tissues of the upper respiratory tract is considered the first barrier to colonization by pathogens, with IgA the major effector of host defense (Mackinnon, 1999). In a study by Gleeson et al. (1999), salivary IgA levels measured in swimmers before individual training sessions showed significant correlations with infection rates, and the number of infections observed in the swimmers was predicted by the preseason and the mean pretraining salivary IgA levels. With runners, sickness rates following a competitive marathon race have been observed to be highest in those exhibiting the lowest salivary IgA levels (Nieman et al., 2001). In two other studies, however, variance in salivary IgA concentration was not related to a history of URTI incidence in elite female rowers or adolescent tennis athletes (Henson et al., 2000; Nehlsen-Cannarella et al., 2000). Thus the data are inconclusive, and research is needed with larger groups of athletes followed for longer periods of time to determine the usefulness of salivary IgA concentration in predicting URTI risk in athletes.

CHANGES IN IMMUNITY FOLLOWING PROLONGED, INTENSIVE EXERCISE

The magnitude of change in immunity that occurs after each bout of prolonged and intensive exercise in athletes may have more clinical significance than training-induced alterations in resting immunity. During this "open window" of altered immunity (which may last between three and 72 hours, depending on the immune measure), viruses and bacteria may gain a foothold, increasing the risk of subclinical and clinical infection. Investigations are currently underway to demonstrate that athletes showing the most extreme immune suppression following heavy exertion are those that contract an infection during the following 1-2 weeks. This link must be established before the "open window" theory can be wholly accepted in humans.

Several studies with animal models have provided important support of the "open window" theory. Davis et al. (1997), for example, have shown that in mice alveolar macrophage antiviral resistance is suppressed 8 h following prolonged strenuous exercise to fatigue, an effect due in part to an increase in circulating adrenal catecholamines.

Many components of the immune system exhibit change after heavy exertion, including the following (for review, see Nieman, 2000a; Mackinnon, 1999):

- Neutrophilia (high blood neutrophil counts) and lymphopenia (low blood lymphocyte counts) induced by high plasma catecholamines, growth hormone, and cortisol.

- Increase in blood granulocyte and monocyte phagocytosis and activation markers (reflecting an inflammatory response due to substances released from injured muscle cells), but a decrease in nasal neutrophil phagocytosis and blood granulocyte oxidative burst activity.

- Decrease in NK cell cytotoxic activity (an important antiviral measure) and mitogen-induced lymphocyte proliferation (a measure of T cell function).

- Decrease in the delayed-type hypersensitivity response (DTH). DTH is a complex immunological process which involves several different cell types (including T lymphocytes) and chemical mediators, and is manifested by firm, red skin indurations.

- Increase in plasma concentrations of pro- and anti-inflammatory cytokines (e.g., tumor necrosis factor alpha (TNF-α), interleukin-6 (IL6), interleukin-10 (IL-10), and interleukin-1 receptor antagonist (IL-1ra)). Cytokines are low molecular-weight proteins and peptides which help control and mediate interactions among cells involved in immune responses. Prolonged and intensive exercise bouts induce muscle cell injury, causing a sequential release of pro- and anti-inflammatory cytokines.

- Decrease in *ex vivo* production of cytokines (interferon γ (IFN-γ), TNF-α, IL-1, IL-2, IL-6, and IL-10) in response to mitogens and endotoxin. This indicates a reduced capacity of the body's immune system to produce cytokines after heavy exertion.

- Decrease in nasal and salivary IgA concentration, and nasal mucociliary clearance. This indicates an impaired ability of the upper respiratory tract to clear external pathogens.

- Blunted major histocompatibility complex (MHC) II expression and antigen presentation in macrophages. The MHC antigens are essential for reactions of immune recognition. After phagocytosis and antigen processing, small antigenic peptides are bound to MHC II and presented to T lymphocytes, an important step in adaptive immunity. These data imply that heavy exertion can blunt macrophage expression of MHC II, negatively affecting the process of antigen presentation to T lymphocytes, and thus their ability to respond to a challenge by viruses.

These data suggest that immune function in several body compartments exhibits signs of stress or suppression for a short period following prolonged endurance exercise. Thus it makes sense that URTI risk may be increased when the endurance athlete goes through repeated cycles of unusually heavy exertion, has been exposed to novel pathogens, and experienced other stressors to the immune system including lack of sleep, severe mental stress, malnutrition, or weight loss. A one-year retrospective study of 852 German athletes showed that risk of URTI was highest in endurance athletes who also reported significant stress and sleep deprivation (Konig et al., 2000). In other words, URTI risk is related to many factors, and when brought together during travel to important competitive events, the athlete may be unusually susceptible.

Guidelines for the Athlete to Reduce the Risk of Infection

To counter this increased risk of URTI, the athlete should consider these guidelines, each of which has a separate connection to the immune system and host protection against pathogens (Mackinnon, 1999; Nieman, 2000b):

- Keep other life stresses to a minimum (mental stress in and of itself has been linked to increased URTI risk).

- Eat a well-balanced diet to keep vitamin and mineral pools in the body at optimal levels.

- Avoid overtraining and chronic fatigue.

- Obtain adequate sleep on a regular schedule (disruption has been linked to suppressed immunity).

- Avoid rapid weight loss (has been related to adverse immune changes).

- Avoid putting the hands to the eyes and nose (a major route of viral self-inoculation).

- Before important race events, avoid sick people and large crowds when possible.

- Influenza vaccination is recommended for athletes competing during the winter months.

REST OR EXERCISE WHEN SICK?

Athletes and fitness enthusiasts are often uncertain of whether they should exercise or rest during sickness. Human studies do not provide definitive answers. Animal studies, however, generally support the finding that one or two periods of exhaustive exercise following injection of the animal with certain types of viruses or bacteria lead to a more frequent appearance of infection and more severe symptoms (Davis et al., 1997; Gross et al., 1998).

With athletes, it is well established that the ability to compete is reduced during sickness (Friman and Ilback, 1998). Also, several case histories have shown that sudden and unexplained downturns in athletic performance can sometimes be traced to a recent bout of sickness. In some athletes, exercising when sick can lead to a severely debilitating state known as "post-viral fatigue syndrome" (Maffulli et al., 1993; Parker et al., 1996). The symptoms can persist for several months, and include weakness, inability to train hard, easy fatiguability, frequent infections, and depression.

Concerning exercising when sick, most clinical authorities in the area of exercise immunology recommend (Friman and Ilback, 1998; Mackinnon, 1999):

- If one has common cold symptoms (e.g., runny nose and sore throat without fever or general body aches and pains), intensive exercise training may be safely resumed a few days after the resolution of symptoms.

- Mild to moderate exercise (e.g., walking) when sick with the common cold does not appear to be harmful. In two studies using nasal sprays of a rhinovirus leading to common cold symptoms, subjects were able to engage in exercise during the course of the illness without any negative effects on severity of symptoms or performance capability (Weidner et al., 1997, 1998).

- With symptoms of fever, extreme tiredness, muscle aches, and swollen lymph glands, 2-4 weeks should probably be allowed before resumption of intensive training.

Nutritional Countermeasures

Nutrition impacts the development of the immune system, both in the growing fetus and in the early months of life. Nutrients are also necessary for the immune response to pathogens so that cells can divide and produce antibodies and cytokines. Many enzymes in immune cells require the presence of micronutrients, and critical roles have been defined for zinc, iron, copper, selenium, vitamins A, B_6, C, and E in the maintenance of optimum immune function (Nieman and Pedersen, 2000). The earliest research on nutrition and immune function focused on malnutrition. It has long been known that malnourished children have a high risk of severe and life-threatening infections. Protein-energy malnutrition adversely affects virtually all components of the immune system.

Although endurance athletes may be at increased infection risk during heavy training or competitive cycles, they must exercise intensively to contend successfully. Athletes appear less interested in reducing training workloads, and more receptive to ingesting drugs or nutrient supplements that have the potential to counter exercise-induced inflammation and immune alterations. There are some preliminary data that various immunomodulator drugs may afford athletes some protection against inflammation, negative immune changes, and infection during competitive cycles, but much more research is needed before any of these can be recommended (Pizza et al., 1999).

The influence of a growing list of nutritional supplements on the immune and infection response to intense and prolonged exercise has been assessed (Nieman and Pedersen, 2000). Supplements studied thus far include zinc, dietary fat, plant sterols, antioxidants (e.g., vitamins C and E, ß-carotene, N-acetylcysteine, and butylated hydroxyanisole), glutamine, and carbohydrate.

Antioxidants

Can antioxidant supplements attenuate exercise-induced changes in immune function and infection risk (Nieman et al., 1997b, 2000c)? Several double-blind placebo studies of South African ultramarathon runners have demonstrated that vitamin C (but not E or ß-carotene) supplementation (about 600 mg/day for three weeks) is related to fewer reports of URTI symptoms (Peters et al., 1993, 1996). This has not been replicated, however, by other research teams. Himmelstein et al. (1998), for example, reported no alteration in URTI incidence among 44 marathon runners and 48 sedentary subjects randomly assigned to a two-month regimen of 1000 mg/day of vitamin C or placebo.

Glutamine

Glutamine, a nonessential amino acid, has attracted much attention by investigators (Mackinnon and Hooper, 1996; Rhode et al., 1998). Glutamine is the most abundant amino acid in the body and is synthesized by skeletal muscle and other tissues. Glutamine is an important fuel for lymphocytes and monocytes, and decreased amounts *in vitro* have a direct effect in lowering proliferation rates of lymphocytes.

Reduced plasma glutamine levels have been observed in response to various stressors, including prolonged exercise. Since skeletal muscle is the major tissue involved in glutamine production and is known to release glutamine into the blood compartment at a high rate, it has been hypothesized that muscle activity may directly influence the immune system by altering the availability of this immune cell fuel substrate.

Whether exercise-induced reductions in plasma glutamine levels are linked to impaired immunity and host protection against viruses in athletes is still unsettled, but the majority of studies have not favored such a relationship (Nieman and Pedersen, 2000). For example, in a crossover, placebo-controlled study of eight males, glutamine supplementation abolished the postexercise decrease in plasma glutamine concentration but still had no influence relative to placebo on exercise-induced decreases in T and natural killer cell function (Rhode et al., 1998).

One problem with the glutamine hypothesis is that plasma concentrations following exercise do not decrease below threshold levels that are detrimental to lymphocyte function as demarcated by *in vitro* experiments. In other words, even marathon-type exertion does not deplete the large body stores of glutamine enough to diminish lymphocyte function.

Carbohydrate Supplements

Research during the 1980s and early 1990s established that a reduction in blood glucose levels was linked to hypothalamic-pituitary-adrenal activation, an increased release of adrenocorticotrophic hormone and cortisol, increased plasma growth hormone, decreased insulin, and a variable effect on blood epinephrine levels (Murray et al., 1991). Given the link between stress hormones and immune responses to prolonged and intensive exercise, carbohydrate compared to placebo ingestion should maintain plasma glucose concentrations, attenuate increases in stress hormones, and thereby diminish changes in immunity (as summarized in the model in Figure 3). Carbohydrate supplementation may also alter immunity following exercise by increasing the availability of energy substrate to immune cells. Glucose is the major energy substrate for immune cells.

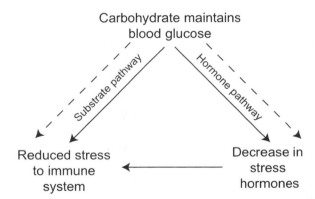

Figure 3. This model suggests that carbohydrate supplementation during prolonged and intensive exercise maintains or elevates plasma glucose concentrations, attenuating the normal rise in stress hormones, and thereby countering negative immune changes. Carbohydrate ingestion may also affect immune function by increasing the availability of glucose as a fuel substrate for immune cells.

Several studies with runners and cyclists have shown that carbohydrate beverage ingestion plays a role in attenuating changes in immunity when the athlete experiences physiologic stress and depletion of carbohydrate stores in response to high intensity (~75-80% VO_{2max}) exercise bouts lasting longer than two hours (Gleeson et al., 1998; Nieman et al., 1997a, 1998a, 1998b). In particular, carbohydrate ingestion (about one liter per hour of a typical sports drink) compared to a placebo has been linked to significantly lower blood cortisol and epinephrine levels, a reduced change in blood immune cell counts, and lower pro- and antiinflammatory cytokines. These data suggest that the endurance athlete ingesting carbohydrate during the race event should experience a much lower perturbation in hormonal and immune measures compared to the athlete largely avoiding carbohydrate.

Conclusions and Recommendations

By far, the most important finding that has emerged from exercise immunology studies is that positive immune changes take place during each bout of moderate physical activity. Over time, this translates to fewer days of sickness with the common cold and other upper respiratory tract infections. This is consistent with public health guidelines urging individuals to engage in near-daily physical activity of 30 minutes or greater.

Risk of upper respiratory tract infections can increase when athletes push beyond normal limits. The infection risk is amplified when other factors related to immune function are present, including exposure to novel pathogens during travel, lack of sleep, severe mental stress, malnutrition, or weight loss.

Many components of the immune system exhibit adverse change after prolonged, heavy exertion lasting longer than 90 minutes. These immune changes occur in several compartments of the immune system and body (e.g., the skin, upper respiratory tract mucosal tissue, lung, blood, and muscle). During this "open window" of impaired immunity (which may last between three and 72 hours, depending on the immune measure), viruses and bacteria may gain a foothold, increasing the risk of subclinical and clinical infection.

Should the athlete exercise when sick? In general, if the symptoms are from the neck up (e.g., the common cold), moderate exercise is probably acceptable and some researchers would argue even beneficial, while bedrest and a gradual progression to normal training are recommended when the illness is systemic (e.g., the flu). If in doubt as to the type of infectious illness, individuals should consult a physician.

The influence of nutritional supplements on the acute immune response to prolonged exercise has been measured in endurance athletes. Antioxidants and glutamine have received much attention, but the data thus far do not support their role in negating immune changes after heavy exertion. At this point, athletes should eat a varied and balanced diet in accordance with the food pyramid and energy needs, and be assured that vitamin and mineral intake is adequate for both health and immune function.

Ingestion of a typical sports drink, about one liter per hour of exertion, has been associated with higher plasma glucose levels, an attenuated cortisol and growth hormone response, fewer perturbations in blood immune cell counts, and a diminished pro- and anti-inflammatory cytokine response. Overall, these data indicate that the physiological stress to the immune system is reduced when endurance athletes use carbohydrate during intense exertion lasting 90 minutes or more.

References

Davis, J.M., M.L. Kohut, L.H. Colbert, D.A. Jackson, A. Ghaffar, and E.P. Mayer. 1997. Exercise, alveolar macrophage function, and susceptibility to respiratory infection. *J. Appl. Physiol.* 83:1461-1466.

Foster, C. (1998). Monitoring training in athletes with reference to overtraining syndrome. *Med. Sci. Sports Exerc.* 30:1164-1168.

Friman, G., and N.G. Ilback. 1998. Acute infection: metabolic responses, effects on performance, interaction with exercise, and myocarditis. *Int. J. Sports Med.* 19(Suppl 3):S172-S182.

Gleeson, M., A.K. Blannin, N.P. Walsh, N.C. Bishop, and A.M. Clark. 1998. Effect of low- and high-carbohydrate diets on the plasma glutamine and circulating leukocyte responses to exercise. *Int. J. Sport Nutr.* 8:49-59.

Gleeson, M., W.A. McDonald, D.B. Pyne, A.W. Cripps, J.L. Francis, P.A. Fricker, and R.L. Clancy. 1999. Salivary IgA levels and infection risk in elite swimmers. *Med. Sci. Sports Exerc.* 31:67-73.

Gross, D.K., K.W. Hinchcliff, P.S. French, S.A. Goclan, K.K. Lahmers, M. Lauderdale, J.A. Ellis, D.M. Haines, R.D. Slemons, and P.S. Morley. 1998. Effect of moderate exercise on the severity of clinical signs associated with influenza virus infection in horses. *Equine Vet. J.* 30:489-497.

Henson, D.A., D.C. Nieman, K.W. Kernodle, G. Sonnenfeld, D. Morton, and M.P. Thompson. 2000. Immune function in adolescent tennis athletes and controls. *J. Sports Med. Phys. Fit.* (in press).

Himmelstein, S.A., R.A. Robergs, K.M. Koehler, S.L. Lewis, and C.R. Qualls. 1998. Vitamin C supplementation and upper respiratory tract infections in marathon runners. *J. Exerc. Physiol. Online* 1(2):1-17.

Konig, D., D. Grathwohl, C. Weinstock, H. Northoff, and A. Berg. 2000. Upper respiratory tract infection in athletes: influence of lifestyle, type of sport, training effort, and immunostimulant intake. *Exerc. Immunol. Rev.* 6:102-120.

Kostka, T., S.E. Berthouze, J. Lacour, and M. Bonnefoy. 2000. The symptomatology of upper respiratory tract infections and exercise in elderly people. *Med. Sci. Sports Exerc.* 32:46-51.

Mackinnon, L.T. 1999. *Advances in Exercise Immunology.* Champaign, IL: Human Kinetics.

Mackinnon, L.T., and S.L. Hooper. 1996. Plasma glutamine and URTI during intensified training in swimmers. *Med. Sci. Sports Exerc.* 28:285-290.

Maffulli, N., V. Testa, and G. Capasso. 1993. Post-viral fatigue syndrome. A longitudinal assessment in varsity athletes. *J. Sports Med. Phys. Fit.* 33:392-399.

Matthews, C.E., I.S. Ockene, P.S. Freedson, M.C. Rosal, J.R. Herbert, and P.A. Merriam. 2000. Physical activity and risk of upper-respiratory tract infection.

Med. Sci. Sports Exerc. 32:S292.

Murray, R., G.L. Paul, J.G. Seifent, and D.E. Eddy. 1991. Responses to varying rates of carbohydrate ingestion during exercise. *Med. Sci. Sports Exerc.* 23:713-718.

Nehlsen-Cannarella, S.L., D.C. Nieman, O.R. Fagoaga, W.J. Kelln, D.A. Henson, M. Shannon, and J.M. Davis. 2000. Salivary immunoglobulins in elite female rowers and controls. *Eur. J. Appl. Physiol.* 81:222-228 .

Nehlsen-Cannarella, S.L., D.C. Nieman, J. Jessen, L. Chang, G. Gusewitch, G.G. Blix, and E. Ashley. 1991. The effects of acute moderate exercise on lymphocyte function and serum immunoglobulins. *Int. J. Sports Med.* 12:391-398.

Nieman, D.C. 2000a. Exercise effects on systemic immunity. *Immunol. Cell Biol.* 78:496-501.

Nieman, D.C. 2000b. Is infection risk linked to exercise workload? *Med. Sci. Sports Exerc.* 32 (suppl 7):S406-S411.

Nieman, D.C., K.S. Buckley, D.A. Henson, B.J. Warren, J. Suttles, J.C. Ahle, S. Simandle, O.R. Fagoaga, and S.L. Nehlsen-Cannarella. 1995. Immune function in marathon runners versus sedentary controls. *Med. Sci. Sports Exerc.* 27:986-992.

Nieman, D.C., O.R. Fagoaga, D.E. Butterworth, B.J. Warren, A. Utter, J.M. Davis, D.A. Henson, and S.L. Nehlsen-Cannarella. 1997a. Carbohydrate supplementation affects granulocyte and monocyte trafficking but not function after 2.5 hours of running. *Am. J. Clin. Nutr.* 66:153-159.

Nieman, D.C., D.A. Henson, D.E. Butterworth, B.J. Warren, J.M. Davis, O.R. Fagoaga, and S.L. Nehlsen-Cannarella. 1997b. Vitamin C supplementation does not alter the immune response to 2.5 hours of running. *Int. J. Sport Nutr.* 7:174-184.

Nieman, D.C., D.A. Henson, O.R. Fagoaga, A.C. Utter, D.M. Vinci, J.M. Davis, and S.L. Nehlsen-Cannarella. 2001. Change in salivary IgA following a competitive marathon race. *Int. J. Sports Med.*

Nieman, D.C., D.A. Henson, G. Gusewitch, B.J. Warren, R.C. Dotson, D.E. Butterworth, and S.L. Nehlsen-Cannarella. 1993. Physical activity and immune function in elderly women. *Med. Sci. Sports Exerc.* 25:823-831.

Nieman, D.C., L.M. Johanssen, J.W. Lee, J. Cermak, and K. Arabatzis. 1990a. Infectious episodes in runners before and after the Los Angeles Marathon. *J. Sports Med. Phys. Fit.* 30: 316-328.

Nieman, D.C., M.W. Kernodle, D.A. Henson, G. Sonnenfeld, and J.M. Davis. 2000a. Acute immune responses to tennis drills in adolescent athletes. *Res. Quart. Exerc. Sport* 71:403-408.

Nieman, D.C., and S.L. Nehlsen-Cannarella. 1994. The immune response to exercise. *Sem. Hematol.* 31:166-179.

Nieman, D.C., S.L. Nehlsen-Cannarella, O.R. Fagoaga, D.A. Henson, M. Shannon, J.M. Davis, M.D. Austin, C. Hisey, J.C. Holbeck, J.M.E. Hjertman, M.R.

Bolton, and B.K. Schilling. 1999. Immune response to two hours of rowing in female elite rowers. *Int. J. Sports Med.* 20:476-481.

Nieman, D.C., S.L. Nehlsen-Cannarella, O.R. Fagoaga, D.A. Henson, M. Shannon, J.M.E. Hjertman, M.R. Bolton, M.D. Austin, B.K. Schilling, R. Schmitt, R. Thorpe. 2000b. Immune function in female elite rowers and nonathletes. *Br. J. Sports Med.* 34:181-187.

Nieman, D.C., S.L. Nehlsen-Cannarella, O.R. Fagoaga, D.A. Henson, A. Utter, J.M. Davis, F. Williams, and D.E. Butterworth. 1998a. Influence of mode and carbohydrate on the cytokine response to heavy exertion. *Med. Sci. Sports Exerc.* 30:671-678.

Nieman, D.C., S.L. Nehlsen-Cannarella, D.A. Henson, D.E. Butterworth, O.R. Fagoaga, and A. Utter. 1998b. Influence of carbohydrate ingestion and mode on the granulocyte and monocyte response to heavy exertion in triathletes. *J. Appl. Physiol.* 84:1252-1259.

Nieman, D.C., S.L. Nehlsen-Cannarella, D.A. Henson A.J. Koch, D.E. Butterworth, O.R. Fagoaga, and A. Utter. 1998c. Immune response to exercise training and/or energy restriction in obese females. *Med. Sci. Sports Exerc.* 30:679-686.

Nieman, D.C., S.L. Nehlsen-Cannarella, P.A. Markoff, A.J. Balk-Lamberton, H. Yang, D.B.W. Chritton, J.W. Lee, and K. Arabatzis. 1990b. The effects of moderate exercise training on natural killer cells and acute upper respiratory tract infections. *Int. J. Sports Med.* 11:467-473.

Nieman, D.C., and B.K. Pedersen. 2000. *Nutrition and Exercise Immunology.* Boca Raton, FL: CRC Press.

Nieman, D.C., E.M. Peters, D.A. Henson, E. Nevines, and M.M. Thompson. 2000c. Influence of vitamin C supplementation on cytokine changes following an ultramarathon. *J. Interferon Cytokine Res.* 20:1029-1035.

Parker, S., P. Brukner, and M. Rosier. 1996. Chronic fatigue syndrome and the athlete. *Sports Med. Train. Rehab.* 6: 269-278.

Peters E.M., J.M. Goetzsche, L.E. Joseph, and T.D. Noakes. 1996. Vitamin C as effective as combinations of anti-oxidant nutrients in reducing symptoms of upper respiratory tract infection in ultramarathon runners. *S. Afr. J. Sports Med.* 11(3):23-27.

Peters E.M., J.M. Goetzsche, B. Grobbelaar, and T.D. Noakes. 1993. Vitamin C supplementation reduces the incidence of postrace symptoms of upper-respiratory-tract infection in ultramarathon runners. *Am. J. Clin. Nutr.* 57:170-174.

Pizza, F.X., D. Cavender, A. Stockard, H. Baylies, and A. Beighle. 1999. Antiinflammatory doses of ibuprofen: effect on neutrophils and exercise-induced muscle injury. *Int. J. Sports Med.* 20:98-102.

Rohde, T., D.A. MacLean, and B.K. Pedersen. 1998. Effect of glutamine supplementation on changes in the immune system induced by repeated exercise. *Med. Sci. Sports Exerc.* 30:856-862.

Shephard, R.J., T. Kavanagh, D.J. Mertens, S. Qureshi, and M. Clark. 1995. Personal health benefits of Masters athletics competition. *Br. J. Sports Med.* 29:35-40.

Tvede, N., J. Steensberg, B. Baslund, J.H. Kristensen, and B.K. Pedersen. 1991. Cellular immunity in highly-trained elite racing cyclists and controls during periods of training with high and low intensity. *Scand. J. Sports Med.* 1:163-166.

Weidner, T.G., B.N. Anderson, L.A. Kaminsky, E.C. Dick, and T. Schurr. 1997. Effect of a rhinovirus-caused upper respiratory illness on pulmonary function test and exercise responses. *Med. Sci. Sports Exerc.* 29:604-609.

Weidner, T., T. Cranston, T. Schurr, and L. Kaminsky. 1998.   The effect of exercise training on the severity and duration of a viral upper respiratory illness. *Med. Sci. Sports Exerc.* 30:1578-1583, 1998.

USE OF NON-STARCH CARBOHYDRATE ENERGY SOURCES IN PERFORMANCE HORSE FEEDS

JAN ERIK LINDBERG
Swedish University of Agricultural Sciences, Uppsala, Sweden

Introduction

Performance is determined by genetic potential, training, and nutrition. An optimal nutrient supply is needed to achieve maximal power output and stamina. The athletic horse is subjected to regular training and competes close to its physiological limits. In contrast, the exercising horse, which may also be trained for successful performance, will not reach its physiological limits during performance. However, the duration and intensity of the work performed by the equine athlete will differ markedly. Racehorses will perform intensive muscular work at high-speed, near-maximal capacity for a couple of minutes, while horses used for three-day events and endurance rides will perform less intensive muscular work at submaximal capacity for many hours. Thus, in the racehorse the causes of fatigue will mainly be related to the depletion of substrates used for energy production and the accumulation of lactate (Frape, 1988; Hiney and Potter, 1996). In contrast, in the endurance horse the causes of fatigue will be related to the heat load and fluid and electrolyte loss, in addition to the depletion of substrates used for energy production (Jansson, 1999).

During exercise the blood flow to the digestive tract decreases, while the blood flow to the locomotor and respiratory muscles increases markedly (Duren, 1998). Interestingly, the pattern of change in blood flow distribution was the same in fasted and fed horses but with significantly higher blood flows in the fed animals. In absolute terms, blood flow (ml/g tissue/min) during exercise is four to five times higher to the locomotor muscles and three to four times higher to the respiratory muscles when compared to blood flow to the digestive organs. This implies that the feeding of the performing athlete has to be made according to a long-term plan and should aim at providing the nutrients necessary for building adequate body nutrient stores. If this is done successfully, it will allow maximal performance with respect to body energy needs and will allow the animal to handle the heat load resulting from extended periods of intensive work. In addition, recovery after exercise will be faster, and this will allow the animal to perform at maximal capacity more regularly.

Digestive Processes and Nutrient Utilization

THE EQUINE DIGESTIVE SYSTEM

Anatomically, horses are classified as nonruminant herbivores or hindgut fermentors (Stevens, 1988). They use endogenous enzymes to digest carbohydrates, protein, and fat in the stomach and small intestine and utilize microflora to ferment organic matter in the hindgut. The stomach is small and composes less than 7% of the empty weight of the digestive system, while the small intestine makes up approximately 27% (Duren, 1998). The hindgut (cecum and colon) is the largest organ system in the gastrointestinal (GI) tract of the horse and accounts for approximately 64% of the empty weight of the system. The small capacity of the upper part of the digestive tract imposes limits on handling large single meals that may overwhelm the digestive capacity and allow undigested feed material to be transported to the hindgut. This may cause excessive and uncontrolled fermentation in the hindgut, with the risk of inducing various digestive problems. However, the design of the digestive tract allows large quantities of fiber-rich feeds to be continuously ingested and utilized by the horse. Due to the anatomical design of the equine GI tract, sufficient quantities of fiber in the diet are a prerequisite for normal function of the hindgut and thus for normal digestion.

HINDGUT DIGESTION

Digestion in the hindgut is extensive in the horse, and proper functioning is necessary to efficiently utilize the fiber-rich part of the diet. The hindgut harbors a vast microflora population that lives in symbiosis with the host animal and is responsible for digestion in this section of the GI tract. A substantial part of the energy in the diet is provided through microbial hindgut digestion (Glinsky et al., 1976), while there appears to be only a marginal absorption of microbial-produced amino acids from the hindgut (McMeniman et al., 1987).

Diet composition (i.e., forage to concentrate ratio, cereal source) and feed processing (i.e., grinding, hydrothermal processing) will affect the partition of digestion between the small intestine and the hindgut and will have an impact on the intensity and extent of digestion. The small intestine is the major site for protein, fat, and soluble carbohydrate digestion, and cell walls are digested in the hindgut (Hintz et al., 1971). The relative importance of hindgut digestion will increase with increased levels of forage in the diet. It has been shown that cecal pH will lower with increased starch intake (Radicke et al., 1991). The effect of starch intake was more pronounced when maize was contributing the starch as compared with oats. This could be explained by the lower small digestibility of maize starch as compared with oat starch (Kienzle, 1994). Willard et al. (1977) showed that when changing from an all-hay diet to an all-concentrate diet the cecal pH was significantly reduced and the molar proportion of acetate was reduced, but the molar proportion of propionate was increased. The dietary-induced changes in hindgut fermentation might influence the extent of hindgut digestion and could explain differences in diet digestibility and nutrient utilization.

Diet Composition

Forages should always be the foundation of an equine diet, with additional concentrate used only to increase the energy density and to supply essential nutrients not contained in the forage. Forages are composed of cell contents (protein, fat, soluble carbohydrates) and cell walls (cellulose, hemicellulose, lignin) and may vary in their relative proportions. The cell content is highly digestible (80-100%) (Fonnesbeck, 1968, 1969), and the true digestibility of the cell wall is more limited (40-50%) (Fonnesbeck, 1968, 1969). Thus, the nutritive value of forages can vary considerably and will largely be determined by the fiber content and the fiber quality. The stage of maturity will have a profound effect on the energy and nutrient content of the forage and on the horse's ability to consume offered quantities. By selecting a high-quality forage (high energy content) rather than a low-quality one, the diet proportions between forage and concentrate can be markedly affected (Table 1) and made more favorable with regards to voluntary feed intake and digestive functions (Willard et al., 1977; Radicke et al., 1991).

Table 1. Diet proportions (dry matter; DM) and total DM intake (DMI) of hay and concentrate, and of cereal grains in a hay:concentrate diet with different hay energy content calculated to cover the energy and protein requirements of a 500-kg mature equine athlete (NRC, 1989).

	Proportion of energy from hay:concentrate	
	Hay:concentrate 25:75[1]	*Hay:concentrate 50:50[2]*
Diet proportions[3]		
Hay, kg DM	4.0	6.6
Concentrate, kg DM	7.0	5.0
Total DMI, kg	11.5	11.6
Cereal grains		
Oats	7.7	5.1
Barley	6.7	4.4
Wheat	6.4	4.2
Maize	6.4	4.2

[1] Hay 8.4 MJ DE/kg DM; 100 g crude protein/kg DM; [2] Hay 10.4 MJ DE/kg DM; 120 g crude protein/kg DM; [3] Concentrate 13.8 MJ DE/kg DM

Concentrate is included in the diets of athletic horses in order to increase the energy density of the diet, thereby making it possible to meet increased energy demands. Cereals, which are characterized by their high starch content, are the major concentrate components. However, feeding excessive amounts of starch can increase the risk of digestive and muscular problems. Total amylase secretion in the equine small intestine is considered to be a limiting factor for starch digestion (Kienzle et al., 1994) and may result in an influx of readily fermentable carbohydrates (i.e., undigested starch) to the hindgut. This could result in colic due to excessive hindgut fermentation (Potter et al., 1992a; Kienzle et al., 1994) and altered microbial activity, leading to unrestrained gas production and a reduction in hindgut pH (Beyer, 1998). Also, gastric ulcers (Beyer, 1998) and tying-up, both sporadic and recurrent exertional rhabdomyolysis (Valberg, 1998), may be related to excessive use of grains and sweet feed in equine rations. Therefore, the replacement of starch-rich cereal grains with non-starch carbohydrate feeds in the equine diet may be an alternative means of avoiding problems related to high starch intakes and undigested starch reaching the hindgut.

The dietary content of starch is markedly affected by the cereal source used in the diet (Table 1), as is the utilization of the cereal carbohydrate part of the diet (Kienzle, 1994). This will change the composition of the digesta reaching the hindgut and will alter hindgut microbial activity.

STARCH UTILIZATION

There are several factors related to the macro- and microstructure of the cereal grain that will affect starch utilization in the horse. The grain macrostructure (i.e., shape, size, husks) will largely determine the utilization of unprocessed cereal grains, but in mechanically processed grains, the macrostructure will be more or less destroyed. The grain microstructure (i.e., structure of starch granules, length and branching of the starch molecule, hydrogen bonds between molecular chains) will to a lesser extent be affected by mechanical processing, and hydrothermal processing (i.e., steam flaking, micronizing, popping, extrusion) may destroy the grain microstructure.

The ileal digestibility of cereal starch varies with grain source and with processing (Kienzle, 1994). In contrast, the total tract digestibility of cereal starches is high and often marginally affected by the grain source and processing (Meyer, 1992). The highest small intestinal starch digestibility is found in oats, and maize starch appears to be less digestible (Kienzle, 1994). The lowest small intestinal starch digestibility has been recorded for barley. A rough mechanical processing of the grain (such as rolling or crushing) does not change the ileal starch digestibility, but fine grinding (<2-mm particle size) will generally improve the ileal starch digestibility. Also, hydrothermal processing (i.e., micronizing, popping) will improve the small intestinal starch digestibility.

In a compilation of data on small intestinal starch digestibility, Kienzle (1994) found a tendency toward lower digestibility with higher starch intakes. The risk of exceeding the small intestinal starch-digesting capacity was dependent on cereal starch source but appeared to occur above an intake of 2 g starch/kg body weight (BW) per meal.

The small intestinal starch digestibility may also be affected by forage source (hay or grass meal), as well as by the proportion of forage and concentrate in the diet (Kienzle, 1994). When the forage source in the diet was grass hay, the small intestinal starch digestibility was lower (20%) than when the forage source in the diet was green meal (47%).

As pointed out by Kienzle (1994), there could be large individual differences in small intestinal starch digestibility in horses, which could partly be explained by differences in small intestinal amylase activity. In addition, individual differences in the eating behavior (i.e., pattern of hay and concentrate ingestion) may be involved in determining the small intestinal starch digestibility.

UTILIZATION OF NON-STARCH CARBOHYDRATE FEEDS

In contrast to cereals, non-starch carbohydrate feeds are characterized by having no starch and a carbohydrate fraction that is composed of sugars and/or dietary fiber. The feeds classified in this category are mainly industrial by-products. The carbohydrate fraction in molasses and syrup contains sugars, and in feeds such as beet pulp and citrus pulp, the major part is made up of dietary fiber.

Simple sugars (glucose and fructose) are effectively utilized by the horse and are absorbed in the small intestine (Meyer, 1992). This is reflected in a rapid increase in plasma glucose values, with a similar response for both glucose and fructose (Bullimore et al., 2000). As shown by Jansson et al. (2002), adult horses have no problem digesting and efficiently utilizing hydrolyzed starch (glucose:maltose:maltotriose proportion of 83:15:2) at levels of 2.5 g/kg BW per day. In contrast, there are limitations in the digestive capacity of certain disaccharides depending on age and the change in secretion of digestive enzymes (Meyer, 1992). Thus, in the foal lactose is effectively utilized due to a high activity of lactase, and sucrose is less efficiently utilized due to a limited activity of sucrase. The situation is reversed in the adult horse. According to Meyer (1992), the upper limit to dietary inclusion of lactose in the adult horse is 1 g/kg BW per day in order to avoid digestive disturbances.

Cellulose and cereal fiber sources are fermented to a limited extent by the equine hindgut microflora (Sunvold et al., 1995a,b). In contrast, fiber-rich feeds containing pectin (sugar beet pulp and citrus pulp), fructooligosaccharides, sugar alcohols, and gums could be expected to be extensively fermented in the hindgut (Sunvold et al., 1995b). However, the rate and extent of fermentation will vary considerably between fiber sources and must be considered when formulating rations for performance horses. For sugar beet pulp, inclusion levels of up to 3.0 g/kg BW per day have been used in adult horses without any negative effects on overall nutrient utilization and performance (Lindberg and Jacobsson, 1992; Lindberg and Palmgren Karlsson, 2001; Palmgren Karlsson et al., 2002).

Non-Starch Carbohydrate Feeds

NUTRITIONAL EFFECTS

Protein digestibility. Replacement of oats with sugar beet pulp (SBP) will result in reduced total tract apparent digestibility of crude protein (CP) at maintained CP content in the diet (Table 2). The reduction observed with SBP inclusion could be explained by an increase in hindgut fermentation due to an increase in the supply of easily fermentable carbohydrates (Moore-Colyer et al., 1997) and the resulting increase in fecal excretion of microbial protein (Sauer et al., 1980; Lindberg and Jacobsson, 1992). Similar effects should be expected with other easily fermentable fiber sources. In contrast, no reduction in the total tract apparent digestibility of CP could be found when barley syrup (BS) replaced oats. The digestion of BS (hydrolyzed barley starch), as well as sugars, will take place in the small intestine and should be expected to be virtually complete when the digesta reaches the hindgut. Consequently, these types of feeds will not contribute to fermentation in the hindgut.

Table 2. Nutritional effects of replacing oats with non-starch carbohydrate energy sources in horse feeds.

		Nutrient content, g/kg DM					Digestibility, %				
Exp.	Diet	Protein	Fat	Starch	Sugars	NDF	Protein	Fat	NDF	Energy	Ref.
I	OLF	109	29	179	50	460	58	22	40	52	1
	OHF	109	55	145	52	461	59	51	42	54	
	SBPLF	111	23	106	49	482	52	-5	42	51	
	SBPHF	109	49	99	50	477	53	40	42	52	
II	Oats	112	25	147	39	491	72	38	40	56	2
	SBP	116	20	86	82	485	67	8	43	54	
III	BS 0	100	26	131	19	426	59	34	42	58	3
	BS 0.5	96	24	109	62	418	54	25	37	55	
	BS 1.0	93	21	84	104	413	55	17	36	54	
	BS 1.5	90	18	61	151	405	58	13	43	60	

1. Lindberg and Palmgren Karlsson (2001). Grass hay:concentrate ratio 0.56:0.35, main concentrate ingredients; OLF (oats), OHF (oats, maize oil), SBPLF (dried unmolassed sugar beet pulp, oats), SBPHF (dried unmolassed sugar beet pulp, oats, maize oil).
2. Palmgren Karlsson et al. (2002). Grass hay:concentrate ratio 0.66:0.34, main concentrate ingredients; Oats (oats), SBP (dried molassed sugar beet pulp, oats).
3. Lindberg (unpublished data) and Jansson et al. (2002). Grass hay:concentrate ratio 0.65:0.35, main concentrate ingredients; BS 0 (oats), BS 0.5 (oats, barley syrup 0.5 kg/d), BS 1.0 (oats, barley syrup 1.0 kg/d), BS 1.5 (oats, barley syrup 1.5 kg/d).

It should be noted that a reduction in total tract digestibility of CP may not give a true reflection of the utilization of dietary CP, due to the influence of hindgut digestion. The absorption of amino acids in the small intestine may be of a similar magnitude despite differences measured in the total tract digestibility. Interestingly, the retention of digested CP and the plasma urea levels remained unchanged when oats were replaced with SBP (Palmgren Karlsson, 2001) or BS (Lindberg, unpublished data), indicating that there were no major differences in CP utilization and nitrogen metabolism between the diets.

Fat digestibility. Replacement of oats with SBP results in a reduction in the total tract apparent digestibility of crude fat (EE). This is caused by a reduction in the dietary fat content (Table 2) and by increased hindgut fermentation. With a lowered dietary fat content, the endogenous fat excretion will make a proportionally larger contribution to the fecal fat content (Meyer, 1992), and with increased hindgut fermentation, a higher endogenous excretion of fat could be expected through enhanced microbial mass (Lindberg and Jacobsson, 1992; Potter et al., 1992b). Also, replacement of oats with BS resulted in a numeric reduction in the total tract apparent digestibility of EE (Table 2) due to the reduction in dietary fat content.

As discussed for CP, a reduction in total tract digestibility of EE may not give a true reflection of the utilization of the dietary fat. It should be expected that the daily intake of fat will greatly influence the crude fat digestibility of the diet (Potter et al., 1992b). Thus, when compiling the digestibility data from diets in which oats were replaced with SBP and BS (Table 3), the crude fat digested was found to be linearly related to the daily intake of fat ($y=0.67x-111$, $r^2=0.91$). The estimated true digestibility of EE (67%) was slightly lower than other published values (Rich et al., 1981; Meyer, 1992). The estimated endogenous fecal excretion of fat in the present data was 13 g/kg DM intake or 237 mg/kg BW. This was considerably higher than values (50-100 mg fat/kg BW) suggested by Meyer (1992) but was within the range of values (9-33 g fat/kg DM intake) reported by Freeman et al. (1968). The discrepancy from the values given by Meyer (1992) may be explained by extensive microbial fermentation in the hindgut and high excretion of microbial mass.

Fiber digestibility. Despite substantial variation in the dietary carbohydrate composition when oats were replaced with SBP and BS (Table 2), the digestibility of neutral detergent fiber (NDF) remained unaffected. If the hindgut digestion was not disturbed by the change in dietary carbohydrate composition, this result should be expected when considering the large NDF contribution from hay in the diets (0.75-0.80 in Exp. I; 0.8 in Exp. II; 0.8-0.9 in Exp. III). Further, the digestibility of NDF in hay:oat diets has been shown to remain unchanged when the dietary proportions have ranged from 100:0 to 60:40 (Palmgren Karlsson et al., 2000). Thus, despite an extensive hindgut digestion of SBP (Longland et al., 1997; Moore-Colyer et al., 1997), its small contribution to the total dietary NDF content (0.14 in Exp. I; 0.06-0.13 in Exp. II) could be expected to result in minor effects on the total tract digestibility of NDF, which would fall within the normal range of variation around the mean (Palmgren Karlsson, 2001).

Energy digestibility and utilization. The digestibility of dietary energy was unaffected when oats were replaced with SBP and BS (Table 2). However, despite limited effects on the digestibility of energy, the excretion of urinary energy (in % of DE) increased (from 4.8-4.9% to 5.3-5.8%) when oats were replaced by SBP (Palmgren Karlsson, 2001). This indicates a negative influence of SBP on the utilization of dietary energy. In contrast, the replacement of oats with BS did not change the extent of urinary energy excretion (Lindberg, unpublished data).

Metabolic Effects

Postprandial glucose response. The replacement of cereal grains with non-starch carbohydrate feeds will reduce the dietary starch content and may alter the glycemic effect of the diet (Stull and Rodiek, 1988). Glucose homeostasis is under strict hormonal control, mainly by insulin, but may also be affected by diet composition. During exercise the glucose supply is primarily provided from body glycogen stores and to a minor extent from gluconeogenesis. In addition, blood glucose levels may be improved by glucose originating from the digestion of dietary starch (Hiney and Potter, 1996). In order to ensure a continuous and sufficient glucose supply for the working muscles, the body glycogen stores have to be filled by proper feeding prior to the onset of exercise. Also, feeding management during the recovery period after exercise may be of importance for the repletion of body glycogen stores (Hiney and Potter, 1996).

Diets resulting in a reduced glucose uptake will be expected to lower peak blood glucose levels and to lower the insulin response, which may have beneficial effects for the exercising horse in maintaining sufficient blood glucose levels (Frape, 1988; Hiney and Potter, 1996). However, available data are not conclusive with respect to the influence of dietary carbohydrate composition on postprandial blood glucose levels. Thus, it has been shown that diets with varying forage to grain ratios fed to ponies (Argenzio and Hintz, 1971; Hintz et al., 1971), as well as diets with varying proportions of alfalfa and corn fed to horses (Stull and Rodiek, 1988), resulted in unchanged blood glucose levels. Similarly, no marked dietary-related effect on postprandial blood glucose was observed (Figure 1) when oats were replaced with molassed SBP (Palmgren Karlsson et al., 2002) or when oats were replaced with BS (Jansson et al., 2002). However, when replacing oats with plain SBP, the postprandial increase in plasma glucose was slower and the peak concentration was lower (Lindberg and Palmgren Karlsson, 2001).

Exercise glucose response. The replacement of oats with SBP had no effect on plasma glucose levels in blood samples taken during an exercise test (ET). The horses completed a distance of 2,600 m on a 2.5% incline (Phase 3) at about 90% of VO_{2max} (~205 beats/min), following a warm-up at submaximal speed for 24 minutes (Phase 1) and a two-hour rest in a box (Phase 2) (Palmgren Karlsson et al., 2002). Also, the replacement of oats with BS had no effect on plasma glucose levels in blood samples taken during an incremental exercise (IE) test performed at a 6.25% incline at four speeds stepwise, increasing from 6 m/s to 9 m/s every second minute, or during a submaximal exercise (SE) test performed on the flat at 50-60% of VO_{2max} (5.5-7.5 m/s) for 40 minutes, which corresponded to a distance of 17 km (Jansson et al., 2002).

Postprandial insulin response. In contrast to blood glucose, a response in postprandial insulin levels is often observed when the availability of dietary carbohydrates is improved due to a change in composition (Hiney and Potter, 1996). This implies that insulin, as compared with glucose, would be a more sensitive and useful indicator of any glycemic effect of the diet.

It has been shown that the postprandial insulin levels were different when feeding the diets with SBP as compared with oats (Figure 1), with a less pronounced insulin response when oats had been replaced with SBP (Lindberg and Palmgren Karlsson, 2001; Palmgren Karlsson et al., 2002). Further, it was also noted that the oat diet resulted in higher plasma insulin values at rest than the diet where oats were replaced with SBP (Palmgren Karlsson et al., 2002). Also, when oats were replaced with BS there was a marked postprandial response in insulin (Jansson et al., 2002). However, in contrast to the studies on SBP, the replacement of oats with BS did not show any differences in insulin response that could be related to the change in dietary carbohydrate composition. These findings can be explained by the change in dietary carbohydrate availability and the resulting change in the site of digestion and absorption of digestion products. The less pronounced insulin response observed with SBP inclusion could be explained by the reduction in dietary starch content and, with a shift in carbohydrate digestion from the small intestine to the hindgut, by an increase in the supply of easily fermentable carbohydrates (Moore-Colyer et al., 1997). In contrast, when oats were replaced with BS the potential availability of the easily available part of the dietary carbohydrate fraction changed, while the composition of fermentable fraction of the diet remained unchanged. Thus, the digestion of BS (hydrolyzed barley starch), as well as of oat starch (Kienzle, 1994), will take place in the small intestine and should be expected to give a similar response in insulin, provided that the digestion of the unprocessed oat starch is virtually complete when the digesta reaches the hindgut. The insulin response suggests a significant influence of diet carbohydrate composition on nutrient utilization in horses and could possibly also have effects on the subsequent performance.

Exercise insulin response. The replacement of oats with SBP had no effect on insulin levels in blood samples taken during the ET (Palmgren Karlsson et al., 2002). Also, the replacement of oats with BS had no effect on insulin levels in blood samples taken during the IE or SE tests (Jansson et al., 2002).

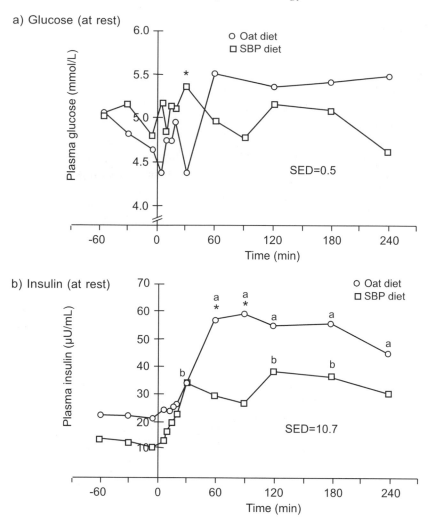

Figure 1. Concentrations of plasma glucose and insulin at rest in Standardbred horses. Oat diet and SBP diet. H = difference between diets (P<0.05). The SED (standard error of difference) refers to the comparison of diets within time. a = Oat diet: value differing significantly (P<0.05) from the preprandial mean value; b = SBP diet: value differing significantly (P<0.05) from the preprandial mean value (Palmgren Karlsson et al., 2002).

Exercise lactate response. The plasma lactate concentration increased following the intensive trots during Phases 1 and 3 of the ET (Figure 2) (Palmgren Karlsson et al., 2002). A higher peak lactate concentration was found at Phases 1 and 3, as well as five minutes after the intensive trot in Phase 1, on the oat diet than on the SBP diet. However, when oats were replaced with BS there were no dietary effects on plasma lactate concentration during the IE or SE tests (Jansson et al., 2002).

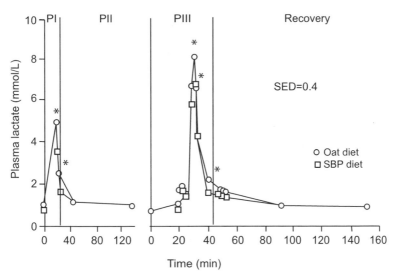

Figure 2. Concentrations of plasma lactate during the exercise test performed in Standardbred horses, where PI = Phase I (warming-up), PII = Phase II (rest) and PIII = Phase III (simulated trotting race). The SED (standard error of difference) refers to the comparison of diets within time (Palmgren Karlsson et al., 2002).

Exercise muscle glycogen and muscle lactate response. When oats were replaced with SBP, the content of muscle glycogen was similar prior to the ET, but it was higher after the ET on the SBP diet (Table 3) (Palmgren Karlsson et al., 2002). Also, the muscle lactate content increased following the ET, and the post-exercise level of muscle lactate was significantly higher on the oat diet than on the SBP diet (Table 3). When oats were replaced with BS, there was a gradual change in muscle glycogen content following the SE test, resulting in more glycogen remaining with increasing replacement of oats (Jansson et al., 2002). It was found that muscle glycogen utilization decreased (r^2=0.96) with increasing proportions of sugar in the diet (Figure 3).

Table 3. Effect of submaximal exercise on muscle glycogen and muscle lactate values (mmol/ kg dry weight) in horses fed diets where oats were replaced with sugar beet pulp (SBP) (Palmgren Karlsson et al., 2002).

		Diet		
	Exercise	*Oats*	*SBP*	*Significance*
Muscle glycogen#	Before	546	597	NS
	After	394	484	P<0.05
Muscle lactate§	Before	10.8	10.4	NS
	After	38.5	22.7	P<0.05

SED 39; § SED 3.8

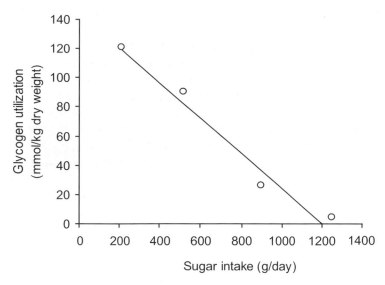

Figure 3. Muscle glycogen utilization (SEM 44) in relation to daily sugar intake (y=143.1-0.12x, R^2=0.96) (Jansson et al., 2002).

Exercise oxygen consumption (VO$_2$) and respiratory quotient (RQ). There was no significant dietary effect with regard to VO$_2$ during the performance of the SE test (Jansson et al., 2002) when oats were replaced with BS, although the VO$_2$ was numerically lowered with increasing replacement of oats. However, for RQ a dietary effect could be verified if the diets were pooled into HIGH (1.8-2.5 g sugar/kg BW per day) and LOW (0.3-1.0 g sugar/kg BW per day) sugar intake. Thus, RQ was consistently higher on HIGH than on LOW (0.83 vs 0.80, 0.83 vs 0.80, 0.81 vs 0.78 and 0.80 vs 0.77 (SD 0.03) at 10, 20, 30, and 40 min, respectively) during the performance of the SE test.

The data presented above show that manipulation of the dietary carbohydrate composition to modify the relative proportions of sugars, starch, and fermentable fiber in the ration could alter energy and glucose metabolism in exercising horses. In accordance with Pagan et al. (1987), a high sugar intake could be expected to augment the metabolism of carbohydrates during submaximal exercise as shown by the increased RQ. Also, as the oxygen consumption was lowered (numerically), it could be expected that a greater proportion of the energy was generated from anaerobic metabolism. However, the plasma lactate levels were not affected by diet, which could be due to the low intensity of the work and that the potential for lactate to be converted into pyruvate by the liver and muscle tissue was not limited. It could be speculated that the increased carbohydrate consumption during the submaximal exercise was due to a high availability of glucose in plasma originating from the liver because muscle glycogen utilization was reduced. This contention is supported in results presented by Pagan et al. (1987), which showed that there is a positive relationship between muscle glycogen content and RQ during low-intensity exercise.

The blood and muscle biopsy data suggest that the rate of glycogenolysis with lactate production can be modified by manipulation of the dietary carbohydrate composition. It appears likely that the dietary proportions of sugars, starch, and fermentable fiber are key elements in understanding this metabolic effect. The glycogen-saving effect of replacing oats with SBP (Palmgren Karlsson et al., 2002) could possibly be explained by a higher production of short-chain fatty acids (SCFA; i.e., acetate, propionate, and butyrate) in the hindgut as a result of the change in diet carbohydrate composition and a shift in digestion from the small intestine to the hindgut, and the subsequent increase in SCFA absorption in the portal blood. After transport into the cell the SCFA will be transformed to acetyl-CoA via specific fatty acyl-CoA ligases, thus resulting in the same key metabolite that is being produced from the beta-oxidation of fat. Therefore, the inclusion of fermentable fiber in the diet may result in a similar glucose-saving (and glycogen-saving) effect as that ascribed to the supply of fat in the equine diet (Potter et al., 1992b) by providing an alternative substrate for the aerobic energy metabolism in the muscle. Another possible, and maybe more likely, explanation to the glycogen-saving effect of replacing oats with SBP (Palmgren Karlsson et al., 2002) could be the increase in sugar intake (increase of about 350 g sugar/day when SBP replaced oats in the diet) and an increased utilization of blood-borne glucose. Acute oral administration of glucose (Geor et al., 2000) and acute ingestion of a glycemic meal (Jose-Cunilleras et al., 2002) prior to submaximal exercise have been shown to cause an augmentation of carbohydrate oxidation and utilization of blood-borne glucose during exercise. This is also supported by the data showing that muscle glycogen utilization decreased with increasing proportions of sugar in the diet (Figure 3) when oats were replaced by BS (Jansson et al., 2002). When oats replaced SBP (Palmgren Karlsson et al., 2002) the decrease in muscle glycogen content was 152 and 113 mmol/kg dry weight on the oat and SBP diets, respectively. The difference between diets (39 mmol/kg dry weight) was comparable to the glycogen-saving effect of increasing sugar intake ($350 \times 0.12 = 42$ mmol/kg dry weight) found by Jansson et al. (2002).

Conclusion

In conclusion, the limited nutritional effects of replacing oats with non-starch carbohydrate feeds suggest that this feeding practice could be used in the horse industry to minimize the risk of digestive disturbances from excessive starch intake without impairing the overall nutrient utilization. Furthermore, a more extensive use of non-starch carbohydrate feeds to allow a manipulation of the dietary carbohydrate composition, aiming at modifying the relative proportions of sugars, starch, and fermentable fiber in the ration, may cause beneficial alterations in the energy and glucose metabolism of the exercising horse.

References

Argenzio, R.A. and H.F. Hintz. 1972. Effect of diet on glucose entry and oxidation rates in ponies. J. Nutr. 102:879-892.

Beyer, M. 1998. Colic. In: Advances in Equine Nutrition, ed. J. D. Pagan, Nottingham University Press, Manor Farm, Trumpton, UK, pp. 483-488.

Bullimore, S.R., J.D. Pagan, P.A. Harris, K.E. Hoekstra, K.A. Roose, S.C. Gardner, and R.J. Geor. 2000. Carbohydrate supplementation of horses during endurance exercise: comparison of fructose and glucose. J. Nutr. 130:1760-1765.

Duren, S.E. 1998. The gut during exercise. In Advances in Equine Nutrition, ed. J. D. Pagan, Nottingham University Press. Pp. 149-159.

Fonnesbeck, P.V. 1968. Digestion of soluble and fibrous carbohydrates of forages by horses. J. Anim. Sci. 27:1336-1344.

Fonnesbeck, P.V. 1969. Partitioning the nutrients of forage for horses. J. Anim. Sci. 28:624-638.

Frape, D.L. 1988. Dietary requirements and athletic performance. Equine Vet. J. 20:163-172.

Freeman, C.P., D.W. Holme, and E.F Annison. 1968. The determination of the true digestibilities of interesterified fats in young pigs. Br. J. Nutr. 22:651-660.

Geor, R.J., K.W. Hinchcliff, L.J. McCutcheon, and R.A. Sams. 2000. Epinephrine inhibits exogenous glucose utilization in exercising horses. J. Appl. Physiol. 88:1777-1790.

Glinsky, M.J., R.M. Smith, H.R. Spires, and C.L. Davis. 1976. Measurement of volatile fatty acid production rates in the cecum of the pony. J. Anim. Sci. 42:1465-1470.

Hiney, K.M. and G.D. Potter. 1996. A review of recent research on nutrition and metabolism in the athletic horse. Nutr. Res. Rew. 9:149-173.

Hintz, H.F., D.E. Hogue, E.F. Walker Jr., J.E. Lowe, and H.F. Schryver. 1971. Apparent digestion in various segments of the digestive tract of ponies fed diets with varying roughage-grain ratios. J. Anim. Sci. 32:245-248.

Jansson, A. 1999. Sodium and potassium regulation-with special reference to the athlethic horse. Swedish University of Agricultural Sciences, Acta Universitatis Agriculturae Sueciae, Agraria 179.

Jansson, A., S. Nyman, A. Lindholm, and J.E. Lindberg. 2002. Effects on exercise metabolism of varying dietary starch and sugar proportions. Equine Vet. J. Suppl. (In press).

Jose-Cunilleras, E., K.W. Hinchcliff, R.A. Sams, S.T. Devor, and J.K. Linderman. 2002. Glycemic index of a meal fed before exercise alters substrate use and glucose flux in exercising horses. J. Appl. Physiol. 92:117-128.

Kienzle, E. 1994. Small intestinal digestion of starch in the horse. Revue Méd. Vét. 145:199-204.

Kienzle, E., S. Radicke, E. Landes, D. Kleffken, M. Illenseer, and H. Meyer. 1994. Activity of amylase in the gastrointestinal tract of the horse. J. Anim. Physiol. Anim. Nutr. 72:234-241.

Lindberg, J.E. and K.G. Jacobsson. 1992. Effects of barley and sugar-beet pulp on digestibility, purine excretion and blood parameters in horses. Pferdeheilkunde 116-118.

Lindberg, J.E. and C. Palmgren Karlsson. 2001. Effect of replacing oats with sugar beet pulp and maize oil on nutrient utilization in horses. Equine Vet. J. 33:585-590.

Longland, A.C., M. Moore-Colyer, J.J. Hyslop, M.S. Dhanoa, and D. Cuddeford, 1997. Comparison of the in sacco degradation of the non-starch polysaccharide and neutral detergent fiber fraction of four sources of dietary fiber by ponies. Proc. 15th Equine Nutr. Physiol. Symp., pp. 120-121.

McMeniman, N.P., R. Elliot, S. Groenendyk, and K.F. Dowsett. 1987. Synthesis and absorption of cysteine from the hindgut of the horse. Equine Vet. J. 19:192-194.

Meyer, H. 1992. Pferdefütterung. 2. Auflage. Verlag Paul Parey, Berlin und Hamburg.

Moore-Colyer, M., J.J. Hyslop, A.C. Longland, and D. Cuddeford, 1997. Degradation of four dietary fiber sources by ponies as measured by the mobile bag technique. Proc. 15th Equine Nutr. Physiol. Symp., pp. 118-119.

NRC, 1989. Nutrient requirements of horses. 5th revised edition. National Academy Press, Washington, D. C., USA.

Pagan, J.D., B. Essén-Gustavsson, A. Lindholm, and J.R. Thornton. 1987. The effect of dietary energy source on excercise performance in Standardbred horses. In Equine Exercise Physiology 2, eds. Gillespie, J. R. & N. E. Robinson, ICEEP Publ. Davis, California, pp. 686-700.

Palmgren Karlsson, C. 2001. Nutrient utilization in horses-Effect of oats replacement on ration digestibility and metabolic parameters. Swedish University of Agricultural Sciences, Acta Universitatis Agriculturae Sueciae, Agraria 270.

Palmgren Karlsson, C., A. Jansson, B. Essén-Gustavsson, and J.E. Lindberg. 2002. Effect of molassed sugar beet pulp on nutrient utilization and metabolic parameters during exercise. Equine Vet. J. Suppl. (In press).

Palmgren Karlsson, C., J.E. Lindberg, and M. Rundgren. 2000. Associative effects on total tract digestibility in horses fed different ratios of grass hay and whole oats. Livest. Prod. Sci. 65:143-153.

Potter, G.D., F.F. Arnold, D.D Householder, D.H. Hansen, and K.M. Brown. 1992a. Digestion of starch in the small or large intestine of the equine. Pferdeheilkunde 107-111.

Potter, G.D., S.L. Hughes, T.R. Julen, and D.L Swinney. 1992b. A review of research on digestion and utilization of fat by the equine. Pferdeheilkunde

119-123.

Radicke, S., E. Kienzle, and H. Meyer. 1991. Preileal apparent digestibility of oats and corn starch and consequences for cecal metabolism. Proceedings of the 12th Equine Nutrition and Physiology Symposium. Calgary, Canada. p. 43.

Rich, G.A., J.P. Fontenot, and T.N. Meacham. 1981. Digestibility of animal, vegetable and blended fats by equines. Proc. 7th Equine Nutr. Physiol. Symp., pp. 30-36.

Sauer, W.C., A. Just, H. Jorgensen, H. Makonen Fekadu, and B. Eggum. 1980. The influence of diet composition on the apparent digestibility of crude protein and amino acids at the terminal ileum and overall in pigs. Acta Agric. Scand. 30:449-468.

Stevens, C. E. 1988. Comparative physiology of the vertebrate digestive system. In Comparative Nutrition, ed. K. Blaxter & I. MacDonald. John Libbey. Pp. 21-36.

Stull, C.L. and A.V. Rodiek. 1988. Responses of blood glucose, insulin and cortisol concentrations to common equine diets. J. Nutr. 118:206-213.

Sunvold, G. D., G.C. Fahey Jr., N.R. Merchen, E.C. Titgemeyer, L.D. Bourquin, L.L. Bauer,and G.A. Reinhart. 1995b. Dietary fiber for dogs: IV. In vitro fermentation of selected fiber sources by dog fecal inoculum and in vivo digestion and metabolism of fiber-supplemented diets. J. Anim. Sci. 73:1099-1109.

Sunvold, G. D., H.S. Hussein, G.C. Fahey Jr., N.R. Merchen, and G.A. Reinhart. 1995a. In vitro fermentation of cellulose, beet pulp, citrus pulp and citrus pectin using fecal inoculum from cats, dogs, horses, humans, and pigs and ruminal fluid from cattle. J. Anim. Sci. 73:3639-3648.

Valberg, S.J. 1998. Exertional rhabdomyolysis in the horse. In: Advances in Equine Nutrition, ed. J. D. Pagan, Nottingham University Press, Manor Farm, Trumpton, UK, pp. 507-512.

Willard, J.G., J.C. Willard, S.A. Wolfram, and J.P. Baker. 1977. Effect of diet on cecal pH and feeding behaviour of horses. J. Anim. Sci. 45:87-93.

EXERCISE AND STRESS—IMPACT ON ADAPTIVE PROCESSES INVOLVING WATER AND ELECTROLYTES

MANFRED COENEN
School of Veterinary Medicine Hannover, Hannover, Germany

Introduction

The widespread use of equines in different situations reflects a simple fact, a general principle for all species which have survived until now: the capacity to react to external influences by adaptation and not by refusal. A key position in this context is the ability of the equine organism–as in other species–to realize a condition as a trigger for such processes; we usually call this "stress response." This implies that any kind of stress stimulates the same principle of answers in the organism. If we take into consideration the capacity to liberate catecholamines and cortisol, there is obviously a common answer, but the real regulating structure in the background is the hypothalamus-pituitary-adrenal axis; this enables the organism to react quite differently depending on the specific kind of stress. Exercise is just such a stressor: enforced circulation, energy mobilization, and maintaining constant body temperature require sensors in a regulatory system to formulate the proper answer (e.g., in the form of lactate or sweat production). Even if specific phenomena such as sweat composition are discussed, it should be taken into account that they are parts of a network. Excellent reviews and collections of papers are available concerning fluids and electrolytes in exercising horses, and the author emphasizes that they are essential in delivering complete information reflecting the current state of knowledge (Carlson, 1987; Meyer, 1987; Meyer, 1990; Jeffcott and Clarke, 1995, 1996, 1999; Hinchcliff, 1998; Kronfeld, 2001a, 2001b, 2001c).

General Reactions to Stressful Conditions

As shown in Figure 1, various situations which upset the current balance of metabolism induce an endocrine response. Signals generated by the gastrointestinal tract or central nervous tissues stimulate communication with the pituitary gland. Direct links exist between the hypothalamus and the adrenal gland to manage heat load by inducing sweating or to prevent hypoglycemia by mobilizing energy reserves.

Mental stress triggers the hypothalamus-pituitary-adrenal axis very effectively–a phenomenon well described in wild animals–but can result in disease and death,

265

mainly due to the associated depression of immune competence. The same principle is present when metabolic stress is induced. Various situations, including increased energy requirement and limited energy supply for a certain period of time, are characterized by an increase in blood cortisol levels (Table 1).

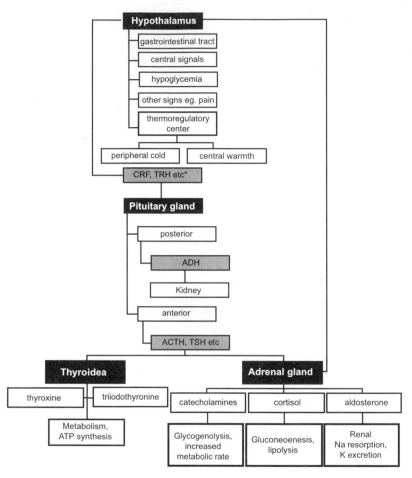

Figure 1. Overview of the hypothalamus-pituitary-adrenal axis (CRF=corticotropin releasing factor; TRH=thyrotropin-releasing hormone; ADH=antidiuretic hormone; ACTH=adrenocorticotropic hormone; TSH= thyrotropic hormone).

Exercise-related activity increases the tonus of the sympathetic nervous system mediated by the catecholamines and ACTH. In contrast to cortisol, which already increases during moderate exercise, changes in circulatory catecholamine levels are only visible during strenuous exercise (Figure 2). The correspondence between workload and catecholamines is demonstrated by the correlation of plasma catecholamines in dependence on lactate (Snow et al., 1992; McKeever 1998;

Table 1. Cortisol in blood plasma (µg/l) of horses under various conditions.

Type of metabolic stress	Control conditions	After load	Authors
Feed withdrawal, 96 h	47	55	Rose and Sampson, 1982
Pack horses, transport uphill, up to 175 kg	29	54	Coenen et al., 1999
Penned, no water, 32 h	80	170	
Transported and watered, 32 h	80	90	Friend, 2000
Transported, no water, 32 h	75	110	
Jumping	60	130	
Cross-country ride	95	155	Linden et al., 1991;
Trotting race	100	190	levels taken from figure
Flat race	80	170	
Distance ride	95	260	
Incremental exercise test	21	30	Nagata et al., 1999
Workload at 105% of VO_{2max}	20	28	
Six consecutive sprints, 1 min, 7 m/s; high fat diet	87	114	Graham-Thiers et al., 2001
Six consecutive sprints, 1 min, 7 m/s; low fat diet	58	83	

Kurosawa et al., 1999; Nagata et al., 1999; Coenen et al., 2001). But the catecholamines also reflect the reaction, meaning the adaptation to training in the form of a lowered reaction to exercise (Figure 2).

Changes in blood flow, increased cardiac output, and stimulation of sweat production are the first consequences of catecholamine liberation. The sensitivity of the sweat rate is clearly demonstrated in normal and anhidrotic horses (Marlin et al., 1999a). The reduced sweat response to adrenaline infusion in anhidrotic horses explains the significance of catecholamines in the adaptive capacity of equines to workloads involving sweat production.

Water and Electrolytes–Impact of Exercise Stress or Stressful Conditions

GENERAL ASPECTS

Body fluids and the electrolytes sodium (Na), potassium (K), and chloride (Cl) hold a key position in the thermoregulation of sweating animals. The intake of water and electrolytes is counteracted in the balanced horse by excretion via urine (chiefly) and feces to keep the balance in a neutral range. As shown in Figure 3, the renal excretion of water and electrolytes is the only dependent variable which reflects differences in intake and/or additional output via sweat (or diarrhea).

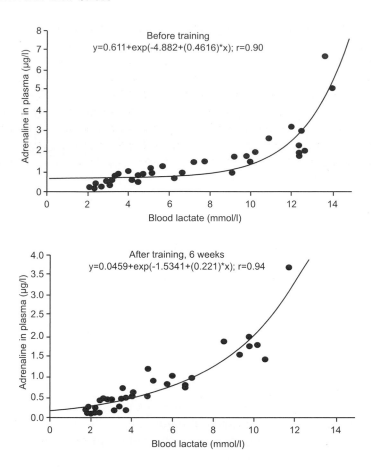

Figure 2. Adrenaline in plasma of trotters in dependance on speed and training status (Coenen et al., 2001)

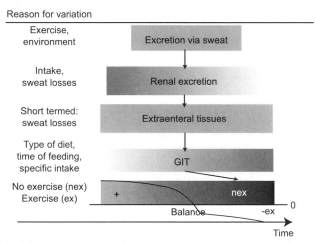

Figure 3. Principle between different compartments exchanging water and electrolytes.

Excretion through sweat itself depends on the duration and intensity of exercise and on environmental conditions, but not on intake. Extraenteral tissues (e.g., extracellular space) can be stressed by temporary depletion if reduced renal excretion does not balance sweat loss. The gastrointestinal tract (GIT) can be involved as a temporary reservoir; regarding that function, its capacity depends on diet and the time between feeding and exercise. Intake, absorption, and fecal and renal excretion are balanced to a steady state. The balance will be at zero after a certain time, but as soon as exercise begins, the balance will drop immediately and turn to the negative side in proportion to sweat losses. This is dictated by thermoregulation.

WATER

Total body water can be estimated at 662 ml/kg BW (Table 2).

Table 2. Fluid volume in the horse (Summary of data from literature).

Compartment	ml/kg BW	n	Method
Total body (TBW)	662	108	Tritium
Extracellular space (ECW)	239	128	Thiocyanate
Plasma volume (PV)	52	163	Evans blue
Extravasal part of ECW (ECWev)	187		ECW-PV
Gastrointestinal tract (GITw)	132	38	Direct weight/slaughtered horses
Intracellular space	291		TBW-(ECW+GITw)

The figures for water distribution are similar to those in other species. The extracellular space includes plasma volume, which varied between breeds. A high variation is also given for water fixed in the GIT, and this depends on the type of feed and the amount of roughage in the ration (Meyer, 1996a; 1996b; 1996c). Water intake reflects the following demands:

* secretion into the GIT,

* transport of dry matter through the GIT,

* dissolution of absorbed nutrients and transport to certain tissues,

* dissolution of substances for renal elimination,

* maintenance of body water space,

* export of heat via sweat and expiration.

The water intake to cover these needs depends on the dry matter of feed, water holding capacity, feed composition, and the environment. Wild horses (*Equus przewalskii*, ~300 kg BW) consume about 1-20 l/day; the main influence is environmental temperature (Figure 4) (Fritsch, 1998).

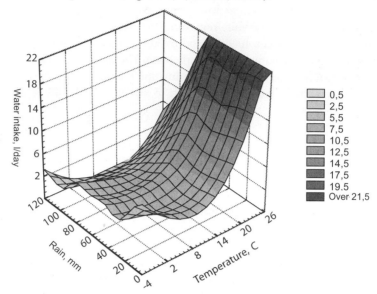

Figure 4. Drinking water intake in *Equus przewalskii* under seminatural conditions (Fritsch, 1998).

At an environmental temperature up to about 15°C, water intake varies for this type of horse at about 2 l/day (<7 ml/kg BW); rain influences water intake associated with feed, but in general this effect seems to be small compared to the dominating role of temperature. At about 20°C, water intake reaches 20 ml/kg BW. Johnson (1998) assumes a daily water consumption rate of 25-80 ml/kg BW. For stabled horses, Meyer et al (1990) measured a daily water intake of 40-75 ml/kg BW. In relation to dry matter (DM) intake, water consumption in horses fed hay and concentrates will vary between 2.5 and 3.5 k/kg DM (Warren et al., 1999).

After feeding and watering, a positive water balance is achieved (Figure 5); water retention increases postprandially for up to about 4-5 hours and begins to decline thereafter. A period of exercise changes water retention dramatically; although there is a decrease in renal water excretion, the rate of fluid loss through sweat during a 2-hour exercise period results in a negative water balance. Limited water intake primarily reduces the amount of water in the GIT (Peters, 1994). A diet low in fiber and feed withdrawal for 12 hours have comparable consequences (Coenen et al., 1990; Coenen, 1991; Meyer et al., 1995). It is not well defined to which degree the GIT contributes to the compensation of exercise-related fluid losses as estimated in some cases (Meyer, 1996a, 1996b, 1996c). There is a lack of clear information, possibly related to the sensitivity of the employed methods.

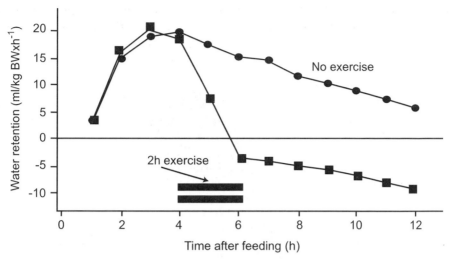

Figure 5. Water retention in horses after ad libitum water availability on days without exercise compared to days with a 2-hour exercise period (Meyer et al., 1990).

Feeding fibrous diets with large amounts of beet pulp may increase water consumption and plasma volume; furosemide treatment, which was used to simulate water losses during exercise in these horses (Warren et al., 1999), induced a greater loss in body weight after ingestion of a diet rich in pectin and a similar decrease in plasma volume compared to feeding a diet low in total fiber and low in soluble fiber (pectin). This "fiber effect" is obviously reduced if a typical source of roughage is fed instead of the highly fermentable pectin from beet pulp. Feeding hay corresponded to higher water intake compared to a hay-grain diet (Pagan and Harris, 1999) but failed to create positive effects on plasma volume.

Sweat production has the greatest influence on water balance and consequently on water intake. As sweat volume varies in relation to exercise conditions, the influence of exercise on sweat production cannot be quantified in a simple figure. Depending on exercise intensity and the environment, the sweat rate varies between 10 and >35 ml/m² x min⁻¹ (Meyer et al., 1990; McCutcheon and Geor, 1998). Exercise-related heat production generally determines the sweat rate. Heat production by the exercising horse depends on total metabolic power (Jones and Carlson, 1995), which is composed of the mass-specific aerobic power (related to oxygen uptake) and the net anaerobic power (lactate accumulation). The metabolic power dictates the increase in body temperature as reflected by the change in pulmonary arterial blood temperature and heat accumulation (Figure 6). As metabolic power reflects the energy expenditure per unit of time, heat production can be estimated assuming that 80% of energy is converted to heat. Sophisticated models describe the routes of heat energy by convection, radiation, conduction, and evaporation (Mostert et al., 1996).

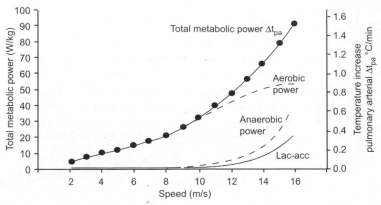

Figure 6. Development of metabolic power in dependence on speed and lactate accumulation and the corresponding increase in body heat indicated by change in temperature of pulmonary arterial blood (Jones and Carlson, 1995).

Neglecting the less significant modes of heat transportation out of the system and assuming that the latent heat of H_2O vaporization is 2428 kJ/l for sweat, calculating 80% of total metabolic power (=energy converted to heat) divided by 2428 delivers a rough impression of the necessary sweat volume and sweat rate respectively. The ability to export remarkably large amounts of heat is essential to maintaining working capacity and depends on environmental temperatures and humidity (Mostert et al., 1996; Jeffcott and Kohn, 1999). Particularly, high humidity reduces the efficiency of evaporation and thus reduces heat export via sweat (Figure 7) (Mostert et al., 1996). In monitoring the complex environmental conditions before and during a competition, the combined measurement of humidity and temperature (expressed in a "wet bulb globe temperature index") specifically recognizes the impact of high humidity on the body's capacity for evaporative energy and is an effective tool in preventing critical heat loads in exercising horses (Schroter et al., 1996).

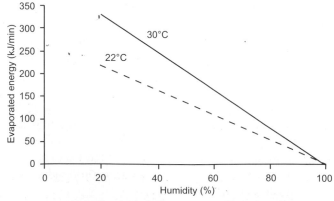

Figure 7. Heat loss via evaporation of sweat during exercise (speed 8.5 m/s) at different temperatures and humidity levels (Mostert et al., 1996).

Regarding variations in workload on the one hand and the complex influence of the environment on cutaneous heat export on the other, average figures for sweat volume or sweat rate are of limited value. However, sweat losses account for ~90% of differences in body weight during the course of exercise (Meyer et al., 1990). As the dry matter of the body remains nearly unchanged, it can be assumed that the conductivity of body mass varies prior to and after exercise; this, in principle, can be measured using the impedance measurement technique. This technique is well-established in human sports, mainly to estimate body fat. Using 5 or 200 kHz (Equistat®), it is possible to estimate horses' fluid compartments; furthermore, there are differences in the impedance before and after exercise, but their relation to changes in body weight due to sweating requires experimental work to establish a model for the calculation of body fluids in exercised horses via impedance measurement. So far, for practical purposes, the change in body weight must be taken as an indicator for sweat. Taking a certain range of sweat rates (Table 3) into account results in body water losses of up to 6.5% and even more under difficult conditions.

Table 3. Sweat rate and total sweat volume and corresponding heat evaporation in a 550-kg horse (TBW 620 ml/kg BW).

Sweat rate ml/kg BW	Total sweat l/horse	% of TBW	Heat export via evaporation, kJ
10	5.5	1.6	13,354
20	11.0	3.2	26,708
30	16.5	4.8	40,062
40	22.0	6.5	53,416

ELECTROLYTES

Exercise induces remarkable changes in the internal balance of several substances such as glycogen, fat, and even calcium (Ca). The drop in ionized Ca, answered by a secretion of parathyroid hormone (PTH), is an example of one of the many reactions in the concert of exercise response (Vervuert et al., 2002). But these reactions do not necessarily (e.g., Ca) change the external balance to a greater degree. Therefore, the influence of exercise on requirements is low.

The acknowledged figures (Table 4) elucidate that cutaneous losses other than for sodium (Na), potassium (K), and chloride (Cl) can be neglected as a factor for the external balance (Meyer, 1987; McCutcheon et al., 1995; McCutcheon and Geor, 1998).

The daily maintenance requirement for Na in a 550-kg horse is calculated to be about 11 g (Table 5). Considering a dry matter (DM) intake of 10 kg/day, it needs on average approximately 1 g Na/kg DM. Many types of roughage contain less than 1 g/kg DM. At least if a horse exercises, original Na contents of feeds are not sufficient to cover the increased requirement. Fecal excretion is less variable compared to renal Na output, which correlates with Na intake. A remarkably high proportion of Na is stored in the skeleton (Table 6).

Table 4. Sweat composition (Meyer 1990; McCutcheon and Geor, 1998).

Major constituents (g/l)		Minor constituents (g/l)		Traces (mg/l)	
				Fe	4.3
Na	2.8	Ca	0.12	Cu	0.3
K	1.4	Mg	0.05	Zn	11.4
Cl	5.3	P	<0.01	Mn	0.16
				Se	<0.005

Table 5. Basic figures for electrolyte requirements (GEH, 1994).

Element	Endogenous losses mg/kg BWxd-1	Utilization %	Requirement maintenance mg/kg BWxd-1	Requirement for exercise	
				net, g/l sweat	total, g/l sweat
Na	18	90	20 (11)*	3.1	3.44
K	40	80	50 (27.5)	1.6	2.0
Cl	5	100	80 (44)**	5.5	5.5

* in brackets: requirement for a 550-kg horse, g/day
** factorial approach not suitable for Cl due to impact on acid base balance if fed according to endogenous losses (Coenen, 1999)

Table 6. Total body electrolytes and the distribution over different tissues (Lindner, 1981; Gürer, 1985; Meyer et al., 1987; Coenen, 1991; Coenen et al., 1991).

	Sodium	Potassium	Chloride
total body store, mg/kg BW			
Whole body mass	1580	2090	1124
partition of several tissues, %			
Muscle	10.8	75.1	19.9
Ingesta	12.4	4.5	14.1
Blood	10.8	2.4	15.5
Skin	8.5	2.6	15.1
GIT tissue	4.3	5.6	6.1
Other organs	2.1	5.0	15.4
Skeleton	51.1	4.7	13.9

Chloride is distributed among several tissue types which contain >15% of total body Cl. Recently ingested portions of Na and Cl are stored in the GIT. This again qualifies the GIT as a temporary reservoir.

The information describing external balance of the specified electrolytes is complete. This includes the fact that within a short time the exercising horse will lose about 8, 3, and 20% of total body Na, K, and Cl, respectively (Table 7). The comparison of these amounts with those in horses suffering from diarrhea (Schott and Hinchcliff, 1998) underlines the fact that only a completely healthy horse can tolerate such high water and electrolyte export rates.

Table 7. Calculated losses of electrolytes via sweat at different sweat rates.

Sweat rate ml/kg BW	Cutaneous losses mg/kg BW			Cutaneous losses in % of total body storage		
	Na	*K*	*Cl*	*Na*	*K*	*Cl*
10	31	16	55	2.0	0.8	4.9
20	62	32	110	3.9	1.5	9.8
30	93	48	165	5.9	2.3	14.7
40	124	64	220	7.8	3.1	19.6

The potassium intake normally greatly exceeds requirements due to the potassium concentrations in most types of roughage (>15 g/kg DM). Muscle tissue contains about three-quarters of total body potassium. Anhidrosis, diarrhea, renal disease, hypocalcaemia, and hyperkalemia are conditions that limit the utilization of a horse's genetically determined exercise capacity (Marlin et al., 1999; McCutcheon et al., 1999; Valberg et al., 1999). Keeping a healthy horse in a high-yielding status requires:

* internal pathways for temporary compensation of a negative electrolyte balance, and

* a specific feeding regime to balance cutaneous water and electrolyte losses.

Can the Horse Regulate Sweat Rate and Sweat Composition to Limit the Negative Balance?

Sweat losses are inevitable losses; they are outside of any regulating influence except the demand for thermoregulation. This has been acknowledged for a long time and demonstrated by the clear relationship between work intensity and sweat rates in various skin regions (Marlin et al., 1999b).

Interestingly, the sensitivity of sweat response decreases in relation to the increase in pulmonary artery temperature (sweat rate sensitivity $g/m^2 xmin-1x°C^{-1}$) from about 18 to ~3 at the neck and from 9 to ~1 in the gluteal region if the workload increases from moderate to strenuous, obviously as a consequence of the altered distribution of blood flow away from the skin towards the excercising muscle (Marlin et al., 1999b). This reaction is not the result of an adaptation to retain water and electrolytes; rather, it reflects the inability to keep sweat production in balance with the need for successful thermoregulation. Even in a state of Na, K, or Cl depletion with the corresponding lowered electrolyte homeostasis, kidney and metabolic consequences, the electrolyte concentrations in sweat remain unchanged (Figure 8, Coenen, 1991). That clearly means the sweat glands cannot (or need not) react to the electrolyte status.

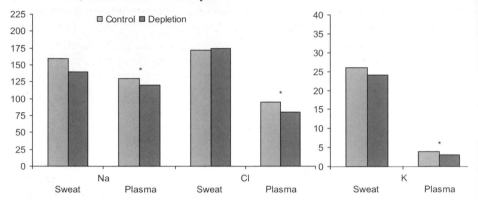

Figure 8. Electrolyte concentrations in sweat and blood plasma in controls and after depleting horses over several weeks (Linder, 1981; Gürer, 1985; Meyer, 1987; Coenen, 1991).

The consequence is a change in electrolyte homeostasis depending on cutaneous losses. To balance these cutaneous losses internally, the horse has the following metabolic tools:

• enforced absorption from the GIT,

• reduced renal output, and

• liberation of electrolytes from certain tissues.

The amounts of water and electrolytes in the GIT are influenced by the type of diet and are obviously reduced in reaction to exercise (Meyer, 1990; Warren et al., 1999). Even if the effect of different dry matter intake is excluded, there still remains an exercise-related intake of water, Na, and Cl but not of K. The conclusion from that result is that the GIT indeed serves as a reservoir. The fact that the amounts of water and electrolytes fixed in the GIT depend on fiber intake (Figure 9) consequently encourages the conclusion that increased roughage consumption–normally meaning hay–could enforce the reservoir function of the GIT. Kronfeld (2001b) criticized the "reservoir hypothesis," taking into consideration the additional load created by extra hay intake, the role of high concentrations of short-chain fatty acids in the hindgut, the heat load caused by fermentation, and, finally, the elevated fecal water output. In his paper, Kronfeld (2001b) emphasizes the advantage of a low-protein, high-fat diet (for stabled horses) containing slowly fermentable fiber (Graham-Thiers et al., 2001). That ration consists of 40% orchard grass hay, 20% oat straw, and in total 40 other feeds such as cereals and oil. Assuming a dry matter intake for an intensively exercising horse of 2.2 kg/100 kg BW x d[-1], the specified diet would result in a daily roughage intake of ~1.3 kg/ 100 kg BW. This is in fact within the same range as the German recommendation of 1-1.2 kg roughage/100 kg BW x d[-1], although the role of the GIT in temporarily contributing to the compensation of sweat losses is one argument in formulating roughage recommendations. However, the integrated examination of roughage and the large intestine in the exercising horse underlines the importance of fiber quality by differentiating between carbohydrate fractions with regard to the end products of fermentation (Hoffman, 2001; Kronfeld, 2001b)–surely a more important aspect than simply the amount of fiber. But the role of heat production by microbial breakdown of carbohydrates seems questionable. In ruminants the heat produced by ruminal fermentation is set at ~4% of gross energy, and the proportion of acetic acid seems to have only a minor effect in altering heat production (Czerkawski, 1980; Orskov et al., 1991). Assuming that the heat liberated by fermentation in the equine hindgut is less than in the rumen, a remarkable reduction might be a disadvantage, posing the risk of destabilizing the intestinal microflora. To allow the gut to perform the function described above, a limit to lactic acid production is necessary (a matter of feed treatment such as extrusion and feed distribution over several meals; maximum of 0.5 kg concentrate/ 100 kg BW per meal, combined with a hay cut just prior to bloom). The role of specific fibrous feeds such as soybean hulls or pectin carriers like sugar beet pulp can be of interest in modifying the proportion of rapidly fermentable fiber (Moore-Colyer and Longland, 2001). But this is an area that deserves further experimental work and much-needed guidelines for incorporating these compounds in a ration.

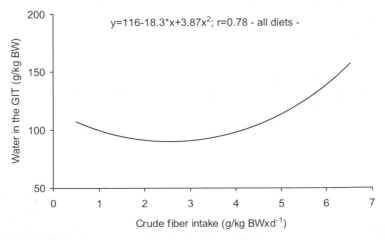

Figure 9. Water in GIT in relation to crude fiber intake (Meyer, 1996a).

Whatever the GIT can yield, the balance during and after exercise remains negative. The kidney may reduce water, Na, and Cl excretion (Schott et al., 1991) but cannot compensate cutaneous losses. As shown for Cl, renal excretion is remarkably reduced, but renal and cutaneous losses still exceed intake, and, further, it takes more than one day to return to the level of renal output which existed prior to exercise (Figure 10). This corresponds with the continued fluid losses and their homeostatic effect following the endurance test (Andrews et al., 1995). The limited renal compensation of sweat losses can possibly be further depressed through a high intake of nitrogen and calcium, as they provoke excretion via the urine.

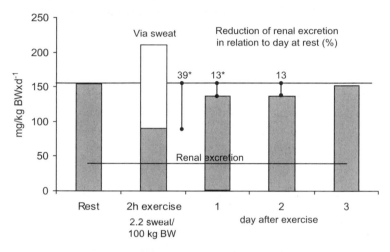

Figure 10. Renal Cl excretion before exercise and the reduction in renal output on the day of exercise and the follow days (Coenen, 1991).

Regarding K balance, the kidney works counterproductively. As a result of the significant transfer of K from the intracellular space to the extracellular space, renal excretion increases in reaction to exercise and thus adds to the K deficit (Meyer, 1987; Schott et al., 1991). The dynamic of the changes in K distribution is often overlooked, and analyses before and after exercise may lead to misinterpretations (Kronfeld, 2001a; Harris and Snow, 1992). Soon after the beginning of exercise, an increase in plasma K occurs, indicating the movement of K from the intracellular space towards the extracellular space (Figure 11). The sweat-related load of K balance is not reflected by plasma concentrations during or immediately after exercise; the measurement of K concentration in plasma a certain time after exercise delivers more information on this aspect.

The third element in handling ongoing sweat losses is tolerance against a temporary depletion of the organism in general (in the case of water) or of certain tissues. The water deficit manifests itself in a reduction of plasma volume and extracellular space. As the hypertonic equine sweat induces hypotonic dehydration, there is a counteracting influx of fluid into the cells (Kronfeld, 2001a); therefore, water export is amplified by a change in water distribution. At what degree does a water deficit become dangerous? The increase in blood viscosity and other hematological changes during exercise (Weiss et al., 1996; Fedde and Erickson, 1998; McKeever, 1998; Funkquist et al., 2001) could prompt the assumption that high sweat losses and, consequently, high water deficits create problems in circulation. The volume itself seems to be less important as long as there is no additional heat storage as a result of decreased fluid volume (Geor and McCutcheon, 1998; Kronfeld, 2001a, 2001b, 2001c). However, because water loss via sweat and electrolyte load as well as energy turnover form a complex concert, a single figure regarding a tolerable volume deficit is of limited value.

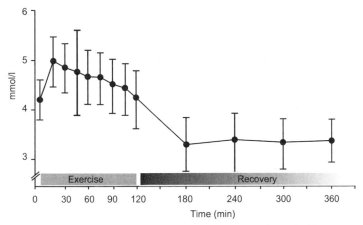

Figure 11. K concentration in the plasma of ponies during a 2-hour exercise and a 4-hour recovery period (2.5-3 m/s) (Coenen, 1991).

The elimination of electrolytes from body stores during exercise is not well-clarified. It can be concluded from depletion experiments that Na levels vary with the fluids, namely plasma volume and extracellular water space. The muscle tissue is additionally involved (Meyer, 1987). In experimentally induced K deficits, a reduction of K in bone occurs (Gürer, 1985). It is not clear whether this takes place during or after exercise in order to compensate for enforced K excretion. Cl again follows water and Na; Cl concentrations are reduced in several tissues by exercise (Coenen, 1999) but interestingly not in muscle. Here there is a strong association with Na ($Na=25.83+61.58$ Cl [$r=0.88$]; mmol/kg muscle DM; Coenen, 1991). During exercise the Cl concentration in muscle increases, obviously due to an increase of the intracellular portion of Cl. Some results from studies on other species suggest that slightly elevated intracellular Cl levels in muscle play a role in limited performance or fatigue (Lindinger and Heigenhauser, 1988). Based on our results, in ponies the portion of Cl shifts towards the intracellular space from 37% prior to exercise to ~12.2% thereafter.

Cl is hardly involved in the acid-base balance, which is described in more detail elsewhere (Kronfeld, 2001a; Hyyppä and Poso, 1998; Kingston and Bayly, 1998). The elimination of CO_2 by expiration depends on the Cl/HCO_{3-} exchange. The decrease in venous plasma Cl partly mirrors its increase in arterial blood (Taylor et al., 1995); the latter, as well as the influence of Cl on breathing (at rest), indicate the demand for Cl in maintaining acid-base balance.

Cl deficiency is clearly correlated to metabolic alkalosis as observed in horses with minimized Cl intake (Coenen, 1991) and in other species (Neathery et al., 1991; Blackmon et al., 1984). That principle is still present during exercise; any burden on Cl homeostasis induces an alkalotic effect (Coenen, 1991).

The different concentrations of electrolytes in sweat result in different answers of electrolyte homeostasis. Figure 12 demonstrates data from the literature, roughly separated into exercise periods with <1h and longer workloads. Regardless of the duration of exercise, the concentrations of Na and K show no major changes, while the Cl concentration drops.

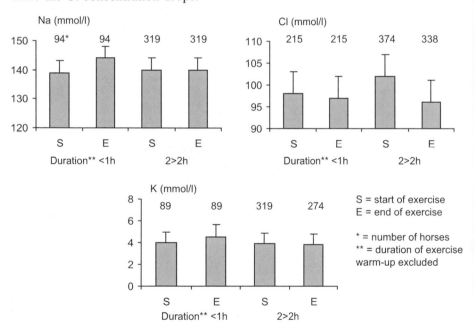

Figure 12. Electrolytes in plasma at start and end of exercise divided in short- and long-lasting workloads (Summary of data from literature).

Strategies in the Care of the Exercising Horse

In an opening comment to students on this aspect, Harold Hintz expressed, "Keep the gut happy." This simply implies the primary role of proper ration planning. Kronfeld (2001a) recommends a ration low in protein–balanced with amino acids– high in fat, and containing slowly fermentable fiber. Reducing protein helps to lower the acidic load for the exercising horse (Graham-Thiers et al., 2001). The rations these authors used contained ~90 g crude protein, mainly from hay and straw. This means protein quality is low if no supplementation with amino acids is implemented. On the other hand, the effect of high- or low-protein diets on performance is small (Miller-Graber et al., 1991; Graham-Thiers et al., 2000). As hay often contains >90 g crude protein, it takes bulky feeds such as straw to keep protein within that range. But especially in the case of high fat in the diet, a more digestible type of roughage than straw should be chosen to maintain sufficient nutrient delivery to the intestinal microflora, even if the protein content of the diet then exceeds requirements.

High levels of fat in the diet are purported to have a number of advantages (Kronfeld, 1998, 2001a, 2001b, 2001c) for exercising horses. Kronfeld et al. recommend up to 12% in the ration for exercising horses in light of muscle glycogen and energetics (1994, 1998). Experimental data from Kronfeld's group indicate that such a high level of fat is still safe (Kronfeld et al., 2001). On the other hand, in cecally fistulated horses fed a semipurified diet consisting of grass meal, starch, sugar, and up to 11% soybean oil, the fat concentration in ileal chyme reached up to 10% of dry matter; in cases with rapid passage, only slight disturbances in fermentation were observed (Coenen, 1986). Zeyner (2001) reported changes in liver enzymes and lipoprotein fractions after using larger amounts of oil. A basic ration design for high-yielding horses with a moderately higher protein concentration compared to the recommendation above includes 6 kg hay, up to ~0.5 kg beet pulp or a combination of beet pulp and soybean hulls, up to 1 kg oil, and ~4 kg processed grain; this feeding concept delivers about 35% of digestible energy (DE) each from roughage and grain and about 26% of DE from fat. The starch intake will be around 2.5 kg/day or even higher. To keep that amount within a safe range, the amount of high-starch concentrates should not exceed 0.5 kg/100 kg BW per meal; this will keep starch intake per meal below 2 g/kg BW (Meyer et al., 1995).

To date there is no conclusive evidence that additives such as niacin or yeast protect the equine microbial system as they do in ruminants.

A main concern in feeding exercising horses, of course, is the challenge regarding the water and electrolyte supply. The question relates not so much to requirements, as these data are sufficiently precise, but more to suitable composition, amounts of supplements, and the proper time for feeding. The general procedure is to stimulate water intake through electrolyte consumption or to use solutions for application via nasogastric tube. There are only small changes in the osmolarity of body fluids (hypotonic dehydration) and, therefore, there is no signal for thirst.

Increasing plasma osmolarity by feeding electrolytes stimulates water intake; our experiments with a salty supplement showed that the stimulation of water consumption completely covered sweat-related weight losses (Coenen, 1991); comparable benefits were observed by Nyman et al. (1996) and Schott et al.

(1999). Application of water alone depresses electrolyte homeostasis, effectively only balancing fluid losses (Hyyppä et al., 1996; Schnermann, 2000). While hypertonic preparations should be avoided, iso- or hypotonic electrolyte solutions are suitable; our experiments revealed no distinct differences in the correction of Na and Cl homeostasis between iso- or hypotonic NaCl solutions (Coenen et al., 1999). Sosa Leon et al. (1995) confirmed the suitability of hypotonic preparations.

Table 8. Mixtures or solutions for supplementation of exercising horses.

Ingredient/units	1	2	3	4	3	4	5	6	7	8
	%	%	g	%	mmol/l	%	%	mmol/l	%	%
Grass meal	47.6									
Sugar beet syrup	33.3									
NaCl	19.1	100	Na 20.2	100		13.2	13.2		88.2	21.1
KCl			K 9			6.8	6.8			8.3
CaCl$_2$			Cl 31.1						6.9	1.8
MgCl$_2$									4.4	1.2
NaH$_2$PO$_4$									0.5	0.14
Glucose										67.4
Glycerol							80			
Commercial product					Na 70, Cl 72, K 31, mmol/l			Na 117, K 40, Cl 130 mmol/l		
Water	free choice	free choice	8.2	101, 0.9 % NaCl	17.5 l	80		6 l	free choice ?	free choice ?
Time of supplementation	during/after	before/during	after	before	before	before/during	before/during	after	before/during	after only
Ref.	1	2	3	4	5	6	6	7	8	8

1) Coenen et al.,1995; 2) Nyman et al., 1996; 3) Hyyppä, 1996; 4) Jasson et al., 1996; 5) Sosa León et al., 1996, additional: phosphate 10, sulfate 10 mmol/l; 6) Schott et al., 1999; 7) Marlin et al., 1998, additional HCO$_3$-, dextrose 30 mmol/l; 8) Kronfeld, 2002.

As the K concentration increases during exercise, an enforced K intake can amplify this reaction and create a certain risk regarding heart function. That is the reason why Kronfeld (2001c) recommends two types of supplements: one without K for use prior to or during exercise and a second one for feeding after exercise. Table 8 shows the composition of different suitable solutions or feeds. Preloading as well as supplementation during exercise or thereafter are investigated and no argument is derived to strictly recommend a specific procedure. The only aspect to consider is that salty feeds prior to exercise must be given with water. As it takes at minimum ~1 hour to achieve an increase in osmolarity, these kinds of supplements should be given about 4 hours before exercise. That allows the horse to consume additional water.

Conclusion

The horse has a high capacity to compensate and to tolerate a load to the thermoregulatory system. But the weakening capacity to eliminate the heat which is produced by strenuous exercise is a performance-limiting factor. A basic ration that depresses the acidic effect of metabolism, lowers heat production itself, and lowers cortisol liberation will be a successful concept. Besides the use of fat (~25% of total DE), fermentable fiber is needed in order to at least prevent a collapse of the microbial system in the hindgut. The influence of fiber types on functioning of intestinal microbes as well as the horse itself needs to be examined in more detail. The water and electrolyte metabolism needs a specific supplement to aid the horse in balancing sweat losses. Dry feeds rich in Na and Cl are easy to handle but must be offered according to an appropriate time schedule to avoid high salt intake without water.

References

Andrews, F.M., D.R. Geiser, et al. 1995. Haematological and biochemical changes in horses competing in a three-star horse trial and three-day event. Equine Vet. J. Suppl. 20:57-63.

Blackmon, D.M., M.W. Neathery, et al. 1984. Clinical aspects of experimentally induced chloride deficiency in Holstein calves. Am J Vet Res 45(8):1638-40.

Carlson, G.P. 1987. Hematology and body fluids in the equine athlete: A review. Equine Exercise Physiology, San Diego 2:393-425.

Coenen, M. 1986. Contributions to digestive physiology of the horse, 13th Communication. J. Anim.Physiol.Anim. Nutr. 56:104-117.

Coenen, M. 1991. Chloride metabolism and chloride requirement in horses. School of Vet. Med. Hannover, Habilitationsschrift.

Coenen, M. 1999. Basics for chloride metabolism and requirement. In: Proc. 16th Equine Nutr. Physiol. Symp., pp. 353-354.

Coenen, M., H. Meyer, and B. Stadermann. 1990. Amount and composition of the GIT content according to type of feed and exercise. Advances in Anim. Physiol. Anim. Nutr. 21:7-20.

Coenen, M., H. Meyer, and B. Steinbrenner. 1995. Effects of NaCl supplementation before exercise on metabolism of water and electrolytes. Equine Vet. J. Suppl. 18:270-273.

Coenen, M., F. Schuckmann, I. Vervuert, and F. von Rennenkampf. 1999. Exercise of pack horses in mountain area. In: Proc. 16th Equine Nutr. Physiol. Symp., pp. 306-307.

Coenen, M., I. Vervuert, J. Harmeyer, U. Wedemeyer, C. Chrobock, and H.P. Sporleder. 2001. Training and type of exercise influence plasma catecholamines in young horses. In: Proc. 17th Equine Nutr. Physiol. Symp., p. 283.

Czerkawski, J.W. 1980. A novel estimate of the magnitude of heat produced in the rumen. Br. J. Nutr. 43(1): 239-43.

Dusterdieck, K.F., H.C. Schott, et al. 1999. Electrolyte and glycerol supplementation improve water intake by horses performing a simulated 60 km endurance ride. Equine Vet. J. Suppl. 30:418-24.

Fedde, M.R., and H.H. Erickson. 1998. Increase in blood viscosity in the sprinting horse: Can it account for the high pulmonary arterial pressure? Equine Vet. J. 30(4):329-34.

Friend, T.H. 2000. Dehydration, stress, and water consumption of horses during long-distance commercial transport. J. Anim. Sci. 78(10):2568-80.

Fritsch, S. 1998. The drinking behaviour of Przewalski horses under seminatural keeping conditions. University Berlin, Thesis.

Funkquist, P., B. Sandhagen, et al. 2001. Effects of phlebotomy on haemodynamic characteristics during exercise in standardbred trotters with red cell hypervolaemia. Equine Vet. J. 33(4):417-24.

Geor, R. J., and L.J. McCutcheon. 1998. Hydration effects on physiological strain of horses during exercise- heat stress. J. Appl. Physiol. 84(6):2042-51.

Gesellschaft für Ernährungsphysiologie der Haustiere, G. 1994. Energie- und Nährstoffbedarf landwirtschaftlicher Nutztiere, Nr. 2: Empfehlungen zur Energie- und Nährstoffversorgung der Pferde. DLG-Verlag, Frankfurt/main; ISBN-3-7690-0517-1.

Graham-Thiers, P. M., D.S. Kronfeld, K.A. Kline, and D.J. Sklan. 2001. Dietary protein restriction and fat supplementation diminish the acidogenic effect of exercise during repeated sprints in horses. J. Nutr. 131:1959-1964.

Graham-Thiers, P. M., D.S. Kronfeld, K.A. Kline, D.J. Sklan, and P.A. Harris 2000. Protein status of exercising Arabian horses fed diets containing 14 % or 7.5 % crude protein fortified with lysine and threonine. J. Equine Vet. Sci. 20:516-521.

Gürer, C. 1985. Untersuchungen zum Kaliumstoffwechsel des Pferdes bei marginaler und zusätzlicher Versorgung. School of Vet. Med. Hannover, Thesis.

Harris, P., and D. H. Snow. 1992. Plasma potassium and lactate concentrations in Thoroughbred horses during exercise of varying intensity. Equine Vet. J. 24(3):220-225.

Hinchcliff, K.W. 1998. Fluids and electrolytes in athletic horses. Vet. Clin. North Am. Equine Pract. 14:1.

Hoffman, R. M., J. A. Wilson, et al. 2001. Hydrolyzable carbohydrates in pasture, hay, and horse feeds: Direct assay and seasonal variation. J. Anim. Sci. 79(2):500-506.

Hyyppä, S., and A.R. Poso. 1998. Fluid, electrolyte, and acid-base responses to exercise in racehorses. Vet. Clin. North. Am. Equine. Pract. 14(1):121-136.

Hyyppä, S., M. Saastamoinen, et al. 1996. Restoration of water and electrolyte balance in horses after repeated exercise in hot and humid conditions. Equine Vet. J. Suppl. (22):108-112.

Jeffcott, L.B., and A.F. Clarke. 1995. Thermoregulatory responses during competitive exercise in the performance horse, Vol I. Equine Vet. J. Suppl. 20.

Jeffcott, L.B., and A.F. Clarke. 1996. Thermoregulatory responses during competitive exercise in the performance horse, Vol II. Equine Vet. J. Suppl. 22.

Jeffcott, L. B., and C. W. Kohn. 1999. Contributions of equine exercise physiology research to the success of the 1996 Equestrian Olympic Games: A review. Equine Vet. J. Suppl. 30:347-355.

Johnson, P.J. 1998. Physiology of body fluids in the horse. Vet. Clin. North Am. Equine Pract. 14(1): 1-22.

Jones, J.H., and G.P. Carlson. 1995. Estimation of metabolic energy cost and heat production during a three-day event. Equine Vet. J. Suppl. 20:23-30.

Kingston, J.K., and W.M. Bayly. 1998. Effect of exercise on acid-base status of horses. Vet. Clin. North Am. Equine Pract. 14(1):61-73.

Kronfeld, D.S. 2001a. Body fluids and exercise: Physiological responses (Part 1). J. Equine Vet. Sci. 21:312-322.

Kronfeld, D.S. 2001b. Body fluids and exercise: Replacement strategies. J. Equine Vet. Sci. 21:368-375.

Kronfeld, D.S. 2001c. Body fluids and exercise: Influences of nutrition and feeding management. J. Equine Vet. Sci. 21:417-428.

Kronfeld, D. S., S.E. Custalow, P.L. Ferrante, L.E. Taylor, J.A. Wilson, and W. Tiegs. 1998. Acid-base responses of fat-adapted horses: Relevance to hard work in the heat. Appl. Anim. Behav. Sci. 59:61-72.

Kronfeld, D.S., P.L. Ferrante, et al. 1994. Optimal nutrition for athletic performance, with emphasis on fat adaptation in dogs and horses. J. Nutr. Suppl. 124:2745S-2753S.

Kronfeld, D.S., J.L. Holland, G.A. Rich, S.E. Custalow, J.P. Fontenot, T.N. Meacham, D.J. Sklan, and P.A. Harris. 2001. Digestibility of fat. In: 17th Proc. Equine Nutr. Physiol. Symp., 156-158.

Kurosawa, M., S. Nagata, et al. 1999. Effects of caffeine and promazine hydrochloride on plasma catecholamines in thoroughbreds at rest and during treadmill exercise. Equine Vet. J. Suppl. 30:596-600.

Lindinger, M. I., and G. J. F. Heigenhauser. 1988. Ion fluxes during tetanic stimulation in isolated perfused rat hindlimb. Am. J. Physiol. 254:R117-R126.

Lindner, A. 1983. Untersuchungen zum Natriumstoffwechsel des Pferdes bei marginaler Versorgung und zusätzlicher Bewegungsbelastung. School of Vet. Med. Hannover, Thesis.

Marlin, D.J., R C. Schroter, et al. 1999. Sweating and skin temperature responses of normal and anhidrotic horses to intravenous adrenaline. Equine Vet. J. Suppl. 30:362-369.

Marlin, D.J., C.M. Scott, et al. 1998. Rehydration following exercise: Effects of administration of water versus an isotonic oral rehydration solution (ORS). Vet. J. 156(1):41-49.

Marlin, D.J., C.M. Scott, et al. 1999. Physiological responses of horses to a treadmill simulated speed and endurance test in high heat and humidity before and after humid heat acclimation. Equine Vet. J. 31(1):31-42.

McCutcheon, L.J., and R. J. Geor. 1996. Sweat fluid and ion losses in horses during training and competition in cool vs. hot ambient conditions: implications for ion supplementation. Equine Vet. J. Suppl. (22):54-62.

McCutcheon, L.J., and R. J. Geor. 1998. Sweating: Fluid and ion losses and replacement. Vet. Clin. North Am. Equine Pract.14(1):75-95.

McCutcheon, L.J., R.J. Geor, et al. 1999. Equine sweating responses to submaximal exercise during 21 days of heat acclimation. J. Appl. Physiol. 87(5):1843-1851.

McCutcheon, L.J., R.J. Geor, et al. 1995. Sweating rate and sweat composition during exercise and recovery in ambient heat and humidity. Equine Vet. J. Suppl. (20):153-157.

McKeever, K.H. 1998. Blood viscosity and its role in the haemodynamic responses to intense exertion. Equine Vet. J. 30(1):3.

Meyer, H. 1987. Nutrition of the equine athlete. Equine Exercise Physiology, 2:644-673.

Meyer, H. 1990. Contribution to water and mineral metabolism of the horse. Adv. Anim. Physiol. Anim. Nutr., 21.

Meyer, H. 1996a. Influence of feed intake and composition, feed and water restriction, and exercise on gastrointestinal fill in horses. Part 1. Equine Practice 18:26-29.

Meyer, H. 1996b. Influence of feed intake and composition, feed and water restriction, and exercise in gastrointestinal fill in horses. Part 2. Equine Practice 18:20-23.

Meyer, H. 1996c. Influence of feed intake and composition, feed and water restriction, and exercise on gastrointestinal fill in horses. Part 3. Equine Practice 18:25-28.

Meyer, H., Y. Gomda, H. Perez-Noriega, M. Heilemann, and A. Hipp-Quarton. 1990. Investigation on the postprandial water metabolism in resting and exercised horses. Adv. Anim. Physiol. Anim. Nutr. 21:35-51.

Meyer, H., M. Heilemann, A. Hipp-Quarton, and H. Perez-Noriega. 1990. Amount and composition of sweat in ponies. Adv. Anim. Physiol. Anim. Nutr. 21:21-34.

Meyer, H., S. Radicke, E. Kienzle, S. Wilke, D. Kleffken, and M. Illenseer 1995. Investigation on preileal digestion of starch from grain, potato, and manioc in horses. J. Vet.Med. A 42:371-381.

Miller-Graber, P.A., L. M. Lawrence, et al. 1991. Dietary protein level and energy metabolism during treadmill exercise in horses. J. Nutr. 121(9):1462-1469.

Montgomery, I., D.M. Jenkinson, et al. 1982. The effects of thermal stimulation on the ultrastructure of the fundus and duct of the equine sweat gland. J. Anat. 135:13-28.

Moore-Colyer, M.J.S., and A.C. Longland. 2001. The effect of plain sugar beet pulp on the in vitro gas production and in vivo apparent digestibility of hay when offered to ponies. In: Proc. 17th Equine Nutr. Physiol. Symp., pp. 145-147.

Mostert, H.J., R.J. Lund, et al. 1996. Integrative model for predicting thermal balance in exercising horses. Equine Vet. J. Suppl. 22:7-15.

Nagata, S., F. Takeda, et al. 1999. Plasma adrenocorticotropin, cortisol and catecholamines response to various exercises. Equine Vet. J. Suppl. 30:570-574.

Neathery, M.W., D.M. Blackmon, et al. 1981. Chloride deficiency in Holstein calves from a low chloride diet and removal of abomasal contents. J. Dairy Sci. 64(11):2220-2233.

Nyman, S., A. Jansson, et al. 1996. Strategies for voluntary rehydration in horses during endurance exercise. Equine Vet. J. Suppl. 22:99-106.

Orskov, E.R., N.A. MacLeod, et al. 1991. Effect of different volatile fatty acids mixtures on energy metabolism in cattle. J. Anim. Sci. 69(8):3389-3397.

Pagan, J.D., and P.A. Harris 1999. The effects of timing and amount of forage and grain on exercise response in Thoroughbred horses. Equine Vet. J. Suppl. 30:451-457.

Peters, H. 1994. Influence of water withdrawal and exercise on amount and content of the intestinal chyme in the horse. School of Vet. Med. Hannover, Thesis.

Rose, R.J., and D. Sampson. 1982. Changes in certain metabolic parameters in horses associated with food deprivation and endurance exercise. Res. Vet. Sci. 32(2):198-202.

Schnermann, J. 2000. Effects of oral administration of glucose or electrolyte supplemention after a standardized exercise test on thermoregulation and electrolyte metabolism in horses. School of Vet. Med. Hannover, Thesis.

Schott, H.C. 1998. Oral fluids for equine diarrhoea: An underutilized treatment for a costly disease? Vet. J. 155(2):119-21.

Schott, H.C., K.F. Dusterdieck, et al. 1999. Effects of electrolyte and glycerol supplementation on recovery from endurance exercise. Equine Vet. J. Suppl. 30:384-393.

Schott, H.C., and K.W. Hinchcliff. 1998. Treatments affecting fluid and electrolyte status during exercise. Vet. Clin. North Am. Equine Pract. 14(1):175-204.

Schott, H.C., D.R. Hodgson, W. Bayly, and P.D. Gollnick. 1991. Renal response

288   *Exercise and Stress*

to high intensity exercise. Equine Exercise Physiology 3, 361-367.

Schroter, R.C., D.J. Marlin, et al. 1996. Use of the wet bulb globe temperature (WBGT) index to quantify environmental heat loads during three-day event competitions. Equine Vet. J. Suppl. 22:3-6.

Snow, D.H., R.C. Harris, et al. 1992. Effects of high-intensity exercise on plasma catecholamines in the Thoroughbred horse. Equine Vet. J. 24(6):462-467.

Sosa Leon, L.A., A.J. Davie, et al. 1995. The effects of tonicity, glucose concentration and temperature of an oral rehydration solution on its absorption and elimination. Equine Vet. J. Suppl. 20:140-146.

Taylor, L.E., P.L. Ferrante, J.A. Wilson, and D.S. Kronfeld. 1995. Arterial and mixed venous acid-base status and strong ion difference during repeated sprints. Equine Vet. J. Suppl. 18:326-330.

Valberg, S.J., J.R. Mickelson, E.M. Gallant, J.M. MacLey, L. Lentz, and F. De La Corte. 1999. Exertinal rhabdomyolysis in Quarter horses and Thoroughbreds: One syndrome, multiple etiologies. Equine Vet. J. Supl. 30:533-538.

Vervuert, I., M. Coenen, U. Wedemeyer, C. Chrobock, J. Harmeyer, and H.P. Sporleder. 2002. Calcium homeostasis and intact plasma parathyroid hormone during exercise and training in young Standardbred horses. Equine Vet. J.

Warren, L.K., L.M. Lawrence, et al. 1999. The effect of dietary fibre on hydration status after dehydration with frusemide. Equine Vet. J. Suppl. 30:508-513.

Weiss, D.J., R.J. Geor, et al. 1996. Effects of furosemide on hemorheologic alterations induced by incremental treadmill exercise in thoroughbreds. Am. J. Vet. Res. 57(6):891-895.

Zeyner, A. 2001. Untersuchungen zum Austausch von stärkereichem Mischfutter durch Sojaöl in Rationen für Reitpferde. Universität Leipzig, Habilitationsschrift.

GROWTH AND DEVELOPMENT

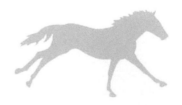

PRINCIPLES OF BONE DEVELOPMENT IN HORSES

LARRY A. LAWRENCE
Kentucky Equine Research, Versailles, Kentucky, USA

Few animals are as precocious as the horse. Within 20 minutes of birth a foal may stand, and within hours can be ready to run at speeds no human athlete will ever achieve. At this stage of life, even with this exceptionally early development, horses have only 17% of their mature bone mineral content, but they also have only 10% of their ultimate body weight. The relationships between growth, nutrition, bone strength and development, body weight, and the forces applied to bone are all orchestrated in a careful balance when optimal growth is achieved.

The selection and breeding of horses for desirable traits have been practiced for over 2000 years. However, most of what we have learned about the growth of horses has been recorded in the past 20-30 years. In 1979 Dr. Harold Hintz reported Windfields Farm's growth data for 1,992 foals from birth to 22 months of age. The records illustrate how quickly foals grow. Thoroughbreds and other light horse breeds will reach 84% of their mature height at six months of age. Assuming a mature Thoroughbred will be 16 hands, the six-month-old weanling will be approximately 13.2 hands. At 12 months that horse will have reached 94% of its adult height or around 15 hands, and at 22 months it has almost finished growing in height, reaching 97% of its full height at approximately 15.2 hands. Mature weight is reached at a slower rate; during the first six months of life, the foal will gain 46% of its mature weight. Assuming a mature weight of 500 kg, the six-month-old will weigh approximately 230 kg. At 12 months it will have reached 65% of its mature weight (325 kg), and at 22 months it should be 90% of its adult weight (450 kg). Average daily gains described by Hintz are the same as those recommended by the National Research Council (NRC) for moderate growth. The NRC reports that six-month-old weanlings with a projected adult weight of 500 kg gained 0.65 kg per day. Twelve-month-old yearlings gained 0.5 kg per day, and 18-month-old long yearlings gained 0.35 kg per day (Table 1).

Radiographic studies on the acquisition of bone mineral in horses from one day of age to 27 years have shown that maximum bone mineral content (BMC) is not achieved until the horse is six years old. If the rate of mineralization of the cannon bone and age are compared, a pattern emerges that is more similar to that of weight gain than height. At six months of age horses have attained 68.5% of the mineral content of an adult horse, and by one year of age they have reached

76% of maximal BMC. Bone is a much more dynamic tissue than it appears to be upon casual observation; however, complete bone mineralization lags behind growth in height and weight.

Table 1. Projected growth parameters for a young horse.

Age	Height	% Mature Height*	Weight	% Mature Weight*
6 months	13.2 h	84%	230 kg	46%
12 months	15.0 h	94%	325 kg	65%
22 months	15.2 h	97%	450 kg	90%

*Estimates based on 16-hand, 500-kg mature horse.

A basic understanding of the process of bone development helps to explain the complicated nature of growth in the horse. There are two anatomical types of bones in the skeleton. Flat bones are generally for protection and include the skull, mandible, and ileum. Long bones are found in the appendicular skeleton and include the metacarpal, humerus, and femur. These bone are different from a functional perspective, and they are developed by two distinctly different processes. The flat bones are developed by intramembranous ossification and the long bones are developed by endochondral ossification. Long bone development is generally of greatest interest because of its impact on the soundness of the horse.

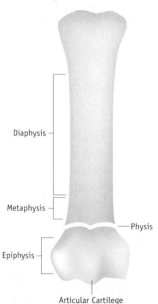

Diaphysis

Metaphysis

Physis

Epiphysis

Articular Cartilege

Figure 1. External examination of the third metacarpal.

External examination of the third metacarpal (Figure 1) shows wide extremities at the ends of the bone (epiphyses), a cylindrical tube tapering to a central waist in the middle (midshaft or diaphysis), and a developmental zone (the metaphysis and physis) between them. In the growing long bone, the physis or growth plate is a layer of proliferating cells and expanding cartilage matrix. The growth plate is calcified, remodeled, and replaced by bone at the end of bone growth. On cross-section the bone marrow cavity is a central cylindrical tube. The waist of long bones contains the most densely calcified area of cortical bone. Looking from the waist to the metaphysis and epiphysis, the cortex becomes thinner and the internal space is filled with a network of thin, calcified trabeculae known as cancellous bone or trabecular bone.

There are two surfaces at which the bone is in contact with soft tissue: an external surface (periosteum) and an internal surface (endosteum). These surfaces are lined with layers of osteogenic cells. The endosteum is more active metabolically because of the structural differences in compact and trabecular bone. Between 80 and 90% of the volume of compact bone is calcified, whereas only 15-20% of the trabecular bone is calcified. Trabecular bone is in close contact with bone marrow, blood vessels, and connective tissue. The endosteal bone surface is 70% of the interface with soft tissues (Baron, 1999). The strength of compact bone helps it fulfill its mostly mechanical function, and trabecular bone is more labile and metabolically active.

Bone is formed by collagen fibers usually oriented in a preferential direction and noncollagenous proteins. Spindle- or plate-shaped crystals of hydroxyapatite $[3\ Ca_3(PO_4)_2](OH_2)$ are found on the collagen fibers within them and in the ground substance. They tend to be oriented in the same direction as the collagen fibers. The orientation of the fibers alternates in mature bone from layer to layer, giving the bone a lamellar structure. When bone is formed rapidly during development, collagen fibers are loosely packed and randomly oriented.

Endochondral ossification occurs in an embryonic cartilage model. Longitudinal growth occurs at the growth plate in a series of zones. The first zone contains resting chondrocytes. The second zone is where chondrocytes divide and synthesize matrix; it is called the proliferative zone. The hypertrophic zone is the site where maturing chodrocyes become larger and produce alkaline phosphate and calcium matrix vesicles. The fourth zone is the calcified zone. The process of mineralization begins when capillaries and osteogenic cells from the diaphysis invade the columns of chondrocytes. The chondrocytes in the newly calcified zone die. Osteogenic cells multiply and differentiate into osteoblasts. Osteoblasts arrange themselves along the remnants of the cartilaginous trabeculae and produce the matrix constituent's collagen and ground substance. Membrane-bound cellular bodies released from chondrocytes and osteoblasts facilitate mineralization. These are known as ECM vesicles and they contain calcium and phosphorus. In addition, they provide enzymes that can degrade inhibitors of mineralization. Alkaline phosphatase hydrolyzes phosphate esters, increasing phosphatase concentration, which in turn increases mineralization. Osteoblasts are transformed into osteocytes or bone cells in calcified matrix. Osteocytes are found embedded deep within bone in osteocytic lacunae. A network of thin canaliculi permeating the entire bone matrix connects osteocytes.

The bone cells associated with resorption of bone are osteoclasts, giant multinucleated cells found in contact with a calcified bone surface lacuna. Osteoclasts resorb bone via lysosomal enzymes (e.g., acid phosphatase and cathepsin K) and collagenase. The enzymes are secreted through a ruffled border. Resorption starts with digestion of the calcium and phosphorus-containing hydroxyapatite crystals. Then the collagen fibers of the matrix are digested by collagenase or by action of cathepsins at low pH.

The process of long bone growth involves the development of bone tissue and the resorption of bone tissue at the same time. As bone develops at the growth plate, it forms the metaphysis. The metaphysis is flared outward with a narrow cortex. Growth must take place within the context of the structural and metabolic functions of the bone. This is accomplished by continual appositional growth on the endosteal side of the bone and active removal of bone by osteoclasts on the periosteal surface.

This brief description of bone development should help clarify the complicated and metabolically sensitive nature of the process. Optimal growth rates may vary somewhat between breeds, but all young horses have several critical considerations for bone growth and development. Extremely rapid growth caused by overfeeding (particularly energy) has been implicated in developmental orthopedic disease (DOD) and unsoundness. Periods of slow or decreased growth followed by rapid growth are particularly dangerous. Imbalanced levels of calcium, phosphorus, and trace minerals have been linked to DOD. Certain types of forced exercise also seem to cause bone development problems.

Bone development begins before birth and continues beyond 18 months of age. The period between three and nine months of age appears to be the most precarious for the foal in terms of DOD. During this time, serious conditions can develop that might restrict the athletic potential of a horse. It is important to monitor growth rates and evaluate the foal's skeletal development. Steady, moderate growth along a typical growth curve appears to provide the best method of reducing developmental problems.

Kentucky Equine Research has been weighing and measuring foals, weanlings, and yearlings monthly in central Kentucky for over 10 years. Those records combined with numbers from universities and Windfields Farm in Canada have resulted in a tremendous vault of comparative growth data. These data have been formulated into software designed to track growth and make comparisons with databases containing records of thousands of foals. Observations from research trials and practical experience have led to the recognition that slow, steady growth is best for horses. Pagan (1998) reported on the incidence of developmental orthopedic disease (DOD) in Thoroughbred foals. A total of 271 foals was monitored. Ten percent of the foals were diagnosed with DOD. Osteochondritis dissecans (OCD) lesions of the fetlock were diagnosed at an average age of 102 days in fillies (2% affected) that were small at 15 days of age (3.18 kg below average). Stifle and shoulder OCD lesions were diagnosed at the average age of 336 days. About 2% of the foals were affected, and they tended to be 5.45 kg above the average weight at 25 days and 31 pounds above average at 120 days. Foals that developed hock OCD lesions tended to be heavier than average at birth and were 8.18 kg above average at 15 days. They had higher average daily gains until 240 days, and they were 15.45 kg above average at that age. Pagan recommends that managers (1) record birth weights; (2) express weights as a percent of a reference; (3) do not allow deviation of 15% or more from the reference weights; (4) keep records of DOD and management changes; (5) weigh monthly; (6) do not overfeed lactating mares; (7) provide adequate turnout; and (8) consider weaning early if foals are growing too fast.

All efforts to support continuous steady growth in foals are important in helping to limit bone development problems. Foals that have had slowed growth followed by large growth spurts are at particular risk for DOD.

References

Baron, R. 1999. Anatomy and ultrastructure of bone. In: J.B. Lain and S.R. Goldring (Eds.) Primer on the Metabolic Diseases and Disorders of Mineral Metabolism. (4th Ed.) p. 3-10. Lippincott, Williams & Wilkins, Philadelphia, PA.

Hintz, H.F., R.L. Hintz, and L.D. van Vleck. 1979. Growth rate of Thoroughbreds: Effect of age of dam, year and month of birth, sex of foal. J. Anim. Sci. 48:480.

Pagan, J.D. 1998. The incidence of developmental orthopedic disease (DOD) on a Kentucky Thoroughbred farm. In: J.D. Pagan (Ed.) Advances in Equine Nutrition. p. 469-475. Nottingham University Press, Nottingham, U.K.

METHODS OF ASSESSING BONE GROWTH AND DEVELOPMENT IN YOUNG HORSES

ELWYN C. FIRTH
Institute of Veterinary, Animal and Biomedical Sciences, Massey University, Palmerston North, New Zealand

Introduction

When raising and training horses we attempt to maximize production and performance capability, while at the same time minimize the possibility of developmental diseases and athletic injury. Improvements in management of growth, conditioning, and training, both systematically and through trial and error, may have had either positive or negative effects. But these effects have rarely been measured directly, preventing comparison between studies and thus delaying discussion and progress.

One of the objectives of most growing and training regimens is to alter orthopedic tissues so they possess greater capability to withstand the rigors of the intended training and competition. There is no research on the relationship between the outcomes, such as reduced bone and joint disease incidence, and the tissue changes we hoped to induce. This is because of the lack of sensitive, noninvasive, and inexpensive methods of monitoring changes, the difficulty of conducting extensive research investigation in commercial practice, and the cost and technical difficulties of long-term epidemiological studies that depend on accurate diagnosis.

It is quite clear that the costs associated with orthopedic growth problems in horses are huge. These include costs of definitive diagnosis of developmental orthopedic disease (DOD), costs of treatment and prevention, withdrawal from sale, reduced sale price, and the costs of continued research to attempt to determine the causes and prevent the diseases. Despite the recognition of various diseases included under the DOD banner and research attempts to determine pathogenesis and prevention, there is little or no substantial rigorous evidence that prevalence and implications of DOD have been reduced for either individuals or industries as a whole. The comment made more than a decade and a half ago, that DOD is the single biggest problem that horse breeders face, probably remains true today.

Although there is some progress on the research front, the way ahead to cure or prevention is not obvious. This is possibly because we do not have abundant rigorous data on some aspects of growth and development as a whole, and certainly in bone growth and development. It is important that such data be acquired for three reasons. First, some DOD is associated with abnormalities of bone tissue, but the sensitivity of the methods we have to detect the disease is not high. Second, some DOD is suggested to be due to bone being of subnormal strength, but we have not ever measured this. Third, nutrition management variations may play a part in the cause of some DOD. The changes in nutrition are introduced by breeders and trainers on a subjective basis, to seek an end point in terms of bone development that is not well defined. For instance, how often does one hear of altered regimens to produce "better bone," "better bone growth," "harder bones," or "higher bone density," when in fact we have little data to know what is normal for these ill-defined parameters at various stages of life or the significance of any change achieved under a particular nutritional management system?

This presentation mentions various ways in which bone can be assessed in the growing horse, and includes a relatively new possibility, peripheral quantitative computed tomography (pQCT), which is the only currently affordable technology that can measure true bone density as well as bone dimension. Some preliminary findings concerning bone development in young pasture-raised horses are also presented.

Noninvasive Methods of Assessing Bone Growth

The reason for any assessment of bone is to estimate its strength so that predictions can be made about its likely capability of function under particular circumstances. There is an absolute requirement for cross-sectional depiction and quantification of bone properties, if understanding of bone physiology in the horse is to increase. This is because, although mineral content has a very large influence on bone strength, it is not only the amount of mineral but the manner in which it is sited in the bone that determines the bone's resistance to the forces which act upon it.

Only three methodologies offer this, namely quantitative ultrasound (QUS), magnetic resonance imaging (MRI), and computed tomography (CT). Although the list below includes techniques which are unable to provide cross-sectional information, emphasis is placed on those that can. More emphasis is placed on CT because research into the validation of QUS is still in progress, and although portable MRI units of suitable resolution are said to be close to market stage, their cost is likely to restrict their use to research institutes for some time, unlike portable CT units.

DIRECT LINEAR MEASUREMENT

Assessment of bone size is possible in some individual limb bones by direct measurement using bony landmarks such as joint margins and is reasonably accurate in the hands of a single observer (Burbidge and Pfeiffer, 1998). Serial measurements of height measure growth of the whole limb column but contribute only indirectly to the study of a particular bone.

BONE MARKERS

Markers expressed during bone synthesis (type I collagen carboxy-terminal propeptide, the bone-specific isoenzyme of alkaline phosphatase, and osteocalcin), bone remodeling (telopeptide of type I collagen and deoxypyrodinoline), and soft tissue turnover (N-terminal propeptide of type III collagen) have been investigated in the horse (Lepage et al., 2001; Price et al., 2001; Carstanjen et al., 2003; Jackson et al., 1996). Markers of bone cell activity and soft tissue turnover follow characteristic patterns of change influenced by age, season, and bodyweight (Price et al., 1995). Markers offer potentially great advantage because their use is relatively noninvasive, and they respond rapidly to changes in the skeleton.

BIOPSY

Postmortem and in vivo ilium biopsy have been used in equine research (Savage et al., 1991a,b) and although invasive appear practical and reliable in investigation of systemic bone responses. Biopsy of distal radius growth plate tissue (Belling and Glade, 1984) does not appear to have been used widely, possibly because of the degree of invasiveness and limited follow-up described. Even when using a much smaller skin incision and biopsy core, and aseptic surgery under general anesthesia (Pearce et al., 1999), biopsy of the distal radial metaphysis, which resulted in little clinically discernible postoperative discomfort, was associated with postoperative slight deviation in the opposite forelimb. Biopsy appears to have little place in growth and development research.

RADIOLOGY

Good-quality radiographs can be examined subjectively, and features of bone assessed to infer features of bone health, such as fracture, periosteal new bone formation, physeal width, cortical width, and patterns of increased or decreased radiodensity. But these are indications of end-stage disease and not development. Radiography is unsuitable for studying abnormal bone development because accuracy is low due to the substantial change required before it is detectable on standard radiographs, and because assessment of presence and significance of the changes is inevitably subjective. Newer technologies of digital radiography and image processing may alter the sensitivity of radiography to detect and quantify more subtle change in bone.

RADIOGRAMMETRY

The measurement of bone dimensions on radiographs allows quantification of the size of parts of the bone. Usually the cortical thickness is measured. The technique has been used previously in metacarpal and other diaphyses in people (Ruiz-Echarri et al., 1996). The method lacks sensitivity and has a precision error of up to 10%, does not account for the implications of intracortical porosity because the latter cannot be recognized, and cannot detect changes in trabecular bone. However, the technique has been employed in the horse (Jeffcott et al., 1988) and most recently in a radiographic index of dorsal and palmar cortical thickness measurements of the third metacarpal, which was considered sufficiently accurate to measure third metacarpal bone shape (Walter and Davies, 2001).

RADIOGRAPHIC ABSORPTIOMETRY

The technique was the first to quantify mineral content and uses an aluminum wedge in the radiographic field, against which attenuation of the x-rays by the bone in question is compared. Standardization is difficult because of factors affecting the radiographic image, although automated image analysis techniques have led to a resurgence of the technique as a cheap screening tool in bones of the human digit. The optical density is proportional to the bone mineral content. In the human digit the method is precise and accurate (Cosman et al., 1991; Yang et al., 1994; Yates et al., 1995).

In horses, the method was originally described by Meakim and coworkers (1981) using excised bones, in which reproducibility was good and correlation with mineral content in the mid-diaphysis of the third metacarpal was between .88 and .94. The technique is used in equine nutritional research despite several sources of error including variability in the radiographic source, scatter radiation, soft tissue surrounding the bone, and limited linear response of radiographic film (Markel, 1996). As well, its use is limited in areas containing cancellous bone because changes in this fraction may be obscured by the overlying cortical bone. The method is planar, and cannot determine the site of mineral in the bone, and thus cannot estimate bone strength directly. Also, in cancellous bone with anisotropic cancellous architecture (e.g., the third carpal bone), even a very small change in radiographic beam angle can lead to significant change in results (Secombe CJ, MVSc thesis, 2000).

QUANTITATIVE ULTRASOUND

The method was used in the third metacarpi of horses to determine velocity of sound through the bone, velocity being highest where the cortex was thickest (Jeffcott and McCartney, 1985). Combined with single photon absorptiometry, transmission velocity was used to estimate bone strength (McCarthy et al., 1988) and was accurate and precise (Buckingham et al., 1992). Glade et al. related ultrasound transmission parameters to biomechanical testing of ex situ equine bone and concluded that the portability, reproducibility, and simplicity of the method lent it great promise (1986). The variation in soft tissue between animals and across time can lead to error.

The ultrasound transmission velocity has a reasonable precision (< 1.5%), but the broadband ultrasound attenuation is less precise (Genant et al., 1996). These two parameters are influenced by bone density and weakly by architecture (trabecular number, orientation, and connectivity) (Nicholson et al., 2001). Faster ultrasound speeds through the outer 3-5 mm of third metacarpal bone shaft were associated with thinner third metacarpal dorsal cortex in different ages of training racehorses (Davies, 2002). Similarly, speed of sound measurements obtained by quantitative ultrasonography in axial transmission mode precisely measured superficial cortical bone properties of third metacarpal and other bones (Lepage et al., 2001; Carstanjen et al., 2002; Carstanjen et al., 2003). The technique appears promising and requires validation for use in detection of appropriate parameters for studying bone growth and development.

PHOTON ABSORPTIOMETRY

The attenuation of low-energy photons emitted by a radionuclide source is determined by a detector opposite the source and is related to bone mineral content per unit length of bone. The technique was potentially useful in the calcaneus (Scotti and Jeffcott, 1988) and third metacarpus (Tomioka et al., 1985; Buckingham et al., 1992). The technical limitations of this technique and its successors, single x-ray absorptiometry and dual photon absorptiometry, led to dual x-ray absorptiometry.

DUAL ENERGY X-RAY ABSORPTIOMETRY (DXA)

The radioisotope source is a dual energy x-ray source. The amount of the two different energy x-rays passing through the patient is determined by the detector opposite the source, and the amounts of fat, lean, and bone tissue in the field can be quantified. DXA is precise and accurate, and is used extensively to measure total body mineral mass or mineral mass of a part in people. DXA is also used extensively in animal model research to detect changes in bone mineral.

From the determination of bone mineral content, and the projected area of bone that has been scanned or defined within the scanned area as a region of interest (ROI), an areal or projectional bone mineral density (BMDa) is produced. The use of the word "density" in this context is a confusing misnomer.

The technique does not discriminate between change in real bone density and bone geometry as the bone alters due to growth, disease, or altered morphology. Increase or decrease in cortical thickness, greater or lesser subperiosteal expansion, greater or lesser apposition or resorption at the endosteal surface, and changes in bone mineral content within the cancellous or cortical compartment within the scanned region cannot usually be discriminated. If the third dimension (parallel to the beam) increases, then BMDa would increase, implying increased strength, although the mechanism for the implication could be either a real (volumetric) density increase, or (third) dimensional increase.

Standard DXA scans provide reliable width and length measurements (Sievanen et al., 1994), and some programs are available for imputing not only geometric parameters but strength indices with some reliability (Carter et al., 1992; Sarin et al., 1999). Such a program is not available for equine limbs.

DXA has been proposed for use in third metacarpal bone mass measurements in racehorses (Grier et al., 1996; Oikawa and Shimazu, 1996). The potential difficulties of the technique have been shown in ex vivo study of equine third metacarpi (Hanson and Markel, 1994; McClure et al., 2001; Carstanjen et al., 2003) in which density obtained was not unexpectedly different when the part was scanned in different projections. The mean BMDa was greater in mediolateral projections than in dorsopalmar or craniocaudal projections. As well, soft tissue disposition can alter findings because the algorithms depend on consistent fat and lean tissue ratios for specific regions in humans. Little attention has been paid to this in the horse as most work has centered on the third metacarpus. When studying bone growth in vivo, the technique is limited.

MAGNETIC RESONANCE IMAGING (MRI)

MRI depends on proton magnetic dipoles generated by the uneven number of protons in hydrogen, the most ubiquitous atom with an odd number of protons, and in other less abundant atoms. The unpaired protons exert a magnetic dipole of measurable strength and vector. When an external magnetic field is applied, the spin vector of the protons aligns with the external applied magnetic field, producing a low-energy or high-energy state; more of the dipoles align into a low-energy state (align with the external applied magnetic field) than into a high-energy state. As the photons absorb energy from exposure to electromagnetic radiation applied as radiofrequency pulses, the proton enters a higher energy state, altering the vector and plane direction of the proton, after which it reverts (relaxes) to the lower energy state. The relaxation characteristics are different for different tissues. The free induction decay data of the excited protons as they lose phase coherence are detected and analyzed to compose two- or three-dimensional images. The borders of cortical bone can be detected, and MRI analysis of cortical bone seems as promising as QCT or pQCT. So far the modality has not been used to study bone development.

PERIPHERAL QUANTITATIVE COMPUTED TOMOGRAPHY (PQCT)

CT has been used mainly for diagnosis in horses. pQCT machines have been developed for imaging the lower arm and leg in people, the purpose being to make only a limited number of cross-sectional images of the limb to obtain bone dimensions. The program quantifies the area of, and the bone mineral content of, the cancellous and cortical bone fractions, and determines the volumetric bone density (BMDv) of each. The density is expressed in volumetric terms since the thickness of the cut is known. This is a tissue density and is the mass of mineral per unit volume of the trabecular or cortical compartment.

Also, a derived strength value can be determined from knowing the center of the bone, the density values, and the distance from the center of all voxels in the slice of bone being examined. Bone that is distributed peripherally in the structural column is more effective in resisting bending and torsion forces.

The stiffness of a structure is a function of the product of some material quality of the bone sampled (such as the elastic modulus), and some parameter expressing the distribution and amount of the tissue (geometric properties of the bone itself). The pQCT does not measure or determine the modulus or intrinsic stiffness, but over a wide range of values the modulus varies linearly with the cortical bone mineral density. The density value of each voxel and its site are determined by CT. The cross-sectional area moment of inertia (CSMI) in either x or y plane expresses the amount of material and its distribution relative to the center of the bone and indicates the efficiency of the cross-sectional architecture of the bone at the level of the slice in resisting bending forces. A similar index expresses resistance to torsion of the longitudinal bone axis and is called polar CSMI. When combined with BMD, such geometric variables are more reliable than either parameter alone in discriminating between strong and weak bones. The product of CSMI and cortical bone density (integrating the pixel area times the square of distance of each pixel from the axis) produces the bone strength index, combining calculation of the geometric properties and the bone material's intrinsic properties at the scan site. This is closely related to the biomechanically determined fracture load of the bone (Ferretti et al., 1996) and is probably the best in vivo estimate available of bone strength.

The radiation source (47 kV and less than 0.3 mA) emits photons which are detected by an array of detectors. The source and detectors move around the limb, which is held in the gantry (140 mm diameter) by supports on either side of it. The limb remains motionless while the detectors and source are moved up or down the limb to take images at other sites as defined in the mask. The mask defines the site of scout scan as well as the voxel size, resolution, number, spacing, and level of the intended scan "slices." The length of the bone is measured from external landmarks, and the level at which the QCT slice is taken is expressed in actual measurement (mm) or in proportional terms (% of bone length) from a reference point. The machine measures the mineral portion of bone by calibration with phantoms of a specific concentration of hydroxyapatite. The attenuation coefficient of each voxel is transformed to a density value in mg/cm^3. Radiation dose is very low.

The system produces a cross-sectional image, and data on the following parameters from each 2-mm slice: bone mineral content, bone area, and bone density separated into cortical and cancellous fractions according to a chosen threshold. Further analysis allows determination of parameters such as cortical thickness, circumference, and strength indices. Regions of interest can be used to quantify properties of particular areas within the slice image. Precision in such machines is 0.3-2% (Augat et al., 1998; Sievanen et al., 1998). Because the density obtained is a volumetric density, meaningful interpretation in growing animals is possible.

Our work so far has required the animal to be anesthetized, a limitation which together with the small gantry size has resulted in production of a vertically oriented machine, with a larger gantry, which allows scanning in the standing animal (Desbrosse, unpublished).

Longitudinal pQCT Scanning in Young Horses

Several foals were scanned from a few weeks of age to 410 days of age, and the results of those scans are presented. The intentions of this pilot study were to determine changes in both diaphyseal and epiphyseal bone and to determine if altering calcium intake affected bone development (Grace et al., 2002).

METHODS

The study group consisted of 17 Thoroughbred foals (nine fillies and eight colts) born to mares kept at pasture for the whole pregnancy, fed supplemental hay in winter, and dosed orally every month with 25 mg of selenium selenate. The foals were born and raised at pasture, were wormed at regular intervals, and were examined and weighed every two weeks. The foals were weaned in two groups, one progressively between May 8 to May 14, and the other group abruptly on May 9, 2000. The colts were castrated at between 15 and 17 months of age.

Calcium intake was increased in some of the foals by feeding a supplement containing calcium for 84 days. All the horses were fed pasture and the three treatment groups were rotationally grazed as a single group in 1.5-2 ha paddocks of ryegrass and white clover pasture starting in late May. To increase calcium intakes equivalent to dietary calcium concentrations of 0.35%, 0.63%, or 1.20% DM, 0.5 kg of a pelleted calcium supplement containing barley meal, malt culums, molasses, soybean oil, and 0%, 8%, or 24% calcium carbonate was fed as a single meal at 0830 h for 84 days to each horse individually; all of the supplement was observed to have been consumed.

The foals underwent a series of pQCT scans (XCT2000, Stratec Medizintechnik, Pforzheim, Germany) at approximately six-week intervals. Each foal had a minimum of six scans, with the exception of one brought-in colt which had only three scans due to its later inclusion in the study group. The foals born early in the breeding season were not scanned until 82 days of age, and foals born later in the breeding season were scanned at younger ages, the youngest being four days old at first scan. Summarized results are presented in Figure 1. The results for phalanx and radius, although not shown here, were similar.

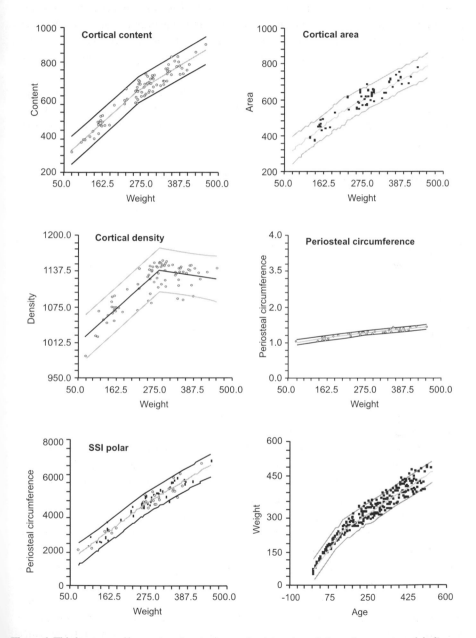

Figure 1. Third metacarpal bone mineral content, area, density, periosteal circumference, strength index, and body weight gain in a group of 17 young horses growing at pasture.

DIAPHYSIS

The bone mineral content and the area it covered in third metacarpal mid-diaphysis increased biphasically, but density plateaued around a mean weight of 275 kg. This indicates that the bone strength (represented as index-expressing resistance to torsion of the bone) increased due to increase in the size of the bone after this weight was achieved, due to continuing increase in periosteal circumference, and not due to density increase. Bone strength was continuing to increase by the end of the study.

There may have been differences between male and female animals, but these are not reported here. The change in bone growth occurred before weaning and long before puberty onset occurs in animals on this breeding farm (Brown-Douglas, PhD thesis 2003). The change in rate of bone growth, as indicated by the inflection points of biphasic growth, was preceded by the most obvious change in body weight growth. This corresponds with current indications that muscle force and bone growth are closely related (Schoenau et al., 2000).

EPIPHYSIS

In early life, the third metacarpal epiphysis cancellous bone is fairly homogeneous, and density was low. By 60 days of age, bone density was already increasing, with dense bone more obvious in areas subjected to highest local articular cartilage contact stress. In the distal third metacarpal epiphysis, by approximately 200 days about 80% of content and area consisted of epiphyseal bone denser than 540 mg/cm^3, a fraction not reached until about 400 days for even denser (>710 mg/cm^3) bone.

CALCIUM

Increasing calcium intake had no significant effect on daily energy intake, dry matter digestibility, or the apparent absorption of calcium, phosphorus, sodium, and potassium. Regardless of calcium intake, the apparent absorption of calcium was 0.56. The apparent absorption of magnesium decreased from 0.50 to 0.38. Perhaps other forms of calcium would increase bone quality at the most susceptible time (post-weaning, winter) or the time of most rapid growth. The scans before and after the calcium supplementation period revealed bone parameter increases attributable to normal age- and season-related bone development, and not due to calcium supplementation, because the changes were common to all groups, with no significant differences between groups (Grace et al., 2002).

References

Augat, P., C.L. Gordon, T.F. Lang, H. Iida, and H.K. Genant. 1998. Accuracy of cortical and trabecular bone measurements with peripheral quantitative computed tomography (pQCT). Phys. Med. Biol. 43:2873-83.

Belling, T.H., and M.J. Glade, 1984. A non-destructive biopsy method allowing rapid removal of live growth-plate cartilage. Vet. Med. 528-531.

Brown-Douglas, C.G. 2003. Aspects of puberty and growth in pasture-raised Thoroughbreds raised in spring and autumn. Massey University.

Buckingham, S.H., L.B. Jeffcott, G.A. Anderson, and R.N. McCartney. 1992. In vivo measurement of bone quality in the horse: Estimates of precision for ultrasound velocity measurement and single photon absorptiometry. Med. Biol. Eng. Comput. 30:41-45.

Burbidge, H.M., and D.U. Pfeiffer. 1998. The accuracy and reliability of linear measurements of the ulna for anthropometrical studies in dogs. Res. Vet. Sci. 65:53-57.

Carstanjen, B., F. Duboeuf, J. Detilleux, and O.M. Lepage. 2003. Equine third metacarpal bone assessment by quantitative ultrasound and dual energy X-ray absorptiometry: An ex vivo study. J. Vet. Med. A Physiol. Pathol. Clin. Med. 50:2-7.

Carstanjen, B., O.M. Lepage, J. Detilleux, F. Duboeuf, and H. Amory. 2002. Use of multisite quantitative ultrasonography for noninvasive assessment of bone in horses. Am. J. Vet. Res. 63:1464-1469.

Carstanjen, B., J. Sulon, H. Banga-Mboko, J.F. Beckers, and B. Remy. 2003. Development and validation of a specific radioimmunoassay for equine osteocalcin. Domest. Anim. Endocrinol. 24:31-41.

Carter, D.R., M.L. Bouxsein, and R. Marcus. 1992. New approaches for interpreting projected bone densitometry data. J. Bone Miner. Res. 7:137-145.

Cosman, F., B. Herrington, S. Himmelstein, and R. Lindsay. 1991. Radiographic absorptiometry: A simple method for determination of bone mass. Osteoporos. Int. 2:34-8.

Davies, H.M. 2002. Dorsal metacarpal cortex ultrasound speed and bone size and shape. Equine Vet. J. Suppl. 337-339.

Ferretti, J.L., R.F. Capozza, and J.R. Zanchetta. 1996. Mechanical validation of a tomographic (pQCT) index for noninvasive estimation of rat femur bending strength. Bone 18:97-102.

Genant, H.K., T.F. Lang, K. Engelke, T. Fuerst, et al. 1996. Advances in the noninvasive assessment of bone density, quality, and structure. Calcif. Tissue Int. 59:10-15.

Glade, M.J., N.K. Luba, and H.F. Schryver. 1986. Effects of age and diet on the development of mechanical strength by the third metacarpal and metatarsal bones of young horses. J. Anim. Sci. 63:1432-1444.

Grace, N.D., E.C. Firth, H.L. Shaw, and E.K. Gee. 2002. Digestible energy intake, dry matter digestibility and effect of increased calcium intake on bone parameters of grazing New Zealand Thoroughbred weanlings. New Zeal. Vet. J. 50:182-185.

Grier, S.J., A.S. Turner, and M.R. Alvis. 1996. The use of dual-energy x-ray absorptiometry in animals. Invest. Radiol. 31:50-62.

Hanson, P.D., and M.D. Markel. (1994) Bone mineral density measurement of equine long bones by dual x-ray absorptiometry. Vet. Surg. 23:402.

Jackson, B., R. Eastell, R.G. Russell, L.E. Lanyon, and J.S. Price. 1996. Measurement of bone specific alkaline phosphatase in the horse: A comparison of two techniques. Res. Vet. Sci. 61:160-164.

Jeffcott, L.B., S.H. Buckingham, R.N. McCarthy, J.C. Cleeland, E. Scotti, and R.N. McCartney. 1988. Non-invasive measurement of bone: A review of clinical and research applications in the horse. Equine Vet. J. Suppl. 71-79.

Jeffcott, L.B., and R.N. McCartney. 1985. Ultrasound as a tool for assessment of bone quality in the horse. Vet. Rec. 116:337-342.

Lepage, O.M., B. Carstanjen, and D. Uebelhart. 2001. Non-invasive assessment of equine bone: An update. Vet. J. 161:10-22.

Markel, M.D. 1996. Fracture healing and its non-invasive assessment. In: A. Nixon (Ed.) Equine Fracture Repair. p. 19-29. WB Saunders, Philadelphia.

McCarthy, R.N., L.B. Jeffcott, and R.N. McCartney. 1988. Ultrasonic transmission velocity and single photon absorptiometric measurement of metacarpal bone strength: An in vitro study in the horse. Equine Vet. J. Suppl. 80-87.

McClure, S.R., L.T. Glickman, N.W. Glickman, and C.M. Weaver. 2001. Evaluation of dual energy x-ray absorptiometry for in situ measurement of bone mineral density of equine metacarpi. Am. J. Vet. Res. 62:752-756.

Meakim, D.W., E.A. Ott, R.L. Asquith, and J.P. Feaster. 1981. Estimation of mineral content of the equine third metacarpal by radiographic photometry. J. Anim. Sci. 53:1019-1026.

Nicholson, P.H., R. Muller, X.G. Cheng, P. Ruegsegger, G. Van Der Perre, J. Dequeker, and S. Boonen. 2001. Quantitative ultrasound and trabecular architecture in the human calcaneus. J. Bone Miner. Res. 16:1886-1892.

Oikawa, M., and K. Shimazu. 1996. In vitro measurement of the bone mineral density of the third metacarpal bone by dual energy x-ray absorptiometry in racehorses: Comparison with single photon absorptiometry. J. Equine Sci. 7:93-96.

Pearce, S.G., E.C. Firth, and W.F. Hunt. 1999. Evaluation of a method for biopsy of the distal radial physeal growth plate in neonatal foals. Vet. Comparative Ortho. Trauma. 12:12.

Price, J.S., B. Jackson, R. Eastell, A.E. Goodship, A. Blumsohn, I. Wright, S. Stoneham, L.E. Lanyon, and R.G. Russell. 1995. Age-related changes in biochemical markers of bone metabolism in horses. Equine Vet. J. 27:201-207.

Price, J.S., B.F. Jackson, J.A. Gray, P.A. Harris, I.M. Wright, D.U. Pfeiffer, S.P. Robins, R. Eastell, and S.W. Ricketts. 2001. Biochemical markers of bone metabolism in growing Thoroughbreds: A longitudinal study. Res. Vet. Sci. 71:37-44.

Ruiz-Echarri, M., A.F. Longas, E. Mayayo, J.I. Labarta, and E. Cancer. 1996. Evaluation of bone mass on X-rays of the left hand and wrist with a magnifying glass. In: E. Schoenau (Ed.) Paediatric Osteology: New Developments in Diagnosis and Therapy.

Sarin, V.K., E.G. Loboa Polefka, G.S. Beaupre, B.J. Kiratli, D.R. Carter, and M.C. van der Meulen. 1999. DXA-derived section modulus and bone mineral content predict long-bone torsional strength. Acta. Orthop. Scand. 70:71-76.

Savage, C.J., L.B. Jeffcott, F. Melsen, and L.C. Ostblom. 1991a. Bone biopsy in the horse. 1. Method using the wing of ilium. Zentralbl Veterinarmed A 38:776-783.

Savage, C.J., L.C. Tidd, F. Melsen, L.B. Jeffcott, and L. Ostblom. 1991b. Bone biopsy in the horse. 2. Evaluation of histomorphometric examination. Zentralbl Veterinarmed A 38:784-792.

Schoenau, E., C.M. Neu, E. Mokov, G. Wassmer, and F. Manz. 2000. Influence of puberty on muscle area and cortical bone area of the forearm in boys and girls. J. Clin. Endocrinol. Metab. 85:1095-1098.

Scotti, E., and L.B. Jeffcott. 1988. The hock as a potential site for non-invasive bone measurement. Equine Vet. J. Suppl. 93-98.

Secombe, C.J. 2000. The quantitative assessment of photodensity of the third carpal bone in the horse. M.V.Sc Thesis. Massey University.

Sievanen, H., P. Kannus, P. Oja, and I. Vuori. 1994. Dual energy x-ray absorptiometry is also an accurate and precise method to measure the dimensions of human long bones. Calcif. Tissue Int. 54:101-105.

Sievanen, H., V. Koskue, A. Rauhio, P. Kannus, A. Heinonen, and I. Vuori. 1998. Peripheral quantitative computed tomography in human long bones: Evaluation of in vitro and in vivo precision. J. Bone Miner. Res. 13:871-882.

Tomioka, Y., M. Kaneko, M. Oikawa, T. Kaenmaru, T. Yoshihara, and R. Wada. 1985. Bone mineral content of the metacarpus in racehorses by photon absorption technique. Bull. Equine Res. Institute 22-29.

Walter, L.J., and H.M. Davies. 2001. Analysis of a radiographic technique for measurement of equine metacarpal bone shape. Equine Vet. J. Suppl. 141-144.

Yang, S.O., S. Hagiwara, K. Engelke, M.S. Dhillon, G. Guglielmi, E.J. Bendavid, O. Soejima, D.L. Nelson, and H.K. Genant. 1994. Radiographic absorptiometry for bone mineral measurement of the phalanges: Precision and accuracy study. Radiology 192:857-859.

NUTRITIONAL ASSESSMENT OF WEANLINGS AND YEARLINGS

LARRY A. LAWRENCE
Kentucky Equine Research, Versailles, Kentucky, USA

Introduction

Height or long bone growth is the developmental priority for young horses. Energy, protein, minerals, and vitamins are first directed to maintenance requirements, and any additional nutrients are used for skeletal growth, specifically long bones (limbs for locomotion) and flat bones (skull, ribs, etc. for protection). Additional nutrients above those needed for optimal bone development are used to fuel more rapid growth, first developing muscle and then producing a heavier and more well-developed young horse. Optimal growth rates may vary somewhat between breeds, but all young horses have several critical considerations for bone growth and development. Extremely rapid growth caused by overfeeding (particularly energy) has been implicated in developmental orthopedic disease (DOD) and unsoundness. Periods of slow followed by rapid growth are of particular concern for developmental disorders.

Optimal bone development is greatly influenced by nutrition. During the first two months of life, the mare's milk contains enough energy, protein, and other essential nutrients to meet the needs for growth. Work in Australia (Kohnke et al., 1999) has shown that a horse maturing to 450-500 kg requires approximately nine kg of milk for each kg of gain at seven days of age, 13 kg at one month of age, and 15 kg at two months of age. Thoroughbred foals may consume up to 18 kg of milk per day. The foals require around 16.4 kg of milk per kg of gain, so they should be gaining just over 1 kg per day. Beyond two months of age, there is a decrease in milk production, and additional nutrients must be supplied by creep feeding until weaning.

Foals begin to nibble grass soon after birth, but they do not develop a functional hindgut that will allow them to extract significant nutrients from forages for months. In contrast, their efficiency of grain utilization is high at three weeks of age.

Contributions of Pasture

Researchers in Australia, New Zealand, and the United States have recently focused on the contribution of pastures to the nutrition of growing horses. Variability in pastures is considerable across regions and seasons of the year. When pastures were analyzed across seasons, researchers at Virginia Tech found that the amount of hydrolyzable and rapidly fermentable carbohydrates could be as much as five times higher during the spring and fall as opposed to winter and summer for cool season forages. While many professional horsemen recognize the importance of pastures to growth and development, pasture care is not often given the attention it requires.

Pastures generally fall into the categories of cool season or warm season and grass or legume. What species are found in a particular area is dependent on the annual rainfall and seasonal variations in temperature. For example, a common pasture for a temperate climate might include bluegrass, orchard grass, and white clover. Pastures subjected to adequate fertilization and rainfall during early spring and fall may produce forage that can support gains in weanlings of up to two pounds per day, although vitamin and mineral supplementation would be necessary. Studies at Virginia Tech have confirmed that even under the best conditions pasture will fall short of some key mineral and vitamin requirements and may vary depending on the location of the farm (Greiwe-Crandell et al., 1997). However, these same pastures during typically hot and dry July and August weather will not provide enough nutrients to support maintenance needs. To avoid the deleterious effects of these drastic swings in available nutrients, producers supply nutrition through carefully fortified rations.

Pasture is one variable of feeding young horses that is constantly changing and must be accounted for to control growth. Changes in weather patterns, for example, may cause a flush of pasture growth and subsequent weight gain, or a drought may leave pastures barren and unable to fulfill nutritional requirements for growth. Researchers at Cornell University illustrated the effects of undernutrition followed by overnutrition. Hintz (1983) fed one group of Standardbred weanlings free-choice feed for eight months, and a second group was given restricted feed for four months and then free-choice feed for four months. Two-thirds of the foals in the restricted-feed group developed contracted tendons within one to four months of being switched to free-access feed.

Several studies of young horses on pasture demonstrate the effects of undernutrition followed by overnutrition. In one project, six-month-old Danish Warmblood colts were fed to gain either 787 or 433 g/head/day until they were 12 months old (McMeniman, 1995). Then, all foals were put in the same pasture to graze. During the first six months of grazing, the colts fed for slow growth rebounded by gaining 138 kg, and colts fed for fast growth gained an average of only 75 kg. This divergence in growth rates describes the compensatory growth expected to increase the incidence of DOD. Researchers also noted that the horses fed for higher gains were significantly heavier and taller with greater cannon bone circumference, even after compensatory growth. The researchers continued the project for two more years. While all the horses were essentially the same height as three-year-olds, the horses fed for more consistent and steady gains were reported to be more vigorous and aggressive.

In a study at the University of Queensland Veterinary Science School, 15 Australian Stock Horse weanlings were divided into three groups (McMeniman, 2000). One group was fed a nutritionally complete pellet diet, a second group was rotationally grazed through three paddocks with the horses being moved every three weeks, and the third group grazed the same paddock throughout the 60-week study. The mean body weight gains of the completely hand-fed group, the rotationally grazed group, and the group that remained on the same pasture were 0.51, 0.37 and 0.34 kg/day, respectively. At the end of the experiment, the horses in the hand-fed group were significantly heavier and had higher body condition scores (system of evaluating the level of fatness of horses) than the horses in the other two groups. The authors indicate height and muscle mass were similar; however, the hand-fed group had more compact (harder or denser) bone between six and 12 months of age. Chemical analysis of the pastures revealed that some had mean crude protein concentrations below those recommended for growing horses, and a high proportion of the pastures were deficient in calcium, copper, and zinc. The pastures with low calcium concentrations also had inverted calcium to phosphorus ratios (below 1:1). Diets containing inverted calcium to phosphorus ratios and low zinc and copper concentrations are associated with the development of DOD.

Energy

The results of pasture studies indicate that foals are eating enough to satisfy energy needs for rapid growth. Foals consuming traditional high-concentrate diets spend less time grazing than similar horses on high-forage diets. It is generally observed that high grain intake reduces forage consumption. This explains how widely dissimilar management systems, some relying heavily on forages and others feeding much more grain, can lead to success in raising horses. The 1989 NRC recommends specific ratios of concentrate to hay for growing horses. The recommended ratio for weanlings is 70% concentrate and 30% hay, while the recommended ratio for yearlings is 60% concentrate and 40% hay.

Gibbs and Cohen (2001) reported the results of a survey of race-bred weanlings and yearlings. They noted that 99% of the farms contacted fed weanlings diets containing less than 70% concentrate, and 62% of the farms fed less concentrate than forage. Turcott and coworkers (2003) placed 24 weanlings on one of three diets with varying concentrate to hay ratios: 70:30, 50:50, and 30:70. The forage fed was 50% alfalfa and 50% timothy grass hay. Diets were balanced to meet all NRC requirements. The weanlings were fed the experimental diets from five to eight months of age. The low-concentrate diet resulted in greater fecal output. The high-concentrate diet had higher protein and ADF digestibilities. The authors state that the study demonstrates weanlings are more efficient at digesting high-concentrate diets and supports the NRC ratio of 70:30 (concentrate:roughage by percent of diet).

Ott and Kivipelto (2003) assigned weanlings to a diet of either 65% concentrate and 35% Bermuda grass hay or 50% concentrate and 50% Bermuda grass hay. The latter diet (50:50) had 3% added fat. The 65:35 group received 1.7 kg/100 kg body weight daily, and the 50:50 group received 1.35 kg/100 kg body weight daily. There were no differences in weight gain, with mean weight gain 0.76 kg/day. The 50:50 group was higher in the withers, had greater heart-girth circumference, and was higher in the hips. Bone mineral deposition was not different; however, weanlings fed the 50:50 diet had the highest values. The authors state the diet containing equal parts concentrate and forage was as effective in promoting growth as the diet that contained more concentrate.

Stephens and coworkers (2003) maintained yearlings in a drylot or on Bermuda grass pasture. Grain was fed to appetite over two 1.5-hour periods per day. There was no difference in intake between the groups. The drylot group received 1.5 kg/100 kg body weight in hay per day. Yearlings housed on pasture were heavier and had greater heart-girth circumference and bone mineral content at 56 and 112 days.

Energy Requirements

All cellular processes require energy. There is an absolute requirement for energy for maintenance, exercise, lactation, and growth. However, there is no single nutrient identified as energy. Energy is derived from nonstructural carbohydrates (starches), structural carbohydrates (cellulose, hemicellulose, etc.), fatty acids, and carbon chains of proteins. Meeting the energy requirements of horses is complicated by the variable contributions of fermentation in the hindgut. Some of the factors affecting fermentation are concentrate to roughage percentages, amount of structural and nonstructural carbohydrates included in the diet, and efficiency of the hindgut in suckling and weanling horses.

Ott (2001) reviewed the energy requirements for growing horses. The energy requirement for growing horses is determined by adding the maintenance requirement to the requirement for tissue energy deposition and efficiency of the conversion of dietary energy to tissue energy. The digestible energy (DE) requirement for maintenance is DE (Mcal) = 1.4 + .03 BW (body weight, kg). When the maintenance formula is combined with the tissue energy deposition and efficiency predictive equation, the daily DE requirement can be predicted by the following equation: DE (Mcal) = [1.4 + 0.03 BW (kg)] + (4.81 + 11.17x - 0.023 x 2) [ADG (kg)].

The desired average daily gain (ADG) drives the energy requirements up or down. The NRC provides a range of growth rates from moderate to rapid. Selecting the appropriate rate of growth is based on the commercial end point and management system. However, the long-range management of the foal must be planned in advance. Growth must be maintained along a moderately steady course.

The NRC suggests that a six-month-old foal with an adult weight of 560 kg gains 0.65 kg/day for moderate growth and 0.85 kg/day for rapid growth. The NRC estimates that the six-month-old weanling would weigh 230 kg.

Pagan (1998) reported growth data collected on Thoroughbred farms in central Kentucky. He found that the foals averaged 0.8 kg ADG, but they weighed 246 kg on average. The NRC DE requirement for a six-month-old foal gaining 0.8 kg/day is 16.2 Mcal. Kentucky Equine Research (KER) estimates the requirement for the same rate of gain to be 16.8 Mcal. The NRC recommends a yearling (12 months old) that will have an adult weight of 560 kg should weigh 350 kg and be gaining 0.5 kg/day for moderate growth and 0.65 kg/day for rapid growth. Pagan (1998) found Kentucky Thoroughbred yearlings weighed 354 kg and were gaining 0.6 kg/day (Tables1-4). The NRC requirement for this yearling would be 21.3 Mcal, while KER would suggest a requirement of 21.6 Mcal.

Table 1. Nutrient requirements for a six-month-old weanling (246 kg) gaining 0.65 kg/day with an estimated mature weight of 560 kg.

	DE (Mcal)	CP (g/day)	Ca (g)	P (g)	Cu (g)	Zn (g)
KER	15.3	764	38.0	25.3	168	504
NRC	15.9	796.6	30.6	16.5	54.9	219.7

Table 2. Nutrient requirements for a six-month-old weanling (246 kg) gaining 0.85 kg/day with an estimated mature weight of 560 kg.

	DE (Mcal)	CP (g/day)	Ca (g)	P (g)	Cu (g)	Zn (g)
KER	17.3	864	44	29.3	168	504
NRC	18.1	906.6	37	20.1	62.5	250.1

Table 3. Nutrient requirements for a twelve-month-old weanling (354 kg) gaining 0.5 kg/day with an estimated mature weight of 560 kg.

	DE (Mcal)	CP (g/day)	Ca (g)	P (g)	Cu (g)	Zn (g)
KER	20	901	47.5	31.7	168	504
NRC	19.8	890	30.2	16	70.7	282.7

Table 4. Nutrient requirements for a twelve-month-old weanling (354 kg) gaining 0.65 kg/day with an estimated mature weight of 560 kg.

	DE (Mcal)	CP (g/day)	Ca (g)	P (g)	Cu (g)	Zn (g)
KER	22.4	1008	52.6	35.1	168	504
NRC	22.1	995	35	18.7	79	316

Dietary energy fed at excessive levels has been implicated as a contributing factor in the onset of DOD (Glade, 1986). Savage et al. (1993) fed a control diet that contained DE at the NRC recommended level and a diet containing 129% of the recommended level to foals 2.5-6.5 months of age for 16-18 weeks. The diets were rice-based pellets. The high-DE diet had approximately 5% added corn oil. Eleven of the 12 foals on the high-DE diet developed multiple dyschondroplasia (DCP) lesions. Only one of the foals on the control diet developed DCP lesions. There were no differences in growth rates between the treatments. The authors indicate there may be an association between high DE and a high incidence of DCP.

Pagan et al. (2001) conducted a field study with 218 Thoroughbred weanlings. A glycemic index was created for each diet fed to horses on six different farms. The incidence of osteochondritis dissecans (OCD) was followed for 6 or 8 months or until the yearlings were sold at auction. Twenty-five of the 218 weanlings (11.5%) had OCD lesions that were treated surgically. The incidence of OCD was significantly higher in foals whose glucose and insulin values were greater than one standard deviation above the entire population when the body weights were compared with the Kentucky average (Pagan, 1998). One farm, which experienced a 32% incidence of OCD, averaged 115% of the reference weight. A second farm, which had no incidence of OCD, averaged 97% of the Kentucky average body weight. The authors suggest that feeding foals a concentrate that produces a low glycemic response may decrease the incidence of OCD.

Protein Requirements

Protein accounts for 80% of the fat-free, moisture-free composition of the body. Amino acids are the building blocks of proteins. The concentration of protein needed in a diet is dependent on how well the amino acid profile matches the needs of the animal. A young growing horse, for example, has a higher requirement for the amino acids needed to build muscle and bone. The amino acid profile varies among different protein sources. Milk protein is superior to soybean meal; soybean meal has been shown to grow weanlings faster than zein, cottonseed meal, and brewers dried grains. When each of these protein sources was supplemented with the amino acid lysine, growth rates improved and were comparable (NRC, 1989). Lysine is the most limiting amino acid and specific requirements have been developed. Threonine is the second most limiting amino acid in the diet.

Ott and Asquith (1986) developed the protein requirements of growing horses based on digestible energy requirements, stating both energy and protein restrictions will reduce the growth of the animal. The crude protein (CP) energy relationship for weanlings is CP (g/day) = 50 g/Mcal DE, and for yearlings it is CP (g/day) = 45 g/Mcal DE. Lysine requirements are also provided on an energy basis. The lysine requirement for weanlings is 2.1 g/Mcal DE per day, and the yearling requirement is 1.9 g/Mcal DE per day.

There have been anecdotal reports of high-protein diets causing DOD. Weanling foals fed 126% of the NRC protein requirement had no greater incidence than foals fed at NRC recommended levels (Savage et al., 1993).

Calcium and Phosphorus Requirements

The importance of calcium and phosphorus to bone mineralization is well known. The ratio of calcium to phosphorus in the bone is 2:1. Horses should be fed diets containing calcium and phosphorus ratios between 3:1 and 1:1. Jordan et al. (1975) fed ratios of 6:1 to pony mares over a four-year period and found narrowing of the cortical area and less bone per unit area of bone. Inverted calcium to phosphorus ratios are not uncommon when high-grain diets are fed with little or poor-quality forages. Nutritional secondary hyperparathyroidism can result from excessive phosphorus intakes in the presence of low calcium. This disease can cause shifting lameness and, in advanced cases, enlargement of the upper and lower jaws (NRC, 1989).

The NRC estimates that a growing horse requires 16 g of calcium/kg of body weight gain. Tables 1-4 compare NRC recommendations for calcium and phosphorus with recommendations developed by KER. The NRC recommends a minimum of 30.6 g/day of calcium for a 246-kg weanling gaining 0.5 kg/day. KER recommends 38 g/day for the same weanling. The NRC minimum phosphorus recommendation for a 246-kg weanling gaining 0.5 kg/day is 16.5 g; the KER optimum recommendation is 25.3 g. For a 246-kg weanling gaining 0.65 kg/day, the NRC recommendation for calcium is 37 g, while the KER recommendation is 44 g. For the same weanling, the NRC recommendation for phosphorus is 20.1, while the KER recommendation is 29.3.

Copper and Zinc

Copper requirements in growing horses have been debated for almost 15 years. Gable et al. (1987) published survey data that they felt indicated an association between copper and DOD. Burton and Hurtig (1991) reported a significant increase in DOD lesions in foals that were fed 8 mg of copper versus foals fed 25 mg/kg. Cymbaluk and Smart (1993) reviewed the literature on copper and its relationship to equine bone disease. They suggested that copper requirement may vary among breeds. They recommended that ponies and draft horses be fed 10 mg/kg and that horses prone to copper deficiency be fed a total of 20-25 mg/kg diet. They also reported a high tolerance to high copper supplementation in the horse. The authors warned against a complicated copper deficiency caused by excessive zinc in the diet competing for the same transportation mechanism as copper. The key to proper copper and zinc nutrition seems to be an optimum ratio of 1:4-5 (copper to zinc). Tables 1-4 indicate copper and zinc requirements for minimum and optimum growth.

Growing horses seem to be able to adapt to a variety of nutritional management systems if adequate nutrients are provided in the correct balance and a moderate rate of growth is maintained throughout the growth phase.

Lierature Cited

Burton, J.H., and M.B. Hurtig. 1991. Dietary copper intake and bone lesions in foals. In: Proc. Equine Nutr. Phys. Symp. 12:67-68.

Cymbaluk, N.F., and M.E. Smart. 1993. A review of possible metabolic relationships of copper to equine bone disease. Equine Vet. J. Suppl. 16:19-29.

Gable, A.A., D.A. Knight, S.M. Reed, J.A. Pultz, J.D. Powers, L.R. Bramlage, and W.J. Tyznik. 1987. Comparison of incidence and severity of developmental orthopedic disease on 17 farms before and after adjustment of ration. In: Proc. Amer. Assoc. Equine Pract. 33:163-169.

Gibbs, P., and N. Cohen. 2001. Early management of race-bred weanlings and yearlings on farms. J. Equine Vet. Sci. 21:279-283.

Glade, M.J. 1986. The control of cartilage growth in osteochondrosis: A review. Equine Vet. Sci. 6:175-187.

Greiwe-Crandell, K.M., D.S. Kronfeld, L.A. Gay, D. Sklan, and P.A. Harris. 1997. Seasonal vitamin A depletion in Thoroughbred mares with retinyl palmitate or B-carotene. J. Anim. Sci. 7:2684.

Hintz, H.F. 1983. Horse Nutrition: A Practical Guide. p. 187. Prentice Hall Press. New York, New York.

Jordan, R.M., V.S. Meyers, B. Yoho, and F.A. Spurrell. 1975. Effects of calcium and phosphorus levels on growth, reproduction and bone development of ponies. J. Anim. Sci. 40:78.

Kohnke, J.R., F. Kelleher, and P. Trevor-Jones. 1999. Feeding Horses in Australia: A Guide for Horse Owners and Managers. RIRDC Publication No. 99/49 RIRDC Project No. UWS -13A. Rural Industries Research and Development Corporation. Barton, ACT.

McMeniman, N.P. 1995. Nutrition of broodmares and growing foals. In: Proc. Equine Nutrition and Pastures for Horses Workshop. Richmond, NSW. p. 48-60.

McMeniman, N.P. 2000. Nutrition of grazing broodmares, their foals, and young horses. In: Report for the Rural Industries Research and Development Corporation. RIRDC Publication No. 00/28 RIRDC Project No. UQ-45A. p. vi.

NRC. 1989. Nutrient Requirements of Horses. (5th Ed.) National Academy Press. Washington, DC.

Ott, E. A. 2001. Energy, protein and amino acid requirements for growth of young horses. In: J.D. Pagan and R.J. Geor (Eds.) Advances in Equine Nutrition II. p. 153-160. Nottingham University Press, Nottingham, U.K.

Ott, E.A., and R.L. Asquith. 1986. Influence of level of feeding and nutrient content of the concentrate on growth and development of yearling horses. J. Anim. Sci. 62:290-299.

Ott, E.A., and J. Kivipelto. 2003. Influence of concentrate:hay ration on growth and development of weanling horses. In: Proc. Equine Nutr. Physiol. Symp. 18:146-147.

Pagan, J.D. 1998. A summary of growth rates of Thoroughbreds in Kentucky. In: J.D. Pagan (Ed.) Advances in Equine Nutrition. p. 449-455. Nottingham University Press, Nottingham, U.K.

Pagan, J.D., R.J. Geor, S.E. Caddel, P.B. Pryor, and K.E. Hoekstra. 2001. The relationship between glycemic response and the incidence of OCD in Thoroughbred weanlings: A field study. In: Proc. Amer. Assoc. Equine Practnr. 47:322-325.

Turcott, S.K., B.D. Nielsen, C. O'Connor, C.D. Skelly, D.S. Rosenstein, and T. Herdt. 2003. The influence of various concentrate to roughage ratios on dietary intake and nutrient digestibilities of weanlings. In: Proc. Equine Nutr. Physiol. Symp. 18:1-2.

Savage, C.J., R.N. McCarthy, and L.B. Jeffcott. 1993. Effects of dietary energy and protein on induction of dyschondroplasia in foals. Equine Vet. J. Suppl. 16:74-79.

Stephens, T.L., E.A. Ott, and J. Kivipelto. 2003. Pasture versus dry lot programs for yearling horses. In: Proc. Equine Nutr. Physiol. Symp. 18:142.

MANAGING GROWTH FOR DIFFERENT COMMERCIAL END POINTS

JOE D. PAGAN

Kentucky Equine Research, Versailles, Kentucky, USA

Introduction

A horse's maximal mature body size is genetically predetermined, but growth rate can be influenced by a number of factors including environment, nutrition, and management. Optimal growth rate results in a desirable body size at a specific age with the least amount of developmental problems. Managing growth in horses becomes a balance between producing a desirable individual for a particular purpose without creating skeletal problems that will reduce a horse's subsequent athletic ability (Figure 1). Growing a foal too slowly results in the risk of it being too small at a particular age or never obtaining maximal mature body size. Growing a foal too quickly results in the risk of developmental orthopedic disease (DOD) such as physitis, angular limb deformities, and osteochondritis dissecans (OCD). There is no single growth rate that is desirable for all types of horses. Therefore, horses should be managed differently for varying growth rates.

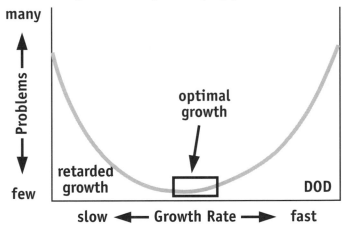

Figure 1. Distribution of growth-related problems during slow and fast growth.

Horses will generally reach physical maturity at around 4-5 years of age. Compared to Thoroughbreds, many breeds such as warmbloods are not expected to compete until later in life, so there is little incentive for rapid growth. Instead, a slow, steady growth rate that will allow the horse to reach maximal mature body size with the fewest problems is desirable. Thoroughbred racehorses are a different story. They are expected to be competitive athletes at two years of age, reaching 85% of mature body weight and 95% of mature height by 24 months of age.

Table 1. Growth rates of Hanoverian and Thoroughbred foals.

	Hanoverian					Thoroughbred				
Age (days)	Body weight (kg)	Body weight (% mature wt[1])	Av. daily gain (kg/d)	Withers height (cm)	Withers height (% mature ht[2])	Body weight (kg)	Body weight (% mature wt[1])	Av. daily gain (kg/d)	Withers height (cm)	Withers height (% mature ht[2])
1	60.0	9%	-	104.0	62%	54.5	10%	-	101.9	62%
15	73.0	11%	0.9	107.0	64%	74.9	13%	1.5	106.8	65%
30	87.3	13%	1.0	110.0	66%	94.9	17%	1.3	111.1	67%
46	103.6	16%	1.1	114.0	68%	116.2	20%	1.3	115.7	70%
60	118.7	18%	1.1	116.0	69%	132.7	23%	1.2	118.8	72%
78	136.6	21%	1.1	120.0	72%	151.2	27%	1.2	122.2	74%
90	152.6	23%	1.1	122.0	73%	165.2	29%	1.0	124.6	76%
106	170.8	26%	1.1	125.0	75%	181.1	32%	1.0	127.3	77%
120	186.4	29%	1.1	128.0	77%	193.7	34%	0.9	129.1	78%
135	202.5	31%	1.0	130.0	78%	207.2	36%	0.9	131.1	79%
150	217.7	33%	1.0	132.0	79%	220.3	39%	0.9	132.7	80%
165	231.9	36%	0.9	134.0	80%	233.4	41%	0.9	134.4	81%
180	244.8	38%	0.9	136.0	81%	245.8	43%	0.8	135.7	82%
193	254.9	39%	0.8	137.0	82%	256.5	45%	0.8	136.8	83%
210	266.8	41%	0.7	138.0	83%	269.1	47%	0.7	138.1	84%

[1]Hanoverian - 650 kg (1,430 lb) mature body weight; Thoroughbred - 570 kg (1,254 lb) mature body weight
[2]Hanoverian - 167 cm (16.1 3/4 hands) mature height; Thoroughbred - 165 cm (16.1 hands) mature height

Warmbloods

In practice, warmbloods grow more slowly than Thoroughbreds. Vervuert et al. (2003) measured body weight and withers height in 629 Hanoverian warmblood foals from birth to 7 months of age. Table 1 compares the growth rates of these foals to the growth rates of thousands of Thoroughbred foals from around the world. To evaluate these data it is useful to view them from two perspectives: (1) in absolute terms as kilograms (kg) of body weight or centimeters (cm) of height, and (2) relative to the horse's mature body size. Thoroughbreds typically have mature body weights of around 570 kg and mature heights of around 165 cm

(16.1 hands). Hanoverians tend to be heavier with mature body weights closer to 650 kg and slightly taller with mature heights of 167 cm (16.1 3/4 hands). Although slightly heavier at birth (60 kg vs. 54.5 kg), the Hanoverian foals grew slower than the Thoroughbreds for the first three months of age and were slightly smaller until 5 months of age. By 7 months of age, the Hanoverian and Thoroughbred foals were practically identical in weight and height.

Without great pressure for early rapid growth, the warmblood breeder should utilize feeding programs that are predominantly forage-based with appropriate protein and mineral fortification to promote sound skeletal development. Table 2 illustrates a sound feeding program for warmblood foals.

Table 2. Suggested feeding program for warmblood foals.

Age (months)	Growth rate (kg/day)	Forage intake (kg/day)	Oats (kg/day)	All-Phase (kg/day)
6	0.8-0.9	4-6	0-2	1
12	0.4-0.6	4-6	0-2	1
18	0.2-0.4	5-7	0-2	1
24	0.1-0.3	5-7	0-2	1

This program depends on large quantities of forage to supply most of the energy and protein to the foal. The source of forage will vary seasonally depending on pasture availability. The extra protein, vitamins, and minerals needed to support optimal skeletal development are provided by All-Phase, a concentrated supplement pellet from Kentucky Equine Research. Oats can be added as needed to supply extra calories to adjust growth rate to a desirable level. Growth monitoring is essential to assess forage intake and to adjust grain intake to maintain a desirable growth rate.

Thoroughbred Racehorses

Because Thoroughbreds begin their athletic careers at an early age, mature body size is not the most important end point that breeders wish to achieve. In fact, there can be several important developmental milestones that must be reached even before a young Thoroughbred enters its first race. Most Thoroughbreds are sold as either weanlings or yearlings at commercial auctions throughout the year. The size of the foal at auction can greatly impact its selling price, so there is strong incentive to market large weanlings and yearlings. Just as important, however, is the foal's skeletal soundness at the time of the sale. A delicate balancing act exists between accelerated growth and skeletal soundness.

The simplest and safest way to deliver a large, mature yearling to the sale is to produce an early foal. Consignors to early sales certainly appreciate this fact and yearlings entered in these sales are largely skewed towards early foaling dates (Table 3). At Keeneland's 2002 select yearling sale held July 15-16 in Kentucky, for instance, 48% of the yearlings offered were born in January or February compared to only 26% of all Thoroughbred foals born in North America in 2001. The Northern Hemisphere's official birth date for Thoroughbreds is January 1.

Table 3. Distribution of month of birth in the Thoroughbred population and in early select yearling sales in North America and Australia.

	Australia			North America	
Birth month	% of total foal crop (2002)	% of Magic Millions sale (2003)	Birth month	% of total foal crop (2001)	% of Keeneland July sale (2002)
August	15	24	January	8	16
September	30	34	February	18	32
October	34	32	March	27	33
November	18	10	April	29	16
December	2	0	May	16	5

At the 2003 Magic Millions select yearling sale held January 9-12 in Queensland, 58% of the yearlings offered were born in August and September compared to 45% of all Thoroughbred foals born in Australia in 2001. The Southern Hemisphere's official birth date for Thoroughbreds is August 1, not July 1, a date that would mirror the Northern Hemisphere birth date. This explains why a larger number of foals are born early in Australia.

Birth date is much more important for foals that will be marketed in early select sales. Table 4 shows the age of yearlings at sale time in early select sales and in later yearling sales in Kentucky and Australia. In Kentucky, a foal born in May would be of similar age at the September yearling sale to a March foal sold in a July yearling sale. A December foal sold as a yearling at the Australian Easter sale would be of similar age to a September foal sold at the Magic Millions sale in January.

Figure 2 summarizes growth measurements from 400 yearlings raised in central Kentucky. These measurements were taken in June, July, and August of the foal's yearling year. January/February foals would be equivalent to Southern Hemisphere August/September foals; March to October foals, April to November foals; and May to December foals. June, July, and August in the Northern Hemisphere would be equivalent to January, February, and March in the Southern Hemisphere.

About 50% of the foals born in January and February and 33% of the foals born in March were sold at select summer sales. In July, January/February foals

Table 4. Age of yearlings at various yearling sales in Kentucky and Australia.

	Australia			North America	
Birth date	*Age at Magic Millions sale (Jan 9)*	*Age at Easter yearling sale (Apr 22)*	*Birth date*	*Age at Keeneland July sale (Jul 15)*	*Age at Keeneland Sept sale (Sept 9)*
Aug 15	513 days	616 days	Jan 15	547 days	603 days
Sept 15	482 days	585 days	Feb 15	516 days	572 days
Oct 15	452 days	555 days	Mar 15	488 days	544 days
Nov 15	421 days	524 days	Apr 15	457 days	513 days
Dec 15	391 days	494 days	May 15	427 days	483 days

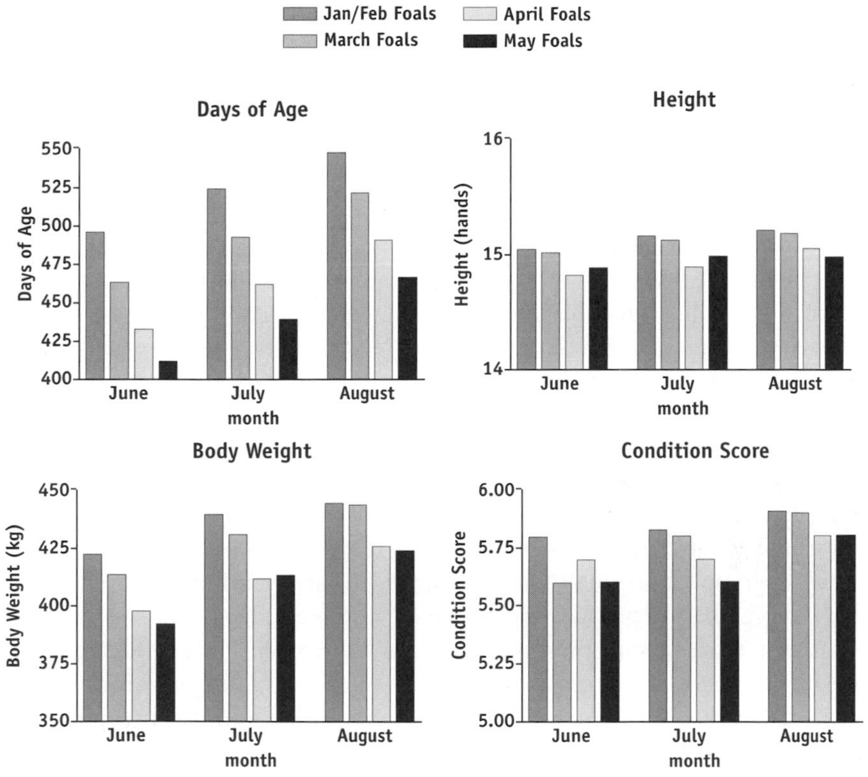

Figure 2. Days of age, height, weight, and condition score of Thoroughbred foals during June, July, and August of their yearling year.

averaged 86 days older than May foals. Withers height averaged around 15 hands in each group and increased only 1-2 cm over the three-month period. There were differences in body weight between groups, but these differences were not as great as might be expected based purely on age. For example, foals born in March had reached about 72.5% of their mature body weight in June when they averaged 462 days of age. When May foals had reached a similar age in August they averaged about 74% of their mature body weights. Therefore, they had grown at a slightly faster rate than the earlier foals. Still, April and May foals were 27 kg lighter than January/February foals at sale time in July. The April and May foals were 72% of their mature body weight in July, while the January/February foals had achieved 77% of their mature body weight by this time.

Interestingly, condition score measured on a scale from 1-9 was very similar in all groups throughout the three-month period. Condition scores averaged from 5.6-5.8 in all groups in July and reached a maximum of 5.8-5.9 in August. This illustrates that the final 60-90 days of sales prepping is not about getting yearlings fat. Rather, these final days are a time to increase the maturity and athletic appearance of yearlings through a combination of nutrition, exercise, and grooming.

In Thoroughbreds destined for the racetrack, there are three different growth rates that might be appropriate depending on when the foal is born and if or when it is to be sold. A pattern of slow early growth (slow growth in Figure 3 and Table 5) may be most appropriate for foals that will not be offered for sale as weanlings or yearlings. Additionally, foals born early in the year that will be sold in later yearling sales may benefit from this type of growth curve. The advantage to slow early growth is that the skeleton is more susceptible to growth-related problems earlier in life. Delaying more rapid growth until after the foal is more mature (>15 months) will reduce the risk of early developmental problems.

Early foals (January/February in the Northern Hemisphere and August/ September in the Southern Hemisphere) can follow the moderate growth pattern shown in Figure 3 and Table 5. This growth curve is also appropriate for later foals that will be marketed at later yearling sales. Such a growth pattern is most commonly followed by Thoroughbred breeders in Kentucky. It produces large yearlings with a limited number of problems. The most aggressive growth program is presented as rapid growth in Figure 3 and Table 5. This growth curve would be most appropriate for late foals that are targeted at early yearling sales. This growth curve is more likely to produce growth skeletal problems but, if properly managed, can result in more mature yearlings earlier in the season. The key to successfully managing this accelerated growth curve is to spread the extra growth over several months rather than trying to add the gain during the traditional prepping period 60-90 days prior to the sale.

Gro-Trac™ and MicroSteed™ are software programs developed by Kentucky Equine Research that allow breeders to accurately track the growth of their foals and develop feeding and management programs that fit the desired rate of growth. Table 6 gives examples of how feeding programs can be tailored to fit a specific growth pattern. Notice that the difference in daily grain intake needed to achieve these different growth rates is only .5 to 1 kg per day. Spread over several months this difference in nutrient intake should result in alterations in growth as depicted

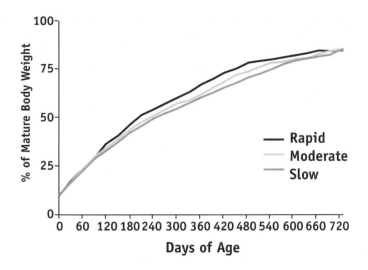

Figure 3. Slow, moderate, and rapid growth rates of Thoroughbred foals.

Table 5. Average daily gains for low, moderate, and rapid growth of Thoroughbred foals.

Age (days)	Slow growth		Moderate growth		Rapid growth	
	Body weight (kg)	*Average daily gain (kg/day)*	*Body weight (kg)*	*Average daily gain (kg/day)*	*Body weight (kg)*	*Average daily gain (kg/day)*
120	190	0.83	194	0.97	203	1.27
181	239	0.80	247	0.87	261	0.95
273	299	0.65	309	0.67	324	0.68
365	344	0.49	352	0.57	380	0.61
455	387	0.48	406	0.50	426	0.51
546	427	0.44	442	0.40	455	0.32
638	461	0.37	467	0.27	472	0.18
730	483	0.24	483	0.17	483	0.12

in Figure 3. Continual growth monitoring is necessary to ensure that the foal has not altered its total nutrient intake by greatly increasing or decreasing forage intake as this will affect growth rate.

In conclusion, the optimal growth rate for an individual foal depends on the foal's intended use and sale date (weanling or yearling). For breeds such as warmbloods that typically do not compete until they have reached their mature size, rapid early growth is not desirable because it may predispose the foal to skeletal problems. For breeds such as Thoroughbreds that will compete as two-year-olds, faster earlier growth is necessary. Foals born later in the year that are

Table 6. Example rations for slow, moderate, and rapid growth.

Age (months)	Desired growth rate	Average daily gain (kg/d)	Pasture (kg/day, 100% DM basis)	Hay (kg/d, as fed basis)	Fortified grain mix (kg/d, as fed basis)
	Slow	0.80	3.0	1.0	2.5
6	Moderate	0.87	3.0	1.0	3.0
	Fast	0.95	3.0	1.0	3.5
	Slow	0.49	3.0	2.0	3.0
12	Moderate	0.57	3.0	2.0	3.5
	Fast	0.61	3.0	2.0	4.0

pointed at early yearling sales need to follow a more aggressive growth curve than early foals or foals that will be sold in late yearling sales. With this type of accelerated program, it is imperative that growth rate is closely monitored and feed intake adjusted to produce acceptable gains. Growth monitoring combined with regular ration evaluations is the safest and most effective way to produce a sound, athletic individual.

Reference

Vervuert, I., M. Coenen, A. Borchers, M. Granel, S. Winkelsett, L. Christmann, O. Distl, E. Bruns, and B. Hertsch. 2003. Growth rates and the incidence of osteochondrotic lesions in Hanoverian warmblood foals. In: Proc. Equine Nutr. Physiol. Soc. Symp. 18:113-114.

CONFORMATION AND SOUNDNESS

C. WAYNE MCILWRAITH
Colorado State University, Fort Collins, Colorado USA

Introduction

The factors that predispose the racehorse to catastrophic injury and musculoskeletal disease continue to be an issue of debate. The cause of racing and training injuries in the horse is considered to be multifactorial, with genetics, racing surface, number of starts, age of the horse, pre-existing disease, biomechanics (conformation), and trauma being implicated as potential etiologic factors (McIlwraith, 1986; Kobluck et al., 1990; Mohammed et al., 1991; Dolvik and Klemetsdale, 1996). Each of these factors needs to be evaluated independently to determine its contribution to the complicated developmental scheme of race injury. Previous experimental studies on the cause of racing injuries in the horse have focused primarily on racing surface (Chaney et al., 1973; Hill et al., 1986), number of starts (Magnusson, 1985; Kobluck et al., 1990; Dolvik and Klemetsdale, 1996), and trauma (Jeffcott et al., 1982; Rossdale et al., 1985).

A controlled experimental study was needed to answer the question of whether conformation plays a role in racing injuries. Two studies were done. The purpose of the first study in racing Thoroughbreds was to make objective measures of conformation and determine if certain limb conformations predispose the racing Thoroughbred to musculoskeletal disease (from minor injury to catastrophic injury). The aim of the racing Quarter Horse study was to make the same determinations.

Materials and Methods

Thoroughbred Study. Included in this study were 115 three-year-old horses bred and reared by the same stable. Photographs were taken of horses with markers placed at designated locations. The slides were scanned, and conformation was measured using a software program (NIH Image Program). Left lateral radiographs, as well as photographs from front and rear, were taken. All photographs had a ruler in place to measure size, and measures could be made of length and angle using points for identification. In addition to lengths and angles, an objective method of grading the degree of offset (bench) knee conformation was also used.

Clinical observations were recorded for each horse, and clinical conditions (including radiographic diagnoses), as well as subjective evaluation of limb rotation, were made. Clinical data were recorded as "event" or "no event." Outcomes with frequencies greater than 5% remained in the data set for statistical analysis, and stepwise (forward) logistic regression analysis was performed to investigate the relationship between the binary response of the clinical outcomes, probability, and the conformation variables by the method of maximum likelihood (Version 6.12, SAS Institute, Inc., Cary, NC). Odds ratios (OR) of 95% confidence intervals were calculated to evaluate relative risk of musculoskeletal problems.

Quarter Horse Study. One hundred sixty-two two-year-old Quarter Horse racehorses in training at Los Alamitos Racecourse, California were included in this study. The horses had no previous racing history or known racing injury or lameness, and all were paid up in two-year-old races (futurities). Data were collected in the same fashion as for the Thoroughbred study, and clinical data were analyzed and odds ratios calculated in the same fashion as previously described.

Results

Clinical outcomes that were significantly (p <.05) associated with conformational variables included effusion of the front fetlocks, effusion of the right carpus, effusion of the carpus, effusion of the hind fetlock, fracture of the right or left carpus, right front fetlock problems, and hind fetlock problems. The odds of having effusion in the front fetlock increased by a factor of 1.3 for every one-inch increase in the bottom line (length of underside) of the neck. The risk of effusion of the right front fetlock increased 1.18 times for every 10% increase in the right offset ratio (a measure of offset knees). For every 10% increase in right offset ratio, the odds of right front fetlock problems increased by a factor of 1.26. For every degree increase in right carpal angle (beyond 180 degrees in a carpal valgus direction), the odds of effusion in the right front carpus decreased by a factor of 0.68. The odds for effusion in the front carpus increased 1.45 for each 10% increase in dorsal:palmar hoof angle ratio. (This is dorsal wall angle:palmar wall angle. If ratio is one, the angles are the same. If greater than one, the heel slope is more, i.e., underslung heels). The risk of effusion in the hind fetlock increased 1.1 times for every degree increase in hind dorsal hoof angle. The odds of sustaining a fracture in the carpus decreased by a factor of 0.53 for every inch increment in scapula length, and, similarly, the odds of a fracture in the front limb were decreased by a factor of 0.5 for every inch increment in scapula length. The risk of right carpal fracture decreased 0.24 times for each one degree increase in carpal valgus angle viewed from the front (increasing carpal valgus). The odds of a fracture in the right forelimb also decreased (OR 0.71) for every degree increase in the carpal valgus angle measured from the front, assuming hoof ratio was held constant. For every 10% increase in the right hoof angle ratio, the odds of a right front limb fracture decreased by a factor of 0.52 with right carpal angle held constant. The dorsal:palmar or dorsal:plantar ratio is the angle of toe in relationship to the angle of the palmar or plantar surface. It can be assumed that the increased odds for carpal effusion reported here are associated with improper hoof balance.

Quarter Horse Study. The length of the humerus was significant for several clinical entities. For every inch increase in the length of the humerus, the odds for a proximal first phalanx chip fragment in the left foreleg increased by a factor of 2.3, and the odds of sustaining synovitis/capsulitis increased by a factor of 1.85 in the left carpus and by 1.7 in the right carpus, all other factors in the model held constant. The length from elbow to ground was found to be significant in both carpi. The odds of sustaining a carpal chip fragment in the left foreleg rose by a factor of 2.06 in the right foreleg and a factor of 2.58 in the left foreleg for every one inch increase in the length from elbow to ground, assuming all other factors in the model held constant. The length of the toe was also significant, as when the length of the toe increased by one inch, the odds of sustaining a carpal chip fracture increased by a factor of 40.33.

For every degree increase in the angle of the shoulder (i.e., more upright), the odds of sustaining a proximal first phalanx chip fragment increased by a factor of 1.48. The odds of sustaining synovitis and capsulitis in the carpus decreased by 0.89 with every degree increase in the angle of the shoulder. For every degree increase in the angle of the left fore pastern (more upright), the odds of sustaining synovitis and capsulitis in the carpus were increased by a factor of 1.09. As the knee offset ratio increased by 10%, the odds of synovitis and capsulitis in both left and right front fetlocks increased by a factor of 2.26.

Discussion

The method used for measuring conformation provided an objective means to investigate the relationship between conformation and clinical conditions, as most reported relationships are based on logical hypotheses and practical experience (Green, 1969; Beeman, 1973; Stashak, 1985). When fetlock problems were grouped together, the right offset knee ratio increased the odds of fetlock problems in the right front fetlock by a factor of 1.26 for every 10% increase, insinuating change of stress in the fetlock joint with an offset knee. It is not surprising that the highest frequency of all clinical outcomes was that of effusion in the front fetlock joints (28% and 31% for right and left, respectively) because many horses in training develop inflammation and synovial effusion, along with varying degrees of lameness (Goodman and Baker, 1990).

The recognition that carpal effusion and incidence of fracture decreased as the carpal angle increased, as viewed from the front, is an important finding in the

Thoroughbred in light of the common desire of a buyer to have a straight leg and the common practice of surgically manipulating carpal valgus to achieve a straighter forelimb. Other significant findings were offset knees being associated with fetlock problems, long toe being associated with carpal problems, and longer scapula length decreasing the likelihood of forelimb fractures.

In the Quarter Horses, many of the odds ratios presented close to 1.0, indicating little importance. However, proximal first phalanx chip fractures, synovitis and capsulitis of the carpus and coffin joint, and carpal chip fractures were associated with conformation variables. It is expected that, with greater numbers, other conformation variables could become significant. The significance of offset knees was supported by the data with an increase in synovitis and capsulitis, as well as carpal chip fragmentation.

Information in this article is provided from "The Role of Conformation in Musculoskeletal Problems in the Racing Thoroughbred and Racing Quarter Horse," by C.W. McIlwraith, T.A. Anderson, P. Douay, N.L. Goodman, and L.R. Overly.

References

Beeman, G.M. 1973. Correlation of defects and conformation to pathology in the horse. In: Proc. Amer. Assoc. Equine Pract. 19:177-198.

Chaney, J.A., C.K. Shen, and J.D. Wheat. 1973. Relationship of racetrack surface to lameness in the Thoroughbred racehorse. Am. J. Vet. Res. 34:1285-1289.

Dolvik, N.I., and Q. Klemetsdale. 1996. The effect of arthritis in the carpal joint on performance in Norwegian cold-blooded trotters. Vet. Res. Comm. 20:505-512.

Goodman, N.L., and B.K. Baker. 1990. Lameness diagnosis and treatment in the Quarter Horse racehorse. In: Vet. Clinics North Am. Equine Pract. 6:85-107.

Green, B.K. 1969. Horse Conformation as to Soundness and Performance. Northland Press.

Hill T., D. Carmichael, Q. Maylin, and L. Krook. 1986. Track condition and racing injuries in Thoroughbred horses. Cornell Vet. 76:361-369.

Jeffcott, L.B., P.D. Rossdale, J. Freestone, C.J. Frank, and P.F. Towers-Clark. 1982. An assessment of wastage in Thoroughbred racing from conception to 4 years of age. Equine Vet. J. 14:185-198.

Johnson, B.J., S.M. Stover, B.M. Daft, H. Kinde, D.H. Read, B.C. Barr, M. Anderson, J. Moore, L. Woods, J. Stoltz, et al. 1994. Causes of death in racehorses over a 2-year period. Equine Vet. J. 26:327-330.

Kobluck, C.N., R.A. Robinson, B.J. Gordon, et al. 1990. The effect of conformation and shoeing: A cohort study of 95 Thoroughbred racehorses. In: Proc. Amer. Assoc. Equine Pract. 35:259-274.

Magnusson, L.E. 1985. Studies on the conformation and related traits of Standardbred trotters in Sweden. Skara, Swedish University of Agricultural Sciences 194.

McIlwraith, C.W. (Ed.) American Quarter Horse Association Developmental Orthopedic Disease Symposium. 1986.

Mohammed, H.O., T. Hill, and J. Lowe. 1991. Risk factors associated with injuries in Thoroughbred horses. Equine Vet. J.23:445-448.

Peloso, J.G., G.D. Mundy, and N.D. Cohen. 1994. Prevalence of, and factors associated with, musculoskeletal racing injuries of Thoroughbreds. J. Am. Vet. Med. Assoc. 204:620-626.

Rossdale, P.D., R. Hopes, N.J. Wingfield-Digby, and K. Offord. 1985. Epidemiological study of wastage among racehorses: 1982 and 1983. Vet. Rec. 116:66-69.

Stashak, T.S. (Ed.) 1985. Lameness in Horses (4th Ed.) Lea & Febriger.

Acknowledgements

With acknowledgements to the Wildenstein Family and Ecurie Wildenstein (Thoroughbred study) and American Quarter Horse Association (Quarter Horse study) for financial support. Disclosure: Dr. McIlwraith has a consultancy arrangement with the Wildenstein Stable.

THE PREVALENCE OF RADIOGRAPHIC CHANGES IN THOROUGHBRED YEARLINGS AND THE EFFECT OF THOSE CHANGES ON FUTURE RACING PERFORMANCE

C. WAYNE MCILWRAITH
Colorado State University, Fort Collins, Colorado, USA

Introduction

Radiographic examination of Thoroughbreds at the time of the yearling sales is common practice in the U.S. Although it is generally accepted that most yearlings have some radiographic changes (judged as normal variation or otherwise), there are few data to estimate the prevalence of these changes in Thoroughbred yearlings at the time of the sales. Howard et al. reported on the occurrence of radiographic abnormalities in 582 yearlings offered for sale during a six-year period (1992). They reported that fore and hind fetlocks were most commonly affected followed by the tarsi, stifles, feet, and carpi. McIntosh et al. followed the development of over 300 yearlings and documented the occurrence of femoropatellar osteochondrosis (1993). The occurrence of selected radiographic changes in clinically normal young horses of other breeds has been investigated in several studies (Sandgren, 1988; Hardy et al., 1991; Carlsten et al., 1993; Sandgren et al., 1993; Grondahl et al., 1994; Grondahl and Engeland, 1995; Jorgensen et al., 1997; Valentino et al., 1999). A better understanding of the prevalence of radiographic changes in Thoroughbred yearlings at the time of sales will help practitioners and researchers focus their work on the most commonly affected sites. These data will also help practitioners that may need further investigation for the complete evaluation of a sale yearling.

The objective of this portion of the Yearling Radiographic Study was to describe the distribution of radiographic changes in yearlings sold at Keeneland and Fasig-Tipton July and September sales from 1993-1996. Changes that tend to be bilateral or biaxial are noted.

Materials and Methods

Radiographs from 1162 pre- and post-sale purchase examinations conducted at the 1993-1996 Keeneland and Fasig-Tipton yearling sales were obtained from a private practice (Morehead) serving buyers and consignors at these sales. Joint examinations included fore fetlocks (DP, flexed LM, DLPMO, and DMPLO views), hind fetlocks (DP, LM, DLPMO, and DMPLO views), carpi (LM, DLPMO, and

333

DMPLO views), tarsi (DP, DLPMO, and DMPLO views), stifles (LM view), and forefeet (DP and LM views). Joint series with missing or non-diagnostic films for any view of a left and right pair were not included in the analysis.

All of the films were evaluated independently by two authors (Kane and Rantanen) and radiographic changes present were categorized by location and type of lesion (e.g., flattening, lucency, fragment, etc.). Discrepancies between these two interpretations were resolved using a third assessment (Park) and the consensus opinion to decide the final categorization of changes. Yearlings were then classified as having a radiographic change if they were present in either the left or right limb. If both limbs were affected, the higher (more severe) category was used to classify the horse.

Fore fetlocks and proximal sesamoid bones were analyzed separately from hind fetlocks and sesamoid bones. Linear defects in the proximal sesamoid bones, discussed here as vascular channels, were categorized as regular (≤ 2 mm in width with parallel sides) or irregular (> 2 mm in width or having nonparallel sides) based on their size and shape. Often a vascular channel ≤ 2 mm in width had parallel sides until it widened into a "V" shape 3-4 mm from the abaxial surface. These were categorized as irregular. Radiopaque "flakes" < 1 mm in size with no corresponding defect associated in a joint margin were not categorized as fragments in any joint. Articular fragments must have had a visible defect in the corresponding joint margin or joint surface. The diameter of subchondral cysts was recorded. Cysts were defined as any lucent areas that extended through the subchondral bone. Flat regions were recorded on several joint surfaces (e.g., condyles or sagittal ridge of the distal third metacarpus, lateral and medial trochlea of the talus, etc.). These areas had to have good radiographic alignment to be categorized as flat because obliquity often makes two partially superimposed curved surfaces seem flattened. Osteophytes in the carpus were measured; in other joints their presence was simply recorded as yes/no. Unless otherwise indicated, percentages reported here are the number of affected yearlings/number of yearlings examined.

Results

The 1162 yearlings included in the study represented 7% of all yearlings sold at the same sales during this time. Six hundred seventy-three (58%) were colts and 489 (42%) were fillies. Most (1074, 92%) of the yearlings were actually sold with only 80 (7%) not reaching their reserve price and eight (1%) being withdrawn prior to entering the sale ring. The typical price of yearlings included in this study (median \$40,000; mean \$70,474 ± 2584 SEM) was higher than for all other yearlings sold at the same sales but not included in the study (median \$20,000; mean \$45,596 ± 676).

There were 1127 fore fetlock, 1102 hind fetlock, 1130 carpal, 1101 tarsal, 660 stifle, and 300 forefeet series that were complete and included in the analyses.

FORE FETLOCKS AND PROXIMAL SESAMOID BONES

Proximal dorsal P1 fragments were present in 18 (1.6%) yearlings and were usually unilateral. Unilateral proximal palmar P1 fragments were found in five (0.5%) yearlings (1 articular, 4 non-articular). Distal third metacarpal or proximal P1 cysts were found in eight (0.7%) yearlings, one of which had bilateral cysts. Three of the cysts recorded were 5 mm in diameter; the others were 2, 6, 7, 10, and 11 mm in diameter. Changes were recorded in the distal dorsal region of the third metacarpus (includes proximal third of the dorsal sagittal ridge) in 380 (33.8%) yearlings. Most of these were a semicircular notch with a well-defined border at the proximal aspect of the dorsal sagittal ridge. Often bilateral, these are usually about 3 mm across (this is often regarded as a "normal" change). However, 22 yearlings (2.0%) had an irregularly shaped lucency (Type I lesion) in this location that was often bilateral (McIlwraith and Vorhees, 1991). Eight horses (0.7%) had fragments (Type II lesion) and one horse (0.1%) had a loose body (Type III lesion) in this location (McIlwraith and Vorhees, 1991). These lesions were all unilateral. Flattening of the distal sagittal ridge of the third metacarpus was noted in 110 (9.8%) yearlings and a lucency was recorded in this location on 196 (17.4%). The lucencies were visible on the DP and/or LM views and were most often bilateral. Flattening of the distal palmar third metacarpus condyles was present in 461 (40.9%) yearlings, but lucencies in this location (often referred to as palmar metacarpal disease or traumatic osteochondrosis) (Pool and Meagher, 1990) were only found in four horses (0.4%). Palmar supracondylar lysis (Pool and Meagher, 1990) of the third metacarpus was present in 54 (4.8%) yearlings with 30 (2.7%) classified as slight and 24 (2.1%) as moderate or extreme. These changes were also usually bilateral. All of the radiographic changes that tended to be unilateral in the fore fetlocks seemed equally distributed between left and right limbs.

Twenty-nine (2.6%) yearlings had elongated proximal sesamoid bones on the forelimbs. Elongation was defined as a greater than 2 mm difference in length between biaxial sesamoids in an attempt to account for the lateral sesamoid which tends to be slightly longer than the medial. Still, elongation of the lateral sesamoid was recorded slightly more frequently than elongation of the medial sesamoid. Independent of sesamoid length, abnormally shaped (proximal, distal, abaxial, or overall enlargement) fore sesamoids were recorded for 34 (3.0%) yearlings and were found almost twice as often on the medial sesamoid compared with the lateral. Forelimb sesamoid fractures (apical, abaxial, basal) were found in 11 (1.0%) yearlings. Only one fracture was of a lateral sesamoid, and two yearlings had bilateral medial sesamoid fractures. Osteophytes were not recorded on any fore sesamoids; however, enthesophytes at the attachments of the suspensory or distal sesamoidean ligaments to the proximal sesamoid bones were recorded on 14 (1.2%) yearlings. Circular lucencies in the sesamoids were found in 164 (14.6%)

yearlings. These were usually only found in one fore sesamoid per animal and were almost twice as common on the medial sesamoid compared with the lateral.

Less than half of all the fore proximal sesamoid bones examined had regular vascular channels and less than 10% had more than three. Regular vascular channels were evenly distributed between limbs and between biaxial pairs of sesamoids. More than half of the fore proximal sesamoid bones examined had irregular vascular channels. (Note that regular and irregular here refers to size and shape, not how frequently the changes occur.) Irregular vascular channels were more common in the medial sesamoid bone. Overall, 26 (2.3%) yearlings were categorized as not having vascular channels in a fore sesamoid, because most had at least one vascular channel in at least one sesamoid.

HIND FETLOCKS AND PROXIMAL SESAMOID BONES

Proximal dorsal P1 fragments were most common on the hind limbs compared with the forelimbs. Thirty-six (3.3%) yearlings had these fragments, and one yearling had bilateral fragments in this location. Proximal plantar fragments were also more common on the hind limbs. Sixty-five yearlings (5.9%) were affected; 20 (1.8%) had non-articular fragments and 45 (4.1%) had articular fragments. Four yearlings had bilateral proximal plantar P1 fragments (2 non-articular and 2 articular). Only two (0.2%) yearlings had distal third metatarsal or proximal P1 cysts in the hind fetlocks. Three hundred thirty-four (30%) yearlings had some changes in the distal dorsal region of the third metatarsus (includes proximal third of the dorsal sagittal ridge). A semicircular notch was noted in 299 (27.1%) yearlings and was often bilateral. Nineteen (1.7%) yearlings had an irregularly shaped lucency (Type I lesion) in this location which was bilateral in four individuals. Twelve (1.1%) yearlings had fragments (2 bilateral, Type II lesion) and four (0.4%) had a loose body (all unilateral, Type III lesion) in this location. In contrast to the third metacarpus, only 20 (1.8%) yearlings had changes in the sagittal ridge of the distal third metatarsus. Two (0.2%) had flattening and 18 (1.6%) had a lucency at this location. Most of these changes were unilateral. Flattening on the distal palmar third metatarsus was found on 71 (6.4%) yearlings examined and one had a lucency in this location. Palmar supracondylar lysis of the distal third metatarsus was not found in any of the yearlings examined.

Elongation of a hind proximal sesamoid was found in eight (0.7%) yearlings and abnormally shaped hind sesamoids were present in 23 yearlings (2.1%). Elongated sesamoids were evenly distributed between left/right and lateral/medial pairs, but medial sesamoids were abnormally shaped more often than lateral sesamoids. Thirty-two (2.9%) yearlings had hind proximal sesamoid fractures. There were 16 fractures of a lateral sesamoid (15 apical and 1 basal) and 24 fractures of a medial sesamoid. In the medial sesamoid 18 apical fractures were recorded with three basal, one abaxial, and two comminuted fractures also recorded. Osteophytes on a hind sesamoid were only found in three (0.3%) yearlings and usually affected more than one hind sesamoid. Enthesophytes were found at the attachments of the suspensory or distal sesamoidean ligaments in 14 (1.3%) yearlings. Circular lucencies in a hind sesamoid were found in 172 (15.6%) yearlings and were more common on the medial sesamoid. Most of those affected had one circular lucency (149, 13.5%) but 21 yearlings (1.9%) had two and two (0.2%) yearlings had three.

Seventy-seven (7.0%) yearlings were categorized as not having any vascular channels in a hind sesamoid. Most had at least one vascular channel in at least one sesamoid. Less than 30% of all hind proximal sesamoid bones examined had regular vascular channels and less than 1% had more than three. Regular vascular channels were evenly distributed between limbs and between biaxial pairs of sesamoids. Irregular vascular channels were found on more than half of the hind proximal sesamoid bones examined. Irregular vascular channels were slightly less common in the medial sesamoid bone.

CARPI

Dorsal medial intercarpal joint disease (characterized by rounded appearance to the radial carpal bone and/or thickened dorsal cortex, proliferative change, enthesophyte, or fragment involving the radial carpal or third carpal bones) was found in 30 (2.7%) of the yearlings examined. These changes were most often unilateral and affected left and right limbs equally. Palmar lucencies in the ulnar carpal bone were detected in 227 (20.1%) yearlings, were usually unilateral, and affected left and right limbs equally. Nine (0.8%) yearlings had carpal fragments that ranged in size from 2 to 10 mm. Nineteen (1.7%) had carpal osteophytes ranging in size from 1 to 4 mm, and three (0.3%) had subchondral cysts in a carpal bone ranging in size from 4 to 10 mm. Carpal fragments, osteophytes, and subchondral bone cysts tended to be evenly distributed between left and right limbs. Accessory carpal fractures affected four (0.4%) yearlings.

HOCKS

Five (0.5%) yearlings had articular lucent areas in the medial malleolus. Fragments or concavities of the distal intermediate ridge of the tibia were found in 48 (4.4%) yearlings and were evenly distributed between left and right limbs. Most of the intermediate ridge lesions were unilateral. One yearling had a flattened lateral trochlear ridge of the talus and 14 (1.3%) had lucencies and/or fragmentation in this location. Flattening of the medial trochlear ridge was more common (12 yearlings, 1.1%), but only seven (0.6%) yearlings had lucencies or fragments on the medial trochlear ridge. "Dewdrop lesions" on the distal medial trochlear ridge were found on 39 (3.5%) of the yearlings examined, and fragments at this location were found in eight (0.7%) yearlings. Osteophytes or enthesophytes at the distal intertarsal or tarsal metatarsal joint margins were found in 80 (7.3%) yearlings.

Wedging or collapse of a distal tarsal bone was present in 13 (1.2%) of the yearlings examined and was usually unilateral.

STIFLES

Thirty-eight (5.8%) yearlings had changes on the lateral trochlear ridge of the femur. Flattening was present in four (0.6%) yearlings and lucencies and/or fragmentation were detected in 34 yearlings (5.1%). Two (0.3%) yearlings had a lucent area with or without a fragment on the medial trochlear ridge. These femoral trochlear ridge lesions tended to be unilateral but also occurred bilaterally. One (0.2%) yearling had a lucent area in the trochlear groove of the femoropatellar joint, two (0.3%) had lucencies in the patella, and one (0.2%) had fragmentation of the distal patella. The medial femoral condyle and proximal tibia could only be visualized in 170 yearlings. No subchondral cysts were detected in these animals.

FOREFEET

Signs of pedal osteitis (proliferation on the dorsal surface of P3, remodeling of the tip of P3) were detected in 33 (11%) of the yearlings with radiographs of the forefeet. Other changes in the forefeet were found in 45 (15%) yearlings. These included 18 (6%) animals with prominent synovial fossae in the navicular bone, 15 (5%) with palmar process fragments, two (0.6%) with spurs on the extensor process of P3, and one (0.3%) with an extensor process fragment.

Discussion

Most yearlings examined in this study had some radiographic changes noted in the fetlocks, proximal sesamoid bones, carpi, tarsi, stifles, or forefeet. Some of the changes recorded are commonly thought to be incidental findings. They were included in this survey for a complete and unbiased assessment of what a practitioner can expect to find when reviewing sale radiographs.

Comparison of the prevalence of changes found in this study with other published work is difficult. Most studies have grouped many specific changes under one broad diagnosis (e.g., OCD of the fetlock). In this study we have kept as much detail as possible in the classification system used to categorize each horse. Another survey of Thoroughbred yearlings in central Kentucky by Howard et al. (1992) used the number of joints examined as a denominator without accounting for the number of horses (e.g., number of fetlocks diagnosed with OCD/number of fore fetlocks examined). Because of this and the rarity of most specific changes, comparison between these studies should be interpreted with caution. Apical fractures of the fore proximal sesamoid (2/2254 joints examined in this study vs.

5/1018 in Howard et al.) seem less common in this study. Proximal dorsal P1 fractures in the hind fetlocks (37/2204 joints examined in this study vs. 24/700 in Howard et al.), and medial malleolus lesions in the tarsi (5/2202 joints examined in this study vs. 5/710 in Howard et al.) all seem to be less common in this study. On the other hand, osteophytes at the joint margins of the distal intertarsal and tarsometatarsal joints (263/2202 joints examined in this study vs. 16/710 in Howard et al.) seem more common in this study. It is unlikely that the differences noted above would be statistically significant if appropriate variance estimates could be included.

Most of the specific radiographic changes observed in this study are rare. This presents unique challenges to clinicians and researchers trying to identify changes that are clinically significant. With thousands of Thoroughbred yearlings sold at auction every year in this country alone, however, even rare changes can present a problem for the sale veterinarian. This study provides data that can be used by researchers and clinicians to help focus their efforts on the most common problem areas and identify yearlings with unusual radiographic changes that may need further investigation.

The Effect of Radiographic Changes in Thoroughbred Yearlings on Future Racing Performance

Radiographic changes found at the time of Thoroughbred yearling sales have a substantial impact on the sale process but can be difficult to interpret. Consignors want to sell their yearlings at a fair market price, and buyers want to identify yearlings with orthopedic problems that are likely to influence future racing performance so new purchases have every chance of reaching their full potential. The sale veterinarian is often asked to identify radiographic changes that could be a future problem without unjustifiably declaring a horse unsuitable for purchase.

There are several reports describing the influence of radiographic changes on future racing performance in Standardbreds. However, comparable information is limited in Thoroughbreds. Spike et al. reported significantly fewer starts and lower total earnings for horses with more than two abnormally shaped linear defects in a proximal sesamoid bone. Most of the interpretation of yearling sale films is still based on clinical experience of the practitioner with horses that have shown clinical signs or required surgery when in race training.

The objectives of this historical cohort study were to identify radiographic changes in the fetlocks, proximal sesamoid bones, carpi, stifles, tarsi, or forefeet of Thoroughbred sales yearlings that are associated with future racing performance; the occurrence of orthopedic problems; and the need for surgery. This abstract is focused on identifying the radiographic changes in Thoroughbred yearlings that are associated with the likelihood of starting at least one race during the two- or three-year-old years.

Materials and Methods

Radiographs from 1162 pre- and post-sale purchase examinations conducted at the 1993-1996 Keeneland and Fasig-Tipton yearling sales were obtained from a private practice (Morehead) serving buyers and consignors at these sales. Joint examinations included fore fetlocks (DP, flexed LM, DLPMO, and DMPLO views), hind fetlocks (DP, LM, DLPMO, and DMPLO views), carpi (LM, DLPMO, and DMPLO views), tarsi (DP, DLPMO, and DMPLO views), stifles (LM view), and forefeet (DP and LM views). Joint series with missing or non-diagnostic films for any view of a left and right pair were not included in the analysis.

All of the films were evaluated independently by two authors (Kane and Rantanen) in a blinded manner and radiographic changes present were categorized by location and type of lesion (e.g., flattening, lucency, fragment, etc.). Discrepancies between these two interpretations were resolved using a third assessment (Park) and the consensus opinion to decide the final categorization of changes. Yearlings were then classified as having a radiographic change if they were present in either the left or right limb. If both limbs were affected, the higher (more severe) category was used to classify the horse. For variables related to vascular channels in the proximal sesamoid bones, the sesamoid with the highest total number of vascular channels (the "worst" sesamoid) was used to classify the yearling. Fore fetlocks and proximal sesamoid bones were analyzed separately from the hind fetlocks and sesamoid bones.

Racing performance data for the two- and three-year old years were obtained from The Jockey Club Information Systems for each horse included in the study. Horses without an official race record were assigned a value of zero starts. The number of race starts during the two- and three-year-old years combined was categorized as YES, the horse started at least one race, or NO, the horse did not start a race during its two- or three-year-old years. Sale price was obtained from Keeneland and Fasig-Tipton sale companies. For yearlings that did not meet their reserve price, the amount of the final bid was used. Yearlings withdrawn from the sale prior to the bidding were assigned a sale price of zero dollars.

Contingency tables were used to crosstabulate horses by radiographic variables and whether the horses started a race during the two- or three-year-old years. Values reported here are the percent of horses that started at least one race and the number of horses that started (starters) divided by the total number of horses with the same radiographic classification. Separate logistic regression models for each variable were used to obtain likelihood ratio chi-square p-values adjusted for sale price to test for an association between the presence or grade of a radiographic change and starting a race while simultaneously controlling for the potential confounding effect of sale price.

Results

The 1162 yearlings included in the study represent 7% of all yearlings sold at the same sales during this time. Six hundred seventy-three (58%) were colts and 489 (42%) were fillies. Most (1074, 92%) of the yearlings were actually sold with only 80 (7%) not reaching their reserve price and eight (1%) being withdrawn prior to entering the sale ring. The typical price of yearlings included in this study (median $40,000; mean $70,474 ± 2584 SEM) was higher than for all other yearlings sold at the same sales but not included in the study (median $20,000; mean $45,596 ± 676).

There were 1127 fore fetlock, 1102 hind fetlock, 1130 carpal, 1101 tarsal, 660 stifle, and 300 forefeet series that were complete and included in the analyses. Overall, approximately 82% of horses without radiographic changes started at least one race during their two- and three-year-old years. (This number provides a convenient reference for comparison with most of the percentages of starters among those yearlings with radiographic changes.)

FORE FETLOCKS AND PROXIMAL SESAMOID BONES

Among radiographic changes observed in the fore fetlock joints, only moderate or extreme palmar supracondylar lysis of the distal palmar third metacarpal had a significant (p = 0.02) effect on the likelihood of starting a race. While 878/1073 (82%) yearlings with no supracondylar lysis and 26/30 (87%) yearlings with slight supracondylar lysis started, only 14/24 (58%) with moderate or severe lesions started a race. Fourteen of 18 (78%) yearlings with proximal dorsal P1 fragments started, and all of the five yearlings with proximal palmar P1 fragments started. More than half of the yearlings with subchondral cysts (5/8, 62%) in the distal third metacarpus or proximal first phalanx started, but with this few cases this was not significantly (p = 0.13) different from the 913/1119 (82%) that started without cysts in this location. Size of the cysts did not appear to affect the likelihood of starting as three of the five cysts in starters were greater than 5 mm in diameter. Radiographic changes of the distal dorsal third metacarpus (includes proximal ridge of the dorsal sagittal ridge) did not have a significant effect on starting (p = 0.28). Compared to the percent (606/749, 81%) of yearlings with no changes at this location that started, 209/347 (84%) yearlings with a "normal" semicircular notch at the most proximal aspect of the dorsal sagittal ridge started, 15/22 (68%) of those with a lucency (Type I lesion) started, and 7/9 (78%) of those with a defect and a fragment or loose body (Type II or III lesion) started (McIlwraith and Vorhees, 1991). Changes recorded on the distal two-thirds of the dorsal sagittal ridge or metacarpal condyles or on the distal palmar sagittal ridge or condyles had little effect on the likelihood of starting a race.

Enthesophytes at the attachments of the suspensory or distal sesamoidean ligaments to the proximal sesamoid bones had a significant (p = 0.04) effect on the likelihood of starting a race. Only 8/14 (57%) yearlings with enthesophytes on the proximal sesamoid bones started compared with 910/1113 (82%) that started without this change. One of two yearlings (50%) with an apical fracture of a proximal sesamoid bone started while 2/3 (67%) with abaxial fractures and 5/6 (83%) with basal fractures started; however, these percentages were not significantly (p = 0.73) different from the percentage of starters among those without sesamoid fractures. There was no significant difference (p > 0.4) in the percentage of yearlings that started with elongated or abnormally shaped proximal sesamoid bones or circular lucencies in the proximal sesamoids compared with yearlings without these changes. Most yearlings in this study had two or three vascular channels (range 0-9) in the "worst" proximal sesamoid bone. No significant (p > 0.40) association was detected between the number of regular (≤ 2 mm and parallel sides) or irregular (> 2 mm or nonparallel sides) vascular channels or the total number of vascular channels and the likelihood of starting a race.

HIND FETLOCKS AND PROXIMAL SESAMOID BONES

Only 25/36 (69%) yearlings with proximal P1 fragments in a hind fetlock started at least one race compared with 874/1066 (82%) that started without these fragments (p = 0.08). Proximal plantar P1 fragments did not appear to have a significant association with starting (p = 0.37), with 18/20 (90%) yearlings with non-articular fragments and 34/45 (76%) yearlings with articular fragments starting. Only two horses had subchondral cysts in the distal third metatarsus or proximal first phalanx, and both started. Similar to the forelimbs, changes of the distal dorsal third metatarsus (includes proximal third of the dorsal sagittal ridge) did not have a significant (p = 0.24) association with starting. Compared to the 619/768 (81%) yearlings with no changes at this location that started, 254/300 (85%) of the yearlings with a "normal" semicircular notch at the most proximal aspect of the dorsal sagittal ridge started, 15/18 (83%) of those with a lucency (Type I lesion) started, and only 11/16 (69%) of those with a defect and a fragment or loose body (Type II or III lesion) started. Both of the horses with a flattened distal sagittal ridge of the third metatarsus and 13/18 (72%) horses with lucency at this location started. Changes found on the distal plantar aspect of the third metatarsus were not associated with starting. Unlike the forelimbs, supracondylar lysis of the plantar distal metatarsus was not observed on the hind limbs.

Similar to the results from the fore proximal sesamoids, a smaller percentage (9/14, 64%) of yearlings with enthesophytes on the hind sesamoid bones started compared with yearlings without this change (890/1088, 82%); however, this difference was not significant (p = 0.13). Yearlings with elongated or abnormally shaped hind proximal sesamoid bones as well as those with osteophytes or circular lucencies in these bones were just as likely (p > 0.47) to start as those without these changes. Fracture of the hind proximal sesamoid bones did not appear to affect the likelihood of starting. Twenty-two of 26 (85%) with apical fractures started and three of four (75%) of those with basal fractures started. Abaxial and comminuted fractures were found in two horses (1 each) and both started. The number of regular and irregular vascular channels as well as the total number of vascular channels in the "worst" hind proximal sesamoid bone were not significantly (p > 0.50) associated with starting. In fact, 87/102 (85%) yearlings with more than four irregular vascular channels in the "worst" sesamoid started.

CARPI

Yearlings with dorsal medial intercarpal joint changes were less likely to start (19/30, 63% started, p = 0.20) compared with those without these changes. A smaller percentage (13/19, 68%) of yearlings with osteophytosis in the carpal joints started compared with the percentage of starters for yearlings without this change (909/1111, 82%); however, this effect was not significant (p = 0.17). The percentage (183/227, 81%) of yearlings starting with circular lucencies in the palmar ulnar carpal bone was nearly identical to that for horses without these lucencies (739/903, 82%, p = 0.68). Seven of nine (78%) of the horses with carpal fragments started; this is similar to the percent (915/1121, 82%) of starters among those without fragments. Two horses with subchondral cysts ≥ 9 mm in diameter in a carpal bone started, and one horse with a 4-mm cyst did not start. Accessory carpal bone fractures were detected in four horses, all of which started at least one race.

TARSI

Yearlings with osteophyte or enthesophyte formation at the distal intertarsal or tarsometatarsal joint margins were significantly (p = 0.03) less likely to start a race (147/193, 76%) compared with those without this lesion (753/908, 83%). Similarly, 61/80 (76%) yearlings with subchondral lucency in these joints started compared with 839/1021 (82%) that started without this change. The effect of subchondral lucency, however, was not significant (p = 0.19). Only 9/13 (69%) yearlings with wedging of the distal tarsal bones started compared with 891/1088 (82%) that started without this lesion (p = 0.25). Most of the tarsal wedging or collapse that was seen in these sales yearlings was slight. There were no significant (p > 0.26) differences in the percentage of starters for yearlings with changes of the medial malleolus, intermediate ridge of the distal tibia, or lateral or medial trochlear ridges of the talus.

STIFLES

All four yearlings with flattening of the lateral trochlear ridge of the distal femur started. However, only 24/34 (71%) with lucency, subchondral defects, and/or fragments at this location started compared with 330/387 (85%) that started without any changes in this location (p = 0.10). Two horses with lucency, subchondral defects, and/or fragments on the medial trochlear ridge started. One of two horses with lucency of the patella and one horse with fragmentation of the distal patella started. Subchondral cysts on the medial femoral condyle or proximal tibia were not found among the 178 yearlings where these locations could be visualized clearly on the LM view.

FOREFEET

There was no significant (p = 0.41) association detected between radiographic changes in the feet and the likelihood of starting a race.

Discussion

This study identified several radiographic changes in the joints of Thoroughbred yearlings that are associated with the probability of starting at least one race during the two- or three-year-old years. It should not be surprising that supracondylar lysis of the distal palmar third metacarpus was associated with decreased probability of starting a race. This lesion is recognized as a sign of chronic inflammation of the fetlock joint (Pool and Meagher, 1990) and has been associated with decreased likelihood of returning to function among a group of older horses examined at a veterinary referral center (Haynes et al., 1983). Enthesophytes are also recognized as an early manifestation of osteoarthritis (Pool, 1996). This is consistent with the results reported here, that yearlings with this lesion are less likely to start a race during their two- and three-year-old years. It is surprising that the number of vascular channels (regular, irregular, or both combined) was not associated with failure to start. A lower average number of starts has been reported for yearlings with more than two abnormal linear defects in a proximal sesamoid bone (Spike et al., 1997). There were, however, only 10 yearlings (2%) in that study that had more than two abnormally shaped linear defects compared with 366/1127 (32%) yearlings in this study. This indicates a substantial difference between the studies in how these criteria were applied. Many of the vascular channels classified as irregular in this study were 2 mm wide with parallel sides for most of their length but widened into a "V" shape 3-4 mm from the abaxial border.

A large effect on the probability of starting a race was seen with dorsal medial intercarpal joint disease (only 63% started with this lesion). These changes were characterized by a rounded appearance to the radial carpal bone and/or a thickened dorsal cortex, proliferative change, enthesophyte or fragment involving the radial carpal or third carpal bones. All of these changes are characteristic of early osteoarthritis, so it should not be surprising that they affect the probability of starting a race. It is somewhat alarming that a radiographic change as common as osteophytosis/enthesopathy of the distal intertarsal and tarsometatarsal joint margins (affected 193/1101 [18%] yearlings overall) was significantly associated with failure to start. The magnitude of the difference in the percent of starters between those with lesions (76%) and without lesions (83%), however, was small.

A significant effect on the ability to start a race was not detected for many radiographic changes that one might expect to influence the future potential of a yearling (e.g., fore fetlock fragments and cysts, sesamoid fractures, OCD lesions of the tarsi or stifles). The reader should recognize, however, that many of these lesions are rare and affected only a few horses in the study. As a result, the ability to detect a significant effect if one truly exists (power of the study) is likely to be low for many of these comparisons.

Results of this study should be used in parallel with a clinical impression based on one's personal experience to best evaluate yearling films. As future studies confirm or refute areas of concern brought to light with this study, a greater foundation of hard evidence on which to base purchase decisions will be built. Further analysis of these and additional data on the development of orthopedic problems and the need for surgery is planned, and a clearer picture of lesions that can be considered significant in the Thoroughbred yearling will develop.

The Yearling Radiographic Study was supported by the American Association of Equine Practitioners (AAEP) with funds provided by the Keeneland Association, the Fasig-Tipton Sales Company, the Ocala Breeders Sales Company, the AAEP Foundation, Barretts Equine Limited, Blood Horse Publications, and The Jockey Club. The authors thank Fred Arnold, Gary Lavin, Jim Becht, Noah Cohen, the AAEP Research Committee, Gary Carpenter, Clay Murray, Mark Adkinson, Bruce Irwin, Donald Butte, Mike King, and the staff of Equine Medical Associates for guidance and technical support.

This paper was first published as Kane, A.J., C.W. McIlwraith, R.D. Park, N.W. Rantanen, J.P. Morehead, and L.R. Bramlage. 2000. The prevalence of radiographic changes in Thoroughbred yearlings. In: Proc. Amer. Assoc. Equine Practnr. 46:365-369, and Kane, A.J., C.W. McIlwraith, R.D. Park, N.W. Rantanen, J.P. Morehead, and L.R. Bramlage. 2000. The effect of radiographic changes in Thoroughbred yearlings on future racing performance. In: Proc. Amer. Assoc. Equine Practnr. 46:370-374.

References

Bramlage, L.R. 1993. Osteochondrosis and the sale horse. In. Proc. Amer. Assoc. Equine Practnr. 39:87-89.
Carlsten, J., B. Sandgren, and G. Dalin. 1993. Development of osteochondrosis in the tarsocrural joint and osteochondral fragments in the fetlock joints of

Standardbred trotters. I. Radiological survey. Equine Vet. J. Suppl. 16:42-47.

Grondahl, A.M., and A. Engeland. 1995. Influence of radiographically detectable orthopedic changes on racing performance in Standardbred trotters. J. Amer. Vet. Med. Assoc. 206:1013-1017.

Grondahl, A.M., G. Gaustad, and A. Engeland. 1994. Progression and association with lameness and racing performance of radiographic changes in the proximal sesamoid bones of young Standardbred trotters. Equine Vet. J. 26:152-155.

Hardy, J., M. Marcoux, and L. Breton. 1991. Clinical relevance of radiographic findings in proximal sesamoid bones of two-year-old Standardbreds in their first year of race training. J. Amer. Vet. Med. Assoc. 198:2089-2094.

Haynes, P.F., C.R. Root, D.L. Clabough, et al. 1983. Palmar supracondylar lysis of the third metacarpal bone. In: Proc. Amer. Assoc. Equine Practnr. 27:185-193.

Howard, B.A., R. Embertson, N.W. Rantanen, et al. 1992. Survey of radiographic findings in Thoroughbred sales yearlings. In: Proc. Amer. Assoc. Equine Practnr. 38:397-402.

Jorgensen, H.S., H. Proschowsky, R.J. Flak, et al. 1997. The significance of routine radiographic findings with respect to subsequent racing performance and longevity in Standardbred trotters. Equine Vet. J. 29:55-59.

Kane, A.J., C.W. McIlwraith, and R.D. Park. 2000. The prevalence of radiographic changes in Thoroughbred yearlings. In. Proc. Amer. Assoc. Equine Practnr. 46:365-369.

McIlwraith, C.W., and M. Vorhees. 1991. Management of osteochondritis dissecans of the dorsal aspect of the distal metacarpus and metatarsus. In: Proc. Amer. Assoc. Equine Practnr. 36:547-550.

McIntosh, S.C., and C.W. McIlwraith. 1993. Natural history of femoropatellar osteochondrosis in three crops of Thoroughbreds. Equine Vet. J. Suppl. 16:54-61.

Pool, R.R. 1996. Pathological manifestations of joint disease in the athletic horse. In: McIlwraith, C.W., and G.W. Trotter (Eds.) Joint Disease in the Horse. p. 87-104. W.B. Saunders, Philadelphia, PA.

Pool, R.R., and D.M. Meagher. 1990. Pathologic findings and pathogenesis of racetrack injuries. Vet. Clinics N. Amer. 6:1-30.

Sandgren, B. 1988. Bony fragments in the tarsocrural and metacarpo- or metatarsophalangeal joints in the Standardbred horse: A radiographic survey. Equine Vet. J. Suppl. 6:66-70.

Sandgren, B., G. Dalin, and J. Carlsten. 1993. Osteochondrosis in the tarsocrural joint and osteochondral fragments in the fetlock joints in Standardbred trotters. I. Epidemiology. Equine Vet. J. Suppl. 16:31-37.

Spike, D.L., L.R. Bramlage, B.A. Howard, et al. 1997. Radiographic proximal sesamoiditis in Thoroughbred sales yearlings. In: Proc. Amer. Assoc. Equine Practnr. 43:132-133.

Valentino, L.W., J.D. Lilich, E.M. Gaughan, et al. 1999. Radiographic prevalence of osteochondrosis in yearling feral horses. Vet. Comp. Orthop. Traumatol. 12:151-155.

INCIDENCE OF RADIOGRAPHIC CHANGES IN THOROUGHBRED YEARLINGS. 755 CASES

N.J. SCOTT, S. HANCE, P. TODHUNTER, P. ADAMS, A.R. ADKINS
Scone Veterinary Hospital, 106 Liverpool Street, Scone, NSW 2337

Introduction

The objective of this retrospective study was to record the incidence of radiographic changes in a proportion of Thoroughbred yearlings being presented for sale in 2003.

Methods and Materials

Reports were gathered from 755 yearling presale radiographic examinations. These reports were composed by A.R. Adkins, S. Hance, P. Todhunter and P. Adams, using similar criteria to that in the Kane et al study of 1162 yearlings. For uniformity, all sets of radiographs were assessed by at least two of the aforementioned veterinarians. Each radiographic examination included a complete set of the 34 views required for the Australian Repository System. For this study each joint was examined separately and as a pair.

Results

See table overleaf.

* Bracketed numbers indicate number of horses affected.

Relevance to Clinical Practice

The results of this study provide a database for ongoing assessment of the significance of particular lesions, evident as radiographic change, in relation to future performance. These results also provide insight into the level of occurrence of certain lesions and hence may be useful in radiographic assessment on an everyday clinical level. Individual breeders may use this information to compare the incidence of lesions occurring on their studs. The presale radiography of yearlings is a relatively new procedure in the Australian Thoroughbred industry and these results in combination with future results may enhance the selection information available to prospective buyers.

FRONT FETLOCKS	% horses affected *	**HIND FETLOCKS**	% horses affected*
SAGITTAL RIDGE OCD		SAGITTAL RIDGE OCD	
- Lysis/Flattening	28.3% (214)	- Lysis/Flattening	5.2% (39)
- Type II (fragmentation)	0.7% (5)	- Type II (fragmentation)	2% (15)
OSTEOCHONDRAL FRACTURES		OSTEOCHONDRAL FRACTURES	
- Dorsal Fetlock Joint	1.7% (13)	- Dorsal Fetlock Joint	3.3% (25)
- Palmar Fetlock Joint	0.5% (4)	- Plantar Fetlock Joint	6.2% (47)
- Sesamoid		- Sesamoid	
• Non-healed	0.5% (4)	• Non-healed	3% (23)
• Healed	0.9% (7)	• Healed	0.6% (5)
DISTAL MCIII CYSTS	2.9% (22)	DISTAL MTIII CYSTS	0.8% (6)
P1/P2 CHANGES		P1/P2 CHANGES	
- Cysts	0.7% (5)	- Cysts	0.4% (3)
- Osteochondral Fractures	0.1% (1)	- Osteochondral Fractures	0.5% (4)
- Osteoarthritis	0.3% (2)	- Osteoarthritis	0.1% (1)
SUPRACONDYLAR LYSIS	1.5% (11)	SUPRACONDYLAR LYSIS	0.1% (1)

CARPI		**TARSI**	
OSTEOCHONDRAL FRACTURE	2.2% (17)	HOCK OCD	
- Radiocarpal Joint	(2)	- Distal Intermediate Ridge	5% (38)
- Dorsal Midcarpal Joint	(8)	- Lateral Trochlear Ridge	2.6% (20)
- Palmar Carpal Joint	(4)	- Medial Trochlear Ridge	0.9% (7)
- Accessory Carpal Bone	(3)	- Medial Malleolus	1.8% (14)
OSTEOPHYTES	2.6% (20)	DISTAL TARSAL JOINT	
CYSTS	0.2% (2)	- Osteophytes	26.5% (200)
		- Collapse	0.6% (5)

STIFLES		**FRONT FEET**	
FEMOROPATELLAR OCD		Dorsal P3 Changes	4.4% (33)
- Lateral Trochlear Ridge	3.8% (29)		
• <2 cm	1.7% (13)	Extensor Process Fractures	0.8% (6)
• 2-4 cm	2% (15)		
• >4 cm	0.1% (1)	Club Feet	0.8% (6)
- Medial Trochlear Ridge	0.8% (6)		
DISTAL PATELLA LYSIS	0.7% (5)	Palmar Process Fractures	0.1% (1)
STIFLE CYSTS			
- Medial Femoral Condyle 5 – 4 mm to 15 – 22 mm	3.4% (26)	Solar Margin Fractures	0.1% (1)
- Lateral Femoral Condyle	0.1% (1)		
FLATTENING			
- Medial Femoral Condyle	7.4% (56)		

THE EFFECT OF GROWTH PROMOTANTS IN YOUNG GROWING HORSES

ANDREW DART
University Veterinary Centre, University of Sydney, Camden, NSW, Australia

Anabolic steroids are compounds that, when administered under certain circumstances, induce an increase in tissue protein from a given amount of digested protein (Vanderwal, 1976). Anabolic steroids have been used successfully as growth promotants in production animals and as therapeutic agents to treat debilitated animals including horses (O'Connor et al., 1973; Snow et al., 1982a). In the belief that certain types of athletic ability are related to muscle development, these anabolic steroids have been used to improve performance in humans and in horses (Ryan, 1976; Dawson and Gersten, 1978) Both steroidal and nonsteroidal compounds are suggested to be capable of producing such an effect. For several years testosterone and its derivatives have been extensively used in many countries in healthy racing animals or foals of all ages in the belief that athletic performance and muscle development are related in some equestrian disciplines (Snow et al., 1982b). However, there is generally a lack of scientific data to support this assumption (Snow et al., 1982a).

Early studies suggesting beneficial effects have not been supported by recent data. Stihl (1968) administered an anabolic steroid to a large group of horses in training. He found an improved appetite, increased body weight, and improved performance in geldings judged to have a weakness in performance. In the same study no beneficial effect could be found in stallions. Relying on an analysis of race results, a study by Dawson and Gersten (1978) claimed improved performance in Thoroughbreds of both sexes after treatment with boldenone undecyclenate.

In contrast Dietz et al. (1974) reported equivocal results in mature Standardbreds of both sexes and immature two-year-old Thoroughbreds treated with anabolic steroids. In a series of studies on healthy sedentary, mature, mixed breed geldings and a group of Thoroughbred geldings undergoing training, the investigators treated horses with weekly injections of nandrolene phenylproprionate. There was no effect of treatment on body weight, body measurements, hematological or serum biochemical variables, skeletal muscle composition, or metabolism that could be associated with improved racing performance (Snow et al., 1982a,b; Nimmo et al., 1982). However, of interest was that nitrogen excretion in treated animals was lower than in control animals during the first training period. There was no difference in the second training period. Weight loss occurred with training in both groups. These results suggest that under some circumstances, nandrolene phenylproprionate may have a protective effect on muscle breakdown, albeit mild.

Results of studies to date would suggest that there is a lack of scientific data indicating that anabolic steroids have any beneficial effects on otherwise normal, healthy horses. It might be construed from the information available that the steroidal anabolics may have a beneficial effect in debilitated animals or animals under stress, particularly associated with transition from stable to paddock or paddock to stable.

In the past 30 years there has been substantial interest in growth hormone (GH) or somatotropin (ST). Reviewing the literature there are over 42,000 references on this hormone between 1966 and 2000. There has been an exponential increase in literature from the mid 1980s when the synthetically produced hormone became available in humans. The commercial availability of recombinant equine somatotropin (eST) has only occurred in the past several years (registered in Australia in May 1998) and created considerable interest in the horse industry for its potential use in performance horses and foals. There is particular interest in treating dysmature foals or foals with early illness and adults with musculoskeletal injuries, wounds, and other performance-limiting diseases. However, it would be naive to ignore the significant interest in treating normal foals to enhance mature height, weight, and muscle bulk and to improve the ergogenic performance of young adult racing animals.

Growth hormone is a small protein produced by the anterior pituitary gland that is responsible for the growth of most body tissues. GH regulates growth through hypertrophy, hyperplasia, or both as a result of tissue differentiation, cell proliferation, and protein synthesis. It also has many specific metabolic effects including increasing the rate of protein synthesis, plasma insulin and glucose concentrations, fatty acid mobilization from adipose tissues, and the use of fatty acids as an energy source. It also decreases the rate of glucose utilization and influences fluid and electrolyte balance. GH is secreted in a pulsatile manner throughout life, declining with age. Stallions have greater frequency and amplitude of secretion, and concentrations are increased during acute exercise. The effects of GH can be mediated either directly through receptors in target tissues or indirectly through the production of somatomedins. The most widely studied somatomedin is somatomedin C or IGF-1 (Smith et al., 1999; Strobil and Thomas, 1996). IGF-1 is primarily produced in the liver but can be produced by a variety of tissues throughout the body. Administration of eST has been shown to increase the serum concentrations of IGF-1 in horses (Smith et al., 1999; Dart et al., 2003).

There has been considerable debate on the cross biological activity of different species forms of eST; it may be best referred to as species limited rather than species specific. Amino acid composition between eST, bovine ST (89.5%), and porcine ST (98.4%) shows considerable homology. Hence, there is some biological activity across these species. In contrast, homology between human ST and eST or bST is less than 67%, and neither bST nor eST is biologically active in humans.

Furthermore, the potential for antibody production against analogous forms of ST used across species is high and potentially dangerous (Gerard, 2001).

eST comes as a sterile white powder, is made into a liquid by diluent, and is administered intramuscularly (EquigenTM, CSL Australia). The manufacturer's recommended dose regimen of eST is 10 μg/kg for 7 days followed by 20 μg/kg for 5 weeks. For the most part studies into the effects of eST have followed this or similar regimens.

The effects of eST administered at 20 μg/kg daily to four-month-old foals for a period of 12 months were evaluated (Capshaw et al., 2001; Kulinski et al., 2002). Treated foals were found to consume similar amounts of feed to controls, and there was no difference in body weight between the groups at any point in time. No difference in body measurements including height at withers, length, width of chest or rump, heart-girth circumference, length of head, or development of the limbs was detected between control and treated foals.

In these studies most organ weights were increased compared to controls, although in notable organs such as the heart these differences were not significant and all measurements were in the reference range for normal organ weights for horses. There were no gross pathological differences between the two groups, and of the tissues evaluated histologically, there were mild inflammatory changes observed in only a few tissues. The loin eye area at the tenth rib was significantly larger in treated animals, which is consistent with findings in pigs treated with pST (Evock et al., 1988). There were no significant hematological or serum biochemical differences between treated and control horses. However, treated horses did have an increased circulating glucose concentration and a tendency towards an increased serum insulin concentration. Increase in glucose and insulin concentrations had been documented in previous reports (Smith et al., 1999; Buonomo et al., 1996).

A biological effect of the injected eST in treated foals was confirmed by the persistent elevation in circulating IGF-1 concentrations compared to untreated foals. The greater response of control foals to challenge by the ST secretagogue compared to treated foals supported the activity. Despite this biological effect, daily treatment of eST at the recommended dose rate of 20 μg/kg failed to have an apparent effect on the growth and development of these foals.

The lack of an effect is somewhat surprising given the results in other species. Long-term treatment in short stature children with human ST increases height, albeit over several years (Sas et al., 1999; Radetti et al., 2000). Shorter term treatment in growing pigs with pST increases carcass length and bone mass (Evock-Clover et al., 1992; Klindt et al., 1992), while in beef cattle bST improves average daily gain, feed efficiency, and lean percentage of carcass, and reduces fat percentage by increasing plasma IGF-1 and enhancing protein synthesis (Schwarz, 1993). It is interesting to note, however, that treatment with pST in newborn pigs until weaning had no effect on plasma IGF-1 concentrations or growth performance (Dunshea et al., 1999).

It is possible that an effect of eST on body characteristics would have been seen if the horses were GH deficient. Treatment of GH-deficient individuals with hST increased lean body mass, decreased body fat, and increased muscle mass (Bengtsson et al., 1993; Nelson, 1995). Alternatively, the dose of eST used in the present experiment may not have been sufficient to stimulate growth in these foals because many of the responses in growing pigs are dose responsive but not necessarily in a parallel fashion (Etherton and Bauman, 1998; Klindt et al., 1992). However, the IGF-1 concentrations in these foals almost doubled suggesting the dose was sufficient to elicit a response. In other studies in horses receiving similar doses, investigators noted elevated circulating leucocytes and subjective analysis of muscle definition but not ultrasound thickness of various muscle groups in aged mares (Malinowski et al., 1997), elevated IFG-1 concentrations in aged geldings and two-year-olds in race training (Smith et al., 1999; Julen Day et al., 1998), and enhanced follicular activity in anovulatory mares (Cochran et al., 1999a,b).

A group of researchers at Sydney University examined the effects of eST on yearling Standardbreds in training (Gerard, 2001; Lambeth, 2001). For 6 weeks Standardbreds received 10 µg/kg daily for 7 days and then 20 µg/kg daily for another 5 weeks while undergoing a 12-week treadmill-training program. The studies found there were small but statistically significant increases in average daily gain and body weight in treated horses compared to controls. The full weight of the gastrointestinal tract (GIT) expressed as a percentage of total body weight was greater in treated horses and probably reflected a greater dry matter intake in treated horses during the last 2 weeks of training. There were no effects on body height at the withers, organ weights, or digestibility of feed. The significant effects were small and considered to be of no consequence in terms of performance of young growing horses in training (Gerard, 2001). These findings were consistent with the previous studies in foals (Capshaw et al., 2001; Kulinski et al., 2002) and with studies in geriatric mares where there was no significant difference in body weight, body condition score, and dry matter intake between treated and untreated horses (Malinowski et al., 1997; Ralston et al., 1997).

There was no effect of eST on exercise capacity (Gerard, 2001). Maximum oxygen consumption, plasma lactate concentrations, heart rates, blood volumes, and run times to fatigue were not significantly different between treated and untreated horses (Gerard, 2001). These findings supported previous studies on aged, untrained geriatric mares that showed aerobic capacity was not improved after eST treatment (McKeever et al., 1998).

The yearlings treated with eST did develop significant decreases in PCV, Hb, MCH, albumin, CK, and AST and there was an increase in WCC, neutrophil, and platelet counts compared to controls. However, all variables remained within normal reference ranges suggesting any change would be of unlikely biological significance (Lambeth, 2001). Histochemical and biochemical analysis of weekly samples of the middle gluteal muscle was performed. There were no differences in muscle composition between eST-treated and control horses. At the completion of the study the weight of the semitendinosus and biceps femoris muscles in relation to body weight of eST-treated animals was compared to untreated controls. Treated horses had a significant increase in the weight of the semitendinosus but not biceps femoris muscle in relation to body weight. An increase in fiber size of the semitendinosus muscle could not be demonstrated in treated horses. Lambeth (2001) concluded there were no significant biological effects on skeletal muscle or hematological or serum biochemical variables associated with eST treatment in young training horses.

Gerard (2001) also evaluated the effect of eST on articular cartilage of the carpus and on the properties of the superficial flexor tendon in yearling horses undergoing training. Ex vivo proteoglycan metabolism of the harvested articular cartilage in treated animals was not different between treated and untreated horses. Biomechanical properties and concentrations of the matrix compound and cartilage oligomeric matrix protein were unchanged following treatment of horses with eST. These reports supported an earlier study finding no difference in the ex vivo biomechanical properties of normal superficial flexor tendons from adult horses treated with eST using the same dose regimen when compared with controls (Dowling et al., 2002a).

Cumulative evidence from these studies indicate that in the young exercising Standardbred horse administration of eST at the manufacturer's recommended dose does not have a major impact in terms of ergogenic augmentation. In addition, there may be limited prophylactic effects of eST on musculoskeletal tissues such as tendons and cartilage under high-intensity exercise. However, it remains possible that higher doses and/or a longer treatment period may have resulted in a different outcome. A study examining the safety margin of eST in the horse found that a single dose up to 5 times the recommended dose caused no untoward side effects (Dart et al., 1998).

Further studies have examined the potential therapeutic benefits of eST in the treatment of musculoskeletal injuries and in wound healing. Dart et al. (2002) examined the effect of eST on the healing of full thickness skin wounds on the distal limb in horses. The study found wounds on horses treated with eST retracted more during treatment and contracted faster after treatment stopped when compared to untreated horses. This is in contrast to a study looking at wounds on the pectoral region of horses where no difference in healing was found (Smith et al., 1999). The implication is that eST appears to modify wound healing of the distal limb. Further study is needed to evaluate whether there is any therapeutic benefit in specific wounds and whether there is potential benefit if eST were administered at strategic times during healing.

Dowling et al. (2002a,b) investigated the effect of eST on the in vitro healing of a tendon using a collagenase model of superficial flexor tendonitis. Tendonitis was induced by injecting the mid-metacarpal region of the tendon with 2000 IU of collagenase. Treatment consisted of eST at 10 µg/kg for 7 days followed by 20 µg/kg for another 5 weeks. Following 6 weeks of treatment, horses were euthanized and tendons harvested for biomechanical testing. Tendons from treated horses had a significantly larger cross-sectional area and lower mean values for ultimate tensile stress and ultimate tensile strain. It was concluded that eST has a negative effect on the biomechanical properties in the early phases of healing superficial digital flexor tendons. Based on this model, eST cannot be recommended for treatment of superficial flexor tendonitis. In contrast a similar study looking at the effects of 10 intralesional injections of 2 µg of recombinant IGF-1 over a 20-day period on a collagenase-induced model of tendonitis in horses showed some biomechanical, cellular, and molecular improvement in healing eight weeks after induction of the lesion (Dahlgren et al., 2002). Other studies have suggested growth factors might modulate the repair process in damaged ligaments and tendons in a variety of species (Abrahamsson et al., 1991a,b; Abrahamsson and Lohmander, 1996; Des Rosiers et al., 1996; Murphy and Nixon, 1997). Given that it has been estimated that only 20-60% of horses sustaining superficial flexor tendonitis will return to racing and even then re-injury is common, further studies are required to evaluate the in vivo effects of growth factors on the ultimate healing and sustainable function under maximal exercise of flexor tendon lesions in the horse (Silver et al., 1983; Bramlage, 1986; Sawdon et al., 1996).

Finally the effect of eST on synovial joint metabolism has been evaluated. Using the manufacturer's recommended dose regimen, horses were treated for 6 weeks and synovial fluid was collected at 6, 8, 11, and 16 weeks. Cartilage was harvested at 16 weeks for analysis. Plasma IGF-1 and synovial fluid GH and IGF-1 were elevated in treated horses and compared to controls. Synovial fluid polysulphated glycosaminoglycans during treatment were significantly lower in treated horses. There was a trend for 3B3(-) epitope:GAG ratio to be higher in treated horses, although this difference was not significant. There was no difference in markers of cartilage metabolism between treated and untreated horses in the cartilage harvested at 12 weeks. The study suggests that eST can modify the joint environment and may achieve concentrations of IGF-1 within the joint used in joint resurfacing studies (Fortier et al., 1999). Further investigation into the role of GH in cartilage metabolism and repair are warranted (Dart et al., In press).

Studies into the role of the steroidal anabolics are limited; however, there appears to be little scientific evidence that there are anabolic effects that might be associated with increased performance of otherwise healthy animals or enhanced development of young horses. These drugs may have application in debilitated horses or in horses that are under stress, particularly in adjusting to the transition from paddock to stable or stable to paddock. It is important that these drugs do not become a treatment panacea, especially when horses may have underlying conditions.

Recombinant growth hormone is a relatively new therapeutic with demonstrated evidence of anabolic effects in a number of species. Recently, equine recombinant growth hormone has become available. To date studies examining the role of eST in the growth and development of foals and the effects of eST on young horses in work have been performed using the manufacturer's recommendations. Evidence would suggest that there is a biological effect when using the recommended dose. Contrary to the results of studies in other species, there appear to be no significant biological effects of eST on the growth and development of young horses. Similarly, there have been no credible effects on horses in training.

Studies looking at the potential therapeutic benefits of eST on the rehabilitation of horses with musculoskeletal injury or wounds are limited. Apart from unsubstantiated observations, there is no valid scientific evidence of a specific application to date. Evidence would suggest that eST may be able to modulate the joint environment. Further investigation of the role of eST in the prevention and healing of osteochondral lesions in the athletic horse may be warranted.

References

Abrahamsson, S.O., G. Lundborg , and L.S. Lohmander. 1991a. Long-term explant culture of rabbit flexor tendon: effects of recombinant human insulin-like growth factor 1 and serum on matrix metabolism. J. Orthop. Res. 9:503-515.

Abrahamsson, S.O., G. Lundborg, and L.S. Lohmander. 1991b. Recombinant human insulin-like growth factor 1 stimulates in vitro matrix synthesis and cell proliferation in rabbit flexor tendon. J. Orthop. Res. 9:495-502.

Abrahamsson, S.O., and L.S. Lohmander. 1996. Differential effects of insulin-like growth factor-1 on matrix and DNA synthesis in various regions and types of rabbit tendon. J. Orthop. Res. 14:370-376.

Bengtsson, B., A.S. Eden, L. Lonn, H. Kvist, A. Stokland, G. Lindstedt, I. Bosaeus, J. Tolli, L. Sjostrom, and O.G. Isaksson. 1993. Treatment of adults with growth hormone (GH) deficiency with recombinant human GH. J. Clin. Endocrinol. Metab. 76:309-317.

Bramlage, L.R. 1986. Superior carpal check ligament desmotomy as a treatment of superficial flexor tendonitis: initial report. In: Proc. Amer. Assoc. Equine Practnr. 32:365.

Buonomo, F.C., J.P. Ruffin, J.J. Brendemeuhl, J.J. Veenhuizen, and J.L. Sartin. 1996. The effects of bovine somatotropin (bST) and porcine somatotropin (pST) on growth factor and metabolic variables in horses. J. Anim. Sci. 74:886-894.

Capshaw, E.L., D.L. Thompson, K.M. Kulinski, C.A. Johnson, and D.D. French. 2001. Daily treatment of horses with equine somatotropin from 4 to 16 months of age. J. Anim. Sci. 79:3137-3147.

Cochran, R.A., D.A. Guitreau, D.A. Hylan, J.A. Carter, H. Johnson, D.L. Thompson, Jr., and R.A. Godke. 1999a. Effects of administration of exogenous eST to seasonally anovulatory mares. In: Proc. Equine Nutr. Physiol. Symp. 16:83.

Cochran, R.A., A.A. Leonardo-Cattolica, M.R. Sullivan, L.A. Kincaid, B.S. Leise, D.L. Thompson, Jr., and R.A. Godke. 1999b. The effects of equine somatotropin (eST) on follicular development and circulating hormone profiles in cyclic mares treated during different stages of the estrous cycle. Domest. Anim. Endocrinol. 16:57-67.

Dahlgren L.A., M.C.H. van der Meulen, J.E.A. Bertram, G.S. Starrak, and A.J. Nixon. 2002. Insulin-like growth factor-I improves cellular and molecular aspects of healing in a collagenase-induced model of flexor tendinitis. J. Orthop. Res. 20:910-919.

Dart, A.J., M. Strong, R.J. Rose, and D.R. Hodgson. 1998. Effects of two large doses of equine recombinant growth hormone on clinical, haematological and serum biochemical variables in adult horses. Aust. Vet. J. 76:6-9.

Dart, A.J., L. Creis, L.B. Jeffcott, D.R.Hodgson, and R.J. Rose. 2002. Effect of equine recombinant growth hormone on second intention wound healing in horses. Vet. Surg. 31:314-319.

Dart, A.J., C.B. Little, C.E. Hughes, et al. 2003. Recombinant equine growth hormone administration: Effects on synovial fluid biomarkers and cartilage metabolism in horses. Equine Vet. J.

Dawson H.A., and K.E. Gersten. 1978. Use of an anabolic steroid in racetrack practice. Mod. Vet. Pract. 59:129-130.

Des Rosiers, E.A., L. Yahia, and C.H. Rivard. 1996. Proliferative and matrix synthesis response of canine anterior cruciate ligament fibroblasts submitted to combine growth factors. J. Orthop. Res. 14:200-208.

Dietz, O., J. Mill, and R. Teutscher. 1974. Experimentelle Untersuchungen zur Andwendung anaboler Steroide bei Sportpferden. Vet. Med. 29:938.

Dowling, B.A., A.J. Dart, D.R. Hodgson, R.J. Rose, and W.R. Walsh. 2002a. Recombinant equine growth hormone does not effect the in vitro biomechanical properties of equine superficial digital flexor tendon. Vet. Surg. 31:325-330.

Dowling, B.A., A.J. Dart, D.R. Hodgson, R.J. Rose, and W.R. Walsh. 2002b. The effect of recombinant growth hormone on the biomechanical properties of healing superficial flexor tendon in horses. Vet. Surg. 31:320-324

Dunshea, F.R., R.H. King, P.C. Owens, and P.E. Walton. 1999. Moderate doses of porcine somatotropin do not increase plasma insulin-like growth factor-1 (IGF-1) or IGF binding protein-3. Domest. Anim. Endicrinol. 16:149-157.

Etherton, T.D., and D.E. Bauman. 1998. Biology of somatotropin in growth and lactation of domestic animals. Physiol. Rev. 78:745-761.

Evock, C.M., T.D. Etherton, C.S. Chung, and R.E. Ivy. 1988. Pituitary porcine growth hormone (PGH) and a recombinant pGH analogue stimulate pig growth performance in a similar manner. J. Anim. Sci. 66:1928-1941.

Evock-Clover, C.M., N.C. Steele, T.J. Caperna, and M.B. Solomon. 1992. Effects of frequency of recombinant porcine somatotropin administration on growth performance, tissue accretion rates, and hormone and metabolite concentrations in pigs. J. Anim. Sci. 70:3709-3720.

Fortier, L.A., G. Lust, H.O. Mohammed, and A.J. Nixon. 1999. Coordinate upregulation of cartilage matrix synthesis in fibrin cultures supplements with exogenous insulin-like growth factor-1. J. Orthop. Res. 17:464-474.

Gerard, M.P. 2001. The effects of equine somatotropin on the physiological response to training in young horses. Ph.D. Thesis. University of Sydney.

Julen Day, T.R., G.D. Potter, E.L. Morris, L.W. Greene, and J.B. Simmons. 1998. Physiologic and skeletal response to exogenous equine somatotropin (eST) in two year old Quarter Horses in race training. J. Equine Vet. Sci. 18:321-328.

Klindt, J., F.C. Buonomo, and J.T. Ten. 1992. Administration of porcine somatotropin by sustained release implant: Growth and endocrine responses in genetically lean and obese barrows and gilts. J. Anim. Sci. 70:3721-3733.

Kulinski, K.M., D.L. Thompson, E.L. Capshaw, D.D French, and J.L. Oliver. 2002. Daily treatment of growing foals with equine somatotropin: Pathologic and endocrinologic assessments at necropsy and residual effects in live animals. J. Anim. Sci. 80:392-400.

Lambeth, R. 2001. The effects of training and administration of equine somatotropin on resting haematology, serum biochemistry and skeletal muscle of Standardbred yearlings. Masters of Veterinary Clinical Studies, University of Sydney.

Malinowski, K., R.A. Christensen, A. Kanopa, C.G. Scanes, and H. Hafs. 1997. Feed intake, body weight, body condition scores, musculation and immunocompetence in aged mares given equine somatotropin. J. Anim. Sci. 75:755-760.

McKeever, K.H., K. Malinowski, R.A. Christensen, and H.D. Hafs. 1999. Chronic recombinant equine somatotropin (eST) administration does not affect aerobic capacity or exercise performance in geriatric mares. Vet. J. 155:19-25.

Murphy, D.J., and A.J. Nixon. 1997. The effects of insulin-like growth factor 1 on intrinsic tenocyte activity in equine flexor tendons. Am. J. Vet. Res. 58:103-109.

Nelson, J.F. 1995. The potential role of selected endocrine systems in aging processes. In: E.J. Masaro (Ed.) Handbook of Physiology. p. 377-394. Oxford University Press, New York.

Nimmo, M.A., C.D. Munro, and D.H. Snow. 1982. Effects of nandrolene phenylproprionate in the horse: (3) Skeletal muscle composition in the exercising animal. Equine Vet. J. 14:229-233.

O'Connor, J.J., M.C. Stillions, W.A. Reynolds, W.H. Linkenheimer, and D.C. Maplesden. 1973. Evaluation of boldenone undecyclenate as an anabolic agent in horses. Can. Vet. J. 14:154-158.

Radetti, G., F. Buzi, C. Pagainini, C. Martelli, and S. Adami. 2000. A four-year dose-response study of recombinant human growth hormone treatment of growth hormone deficient children: Effects on growth, bone growth and growth mineralization. Eur. J. Endocrinol. 142:42-46.

Ralston, S.L., K. Malinowski, and R.A. Christensen. 1997. Body weight, condition and postprandial energy metabolites in aged mares following daily injection with equine somatotropin. J. Anim. Sci. 75:275.

Ryan, A.J. 1976. Anabolic-androgenic steroids. Handbook of Experimental Pharmacology. Spronger-Verlag, Berlin. 142-515-534.

Sas, T., W. de Waal, P. Mulder, M. Houdijk, M. Jansen, M. Reeser, and A. Hokken-Koelega. 1999. Growth hormone treatment in young children with short stature born small for gestational age: 5-year results of a randomized double blind, dose-response trial. J. Clin. Endocrinol. Metab. 84:3064-3070.

Sawdon, H., J.V. Yovich, and T. Booth. 1996. Superficial flexor tendonitis in racehorses: Long-term follow-up of conservatively managed cases. Aust. Equine Vet. 14:21-25.

Schwarz, F.J.D., R. Schams, R. Ropke, et al. 1993. Effects of somatotropin treatment on growth performance, carcass traits, and the endocrine system in finishing beef heifers. J. Anim. Sci. 77:2721-2731.

Silver, I.A., P.M. Brown, and A.E. Goodship. 1983. A clinical and experimental study of tendon injury, healing and treatment in the horse. Equine Vet. J. Supp. 1:1-43.

Smith, L.A., D.L. Thompson, D.D. French, and B.S. Leise. 1999. Effects of recombinant equine somatotropin on wound healing, carbohydrate and lipid metabolism, and endogenous somatotropin response to secretagogues in gelding. J. Anim. Sci. 77:1815-1822.

Snow, D.H., C.D. Munro, and M.A. Nimmo. 1982a. Effects of nandrolene phenylproprionate in the horse: (1) Resting animal. Equine Vet. J. 14:219-223.

Snow, D.H., C.D. Munro, and M.A. Nimmo. 1982b. Effects of nandrolene phenylproprionate in the horse: (2) General effects in animals undergoing training. Equine Vet. J. 14:224-228.

Stihl, H.G. 1968. Uber die Anwendung eines anabolin steroids in der Pferdepraxis. Berl. Munch. Tieratzl. Wschr. 81:378-382.

Strobil, J.S., and M.J. Thomas. 1996. Human growth hormone. J. Amer. Soc. Pharm. Ther. 46:1-34.

Vanderwal, P. 1976. Anabolic agents in animal production. FAO/WHO Symposium. F. Coulston and F. Korte (Eds.) George Thieme, Stuttgart 60-78.

NUTRITIONAL CHALLENGES OF FEEDING THE TWO-YEAR-OLD

JOE D. PAGAN
Kentucky Equine Research, Versailles, Kentucky, USA

Introduction

Many horses begin their athletic careers long before they have reached maturity. Thoroughbreds enter race training as young as 18 months of age and may race before they have reached two years of age. Feeding this type of young horse is challenging because nutrients must be supplied for both growth and exercise. Additionally, little research has been done to quantify the nutrient requirements of horses this age. This paper will compare the nutrient requirements of growing horses, two-year-olds, and mature racehorses and give recommendations for feeding the two-year-old.

The energy, protein, and lysine requirements of long yearlings, two-year-olds, and adult racehorses are listed in Table 1. The requirements for two-year-olds are derived largely from combining information about requirements for growth and performance as few studies have been conducted with two-year-olds to quantify their requirements. Below is a brief explanation of how each requirement was calculated.

Digestible Energy

The energy requirements of horses are generally expressed in terms of digestible energy (DE) as either Mcal/day or MJ/day. For growing horses, the DE requirement is the sum of the maintenance energy requirement (DE Mcal/d) = 1.4 x (.03 x BW) plus a DE requirement for growth, where the efficiency of utilization of DE for growth equals 18.4 Mcal/kg gain in yearlings and 19.6 Mcal/kg gain in two-year-olds. Therefore, a long yearling that weighs 425 kg with an average daily gain of 0.4 kg/d would have a DE requirement of 14.1 Mcal (maintenance) + 7.4 Mcal (growth) = 21.5 Mcal DE/day. The two-year-old that weighs 485 kg and has an ADG of 0.25 kg/d would have a higher maintenance requirement because it is heavier (16 Mcal/d) but would have a smaller requirement for growth since its average daily gain (ADG) is slower (4.9 Mcal/d). Its daily DE requirement with no exercise would equal 21 Mcal/d.

Table 1. Digestible energy (DE), crude protein (CP), and lysine requirements of long yearlings, two-year-olds, and adult racehorses.

	Long Yearling	Two-year old				Adult Racehorse
Training	No	No	Light	Moderate	Heavy	Heavy
Age (months)	18	24	24	24	24	Mature
BW (kg)	425	485	485	485	485	500
ADG (kg/d)	0.4	0.25	0.25	0.25	0.25	0
DE (Mcal/d)	20.6	21	24.9	28.9	36.9	32.8
CP (g/d)	925	890	980	1070	1160	906
Lysine (g/d)	39	36	39	47	61	32

The DE requirement for exercise is defined as a multiple of maintenance. Light, moderate, and heavy work are assumed to increase a horse's DE requirement to levels equal to 1.25, 1.50, and 2.0 times maintenance, respectively. For a two-year-old, this would equal 20, 24, and 32 Mcal/d. Adding the DE for growth (4.9 Mcal/d) to the requirement for maintenance and exercise yields requirements of 24.9, 28.9, and 36.9 Mcal DE/day for two-year-olds in light, moderate, and heavy work, respectively.

Crude Protein

The crude protein (CP) requirements for growth and maintenance are based on a CP:DE ratio. The maintenance CP requirement equals 40 g CP/Mcal DE. The CP requirement for yearlings equals 45 g CP/Mcal DE, and the CP requirement for two-year-olds equals 42.5 g CP/Mcal DE. The NRC (1989) suggests that the maintenance CP:DE ratio is appropriate for exercise as well, but I believe that this overestimates the CP requirement at higher work intensities. Instead, I recommend that CP intakes increase to 110%, 120%, and 130% at light, moderate, and high work intensities in both two-year-olds and adult performance horses.

Lysine

The first limiting amino acid for growth in horses is lysine. The lysine requirement of long yearlings is equal to (1.9)(Mcal DE/day). For idle two-year-olds, the requirement equals (1.7)(Mcal DE/day), and for mature horses, the lysine equals 3.5% of daily CP intake. Lysine requirements for exercise increase at a similar rate as CP requirements.

Comparative Digestibilities

Kentucky Equine Research has conducted dozens of digestibility studies with mature horses that evaluate the apparent digestibility of a number of nutrients. A summary of many of these trials has been published (Pagan, 1998). Table 2 summarizes the results of these trials compared to a recent trial in which eight Thoroughbred two-year-olds were studied. These two-year-olds were fed grass hay, sweet feed, and a supplement pellet at an average daily dry matter intake of 8.3 kg. The apparent digestibility of most nutrients was similar between both groups. A notable exception was phosphorus, which was much more digestible in the two-year-olds. It is also interesting to note that zinc digestibility was very low (7% and 9%) in both groups.

Table 2. Comparative digestibilities of nutrients by two-year-olds and mature horses.

Nutrient	Two-year-olds (8.3 kg DM/day)		Mature horses (7.1 kg DM/day)	
	Concentration	Apparent digestibility (%)	Concentration	Apparent digestibility (%)
DM	100%	59%	100%	62%
CP	12.6%	64%	13.1%	71%
ADF	25.8%	32%	28.8%	40%
NDF	43.3%	39%	46.9%	45%
HEMI	17.5%	50%	18.1%	52%
Fat	4.1%	70%	3.6%	58%
Ash	6.1%	37%	7.5%	43%
NSC	34.0%	84%	28.9%	89%
Ca	0.58%	41%	0.89%	44%
P	0.45%	24%	0.39%	9%
Mg	0.19%	37%	0.22%	37%
K	1.7%	63%	1.6%	75%
Zn	60 ppm	7%	84 ppm	9%
Cu	18 ppm	40%	22 ppm	30%
Mn	107 ppm	27%	83 ppm	9%

Calcium, Phosphorus, and Magnesium Balance

The major minerals required for skeletal development are calcium, phosphorus, and magnesium. The two-year-olds in this study were fed calcium, phosphorus, and magnesium intakes equal to 48 g/d, 37.3 g/d, and 15.8 g/d, respectively. The two-year-olds retained an average of 5.2 g calcium, 5.9 g phosphorus, and 3.2 g magnesium per day (Figure 1). Fecal calcium and phosphorus excretion equaled 30 g/day. The horses excreted very little phosphorus or magnesium in their urine, but urinary calcium excretion averaged 12.7 g/day.

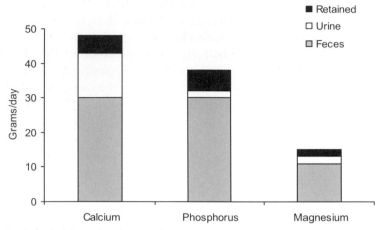

Figure 1. Amount of calcium, phosphorus,and magnesium retained or excreted in the feces or urine.

A real concern for trainers is how differently to feed two-year-olds compared to older horses in the stable. Table 3 contains a typical feeding program for an adult Thoroughbred in race training along with a feeding program for a two-year-old in moderate work using the same hay and grain mix. Both horses are fed 6 kg of timothy hay and a 12.0% protein grain mix that supplies 3.1 Mcal DE/kg. The adult racehorse would require 6.5 kg of grain to meet its energy requirement, while the two-year-old requires 5.25 kg/day.

Table 3. Feeding programs for adult racehorses and two-year-olds in training.

	Timothy hay	Grain mix	Timothy hay	Grain mix	Timothy hay	Grain mix
			Adult racehorse		*Two-year-old*	
	Composition		*Daily intake*		*Daily intake*	
DM	93.9%	88.0%	6.0 kg	6.5 kg	6.0 kg	5.25 kg
DE	2.1 Mcal/kg	3.1 Mcal/kg	12.5 Mcal	20.3 Mcal	12.5 Mcal	16.4 Mcal
CP	8.0%	12.0%	480 g	785 g	480 g	634 g
Lysine	0.24%	0.65%	14.4%	34.7%	14.4%	34.3%
Calcium	0.34%	0.60%	20.4%	39.2 g	20.4 g	31.7 g
Phosphorus	0.21%	0.52%	12.6%	34.0 g	12.6 g	27.5 g

Figures 2 and 3 show how well these rations meet the nutrient requirements of the two types of horses. Although the hay and grain are not excessively high in protein or minerals, the adult racehorse's ration supplies more protein, lysine, calcium, and phosphorus than needed because of the high level of intake required to meet the racehorse's energy requirement. A ration using the same hay and grain mix also meets the nutrient requirements of the two-year-old in moderate work. Again, a fairly high level of intake provides adequate nutrients from feedstuffs containing fairly low concentrations of protein and minerals. The bottom line from this comparison is that most rations fed to adult racehorses contain adequate protein, calcium, and phosphorus for two-year-olds. If caloric intake must be restricted in a two-year-old, higher levels of fortification may be needed.

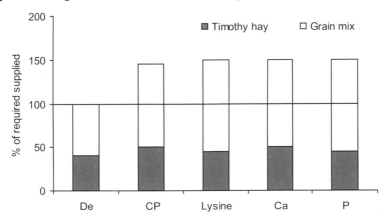

Figure 2. Nutrients supplied from a ration consisting of timothy hay and grain mix for an adult racehorse.

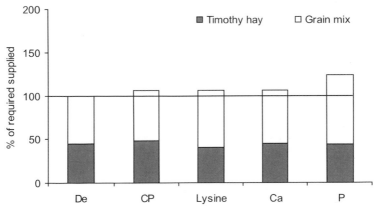

Figure 3. Nutrients supplied from a ration consisting of timothy hay and grain mix for a two-year-old in moderate work.

In conclusion, the nutrient requirements of the two-year-old are intermediate between the growing foal and the adult performance horse. If the two-year-old is in training, it can be fed feeds that are typically formulated for adult performance horses because the elevated level of feed intake required to meet the energy required for exercise will provide the extra protein and minerals needed for growth.

References

NRC. 1989. Nutrient Requirements of Horses (5th Ed.). National Academy Press, Washington, DC.

Pagan, J.D. 1998. Nutrient digestibility in horses. In: J.D. Pagan (Ed.) Advances in Equine Nutrition, Nottingham University Press, Nottingham, UK.

PATHOLOGICAL CONDITIONS

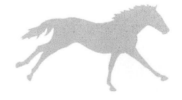

PATHOLOGICAL COMPLIC

OVERVIEW OF BONE DISEASE

C. WAYNE MCILWRAITH
Colorado State University, Fort Collins, Colorado, USA

Introduction

Bone is a critical component of the equine musculoskeletal system. It not only provides strength to the legs, but also acts as the foundation for cartilage in the moveable joints. Much of the clinical disease in the horse associated with bone involves the subchondral bone immediately under the articular cartilage leading to problems in the joint. These conditions can be divided into developmental problems of bone and traumatic problems of bone. They will be considered separately.

Developmental Problems of Bone

The term developmental orthopaedic disease (DOD) was coined in 1986 to encompass all orthopaedic problems seen in the growing foal (McIlwraith 1986) and is a term that encompasses all general growth disturbances of horses and is therefore nonspecific. The term should not be used synonymously with osteochondrosis, and it is inappropriate for subchondral cystic lesions, physitis, angular limb deformities, and cervical vertebral malformations all to be presumed as manifestations of osteochondrosis. When the term developmental orthopaedic disease was first coined, it was categorized to include the following:

- Osteochondrosis—Osteochondrosis is a defect in endochondral ossification that can result in a number of different manifestations depending on the site of the endochondral ossification defect. These manifestations include osteochondritis dissecans (OCD) and *some* subchondral cystic lesions—not all subchondral cystic lesions or osseous cyst-like lesions are necessarily manifestations of osteochondrosis. Another manifestation is some physitis (but we now recognize that most clinical swelling associated with the physis has no pathologic change involving the physis itself).

- Acquired angular limb deformities.

- Physitis.

- Subchondral cystic lesions.

- Flexural deformities.

- Cuboidal bone malformation.

Osteochondrosis

Osteochondrosis (dyschondroplasia) was initially defined as a disturbance of cellular differentiation in the growing cartilage (Olsson, 1978). Osteochondrosis is considered to be the result of a failure of endochondral ossification and, therefore, may affect either the articular epiphyseal cartilage complex or the metaphyseal growth cartilage. It is usually in the articular epiphyseal cartilage. It can have three consequences:

1. These areas of retained cartilage, due to a lack of endochondral ossification, can heal.

2. They can break out and form flaps of cartilage and bone or fragments of cartilage and bone (called osteochondritis dissecans or OCD).

3. The retained cartilage can undergo necrosis and form a subchondral cystic lesion (subchondral bone cyst).

The majority of cases of OCD and subchondral bone cysts are considered to be the result of necrosis occurring in the basal layers of the thickened retained cartilage with subsequent pressure and strain within the joint giving rise to fissures in the damaged cartilage.

Osteochondritis Dissecans

There is a general agreement that this condition involves a dissecting lesion with the formation of a chondral or osteochondral flap. Flaps may become detached and form joint mice. In some instances, lesions have been found at arthroscopy that consist of cartilage separated from bone, and the cartilage does not appear to be thickened (McIlwraith, 1993). Based on these observations, the author questions whether persistence of hypertrophied cartilage is a necessary event prior to the development of an OCD lesion. This question is based on instances seen at arthroscopic examination or in follow-up histologic examination where dissection or separation occurs close to the cartilage-bone interface, rather than in the underlying cancellous bone between normal cartilage and a normal bone-cartilage junction, as it commonly does in humans. The clinical manifestations and treatment of the common entities of OCD are discussed in a separate lecture.

Subchondral Cystic Lesions

Subchondral bone cysts were first reported as a clinical entity in 1968 (Pettersson and Sevelius, 1968). Subchondral cystic lesions have also been proposed as manifestations of osteochondrosis by a number of authors (Stromberg, 1979; Rooney, 1975), and there is some pathologic support for this (Rejno and Stromberg, 1978). However, more recent work has demonstrated that subchondral cystic lesions can be produced from a small defect in the bone (Ray et al., 1997), and other work has shown that the lining of clinical subchondral cystic lesions contained increased quantities of neutral metalloproteinases, PGE-2 and interleukin-1, and also are capable of osteoclastic resorption of bone.

The Cause of OCD

Despite the instances where there is no evidence of thickened cartilage, it is generally accepted that most OCD lesions are manifestations of osteochondrosis. In the one- to two-year-old horse, most cases of subchondral cystic lesions are also related to osteochondrosis. For that reason, the following discussion is on various etiologic factors associated with osteochondrosis.

GENETIC PREDISPOSITION

There have been a number of genetic studies on the heredity of OCD in the hock in Standardbreds and Scandinavian cold-blooded horses. A radiographic survey by Hoppe and Phillipson (1985) in Standardbred trotters and Swedish Warmbloods showed that one stallion of each breed had a significantly higher frequency of OCD among its progeny, compared with the progeny groups of the other stallions ($p<0.001$). In another study, Shougaard et al. (1990) showed radiographic evidence of a significantly higher proportion of OCD in the progeny of one of eight stallions, even though the stallion itself did not show radiographic signs of OCD. Since that time, there have been two additional studies (Grondahl and Dolvik, 1992; Phillipson et al., 1993) on the heritability of osteochondrosis in the tibiotarsal joint. Both of these studies were in Standardbred trotters, but did show significant heritability with OCD. Studies in other breeds are markedly lacking. In the Dutch Warmblood, there has been a protocol preventing breeding of stallions with any OCD for ten years, but whether this has lowered the incidence of the disease is questionable.

GROWTH AND BODY SIZE

An association has been made between body weight and OCD by Pagan and Jackson. Foals in Kentucky that had to have arthroscopic surgery for OCD were significantly heavier than foals that did not have OCD.

MECHANICAL STRESS AND TRAUMA

It has long been recognized clinically that mechanical stresses precipitate the onset of clinical signs, presumably by avulsing an OCD flap or fragment (McIlwraith, 1987). The role of trauma as a primary initiator of a lesion is more controversial. Pool pointed out that there are no unique histologic features that will consistently distinguish the lesion of osteochondrosis from that of trauma at a developing osteochondral junction, and that the radial vessels supplying the chondrocytes in the epiphyseal physis may be sheared and cause a primary osteochondrosis lesion (Pool, 1986). He felt that biomechanical forces are an important factor and are superimposed upon an idiopathic lesion to produce defective cartilage. Reflection back to the classic paper by Konig in 1887 is appropriate in considering the potential role of trauma in the pathogenesis. He claimed that loose bodies in the knee joints of young people had three causes: a) very severe trauma, b) lesser trauma causing contusion and necrosis and c) minimal trauma acting on an underlying lesion—for which he suggested the name "osteochondritis dissecans" (and for which he is considered the originator) (Barrie, 1987). I feel that these three different syndromes can be seen in the horse.

DEFECTS IN VASCULARIZATION

OCD was initially described as being caused by a vascular or ischemic necrosis of the subchondral bone (Adams, 1974; Schevitz, 1966). Although recent work in the pig suggested that the viability of epiphyseal cartilage and the articular epiphyseal cartilage complex is highly dependent on adequate blood supply from cartilage canal vessels and implicates a defect in blood supply in the pathogenesis of osteochondrosis (Carlson et al., 1991), there is no evidence yet documented in the horse.

NUTRITION

Osteochondrosis-like lesions have been induced in horses by feeding 130% of National Research Council (NRC) carbohydrate and protein (Glade and Belling, 1986). More recently, further work has defined that 130% of NRC digestible energy will certainly significantly increase the incidence of osteochondrosis lesions, but increasing the protein content does not (Savage et al., 1993).

MINERAL IMBALANCES

Various mineral imbalances have been implicated in the pathogenesis, including high calcium, high phosphorus, low copper and high zinc. There is no good equine-specific support for high calcium causing problems, but three times the

NRC levels of phosphorus significantly increased the number of OCD lesions (Savage et al., 1993).

Low copper has been implicated as a cause. In experimental studies, it has been reported that a marked copper deficiency (1.7 ppm) produced both flexural deformities and osteochondrosis-like lesions (Bridges and Harris, 1988). Bridges and Harris also noticed a softening of articular cartilage and suggested that the low copper status may lead to reduced cross-linking of collagen by lysyl oxidase, predisposing to physeal and articular fractures. Hurtig et al. conducted a controlled experiment with high (30 ppm) and low (7 ppm) copper diets (1990). A much higher incidence of lesions of osteochondrosis was seen in the foals fed the low copper diet. Many of the changes were present in the cervical spine. Hurtig considered the lesions as one of reduced structural strength rather than arrested or abnormal endochondral ossification. Further work has been done in copper by Pearce et al. in New Zealand. The absolute levels of copper at which OCD can be produced have been questioned, or at least it appears clear that there are differences between different countries. Professor Elwyn Firth's group failed to produce significant clinical OCD with low copper diets. They also showed that, while oral supplementation of mares could enhance the foals' copper status, parental administration could not.

Excessive zinc intake has been related to equine osteochondrosis (Messer, 1981). The effects of environmental exposure to zinc and cadmium were studied in pregnant pony mares, following observations of lameness, swollen joints, and unthriftiness, particularly in foals (Gunson et al., 1982).

ENDOCRINE FACTORS

It has been postulated by Glade that the production of osteochondrosis lesions in association with overfeeding is mediated by the endocrine system (Glade and Belling, 1986). Glade has proposed that feeding initiates increased concentrations of insulin and T_4, and high concentrations of insulin could inhibit growth hormone, although the exact mechanism is not known (Glade, 1986). A long-term administration of dexamethasone has been associated with the production of osteochondrosis-like lesions (Glade and Krook, 1983). More recent work showing an association between high-glycemic feed, insulin secretion, and osteochondrosis has been made by Ralston and Pagan.

SITE VULNERABILITY

Because the lesions of equine osteochondrosis occur at specific anatomic sites, this does suggest vulnerability that could be related back to trauma or excessive stress and interference with blood supply as originally suggested by Pool (1986). Lesions are frequently bilateral in the femoropatellar and tarsocrural joints and quadrilateral in the fetlock joint, although they infrequently involve different joints in the same animal. This observation could perhaps suggest a "window of vulnerability" in the endochondral ossification of that specific joint at that specific location.

Natural History of Osteochondrosis Lesions

Recent work done by the workers at Utrecht (van Weeran and Barneveld, 1999) has shown that many lesions in the stifle and the hock will heal. In this study, foals were radiographed every month, and lesions developed (defects developed, signifying a lack of endochondral ossification) and then the lesions healed. Relatively few of them became clinical, but the times at which they were going to persist were established. This study emphasized that we need to be careful of radiographic surveys in deciding that we have a problem with OCD. This author feels that only when we have clinical signs associated with it should we be intervening. This study also clarified the age at which surgical treatment was appropriate. If surgical intervention is carried out at a very young age, it is likely that it is unnecessary in many instances.

Further work by McIntosh and McIlwraith (1993) showed that it was certainly possible to have lesions heal beyond this time if foals were confined. Definition of what lesions can heal with conservative management has greatly progressed treatment, and this is discussed elsewhere.

Traumatic Lesions of the Subchondral Bone

In recent years, good evidence has been provided that intra-articular fractures are preceded by subchondral bone disease. This subchondral bone disease consists of a spectrum of microcracks, diffuse microdamage, cell loss (apoptosis or necrosis) and accompanying subchondral bone sclerosis (Kawcak et al., 2000; Kawcak et al., 2001).

Cause of Subchondral Bone Disease

The development of microdamage is presumed to be associated as a consequence of cyclic trauma. The repeated wear and tear has been noted with radiographic study and, more recently, CT to contribute to subchondral bone sclerosis. However, the direct association between sclerosis leading to the necrosis of bone has not been totally demonstrated. The development of lytic lesions in the subchondral bone, however, is presumed to be associated with microdamage. Factors involved in the predisposition of horses to damage based on the cyclic trauma of an athletic career include racetrack or arena surface, conformation, genetic predisposition, as well as a destabilizing traumatic injury.

Consequences of Traumatic Subchondral Bone Disease

Subchondral bone disease creates an environment for pathologic fractures. The most common manifestation are osteochondral chip fractures, which can be career-ending if not treated successfully. However, the overall success with arthroscopic surgery is high. Slab fractures represent a more severe injury requiring internal fixation. Some of these cases can return to athletic activities. However, in other instances, such as collapsing slab fractures in the carpus, the failure to treat adequately can lead to loss of life. The third level of fracture injury in terms of severity are the catastrophic injuries that can be life-threatening. Surgical treatments of such conditions are salvage procedures.

Diagnosis

Early diagnosis is critical. The recognition that early disease in the subchondral bone can lead to fractures has resulted in research efforts to diagnose bone disease early.

References

Adams OR. Lameness in horses. 3rd ed. Philadelphia: Lea and Febiger, 1974.

Barrie HJ. Osteochondritis dissecans. 1887-1987. A centennial look at Konig's memorable phrase. J Bone Jt Surg 1987;69-B:693-695.

Bridges CH, Harris ED. Experimentally induced cartilaginous fractures (osteochondritis dissecans) in foals fed low-copper diets. J Am Vet Med Assoc 1988;193:215-221.

Carlson CS, Meuten DJ, Richardson DC. Ischemic necrosis of cartilage in spontaneous and experimental lesions of osteochondrosis. J Orthop Res 1991;9:317-329.

Glade MJ, Belling TH. A dietary etiology for osteochondrotic cartilage. J Equine Vet Sci 1986;6:151-155.

Glade MJ, Krook L, Schryver HF, et al. Morphologic and biochemical changes in cartilage of foals treated with dexamethasone. Cornell Vet 1983;73:170-192.

Glade MJ. Control of cartilage growth in osteochondrosis: a review. J Equine Vet Sci 1986;6:175-187.

Gunson DE, Kowalczyk DF, Shoop CR et al. Environmental zinc and cadmium pollution associated with generalized osteochondrosis, osteoporosis and nephrocalcinosis in horses. J Am Vet Med Assoc 1982;180:295-299.

Hintz HF, Hintz RL, Van Vleck LD. Growth rate of Thoroughbreds, effect of age of dam, year and month of birth and sex of foal. J Anim Sci 1979;48:480-487.

Hoppe F, Phillipsson J. A genetic study of osteochondrosis in Swedish horses. Equine Pract 1985;7:7-15.

Hurtig MB, Green SL, Dobson H et al. Defective bone and cartilage in foals fed a low copper diet, in Proc 35th Annual Conv Am Assoc Equine Practnr 1990;637-643.

Kawcak CE, McIlwraith CW, Norrdin RW, Park RD, James SP. The role of subchondral bone and joint disease: a review. Equine Vet J 2001;33:120-126.

Kawcak CE, McIlwraith CW, Norrdin RW, Park RD, Steyn PS. Clinical effects of exercise on subchondral bone of carpal and metacarpophalangeal joints in horses. Am J Vet Res 2000;61:1252-1258.

Kawcak CE, Norrdin RW, Frisbie DD, McIlwraith CW, Trotter GW. Effects of osteochondral fragmentation and intra-articular triamcinalone acetonide treatment on subchondral bone in the equine carpus. Equine Vet J 1997;30:66-71.

McIlwraith CW, ed. AQHA Developmental Orthopedic Disease Symposium. Amarillo, TX: American Quarter Horse Association 1986;1-77.

McIlwraith CW. Inferences from referred clinical cases of osteochondritis dissecans. Equine Vet J Supplement 1993;16:27-30.

McIlwraith CW. Osteochondrosis. In: Stashak TS, ed. Adams' Lameness in Horses, 4th ed. Philadelphia: Lea and Febriger, 1987;396-410.

McIlwraith CW. What is developmental orthopaedic disease, osteochondrosis, osteochondritis, metabolic bone disease? Proc 39th Annual Convention AAEP 1993;35-44.

Messer NT. Tibiotarsal effusion associated with chronic zinc intoxication in three horses. J Am Vet Med Assoc 1981;178:294.

Norrdin RW, Kawcak CE, Capwell BA, McIlwraith CW. Subchondral bone failure in an equine model of overload arthrosis. Bone 1998;22:133-139.

Olsson SE. Introduction. Acta Radiol Supp 1978;358:9-14.

Pettersson H, Sevelius F. Subchondral bone cysts in the horse: a clinical study. Equine Vet J 1968;1:75.

Pool RR. Pathologic manifestations of osteochondrosis. In: McIlwraith CW, ed. AQHA Developmental Orthopedic Disease Symposium. Amarillo, TX: American Quarter Horse Association, 1986;3-7.

Rejno S, Stromberg B. Osteochondrosis in the horse. II. Pathology. Acta Radiol Suppl 1978;358:153-178.

Rooney JR. Osteochondrosis in the horse. Mod Vet Pract 1975;56:41-43 and 113-116.

Schougaard H, Falk-Ronne J, Phillipsson J. A radiographic survey of tibiotarsal osteochondrosis in a selected population of trotting horses in Denmark and its possible genetic significance. Equine Vet J 1990;22:288-289.

Stromberg J. A review of the salient features of osteochondrosis in the horses. Equine Vet J 1979;11:211-214.

ADVANCED TECHNIQUES IN THE DIAGNOSIS OF BONE DISEASE

C. WAYNE MCILWRAITH
Colorado State University, Fort Collins, Colorado, USA

Introduction

It is now recognized that early disease in the subchondral bone (including microdamage, microcracks, apoptosis and inappropriate remodeling) all contribute to the development of osteochondral fractures. An ability to recognize this change early could potentially prevent many osteochondral fractures, as well as more severe fractures (including catastrophic ones). It is also recognized that stress fractures are commonly the result of bone remodeling. All of the initiators to bone remodeling are still not clarified, but it is recognized that stress fractures in the rehabilitation phase of horses coming back after surgery or lay-up can lead to catastrophic fractures requiring euthanasia. Early diagnosis of bone disease is key to the prevention of such injuries. It is also important to recognize that adaptation and pathologic change are very similar processes. Differentiation of these changes is also a key to early diagnosis.

The purpose of this paper is to outline some of these newer techniques, and compare what they can do to what is currently available.

Radiography and Computed Radiography

Radiography has been the standard clinical technique the veterinarian uses to diagnose fractures and obvious bone disease. The advent of computed radiography has improved the definition of the bone in many of these conditions. However, there are still major limitations to radiography, in that we need 30-50% loss in bone density for it to be apparent on a radiograph and do not get the best definition of early subchondral bone disease. We do not get definition of articular cartilage disease or definition of disease of other soft tissue such as ligaments and menisci.

Nuclear Imaging

There will be increased uptake of technetium in areas of early subchondral bone disease (Kawcak et al 2000). It is therefore useful as a sensitive diagnostic technique for early bone disease, but is relatively non-specific. It is also often unrewarding for chronic problems. Nuclear scintigraphy has been extremely useful for the early recognition of stress fractures, and this has definitely decreased the number of catastrophic injuries resulting from stress fractures in athletes.

In southern California, the modality is available at the racetracks. If a horse has a hind-limb lameness that cannot be localized lower down, a nuclear scan is done, and typically will reveal a local area of uptake, representing a stress fracture. In many instances, this fracture cannot be defined with radiography. At the moment, nuclear scintigraphy is the gold standard for diagnosing stress fractures (it is now recognized that stress fractures lead to more severe fractures, so this serves as a huge prevention for catastrophic injury). The typical locations for these stress fractures are in the tibia, femur, pelvis, and humerus (in the forelimb).

Computed Tomography (CAT Scan/CT)

We have used this modality as a resource tool for a number of years, as has the Equine Research Group at Massey University (Prof. Elwyn Firth). In the work done by Dr. Chris Kawcak in our laboratory, we were able to show the development of subchondral bone sclerosis, as well as later development of subchondral bone necrosis using quantitated CT (osteoabsorptiometry). Prof. Firth's group similarly documented changes in the bone with exercise using a peripheral (portable) qCT unit and lowered bone mineral density (BMD) with OCD (Firth et al., 1999). A portable CT that can be used in the standing horse has recently been developed and is currently undergoing investigation. This could offer a practical means of monitoring bone density (or changes in bone density) with exercise in a clinical horse population. The use of CT, combined with modeling, is now a useful surgical tool for diagnosing fractures in more than one direction.

MRI

Most MRI usage, up until now, has been limited to the distal limb. However, the technology is becoming available to do limbs at least up to the carpus and tarsus. MRI will be extremely valuable for documentation of subtle changes in the bone, as well as other soft tissues of joints. There is a standing MRI (Hallmarq) that is being marketed from England. It will provide reasonable images of the distal phalanges and can image hind fetlocks (but not front fetlocks). At this stage, we are investing in an extremity MRI scanner (ONI) that will require anesthesia, but has the power to provide excellent images.

Optical Coherence Tomography

This is useful for evaluation of articular cartilage in vivo. It is currently being used as a research technique, but could be adapted in the future.

Fourier Transformed Infrared Imaging (FT-IR)

This is used on sections of bone. Infrared irradiation is directed toward a sample, and some passes through. The resulting spectrum represents the molecular absorption and transmission and an absorption spectrum is unique for each molecular structure. It has been used by the Utrecht group for examination of articular cartilage and evaluation of proteoglycan content.

Diagnostic Arthroscopy

The use of diagnostic arthroscopy has always been the gold standard technique for diagnosing and defining articular cartilage damage. However, it also needs to be recognized that it has been extremely useful in diagnosing and defining subchondral bone disease. Because of the focal nature of subchondral bone disease in some locations, specific localization of this problem is often only possible with the arthroscope. Scintigraphy can lead to the affected joint, but is not specific in location within that joint. CT can help define many of these when it is a practically available technique. Obviously, diagnostic arthroscopy requires anesthetic and is a minimally invasive procedure. At the present time, it is an important part of our armamentarium, however. The other advantage with arthroscopy is that, at the same time, we can commonly treat these subchondral lesions.

Synovial Fluid and Serum Biomarkers

The development of synovial fluid and serum biomarkers offers great potential for the early diagnosis of articular cartilage, bone, and tendon disease. Considerable work has been done with these biomarkers in various diseases and will be detailed below.

Principle of Biomarkers

The term "biomarker," "biochemical marker," and "molecular marker" have all been used to describe either direct or indirect indicators of abnormal skeletal tissue turnover. These markers are generally molecules that are the normal products and by-products of the metabolic processes occurring within the skeleton. Alterations occur in the balance between the anabolic and catabolic processes in disease, and, therefore, the concentrations of biomarkers may either increase or decrease. In joint disease, such molecules typically appear in the synovial fluid of affected joints. If the underlying subchondral bone is involved, the molecules of osseous origin will usually be cleared directly into the bloodstream.

Biomarkers can be used in one of the following ways:

1.   As a diagnostic test to differentiate between affected and non-affected joints/ animals.

2.   As a prognostic test to identify joints/animals likely to show rapid progression or to predict response to therapy.

3.   As an evaluative test to assess the severity, monitor change in disease status, or monitor response to therapy.

Cartilage Degradation Markers

AGGRECAN ASSAYS

Sulfated glycosaminoglycan (sGAG)—this is typically measured with a biochemical assay that uses the dimetylmethylene blue (DMMB). This assay identifies all sGAGs present in synovial fluid, regardless of their origin.

Chondroitin sulfate (CS)—by-products of aggrecan degradation have been measured, including proteoglycan fragments that contain "epitopes" that allow for their immunologic detection with antibodies. Antibodies have been developed to recognize both native epitopes in chondroitin sulfate and neoepitopes (new epitopes) created by the digestion of CS with enzymes. There has been little work done with these in horses.

Keratan sulfate (KS)—conflicting reports have been published concerning the relationship of KS in equine body fluids and joint disease. In a study in our laboratory, it was not useful.

Aggrecan core protein—antibodies have been developed against native epitopes in the protein core of aggrecan and against neoepitopes created by the digestion of the aggrecan core matrix, metalloproteinases (MMPs), and aggrecanases. Both of these enzymes are involved in the metabolic turnover of aggrecan in health and disease.

COLLAGEN ASSAYS

Cleaved Type II Collagen—initial degradation of fibrillar collagens occurs as a result of the action of collagenases. This digestion results in two collagen fragments of ¾ and ¼ length with newly created ends at the cleavage site. The COL2-¾Cshort antibody recognizes collagenase-cleaved fragments of both Type I and Type II collagen so is not specific to cartilage collagen. However, an antibody named 2¾CEQ has been developed in our laboratory that is specific for the collagenase-cleaved ¾ fragments of Type II collagen of the horse, and preliminary studies suggest that it may prove useful in assaying equine body fluids for abnormalities in Type II collagen turnover, as may occur in osteochondrosis.

Collagen cross-links—although mature collagen molecules possess cross-links that provide cohesiveness and stability to the collagenous framework, with collagen degradation, these cross-links are released from the tissue. Although pyridinolone (PYD) cross-links predominate in cartilage, because they are major cross-links in all connective tissues, they do not provide specificity as a cartilage degradation marker. Another pyridinium crosslink called dioxypyridinolone (DPYD) is found in small amounts in mineralized tissue and will be described below as a marker of bone collagen degradation.

Cartilage Synthesis Markers

COLLAGEN ASSAYS

Type II procollagen peptide—Type II collagen is secreted by chondrocytes as individual procollagen chains that are further processed after triple helix formation by the enzymatic cleavage of the propeptides of both ends of the procollagen chain. It has been shown that the rate of release of the propeptide at the carboxi-terminus, the C-propeptide, is proportional to the rate of Type II collagen synthesis. We have seen increased levels of this C-propeptide in both synovial fluid and serum of horses with osteochondral fragmentation and also in the synovial fluids and sera of horses with osteochondrosis. We also showed a direct relationship between the levels of CPII and the severity of disease.

AGGRECAN ASSAYS

Chondroitin sulfate—large, newly synthesized aggrecan molecules have an epitope called 846 that can be measured to monitor aggrecan synthesis. This epitope progressively disappears from cartilage with aging, but reappears in joints with osteoarthritis. In horses with osteochondral fragmentation, significantly higher synovial fluid and serum levels of the 846 epitope were found compared with control horses.

Bone Degradation Markers

Bone markers have been found useful in diagnosis of osteochondrosis, as well as predicting progression and monitoring response to treatment. Bone markers may also be important in assessing bone remodeling in training, identifying abnormalities in the bones of exercising horses before they progress into potentially serious injuries, such as fractures.

COLLAGEN ASSAYS

Cleaved Type II Collagen—the COL2¾Cshort antibody recognizes collagenase-cleaved fragments of both Type I and Type II collagen, so it is not specific to bone collagen, but when this antibody is used in combination with the previously described 2¾CEQ antibody that is specific for equine Type II collagen, a clear picture emerges in the relative breakdown of Type I collagen. Its use in equine studies has been restricted to measurement of serum levels in foals predisposed to osteochondrosis, where significantly increased levels of Type I collagen and less Type II collagen turnover during the first five months of life in those foals occurred when they had more severe or more numerous OCD lesions.

Collagen cross-links—the DPYD cross-links are almost exclusively found in bone, and may therefore be the best cross-link to monitor bone turnover. They have not been very rewarding in the horse. Another product of Type I collagen degradation are the cross-linked ends or "telopeptides" that can be measured in serum by using commercially available immunoassays. An assay for the carboxy-terminal link telopeptide of Type I collagen (ICTP) has been used in equine studies to show that serum ICTP levels decrease with age and differ between breeds. Increased levels have been reported in horses with DOD compared with age-matched controls.

Another cross-link assay that can be used in horses is the C-telopeptide cross-link (CTx) assay. Unlike most other bone markers, serum CTx levels appear to increase in foals with increasing age. More studies that assay CTx levels need to be performed in the horse to determine its value as a biomarker of joint disease.

Non-collagenous protein assays—potential non-collagenous protein markers of bone degradation exist, including bone sialoprotein (BSP) and tartrate-resistant acid phosophotase (TRAP), but no assays are currently available for their detection in the horse.

Bone Synthesis Markers

COLLAGEN ASSAYS

Type I procollagen propeptide—as with Type II collagen, Type I procollagen of bone also possesses propeptides that are cleaved and released from the collagen molecules upon fibril formation. Assays exist for both the N-terminal (PINP) and C-terminal (PICP) propeptides, but only the latter is currently applicable to horses. Serum PICP levels decrease with age and increase with exercise. Reduced serum levels were detected in horses with DOD compared with age-matched controls.

NON-COLLAGENOUS PROTEIN ASSAYS

Bone-specific alkaline phosphatase—as with PICP, an inverse relationship exists between age and the serum levels of bone-specific alkaline phosophotase (BALP) in the horse, and serum levels increase with exercise. Higher levels have been reported in clinically affected OA joints than the contralateral control joints with a strong positive correlation between BALP levels and the degree of articular cartilage damage.

Osteocalcin—osteocalcin is also produced by the osteoblasts and is an accepted marker of bone formation. Preliminary studies in osteochondrosis and osteochondral fragmentation suggest limited value in these conditions.

Use of Markers to Aid in Diagnosis of Early Joint Disease

CS 846 and CP-II were shown to be of use in diagnosing osteochondral damage in the horse (Frisbie et al., AJVR 1999). Synovial fluid and serum concentrations were evaluated in 38 horses with unilateral carpal osteochondral fragmentation, compared to 25 unaffected joints and also fluids from normal control horses. Synovial fluid marker changes with OCF included the total protein being significantly higher, the CS-846 being significantly higher, CP-II not being significantly higher (p=.06), keratan sulfate being not significantly higher (p=.28), and white blood cell count being not significantly higher. There was a significant linear increase with grade of fragmentation in both total protein and CS-846 and no significant increase in CP-II or KS. With serum markers, CS-846 and CP-II were both significantly higher, but KS was still not significantly higher. It was concluded that CS-846 and CP-II were useful markers in synovial fluid and serum, and that using these markers predicted the presence or absence of OCF in 80% of cases.

ALTERATIONS IN SERUM BIOMARKERS IN EQUINE
OSTEOCHONDROSIS

Looking at osteochondrosis foals from zero to five months compared with foals with low scores, they have high levels of CP-II, high levels of COL2¾Cshort and lower levels of 2¾CEQ (Billinghurst et al., AJVR 2001).

Use of Markers in In-Vitro Studies

We have used markers to monitor degradation in IL-1/cartilage explant systems (Billinghurst et al., 1999). Articular cartilage degradation was inhibited by an MMP-inhibitor. A concentration of 100nM decreased collagenase-cleaved Type 2 collagen fragment generation and release, decreased proteoglycan release, and increased proteoglycan synthesis and DNA content.

Use of Markers to Distinguish Effects of Exercise versus Pathologic Change During Exercise

In this study, a number of synovial fluid and serum markers were assessed in a group of horses exercised on a treadmill, compared to a group of horses with osteoarthritis exercised on a treadmill. Levels of bone markers were higher in serum than synovial fluid samples, whereas the level of articular cartilage markers was higher in synovial fluid than in serum.   In osteoarthritis, cartilage metabolism preceded bone metabolism based on biomarker results. There was significant correlation between articular cartilage bone markers in the clinical examination, as well as gross and histologic changes of articular cartilage. The level of biomarkers was higher as a result of OA compared to exercise. This increase was seen in all bone markers except serum CTx-I and 2¾CEQ (Al-Soyabil F. Ph.D. Dissertation, Colorado State University, 2002).

Use of Markers in Detection of Osteomyelitis

Biomarkers seem to be of potential value in differentiating infected nonunion and aseptic nonunion fractures (Southwood et al., 2003).

References

Billinghurst RC. Biomarkers of joint disease.   In Robinson EW (ed) Current
    Equine Therapy: 513-520.
Billinghurst RC, Buckston EM, Edwards MG, McGraw BS, McIlwraith CW. Use
    of an antineoepitope antibody for identification of Type II collagen
    degradation in articular cartilage. Am J Vet Res 2001; 62: 1031-1039.
Billinghurst RC, O'Brien K, Poole AR, McIlwraith CW. Inhibition of articular
    cartilage degradation in culture by a novel, non-peptitic matrix
    metalloproteinase inhibitor. Inhabition of matrix metalloproteinases. New
    York Acad Sci 1999; 878: 594-597.
Brown NAT, Kawcak CE, Pandy MG, McIlwraith CW. Moment arms of muscles
    about the carpo- and metacarpophalangeal joints in the equine forelimb.
    Am J Vet Res 2003; 64: 351-358.
Firth EC, van Weeren PR, Pfeiffer DU et al. Effective age, exercise and growth
    rate on bone mineral density (BMD) in third carpal bone in distal radius of
    Dutch Warmblood foals with osteochondrosis. Equine Vet J: Supplement
    1999; 31: 74-78.
Frisbie DD, Ray CS, Ionescu M, Poole AR, Chapman DL, McIlwraith CW.
    Measurement of synovial fluid in serum concentrations of the 846 epitope
    of chondroitin sulfate and of carboxipropeptides of Type II procollagen
    for diagnosis of osteochondral fragmentation in horses. Am J Vet Res 1999;
    60: 306-309.
Kawcak CE, McIlwraith CW, Norrdin RW, Park RD, James SP. The role of
    subchondral bone in joint disease: A review. Equine Vet J 2001; 33: 120-
    126.
Kawcak CE, McIlwraith CW, Norrdin RW, Park RD, Stein PS. Clinical effects
    of exercise on subchondral bone of carpo- and metacarpophalangeal joints

in horses. Am J Vet Res 2000; 61: 1252-1258.

Lepage OM, Carstanjen B, Uebelhart D. Non-invasive assessment of equine bone: An update. Equine Vet J 2001; 161:10-22.

Price JS, Jackson BF, Grey JA, Paris PA et al. Biochemical markers of bone metabolism in growing Thoroughbreds: A longitudinal study. Research Vet Science 2001; 71: 37-44.

Ray CS, Poole AR, McIlwraith CW. Use of synovial fluid and serum markers in articular disease. In: McIlwraith CW, Trotter GW (eds): Joint Disease in the Horse, Philadelphia, WB Saunders 1996.

Southwood LL, Kawcak CE, McIlwraith CW, Frisbie DD. Evaluation of serum biochemical markers of bone metabolism for early diagnosis of non-union and infected non-union fractures in rabbits. Am J Vet Res 2003; 64: 727-735.

Southwood LL, Kawcak CE, McIlwraith CW, Stein P, Frisbie DD. Use of scintigraphy for assessment of fracture healing and early diagnosis of osteomyelitis following fracture repair in rabbits. Am J Vet Res 2003; 64: 736-745.

SURGICAL AND MEDICAL MANAGEMENT OF OSTEOCHONDRITIS DISSECANS (OCD)

C. WAYNE MCILWRAITH
Colorado State University, Fort Collins, Colorado, USA

Introduction

Osteochondritis dissecans (OCD) is an important entity within the developmental orthopedic disease complex. It is a frequent cause of lameness in young athletic horses and is the most frequent condition of the complex requiring surgical intervention. OCD has been classically considered as a manifestation of osteochondrosis (McIlwraith, 1993b). Rejno and Stromberg described the first stage of osteochondrosis as a disturbance of cellular differentiation in the growing cartilage, and the second as involving necrosis of the basal layers of the thickened retained cartilage with subsequent pressure and strain within the joint, giving rise to fissures in the damaged cartilage (1978). The terms osteochondrosis, osteochondritis dissecans, and osteochondrosis dissecans have been regularly used as synonyms, and their meaning is still somewhat controversial. The terms have been distinguished as follows: osteochondrosis is the disease, osteochondritis is the inflammatory response to the disease, and OCD is the condition in which a flap can be demonstrated (Poulos, 1986). This is a simple but fairly appropriate representation. This presentation addresses the clinical aspects of OCD, including the clinical signs and diagnosis, as well as treatment options and prognosis. Although arthroscopic surgery is the most commonly recommended treatment to achieve athletic activity and prevent degenerative joint disease, certain situations in which conservative treatment is successful have been recognized.

Three categories of OCD lesions are recognized: (1) those showing clinical and radiographic signs, (2) those showing clinical without radiographic (but arthroscopic) signs, and (3) those showing radiographic but no clinical signs. Data from the first two categories of disease have been tabulated for the most commonly selected joints from the author's surgical case reports (McIlwraith, 1993a). The relative incidence of clinical signs versus radiographic lesions has also been documented in the femoropatellar joint by McIntosh and McIlwraith (1993). Similar data in other joints are needed.

The clinical aspects of OCD are presented next for the individual joints in which OCD is most common.

Osteochondritis Dissecans of the Femoropatellar Joint

OCD was first described in the femoropatellar joint in the horse by Nilsson in 1947 (Nilsson, 1947). The lesion described by Nilsson is believed to be similar to lesions currently referred to as OCD. Similar lesions were described as osteochondral fractures in 1973 (O'Brien, 1973). Since that time there have been a number of reports concerning pathologic and surgical aspects of the condition (Moore and McIlwraith, 1977; Wyburn, 1977; Rejno, 1978; Stromberg and Rejno, 1978; Trotter et al., 1983; Pascoe et al., 1984; McIlwraith and Martin, 1985; Foland et al., 1992; McIlwraith, 1987; Wright and Pickles, 1991). The clinical signs have been well defined, but the treatment is more controversial. The femoropatellar joint is one of the principal sites of OCD in the horse.

INCIDENCE AND CLINICAL SIGNS

In a recent study, more than 50% of the horses operated upon for femoropatellar OCD were Thoroughbreds (Table 1) (Foland et al., 1992). There were 53 females in the same group and 108 males (82 intact and 26 gelded). The age distribution of 161 horses presented for femoropatellar OCD is presented in Table 2.

Table 1. Breed disposition of 161 horses operated on for femoropatellar osteochondritis dissecans (Foland et al., 1992).

Breed	Number	Percentage
Thoroughbred	82	50.9
Quarter Horse	39	24.2
Arabian	16	9.9
Warmblood	9	5.6
Crossbred	5	3.1
Paint Horse	3	1.9
Appaloosa	3	1.9
Other	4	2.5

Table 2. Age distribution of 161 horses presented for femoropatellar osteochondritis dissecans (Foland et al., 1992).

Age (Years)	Number	Percentage
<1	22	13.7
1	68	42.2
2	36	22.4
3	21	13.0
≥4	14	8.7

Approximately 55% of the horses were 1 year of age or less at presentation, and the younger animals tended to have more severe lesions (Foland et al., 1992).

Clinical signs may develop at any age. More mature animals frequently present with a sudden onset of clinical signs thought to be associated with the displacement of osteochondral fragments. Less frequently, clinically silent lesions may be identified in mature horses, and a sudden onset of clinical signs may also occasionally be seen in cases in which fragmentation has not yet developed. In one study on one farm, the average age of identification of femoropatellar OCD problems was 12.6, 9, and 6 months in 3 consecutive years (McIntosh and McIlwraith, 1993).

Horses with OCD of the femoropatellar joint usually present with differing degrees of distension of the femoropatellar joint and differing degrees of lameness, depending on the severity of the lesions. Distension of the femoropatellar joint is the more consistent presenting sign. However, the clinicopathologic changes in the synovial fluid are usually minor. Lameness varies from nondiscernible to severe. Other common abnormalities of gait include reduced cranial phase to the stride and lowered foot arc. In young animals with severe lesions, there may be difficulty in rising. Concurrent flexural deformities have also been reported (Moore, 1977; McIlwraith and Martin, 1985). Lateral luxation of the patella in association with OCD of the lateral trochlear ridge of the femur has been seen (McIlwraith, 1987). Unilaterally affected animals are often asymmetrically muscled, whereas bilateral cases frequently exhibit poor hind limb muscle development (Wright and Pickles, 1991). The disease is commonly bilateral. In one recent series, 91 horses (57%) were bilaterally affected and 70 horses (43%) had unilateral disease (Foland et al., 1992).

Lateromedial radiographs provide the most useful information with regard to the location and nature of the lesions. Caudolateral to craniomedial oblique projections may also provide additional information with regard to the depth of the lesion on the lateral trochlear ridge of the femur. The most common defect seen radiographically is an irregularity or flattening in the subchondral bone of the lateral trochlear ridge of the femur that may be localized or generalized. In either situation, the area of the lateral trochlear ridge that articulates with the distal aspect of the patella in the standing position is involved. Lesions manifesting as defects on radiographs usually manifest with an OCD flap or elevated cartilage. Partially mineralized flaps may be observed radiographically in some instances. There are islands of mineralized tissue in other defects. Mineralized free bodies or joint mice that have detached from the primary defect may be present loose within the joint or attached to synovial membrane. The presence of irregular subchondral defects without joint mice tends to be seen in younger horses. Cystic lesions and undermined lytic lesions within the subchondral bone are observed in other instances. Similar lesions may be seen on the medial trochlear ridge but are usually limited to irregularities of contour and are not as extensive. In a number of instances, a separation of cartilage from the medial trochlear ridge without any defect in the subchondral bone (and therefore no radiographic signs) is seen at surgery. Primary OCD of the patella is relatively rare but is seen in some instances. Articular cartilage degenerative changes may be seen secondary to severe OCD of the lateral trochlear ridge of the femur (usually on the lateral facet of patella). In severe cases of OCD of the trochlear ridges, remodeling of the patellar contour may be visible. Localized defects of the patellar contour visualized on radiographs may represent primary osteochondrosis or secondary changes. Care must be taken not to diagnose the radiographic changes of endochondral ossification on the trochlear ridges of young foals as OCD lesions (Adams and Thilsted, 1985).

The most common location for OCD lesions is the lateral trochlear ridge of the femur. The overall incidence in a series of cases (Foland et al., 1992) is presented in Table 3. Thirty-two horses had loose bodies in at least one joint in this series. Grades as determined from surgery reports were equal to the radiographic grades in 111 cases, but at surgery 46 horses had lesions that were worse than those seen radiographically. In a related study, the radiographs of 72 femoropatellar and femorotibial joints from 50 horses that had arthroscopic surgery were evaluated (Steinheimer et al., 1996). Ninety-four arthroscopically evaluated areas were graded according to a predetermined system (based on surgery reports).

Table 3. Location of osteochondritis dissecans lesions in 252 femoropatellar joints (Foland et al., 1992).

Location	No. of joints affected
LTR	161
LTR and patella	31
MTR	17
LTR and MTR	17
LTR, patella and TG	4
LTR, MTR and patella	3
MTR and patella	3
Patella	3
LTR, MTR, TG and patella	3
LTR and TG	3
LTR, MTR and TG	3
MTR and TG	3
TG	1

LTR = lateral trochlear ridge; MTR = medial trochlear ridge ; TG = trochlear groove.

The radiographic grade was then compared with arthroscopic findings in the same location and statistical analysis performed to determine the association between radiographic subchondral bone changes and arthroscopic findings. Radiographically normal areas in the femoropatellar joint were arthroscopically positive for cartilaginous changes in 40% of the femoropatellar joints. Areas of mild subchondral bone flattening (grade I) in the lateral trochlear ridge of the femur were arthroscopically positive for cartilage changes 78% of the time. Ninety-six percent of moderate to severe subchondral bone changes (grades II to V) were arthroscopically positive for cartilage damage. This research demonstrated that (1) a significant number of radiographically normal joints have cartilage changes, (2) areas of mild subchondral bone flattening have cartilage changes in most cases, and (3) areas of moderate to severe subchondral bone change have arthroscopically detectable cartilage changes.

Lesions of OCD in joints other than the femoropatellar joint may occur at the same time. In the previously mentioned series of 161 horses, 10 horses underwent surgery for other OCD lesions at the time of the femoropatellar arthroscopy (Foland et al., 1992). Five had OCD of both metatarsophalangeal joints, four had OCD of the tarsocrural joint, and one had OCD of the scapulohumeral joint. Two other horses had subchondral cystic lesions of the medial femoral condyle.

TREATMENT

Conflicting reports have been published concerning the management of OCD of the equine femoropatellar joint. In 1977, Wyburn reported that satisfactory results were achieved with conservative therapy if osteochondral fragments were not seen radiographically, but that surgery was indicated if free bodies were noted (Wyburn, 1977). However, two later reports showed that at surgery fragments that could not be detected radiographically were often found (Pasco et al., 1984; McIlwraith, 1985). Another group of authors also felt that 54% of horses with stifle problems (OCD of the femoropatellar joint and subchondral cystic lesions of the femorotibial joint were not distinguished) were improved after conservative therapy (Rose et al., 1985), but an examination shows the results to be inferior to those reported with surgery (Foland et al., 1992). Stromberg and Rejno reported radiographic evidence that young horses that had large subchondral defects and were not treated surgically developed degenerative joint disease (1978). Steenhaut et al. also considered the outcome without surgical treatment to be poor (1982). Favorable results after surgical treatment using arthrotomy have been reported (Stromberg and Rejno, 1978; Pasco et al., 1984). The advantages of using arthroscopic surgery to treat femoropatellar OCD are now well recognized, and the results of surgery with this technique have been published (McIlwraith, 1985; Foland et al., 1992; Martin and McIlwraith, 1985).

More recent work indicates that conservative treatment can be appropriate in some instances. A recent study demonstrated considerable success in Thoroughbreds (based on subsequent racing performance) with conservative treatments. In this study a careful assessment of foals led to the detection of lesions at an early age, and it was concluded that with confinement early radiographic lesions of OCD (subchondral bone contour irregularity and subchondral lysis) are potentially reversible. On a farm affected with a high incidence of femoropatellar OCD, three crops of foals were evaluated. Of 11 horses not operated on in 1989 (some other horses were operated on), 6 raced, 3 had no follow-up, 1 became a jumper, and 1 was operated on later. In 1990, 9 foals with clinical and radiographic lesions of OCD were treated conservatively; at the time of the report, 2 had raced, 2 were still unraced, 3 had lameness, and 2 were used for nonracing careers. In 1991, 10 cases were diagnosed (5 horses had no radiographic lesions initially but subsequently developed them, and 1 never had a radiographic lesion but had persistent synovial effusion). Of these 16, 4 horses were sold as yearlings, reportedly without synovial effusion or lameness, 1 died of unrelated causes, 10 are currently racing or training, and 1 subsequently developed OCD of the metatarsophalangeal joints. There was a trend in these data to indicate that lesser lesions healed with conservative treatment and more severe ones persisted in having clinical signs. There were two exceptions (successful results when the lesion was large) to this rule.

A case can be made for arthroscopy in all cases in that unsuspected intra-articular pathologic changes are often found, and early management of these problems can be instituted. It has been stated that once a radiographic diagnosis of OCD has been made in humans, arthroscopic staging of the disease and treatment are the next logical steps and that conservative treatment by casting, immobilization, and limitations of activities (particularly in children) should be tried initially before resorting to surgery (Ewing and Voto, 1988). It was noted that it is still difficult to predict when a lesion will heal and when a lesion will persist, particularly if arthroscopy is not done (Ewing and Voto, 1988). If conservative treatment is to be attempted, restriction of exercise with confinement is the critical factor. Restricted activity is the basis for the conservative management of human juvenile OCD but is not consistently successful (Aglietti et al., 1994).

The treatment of femoropatellar OCD with arthroscopic surgery has been extensively described elsewhere (Martin and McIlwraith, 1985; McIlwraith and Martin, 1985; McIlwraith, 1990; Foland et al., 1992).

Evaluation of the lesion in the joint is carried out thoroughly as not all lesions are detected radiographically, and each lesion is assessed with a probe. Elevators are used to separate OCD flaps. The flaps are generally removed with rongeurs, and the underlying lesions are debrided with curets, motorized equipment, or both. Loose bodies are also removed. Debridement of all pathologic tissue is necessary.

The results of arthroscopic surgery for the treatment of OCD of the femoropatellar joint have been reported in 252 femoropatellar joints in 161 horses (Foland et al., 1992). Follow-up information was obtained on 134 horses, including 79 racehorses and 55 nonracehorses. Eighty-six (64%) of these 134 horses returned to their intended use, 9 (7%) were in training, 21 (16%) were unsuccessful, and 18 (13%) were unsuccessful because of other defined reasons. Of the 18 horses that were unsuccessful because of other reasons, 14 developed unassociated lameness (10 forelimb and 4 hindlimb), 1 died of colic, 1 became a wobbler, 1 developed a fatal case of enteritis, and 1 died under anesthesia during surgery for an unrelated problem in another clinic. The time from surgery until the horses started training was dictated in many cases by the age of the horse. Those horses that had already performed or trained before surgery returned to training 4 to 6 months after surgery. Sufficient follow-up was available for 11 of the 12 horses that had surgery for OCD in other joints at the time of femoropatellar surgery. Six of these horses (55%) were successful, 3 (27%) were unsuccessful, and 2 (18%) were unsuccessful because of other reasons.

There was a significant effect of lesion size on prognosis. Horses with grade 1 lesions (<2 cm in length) had a significantly higher success rate (78%) than horses with grade 2 (2 to 4 cm) or grade 3 (>4 cm) lesions (63 and 54% success rates, respectively) (Foland et al., 1992). A significantly higher success was also noted for horses operated on at 3 years compared with the remainder of the study population. A significantly lower success rate was noted for yearlings than for the remainder of the population. It was felt that the lowest success rate in horses operated on as yearlings is probably associated with the fact that more severe lesions occurred in the yearling horses (16% grade I, 13% grade II, 46% grade III) and less severe lesions occurred in the 3-year-old group (52% grade I, 38% grade II, 10% grade III). There was no significant difference in outcome related to the sex of the animal involved; racehorse versus nonracehorse; the lesion location; unilateral versus bilateral involvement; the presence or absence of patellar or trochlear groove lesions; or the presence or absence of loose bodies.

Although the results of this study may at first seem somewhat discouraging in that only 64% of the horses returned to or achieved the intended level of performance, many of these horses were operated on at relatively young ages and consequently had not yet proved themselves as athletes (over 50% were 1 year of age or younger). A study on racing performance in Thoroughbreds born in 1984 indicated that approximately 60% of all named foals should start a race (Dink, 1990). The inclusion of only named foals (registered with The Jockey Club) would exclude those that showed no potential or developed other problems at a young age and were consequently not registered. In our study, many of the horses had surgery before they were named, and this led us to believe that a 64% success rate is comparable with successful performance in the normal population of racing Thoroughbreds (Foland et al., 1992).

Although a permanent clinical cure can often be associated with surgery, limited data show that the nature of the healing tissue is different from that of normal osteochondral tissue (McIlwraith, 1990) on the basis of long-term follow-up radiographs of sound horses operated on by the author. Irregular subchondral contours frequently persist, and this suggests that subchondral bone remodeling does not take place in the femoral trochlear ridges. In humans, OCD may affect the trochlear ridges but more commonly affects the femoral condyles (Smith, 1990). Surgical treatments include the removal of flaps, drilling through the lesion into bone, and fixation of the flap (Ewing and Voto, 1988; Smith, 1990; Aglietti et al., 1994).

Osteochondritis Dissecans of the Femorotibial Joints

Subchondral cystic lesions are the most common developmental orthopedic disease involving the femoral condyles. However, cases of OCD of the femoral condyles have been encountered. Lesions of OCD may accompany subchondral cystic lesions or occur on their own (most commonly in Thoroughbreds). The lesions manifest radiographically as an irregular defect in the subchondral bone, best seen on a flexed lateral view. They appear arthroscopically as typical OCD lesions and have responded to surgical treatment. A series of lesions of the femoral condyle, some of which may be lesions of osteochondrosis, was also recently reported. Because these cases have been recognized infrequently, figures for prognosis do not exist.

Osteochondritis Dissecans of the Tibiotarsal (Tarsocrural) Joint

OCD of the tarsocrural joint was first described in the horse in 1972 (DeMoor, 1972). Before this, however, seven cases of a condition that appears identical to OCD were described by Birkeland and Haakenstad as intracapsular bony fragments of the distal tibia (1968). These authors later described the lesions as OCD (Birkeland and Haakenstad, 1974). In 1978 Stromberg and Rejno also reported OCD lesions in 61 tarsocrural joints in 49 horses (Stromberg and Rejno, 1978). There have been a number of recent reports documenting the incidence, clinical signs, and results of treatment of OCD of the tarsocrural joint (Hoppe, 1984a,b; Sandgren, 1988; Alvarado, 1989; Grondahl, 1991; McIlwraith et al., 1991; Carlsten et al., 1993; Laws et al., 1993; Beard et al., 1994).

INCIDENCE, CLINICAL SIGNS, AND DIAGNOSIS

OCD of the tarsocrural joint is seen most frequently in Standardbred horses (Birkeland and Haakenstad, 1968, 1974; DeMoor, 1972; Stromberg and Rejno, 1978; Hoppe, 1984a,b; Sandgren, 1988; Alvarado, 1989; Grondahl, 1991; McIlwraith et al., 1991; Carlsten et al., 1993). In the largest series of clinical cases published to date, 154 of 225 horses were intended for racing (106 Standardbreds, 30 Thoroughbreds, 18 Quarter Horses), and the remaining 71 comprised 20 Arabians, 18 Quarter Horses, 13 warmbloods, 4 American Saddlebreds, 4 Appaloosas, 4 Thoroughbreds, 3 draft horses (1 Clydesdale, 1 Percheron, 1 Shire), 2 American Paint Horses, 1 Morgan, 1 National Show Horse, and 1 Lipizzaner (McIlwraith, 1991).

The presenting clinical signs were synovial effusion of the tarsocrural (tibiotarsal) joint and lameness. Synovial effusion of the joint is the most common reason for cases being presented, particularly in animals presented before being put into training. Obvious lameness is often not observed. Older horses (>2 years) or racehorses may be presented for lameness. Of 303 joints with tarsocrural OCD in which the presence or absence of synovial effusion was recorded, synovial effusion was the presenting clinical sign in 261 joints (86.1%) (McIlwraith, 1991). In racehorses, effusion was present in 166 joints (81%) and absent in 39 joints. In nonracehorses, effusion was present in 95 joints (96.9%) and absent in 3 joints. The degree of lameness was not recorded consistently but was usually designated as mild. The exception was when severe lesions were present on the lateral trochlear ridge of the talus (lesions involving the entire visible portion of the lateral trochlear ridge of the talus when viewed arthroscopically in the flexed position). Racehorses presented most often at 2 years of age, having trained or raced, whereas nonracehorses presented most often as yearlings before training (Table 4) (McIlwraith, 1991). The age range was from yearling or less up to 14 years of age. Lesions of OCD of the distal articular surface of the tibia have been reported at postmortem in a 3-day-old foal euthanized for neonatal maladjustment syndrome (Rejno and Stromberg, 1978).

Table 4. Age of racehorses and nonracehorses at time of presentation with tarsocrural osteochondritis dissecans (McIlwraith et al., 1991).

Type	Age (years)	Number	Percentage
Racehorse	1	34	22.1
	2	68	44.2
	3	36	23.4
	4	8	5.2
	5	4	2.6
	6	1	0.6
	7	2	1.3
	9	1	0.6
Nonracehorse	1	33	46.5
	2	18	25.3
	3	6	8.5
	4	6	8.5
	5	1	1.4
	7	1	1.4
	8	1	1.4
	9	1	1.4
	10	1	1.4
	13	2	2.8
	14	1	1.4

The radiographic manifestations depend on the location of the lesions. In a series of 318 joints, lesions were seen most frequently in the intermediate ridge of the distal tibia, followed by the lateral trochlear ridge of the talus and the medial malleolus, respectively (Table 5) (McIlwraith, 1991). Lesions were also seen in multiple sites in 22 joints, and loose bodies were present in eight joints. Five of these had separated from intermediate ridge lesions, and three had separated from lateral trochlear ridge lesions. The lesions on the distal intermediate ridge of the tibia commonly consist of separation of a bony fragment from the dorsal aspect of the intermediate ridge and are best demonstrated on the dorsomedial-plantarolateral oblique radiograph. OCD lesions of the intermediate ridge of the tibia have been rated on a scale of 0 to 5, according to the defects and the presence and size of the fragments within them (Hoppe, 1984b). Most of the author's surgical cases are either grade 4 or grade 5 (some grade 3) with this classification, and Hoppe grade 1 and 2 lesions (defect but no fragment) are rare, at least in cases with clinical signs. In a separate study, intermediate ridge lesions were classified into three sizes to evaluate the possibility that the size of the fragment affects the prognosis (McIlwraith, 1991). Fragment size did not influence prognosis, and the usefulness of such a grading system is questionable. Lesions on the lateral trochlear ridge are best demonstrated with dorsomedial-plantarolateral oblique radiographs.

Table 5. Location of osteochondritis dissecans lesions in 318 tarsocrural joints (McIlwraith et al., 1991).

No. of joints	Location
244	Intermediate ridge (dorsal aspect) of distal tibia
37	Lateral trochlear ridge of talus
12	Medial malleolus (dorsal aspect) of tibia
11	Intermediate ridge of tibia plus lateral trochlear ridge of talus
4	Intermediate ridge plus medial malleolus of tibia
3	Intermediate ridge plus medial trochlear ridge of talus
3	Medial trochlear ridge of talus
3	Lateral trochlear ridge of talus plus medial malleolus of tibia
1	Lateral and medial trochlear ridge of talus
Total 318	

The lesions may consist of areas of lucency in the bone with or without osseous flaps or fragments visible on the radiographs. Loose bodies may be quite remote and on the medial side of the joint. Radiographs may not accurately depict the amount of articular cartilage dissection extending beyond the subchondral bone defect in some lateral trochlear ridge lesions (McIlwraith, 1991). Lesions of the medial malleolus of the tibia may be demonstrated with a dorsoplantar or dorsolateral-plantaromedial oblique radiograph. These lesions are depicted relatively accurately by radiographs. Lesions of the trochlear ridge of the talus may be demonstrated with dorsolateral-plantaromedial oblique or lateromedial radiographs.

A longitudinal study of 77 Standardbred foals examined and radiographed six times from birth to the age of 16 months provides information on the timing of the development of radiographic lesions (Sandgren, 1988). Eight horses (10.4%) showed lesions of OCD in the tarsocrural joints at the age of 12 months (considered to have permanent OCD). These eight horses all showed abnormal ossification and/or OCD before 3 months of age, and in four of these the lesions were present before 1 month of age. At the sites of predilection for hock OCD the authors also recognized abnormal endochondral ossification of the subchondral bone that reverted to normal in 11 other horses. All of these were radiographically normal after the examination at 7 or 8 months, and there were no other lesions at examination at 16 months. In another study in Norway, radiographs were taken of the tarsocrural joints in 753 Norwegian Standardbred trotters, all yearlings (Grondahl, 1991). OCD lesions of the intermediate ridge of the distal tibia and/or the lateral trochlear ridge of the talus were diagnosed in 108 (14.3%) horses. The lesional changes were bilateral in 49 (45.4%) affected horses. Radiographs were repeated in 79 horses after 6 to 18 months and revealed OCD in only one additional joint. No clinical evaluation was reported in this latter study.

Lesions that were not apparent on radiographs may also be identified during arthroscopy. In one study, in 13 joints OCD lesions were present at arthroscopy without being identified by radiographic examination (McIlwraith, 1991). In four of these cases, there was synovial effusion without radiographic change in the joint contralateral to the one with the radiographic lesion (three on the distal intermediate ridge and one on the medial malleolus). In nine other cases, the lesions (four medial malleolus, three lateral trochlear ridge, and two medial trochlear ridge) were found during arthroscopy of a joint with other radiographically apparent lesions. Loose bodies were detected by different radiographic views, depending on their location. It is also important to recognize that OCD can be diagnosed frequently on radiographs when no clinical signs are present (Hoppe, 1984a; Sandgren, 1988; Alvarado et al., 1989; Grondahl, 1990; Carlsten et al., 1993). Distinction of these cases from ones with clinical signs is important when assessing the need for surgery or the results of conservative treatment (Hoppe, 1984a; Alvarado et al., 1989; Carlsten et al., 1993; Laws et al., 1993; Beard et al., 1994).

In hocks, observable radiographic changes that are not lesions of OCD include spurs or fragments (dewdrop lesions) of the distal end of the medial trochlear ridge of the talus, an irregularly shaped depression (synovial fossa) in the central region of the intertrochlear groove of the talus, and a degree of flattening of the medial trochlear ridge centrally that may be seen particularly in heavy horses (Shelley and Dyson, 1984). Separated OCD fragments can occasionally lodge in the proximal intertarsal joint.

TREATMENT

The need for surgery on individual cases of OCD of the tarsocrural joint is still questioned by some, but the literature supports a surgical approach (Birkeland and Haakenstad, 1968; DeMoor et al., 1972; Stromberg and Rejno, 1978; McIlwraith, 1991). In a study comparing 25 horses treated conservatively with 23 horses operated on with arthrotomy, it was concluded that lesions of the hock were of clinical significance and that surgical removal of the fragment seemed to give a better result than conservative treatment (Stromberg and Rejno, 1978). Hoppe found that horses affected with OCD seemed to have a poorer performance capacity than normal horses, but their performance was improved by surgical treatment (1984a). One reason for a discrepancy in opinions is that some radiographic surveys are without any clinical data (Alvarado et al., 1989; Grondahl, 1991).

When clinical signs are present, surgical treatment is preferred, particularly if an athletic career is planned (McIlwraith, 1991). Arthroscopic surgery is used, and follow-up results support its value (McIlwraith, 1991; Beard et al., 1994). It is recognized that some horses have had full athletic careers despite lesions being present radiographically, and it is presumed that the lack of clinical signs is associated with some form of stability between the lesion and parent bone. In contrast, horses often develop problems when in training, and lameness is a factor in many of these cases. Resolution of synovial effusion is also of particular importance to nonracehorse owners. Case selection is important, however. The presence of radiographic changes in the distal tarsal joints (such changes are seen quite often) should be noted when prognosis is discussed. As mentioned above, dewdrop lesions or the presence of calcified fragments at the distal end of the medial trochlear ridge of the talus are not indications for surgery, as they are usually extra-articular. If a free OCD fragment is present in the proximal intertarsal joint, then removal is indicated. Lateral malleolus fragments are usually traumatic in origin and are rarely a manifestation of OCD.

Arthroscopic surgery provides definite advantages over arthrotomy, and techniques have been described extensively elsewhere (Martin and McIlwraith, 1985; McIlwraith, 1991). The overall functional ability and cosmetic appearance of the limbs are excellent. In a study in which postsurgical follow-up was obtained for 183 horses, 140 (76.5%) raced successfully or performed their intended use after surgery (McIlwraith, 1991). Of the remaining 43, 11 were considered to still have a tarsocrural joint problem. Nineteen developed other problems precluding successful performance. Eight were considered poor racehorses without any lameness problems identified, three were killed because of septic arthritis, and two died from other causes. There was no effect of age, sex, or limb involvement on the outcome. The success rate relative to location of the lesion was 139 of 177 (78.5%) for the distal intermediate ridge of the tibia, 24 of 31 (77.4%) for the lateral trochlear ridge of the talus, 7 of 9 (77.8%) for the medial malleolus of the tibia, 3 of 3 (100%) for the medial trochlear ridge of the talus, and 17 of 22 (77.3%) pooled for multiple lesions (no significant differences). The success rate relative to the three size groups for intermediate ridge lesions was 27 of 33 (81.8%) for lesions 1 to 9 mm in width, 86 of 116 (74.1%) for lesions 10 to 19 mm in width, and 41 of 47 (87.2%) for lesions 20 mm or greater in width.

When the success rate was considered relative to the findings of additional lesions at arthroscopy, 16 of 19 (84.2%) with articular cartilage fibrillation, 5 of 10 (50%) with articular cartilage degeneration or erosion, 3 of 5 (60%) with loose fragments, 0 of 2 with proliferative synovitis, and 0 of 1 with joint capsule mineralization were successful. There was a significantly inferior outcome in racehorses with articular cartilage degeneration or erosion (p < 0.05). The presence of articular cartilage fibrillation did not affect the prognosis. The results with proliferative synovitis and joint capsule mineralization were poor, but there were insufficient numbers to determine the significance.

Follow-up data on the degree of synovial effusion resolution were obtained for 217 joints that had effusion preoperatively (McIlwraith, 1991). The synovial effusion resolved in 117 of 131 racehorse joints (89.3%) and 64 of 86 nonracehorse joints (74.4%). Of the 22 nonracehorse joints in which resolution did not occur, the owner calculated that 75% resolution had occurred in 12 and 50% resolution had occurred in another four. The resolution of synovial effusion was also documented relative to the location of the lesion. The outcome for synovial fluid resolution was significantly inferior (p < 0.05) for lesions of the lateral trochlear ridge of the talus or medial malleolus of the tibia compared with lesions of the distal intermediate ridge of the tibia.

There was no relationship between postoperative performance and the resolution of effusion (McIlwraith, 1991). In 165 horses in which effusion was resolved, 141 (85.4%) raced or performed successfully. Of the 30 horses in which effusion was not resolved, 25 (83.3%) raced or performed successfully. Five horses that had OCD in the tarsocrural joint also had proximal plantar lesions of the first phalanx (four had successful results and one was lost to follow-up). Two horses had lesions of the lateral trochlear ridge of the femur (one was successful and one was lost to follow-up). One horse had a proximodorsal lesion of the distal sagittal ridge, and no follow-up was available.

Recently the results of treatment of 64 Thoroughbreds and 45 Standardbred horses treated for OCD of the tarsocrural joint with arthroscopic surgery before 2 years of age were reported, and the results were compared with those of other foals from the dams of the surgically treated horses (siblings) (Bears et al., 1994). Racing data, including the number of starts and money won during the 2 and 3-year-old racing years, were obtained for affected horses and their siblings. Statistical analysis was performed to test the hypothesis that there is no difference between the racing performance of horses with OCD of the tarsocrural joint that have been surgically treated by means of arthroscopic removal of the fragments before racing and that of their siblings. In 109 horses, 174 lesions were recorded. The distribution of lesions was similar to that previously reported (McIlwraith, 1991). For the Standardbreds, 22% of those that had surgery raced as 2-year-olds and 43% raced as 3-year-olds, compared with 42 and 50% of the siblings that raced as 2- and 3-year-olds, respectively. For the Thoroughbreds, 43% of those that had surgery raced as 2-year-olds and 78% raced as 3-year-olds, compared with 48% and 72%

of the siblings that raced as 2- and 3-year-olds, respectively. The median number of starts for surgically treated horses was decreased compared with the median number of starts for siblings for all groups except 3-year-old Thoroughbreds. Median earnings were lower for affected horses than for siblings for both breeds and both age groups. Among affected horses, the ability to start at least one race was not associated with lesion location or unilateral versus bilateral involvement. There was a tendency for horses with multiple lesions to be less likely to start a race than horses with only a single lesion; however, the difference was significant only for 2-year-old Standardbreds. Affected Standardbreds and Thoroughbreds were less likely to race as 2-year-olds than were their siblings (Beard et al., 1994). The authors noted that although the percentage of horses that raced was lower than that previously reported (McIlwraith, 1991), it was inappropriate to compare this study with previous studies because selection criteria and control groups were different and racing performance was not analyzed by year in previous studies. In the previous studies, older horses that had already raced were included. For other performance-limiting injuries such as apical sesamoid fractures, the prognosis after surgical treatment is better for horses that have already proved themselves capable of racing than for horses that have never raced (Spurlock and Gabel, 1983). The authors recognized the stringent definition for outcome in that horses that lived to racing age and did not compete were counted as failures, regardless of whether the reasons the horses did not compete were related or unrelated to the surgery. The authors stated that they currently recommended removal of any osteochondral fragment associated with joint effusion but warned owners that affected foals may already have or may develop other orthopedic conditions that could limit their performance. In another study it was shown that horses treated for osteochondrosis of the cranial intermediate ridge of the tibia performed as well as matched controls (Laws et al., 1993).

Osteochondritis Dissecans of the Metacarpophalangeal and Metatarsophalangeal Joints

There is some divergence of opinion as to what is considered OCD within the fetlock and also those entities that might be considered appropriate to include within developmental orthopedic disease (Yovich et al., 1985; Barclay et al., 1987; Foerner et al., 1987; McIlwraith and Vorhees, 1990; Grondahl, 1992b; McIlwraith, 1993b) The following conditions should be addressed:

1.   *OCD of the dorsal aspect of the distal metacarpus and metatarsus.*

      It is undisputed that this is a manifestation of OCD (Yovich et al., 1985; McIlwraith, 1987; McIlwraith and Vorhees, 1990). The condition was initially described as OCD of the sagittal ridge of the third metacarpal and metatarsal bones (Yovich et al., 1985), but the term has been modified after recognition that the disease process commonly extends onto the condyles of the metacarpus and metatarsus (McIlwraith and Vorhees, 1990). In one radiographic study, OCD changes in the dorsal aspect of the sagittal ridge of the third metacarpus or metatarsus were seen in 118 of 753 yearling Standardbred trotters, with 61 forelimbs and 147 hind limbs affected (Grondahl, 1992b). In a second study in which horses were evaluated and treated on the basis of having clinical signs, the problem was assessed in 65 horses (McIlwraith and Vorhees, 1990). These lesions usually involve the proximal aspect of the distal dorsal metacarpus or metatarsus. In some instances the most distal aspect of the metacarpus or metatarsus is involved (McIlwraith and Vorhees, 1990). When this is the case, the lesion is within the metacarpophalangeal or metatarsophalangeal articulation.

2. *Proximal palmar or plantar first-phalanx fragments.*

Bony fragments associated with the palmar or plantar part of the metacarpo- and metatarsophalangeal joints were first described in 1972 by Birkeland (Birkeland, 1972). Opinions differ as to whether these fragments are the results of fractures (Birkeland, 1972; Pettersson and Ryden, 1982; Bukowiecki et al., 1986) or osteochondrosis (Foerner et al., 1987; Roneus and Carlsten, 1989; Nixon, 1990). Because follow-up radiographic examination showed that such fragments seldom develop in horses beyond 1 year of age, it was considered that this condition is a manifestation of developmental orthopedic disease (Grondahl, 1992b; Carlsten et al., 1993). More recent studies suggest that although these fragments do indeed show up in young horses, they are the results of a traumatic avulsion associated with the short distal sesamoidean ligament (Dalin et al., 1993). Lameness caused by the bony fragments has been reported to be evident only at the horse's maximal performance (Barclay et al., 1987; Foerner et al., 1987; McIlwraith, 1990) and some fragments at this site do not cause lameness (Barclay et al., 1987; Hardy et al., 1987; Grondahl, 1991). In one radiographic study, these fragments were observed in the palmar or plantar aspect of the metacarpo- and metatarsophalangeal joints in 89 of 753 (11.8%) yearling trotters (Grondahl, 1992b). Fragments were recorded in 7 forelimbs and 86 hind limbs, and bilateral occurrence was observed in the hind limbs of 11 horses. Eleven of 77 foals developed palmar or plantar fragments in another study (Carlsten et al., 1993).

3. *Proximodorsal first-phalanx fragments.*

These fragments, at least in racehorses, have long been considered traumatic in origin and to cause lameness (Yovich and McIlwraith, 1986; McIlwraith, 1987). One group has proposed that these fractures in Thoroughbred racehorses are manifestations of osteochondrosis (Krook and Maylin, 1988), but this is not generally accepted, at least in Thoroughbreds. However, dorsal bony fragments in the metacarpo- and metatarsophalangeal joints were diagnosed in 36 of 753 (4.8%) yearling Standardbred trotters in a radiographic survey (Grondahl, 1992b); 11 horses had two affected joints, and 1 horse had three affected joints. The condition was seen in 35 forelimbs and 14 hind limbs. The author also considered these to be manifestations of developmental orthopedic disease. Similar fragments may be found in warmblood horses as well, and some of these fragments could be osteochondrosis-related. The majority of clinical conditions, however, are considered to be traumatic in origin.

The fourth condition that has been labeled as OCD is the condition that was initially described as OCD of the palmar metacarpus (Hornof et al., 1981). This condition is now generally accepted to be a traumatic entity and not a syndrome of osteochondrosis (Pool and Meagher, 1990).

Osteochondritis Dissecans of the Dorsal Aspect of the Distal Metacarpus and Metatarsus

INCIDENCE, CLINICAL SIGNS, AND DIAGNOSIS

Figures on the incidence of this condition are mentioned in the previous section. Synovial effusion is usually the first indication of a problem. The degree of associated lameness varies, but flexion of the fetlock usually provokes lameness (Yovich et al., 1985; McIlwraith and Vorhees, 1990). Confirmation of OCD is made by radiography. If OCD is diagnosed in one fetlock, the other three are radiographed, because clinically silent lesions are commonly found. Although there may be no synovial effusion in these latter joints and lameness is inapparent, a positive response is often induced with flexion.

For purposes of treatment decision and prognosis, the lesions have been divided into three types: Type I is that in which a defect or flattening is the only visible radiographic lesion; Type II is that in which a defect or flattening with fragmentation is associated with the defect; Type III is that in which there is a defect or flattening with or without fragmentation plus one or more loose bodies.

Oblique radiographs should be taken as well as dorsopalmar (-plantar) and lateral radiographs for the purposes of discerning involvement of the medial or lateral condyles of the distal metacarpus or metatarsus (McIlwraith and Vorhees, 1990).

TREATMENT

When this condition was first reported, there were eight horses in the series (Yovich et al., 1985). Two horses with Type II OCD were euthanized, four horses with

Type I OCD were treated conservatively, one horse with Type II OCD was treated conservatively, and one horse with Type II OCD was operated on arthroscopically. Based on these small numbers, a working hypothesis was made that if the defects are without fragmentation (Type I lesion), conservative treatment will generally be successful. In contrast, it was hypothesized that defects with fragmentation need surgery. This hypothesis has turned into our current recommendations for treatment based on follow-up data (McIlwraith and Vorhees, 1990).

Of 15 horses with Type I lesions that were treated conservatively, 12 resolved clinically, and 8 of these showed remodeling of the lesions with improvement on radiographic examination. In 3 horses, the clinical signs persisted. In 2 of these cases, the radiographs showed no change and the horses eventually underwent surgery. In the other case, the clinical and radiographic signs progressed but the horse was not operated on. In 8 horses with Type II lesions in which owners requested conservative management, 2 eventually underwent surgery because of the persistence of clinical signs. Clinical signs persisted in 5 other horses, but surgery was not performed. The clinical signs improved in only 1 horse. In most of the cases in which clinical signs persisted, the fragmentation also progressed radiographically or at least did not resolve. It was also clear in this study that clinical signs of effusion may appear before definitive radiographic changes. Progression of some Type I lesions was noted. Such joints do not develop osseous fragmentation, but the lesions progressed to become larger defects, particularly on the condyles (seen on oblique-view radiographs). A few cases of Type II lesions improved radiographically. These were generally joints with small fragments, and the fragment fused in place, resulting in a bony protuberance at this location. In the above group of conservatively managed horses, most horses were 1988 foals. At that time, the horses on the farm were followed radiographically without any particular management change. In 1989, creep feed was discontinued in foals in which any swelling developed, and this was successful in reducing problems. During 1990, the energy intake was routinely restricted, with an apparent decrease in problems.

Surgery is usually recommended for Type II or Type III lesions. Most of the cases in a series of 42 horses operated on with arthroscopic surgery and previously reported were Type II or Type III lesions (McIlwraith and Vorhees, 1990). Some Type I lesions were operated on if they had not responded to conservative management. In other instances, Type I lesions were operated on in individual joints if a Type II or Type III lesion was present in another fetlock joint in the same horse. This was before our retrospective data with conservative cases recognized that Type I lesions do not usually require surgical treatment. The technique for arthroscopic surgery for the treatment of this condition has been described elsewhere (McIlwraith, 1990). The series of 42 horses previously reported included 20 Thoroughbreds, 8 Quarter Horses, 7 Arabians, 4 warmbloods, 1 Standardbred, 1 Percheron, and 1 Appaloosa (McIlwraith and Vorhees, 1990). There were 18 fillies, 15 colts, and 9 geldings. The forelimbs were involved in 10 horses, the hind limbs in 15, and both forelimbs and hind limbs in 17. Surgery was done on one fetlock in 10 horses, two fetlocks in 17, three fetlocks in 1, and four fetlocks in 14. In 48 joints, the proximal 2 cm of the sagittal ridge was involved, whereas in 11 joints the lesions extended distal for more than 2 cm. In 14 joints, the lesions involved the lateral or medial condyles of the metacarpus or metatarsus with or without lesions of the sagittal ridge.

Of the 42 horses operated on, follow-up was obtained in 28 (McIlwraith and Vorhees, 1990). Eight horses were convalescing, and in six horses follow-up was unavailable. Surgery was successful in 16 horses (57.1 %) and unsuccessful in 12 horses (42.8%). Of the 12 unsuccessful cases, 7 horses were considered still to have a problem in the fetlock (25%); in 3 horses, treatment was unsuccessful because of other reasons; in 1 horse, treatment was unsuccessful for unidentified reasons but the fetlock joint was considered to be normal; and 1 horse died. The success rate was found to be related to certain other factors. There was a trend for the success rate to be higher for surgery in hindlimbs than in forelimbs (p = 0.09). The lack of statistical significance in some instances is probably related to low overall numbers. In the forelimbs only 2 cases were successful, whereas 6 were unsuccessful. In the hind limbs 7 cases were successful and 3 were unsuccessful. When both forelimbs and hind limbs were involved, there were 7 successes and 3 failures. Type III lesions had 4 successes and 4 failures, whereas Type II lesions had 10 successes and 4 failures. The difference, however, was not statistically significant (p = 0.25). There was no statistical difference between proximal and distal lesions. In contrast, there were statistical differences in the success rate depending on whether there was articular cartilage erosion or wear lines on the articular surfaces. Only 3 of 12 cases with erosions or wear lines were successful, whereas 13 of 16 with no erosions were successful (p = 0.0029). There was also a significantly inferior result when a defect was visible on the condyle on oblique radiographs. When a defect was visible, 6 of 13 were successful, whereas if a defect was not visible, 10 of 15 were successful (p = 0.0274). Osteophytes were also negative prognostic indicators: 3 of 9 with osteophytes present on the first phalanx were successful, whereas 13 of 19 with no osteophytes were successful (p = 0.1792).

It was concluded that surgical management of Type II and Type III lesions will allow athletic activity in most cases, but clinical signs will persist in 25%. Whether surgery will be successful or not will be affected by the extent of the lesions as evident arthroscopically (and in some instances radiographically), as well as the presence of osteophytes and the presence of erosion and wear lines.

Proximal Palmar or Plantar First-Phalanx Fragments

INCIDENCE, CLINICAL SIGNS, AND DIAGNOSIS

Two types of fragments have been described: (1) Type I osteochondral fragments of the palmar or plantar aspect of the first phalanx (Barclay et al., 1987; Foerner et al., 1987), also called bony fragments of the palmar or plantar part of the metacarpo- and metatarsophalangeal joints (Grondahl, 1992b), and (2) Type II osteochondral fragments of the palmar or plantar aspect of the fetlock joint (Foerner et al., 1987) also called ununited proximoplantar tuberosity (Grondahl, 1992a) or united plantar eminence (Carlsten et al., 1993) of the proximal phalanx. As discussed previously, these fragments have been found frequently on radiographs of yearling trotters (Grondahl, 1992b).

Type I fragments usually occur in the hind fetlock joints, and the consistent complaint is that the horse has a hind limb problem that occurred at the upper level of the horse's performance ability and prevented the horse from competing successfully. Metatarsophalangeal joint distension is uncommon (Barclay et al., 1987; Foerner et al., 1987). There may be a response to flexion tests, and intra-articular anesthesia usually eliminates the existing lameness or response to flexion. Fragments are best demonstrated on lateromedial oblique and dorsal 20° proximal 75° lateral-plantarodistomedial views. Dorsoplantar radiographs may also demonstrate the fragments. In one series of clinical cases the fragments were most commonly seen medially (Table 6).

Table 6. Location of proximal palmar (plantar) fragments of first phalanx in a clinical series of 119 horses (146 joints) operated on arthroscopically (Fortier et al., 1995).

Limb	Medial	Lateral	Total
Left rear	72	20	92
Left fore	5	1	6
Right rear	42	21	63
Right fore	1	2	3
Total	120	44	164

Lameness may develop in association with Type II fragments but is uncommon. These fragments are easily recognized on conventional oblique radiographs (Grondahl, 1992a).

In a longitudinal study of 77 Standardbred foals examined and radiographed six times from birth to the age of 16 months, 11 foals (14.3%) showed either palmar (or plantar) fragments (or bony defects greater than 5 mm at the site of attachment of the short sesamoidean ligaments to the proximal phalanx) or ununited palmar (or plantar) eminences of the proximal phalanx (Carlsten et al., 1993). At four or more examinations from birth to 16 months, some were considered to have permanent lesions. All of these 11 foals had the lesions identified before the age of 5 months and six before the age of 3 months. In seven horses, early radiographic changes reverted to a normal appearance before the age of 8 months. It was noted that the extra-articular osteochondral fragments of ununited proximal and united plantar eminences cannot be considered permanent until after the age of 1 to 2 years because these fragments may unite to the proximal eminence of the proximal phalanx after 2 years of age, but in such cases early signs of unification are seen after 12 months of age.

TREATMENT

If Type I osteochondral fragments are incidental findings at radiography, treatment is not usually indicated. To be considered a surgical candidate, the patient must have demonstrable lameness referable to the fetlock in addition to a radiographically demonstrable lesion. In these cases, arthroscopic surgery is an effective method of treatment (Foerner et al., 1987; McIlwraith, 1990) In one series of 19 horses, 10 were treated with arthrotomy and all of these returned to full use of the joint (Foerner et al., 1987). Seven horses were treated intra-articularly with corticosteroids, and only one of these horses was able to return to full use of the joint. Successful results have been obtained more recently with arthroscopic surgery (Foerner et al., 1987; McIlwraith, 1990; Fortier et al., 1995). In 55 of 87 (63%) racehorses and in 100% of 9 nonracehorses, performance returned to preoperative levels after surgery (Fortier et al., 1995). Standardbred racehorses constituted 109 of the 119 (92%) horses. At surgery, evidence of full-thickness cartilage fibrillation was noticed in nine metatarsophalangeal joints but was not found in any metacarpophalangeal joints. Synovial proliferation in the area of and immediately adjacent to the fragment was recorded in an additional four metatarsophalangeal joints. A significant ($p < 0.0001$) association between abnormal surgical findings and unsuccessful outcome was found with 10 of 32 (31%) unsuccessful horses with evidence of articular cartilage loss or synovial proliferation. Only 1 of 55 (2%) successful horses had synovial proliferation evident at surgery, and none had evidence of articular cartilage damage (Fortier et al., 1995). All osteochondral fragments removed in this study were Type I fragments.

With Type II osteochondral fragments (or ununited proximoplantar tuberosity [UPT] of the proximal phalanx), surgery is rarely indicated. UPT was seen radiographically in 18 (2.4%) of 753 Standardbred yearlings in one report (Grondahl, 1992a). All fragments were in the pelvic limb. The condition was seen laterally in 16 horses, whereas one horse had a medial and lateral tuberosity affected and another only one medial tuberosity. Lameness was not observed in any horse before the first examination. On follow-up examination, 12 UPTs in 11 horses had united to the proximal phalanx after 6 to 12 months. One horse was unchanged at 7 months, and the remaining four had a radiographic worsening of the condition, with the UPT more dislocated. Three of these four horses also had calcification of the distal sesamoidean ligaments and periosteal proliferation. Two of the horses with the most severe radiographic changes developed lameness and subsequently underwent surgery to remove the fragment. This gives an incidence of clinically significant disease for UPT in 2 of 16 horses (12.5%) diagnosed and followed. It is also to be noted that in 11 of 18 horses, Type I osteochondral fragments of the plantar part of the metacarpophalangeal joint were seen together with UPT in the same pelvic limb. Occurrence of the latter condition may be an indication for surgery. A common etiologic factor could explain the incidence of the simultaneous occurrence of these two conditions. It has been proposed that clinical signs in conjunction with a UPT may have been caused by tension on the distal sesamoidean ligaments with training (Grondahl, 1992a). Wear and tear of the attachment of these ligaments was considered to possibly stimulate dislocation of the fragment, ligamentous calcification, or periosteal proliferation, and the author therefore recommended restricted training of horses with radiographic evidence of the disease (Grondahl, 1992a). The author also recommended that owners of these horses have them radiographed regularly (every 4 months) and consider surgery if radiographic or clinical evidence indicates progression of the condition. Such cases are unusual.

Osteochondritis Dissecans of the Scapulohumeral Joint

OCD of the shoulder is the most severely debilitating form of OCD seen in the horse. It is, however, less common than the previously discussed entities. Primary lesions of OCD occur on the glenoid as well as the humeral head, and the disease often affects a major part of the joint surfaces. Severe diffuse OCD lesions as well as single or multiple cystic lesions may occur on the glenoid. Secondary degenerative joint disease was recorded in 35 of 54 cases (Nyack et al., 1981).

INCIDENCE, CLINICAL SIGNS, AND DIAGNOSIS

As mentioned above, OCD of the shoulder is less common than that of the femoropatellar, tarsocrural, or fetlock joints. A series of 54 cases has been reported (Nyack et al., 1981). In a series of 59 joints in 48 horses operated on by the author, there were 19 Quarter Horses, 14 Thoroughbreds, 6 crossbreds, 3 Arabians, 3 warmbloods, 2 Morgans, and 1 American Paint Horse (Howard and McIlwraith, unpublished data). The problem was unilateral in 38 horses and bilateral in 10. The humeral head was involved in 12 horses, the glenoid was involved in 11, and both the humeral head and the glenoid were involved in the 26 other joints that had arthroscopic surgery.

Most cases of OCD of the shoulder present as yearlings or younger (it has been reported at 3 months) and manifest with a history of intermittent forelimb lameness of insidious onset. The forelimb lameness often exhibits a swinging component, with reduced limb protraction a common finding. It is common to see muscle atrophy over the shoulder, and pain may be demonstrated by using direct pressure over the joint or by pulling the leg upward and craniad, caudad, or into an adducted position. Stumbling may occur as a result of inadequate foot clearance and the shortened anterior phase of stride. A small foot with a long heel and club-footed appearance often develops in the affected limb because of the altered gait. Synovial effusion cannot usually be detected because of the muscles and tendons overlying the scapulohumeral joint. When chronicity is evidenced by a smaller foot and when there is muscle atrophy over the shoulder, we consider the presentation of a horse 1 year old or younger for forelimb lameness to be sufficient reason for taking standing radiographs of the shoulder.

The problem may be localized to the shoulder using intra-articular analgesia. This diagnostic aid is important, as the condition can often be diagnosed definitively only by taking radiographs with the horse under general anesthesia. A 3-inch, 18-gauge spinal needle is used for intra-articular analgesia of the shoulder. The needle is inserted cranial to the infraspinatus tendon at the level of the greater tuberosity of the humerus. The needle is inserted slightly caudad and ventrad. Mepivacaine or lidocaine 2% (20 ml) is injected. A 100% response to the block is not necessary to consider the test positive. It is relatively common for an OCD lesion in the shoulder to have intact cartilage at the surface and a dissection plane with subchondral cavitation beneath when it is evaluated arthroscopically. A dramatic response to local analgesia cannot be expected in such cases.

When OCD involves the humeral head, the most common radiographic change is flattening or indentation of the caudal aspect of the humeral head. Lesions in the glenoid manifest either as diffuse areas of subchondral lucency or as cystic lesions (usually multiple). Subchondral bone irregularities are a significant sign in either the humeral head or the glenoid. Lesions may occur in both locations in the same joint. Osteophyte formation (caudal humeral head) is reasonably common, and subchondral sclerosis may also be seen. Cystic lesions in the glenoid have been seen as solitary lesions. Free bony fragments are rare.

TREATMENT

Conservative nonsurgical treatment of osteochondrosis of the shoulder has met with minimal success with respect to athletic performance (Meagher et al., 1973; Nyack et al., 1981; Rose et al., 1985). Animals have been treated successfully with arthrotomy (Schmidt et al., 1975; Mason and McLean, 1977; DeBowes et al., 1982; Nixon et al., 1984). Extensive soft tissue dissection is necessary, however, and the craniomedial aspect of the joint may not be visualized (Schmidt et al., 1975). The development of arthroscopic surgery techniques has provided advantages over arthrotomy in both avoiding these complications and providing additional benefits, particularly improved visualization of the whole joint and a lack of surgical morbidity (Bertone and McIlwraith, 1987a,b; Bertone et al., 1987; Nixon, 1987; McIlwraith, 1990); however, the arthroscopic technique is not easy and becomes extremely difficult in an adult horse.

Because of the generalized pathologic changes present in many instances, surgical cases should be selected carefully. However, surgery will benefit some horses even when secondary degenerative changes are present (Bertone et al., 1987). Although the ability of the young equine joint to heal after curettage of major defects is impressive, we still lack sufficient numbers to give realistic percentages. With very severe cases, a poor prognosis is offered and surgery is not recommended.

At arthroscopic surgery the lesions are usually more extensive than could be surmised from the radiographs (Bertone et al., 1987). In most instances, the cartilaginous changes extend beyond the limits of the subchondral bone abnormalities observed on radiographs, particularly in the glenoid. In some horses in which a lesion is limited radiographically to the glenoid or the humeral head, additional lesions are found arthroscopically on the opposing articular surface. The most common arthroscopic abnormalities of the humeral head are cartilage discoloration with undermining or erosion down to subchondral bone on the caudal aspect of the articular surface. In some instances, a lesion is not visible initially and probing is required to ascertain the area of undermined cartilage. The most common arthroscopic abnormality in the glenoid is cracked and undermined articular cartilage with fissure formation and fibrillation. An additional common finding is defective, friable subchondral bone, and these lesions may extend quite deeply (young horses do have subchondral bone of a softer consistency, and it is sometimes difficult to differentiate pathologic from nonpathologic bone). Problems with arthroscopic surgery in the shoulder include difficulty with arthroscopic placement, difficulty establishing triangulation with the instrument portal, extravasation of fluids, difficulty in reaching potential lesions, and damage to instruments (Bertone et al., 1987; Nixon, 1987).

The results of arthroscopic surgery for OCD and subchondral cystic lesions of the shoulder were initially described for 13 shoulders in 11 horses (Bertone et al., 1987). The lameness decreased in all 11 horses after surgery, with 9 of the 11 horses reported as becoming sound, and 2 remaining lame at short-term follow-up. On long-term follow-up, five horses were athletically sound and were being shown, ridden, or raced after 5 to 20 months. A sixth horse was sound when beginning race training. A seventh horse was pasture-sound and was to begin race training in several months at the time of the report. An eighth horse showed well in halter for 12 months, but shoulder lameness returned; this horse was donated and necropsy was performed. The ninth, tenth, and eleventh horses remained lame. Complications included the development of subchondral cyst-like lesions and signs of degenerative joint disease. Follow-up radiographic assessment of 6 of the 9 sound horses revealed improvement in the contour of the humeral head and joint space and more even density of the humeral epiphysis and glenoid of the scapula in 6 horses. One of these horses showed marked improvement in subchondral bone density and the surface contour of the glenoid cavity. In two of the remaining five horses, the caudal border of the glenoid cavity had remodeled to appear more like the contralateral joint. In the fourth of the six sound horses, radiographs obtained 1 year later showed a subchondral cystic lesion in the bone adjacent to the scapula that had definitely not been present previously, but the horse was still sound and remained so. The contour of the glenoid articular surface on its caudal border was smoother postoperatively, the subchondral osteosclerosis was reduced in thickness, and the horse was athletically sound. In the fifth horse in this group, an osteophyte on the humerus had enlarged, but definite improvement was noted in the joint contour of both the humeral head and the glenoid cavity. Radiographs obtained from one of the two horses that improved but was still lame showed no improvement in the glenoid lesion radiographically. In the horse that deteriorated clinically, in which euthanasia was chosen, the humeral epiphysis was severely deformed with a defect in the articular surface contour, a subchondral cystic lesion, and a small intra-articular fracture of the cranial margin of the glenoid cavity.

A larger, long-term follow-up study has recently been completed. Of 49 horses operated on by the author, complete follow-up was obtained in 35. Sixteen operations were successful (45.7%) and 19 unsuccessful (54.3%). Five additional horses were in various stages of convalescence or training, and nine horses were lost to follow-up. An alternative arthroscopic technique has been reported in nine normal horses and two cases of osteochondrosis (Nixon, 1987).

References

Adams, W.H., and J.P. Thilsted. 1985. Radiographic appearance of the equine stifle from birth to six months. Vet. Radio. 26:126-132.

Aglietti, P., R. Buzzi, P.B. Bassi, and M. Fioriti. 1994. Arthroscopic drilling in juvenile osteochondritis dissecans of the medial femoral condyle. J. Arthroscopy Rel. Surg. 10:286-191.

Alvarado, A.F., M. Marcoux, and L. Breton. 1989. The incidence of osteochondrosis on a Standardbred breeding farm in Quebec. In: Proc. Amer. Vet. Med. Assoc. Equine Practnr. 35:293-307.

Barclay, W.P., J.J. Foerner, and T.N. Phillips. 1987. Lameness attributable to osteochondral fragmentation of the plantar aspect of the proximal phalanx in horses: 19 cases (1981-1985). J. Amer. Vet. Med. Assoc. 191:855-857.

Beard, W.L., L.R. Bramlage, R.K. Scheider, and R.M. Embertson. 1994. Postoperative racing performance in Standardbreds and Thoroughbreds with osteochondrosis of the tarsocrural joint: 109 cases. J. Amer. Vet. Med. Assoc. 204:1655-1659.

Bertone, A.L., and C.W. McIlwraith. 1987a. Arthroscopic approaches in intra-articular anatomy of the equine shoulder joint. Vet. Surg. 16:317-322.

Bertone, A.L., and C.W. McIlwraith. 1987b. Osteochondrosis of the equine shoulder: Treatment with arthroscopic surgery. In: Proc. Amer. Assoc. Equine Practnr. 33:683-686.

Bertone, A.L., C.W. McIlwraith, B.E. Powers, et al. 1987. Arthroscopic surgery for treatment of osteochondrosis in the equine shoulder joint. Vet. Surg. 16:303-311.

Birkeland, R. 1972. Chip fractures of the first phalanx in the metatarsophalangeal joint of a horse. Acta. Radiol. Suppl. 29:73-77.

Birkeland, R., and L.H. Haakenstad. 1968. Intracapsular bony fragments of the distal tibia of the horse. Equine Vet. J. 152:1526-1529.

Birkeland, R., and L.H. Haakenstad. 1974. Osteochondritis dissecans. Ii heseledtet hos hust. Kirurgiskog konservativ behandling. In: Proc. Nord. Vet. Cong. Reykjavik 34.

Bukowiecki, C.F., L.R. Bramlage, and A.A. Gabel. 1986. Palmar/plantar process fractures of the proximal phalanx in 15 horses. Vet. Surg. 15:383-388.

Carlsten, J., B. Sandgren, and G. Dalin. 1993. Development of osteochondrosis in the tarsocrural joint and osteochondral fragments in the fetlock joints of Standardbred trotters: I. A radiological study. Equine Vet. J. Suppl. 16:42-47.

Dalin, G., B. Sandgren, and J. Carlsten. 1993. Plantar osteochondral fragmentation in the fetlock joints of Standardbreds: Results of osteochondrosis or trauma? Equine Vet. J. Suppl. 16:62-65.

DeBowes, R.M., P.C. Wagner, and B.D. Grant. 1982. Surgical approach to the equine scapulohumeral joint through a longitudinal infraspinatus tenotomy. Vet. Surg. 11:125-128.

DeMoor, A., F. Verschooten, P. Desmet, et al. 1972. Osteochondritis dissecans of the tibiotarsal joint of the horse. Equine Vet. J. 4:139-143.

Dink, D. 1990. Advantages of a February foal. Thoroughbred Times 18:28-32.

Ewing, J.W., and S.J. Soto. 1988. Arthroscopic surgical management of osteochondritis dissecans of the knee. J. Arthroscopic Rel. Surg. 4:37-44.

Foerner, J.J., W.P. Barclay, T.N. Phillips, et al. 1987. Osteochondral fragments of the palmar/plantar aspect of the fetlock joints. In. Proc. Amer. Assoc. Equine Practnr. 33:739-744.

Foland, J.W., C.W. McIlwraith, and G.W. Trotter. 1992. Osteochondritis dissecans of the femoropatellar joint: Results of treatment with arthroscopic surgery. Equine Vet. J. 24:419-423.

Fortier, L.A., J.J. Foerner, and A.J. Nixon. 1995. Arthroscopic removal of axial osteochondral fragments of the plantar/palmar proximal aspect of the proximal phalanx in horses: 119 cases (1988-1992). J. Amer. Vet. Assoc. 206:71-74.

Grondahl, A.M. 1991. The incidence of osteochondrosis in the tibiotarsal joint of Norwegian Standardbred trotters: A radiographic study. J. Equine. Vet. Sci. 11:272-274.

Grondahl, A.M. 1992a. Incidence and development of ununited proximoplantar tuberosity of the proximal phalanx in Standardbred trotters. Vet. Radiol. Ultrasound 33:18-21.

Grondahl, A.M. 1992b. The incidence of bony fragments in osteochondrosis in the metacarpometatarsophalangeal joints of Standardbred trotters: A radiographic study. J. Equine Vet. Sci. 12:81-85.

Hance, S.R., R.K. Schneider, R.M. Embertson, et al. 1993. Lesions of the caudal aspect of the femoral condyles in foals: 20 cases (1980-1990). J. Amer. Vet. Med. Assoc. 202:637-646,

Hardy, J., M. Marcoux, and L. Breton. 1987. Prevalence et des fragments articulaires retrouves au boulet chez le chevel Standardbred. Med. Vet. Quebec 17:57-61.

Hoppe, F. 1984a. Osteochondrosis in Swedish horses: A radiographic and epidemiological study with special reference to frequency and heredity. Thesis. University at Uppsala, Sweden.

Hoppe, F. 1984b. Radiological investigations of osteochondrosis dissecans in Standardbred trotters and Swedish Warmblood horses. Equine Vet. J. 16:425-429.

Hornof, W.H., T.R. O'Brien, and R.R. Pool. 1981. Osteochondritis dissecans of the distal metacarpus in the adult racing Thoroughbred horse. Vet. Radiol. 22:98-106.

Howard, R.D., and C.W. McIlwraith. Unpublished data.

Krook, L., and G.A. Maylin. 1988. Fractures in Thoroughbred racehorses. Cornell Vet. 78:5-47.

Laws, E.G., D.W. Richardson, M.W. Ross, et al. 1993. Racing performance in Standardbreds following conservative and surgical treatment for tarsocrural osteochondrosis. Equine Vet. J. 25:199-202.

Martin, G.S., and C.W. McIlwraith. 1985. Arthroscopic anatomy of the equine femoropatellar joint and approaches for the treatment of osteochondritis dissecans. Vet. Surg. 14:99-104.

Mason, A., and A.A. McLean. 1977. Osteochondrosis dissecans of the head of the humerus in two foals. Equine. Vet. J. 9:189-191.

McIlwraith, C.W. 1987. Disease of joints, tendons, ligaments and related structures. In: Stashak, T.S. (Ed.) Adams' Lameness in Horses (4th Ed.). p. 339-447. Lee and Febiger, Philadelphia.

McIlwraith, C.W. 1990. Diagnostic and Surgical Arthroscopy in the Horse. p. 113-159. Lee and Febiger, Philadelphia.

McIlwraith, C.W. 1993a. Inferences from referred clinical cases of osteochondritis dissecans. Equine Vet. J. 16:27-30.

McIlwraith, C.W. 1993b. What is developmental orthopedic disease, osteochondrosis, osteochondritis, metabolic bone disease? In: Proc. Amer. Assoc. Equine Practnr. 39:35-44.

McIlwraith, C.W., and G.S. Martin. 1985. Arthroscopic surgery for the treatment of osteochondritis dissecans of the equine femoropatellar joint. Vet. Surg. 14:105-116.

McIlwraith, C.W., and M. Vorhees. 1990. Management of osteochondritis dissecans of the dorsal aspect of the distal metacarpus and metatarsus. In: Proc. Amer. Assoc. Equine Practnr. 35:547-550.

McIlwraith, C.W., J.J. Foerner, and M. Davis. 1991. Osteochondritis dissecans of the tarsocrural joint: Results of treatment with arthroscopic surgery. Equine

Vet. J. 23:155-162.

McIntosh, S.C., and C.W. McIlwraith. 1993. Natural history of femoropatellar osteochondrosis in three crops of Thoroughbreds. Equine Vet. J. 16:54-61.

Meagher, D.M., R.R. Pool, and T.R. O'Brien. 1973. Osteochondritis dissecans of the shoulder joint in the horse. In: Proc. Amer. Assoc. Equine Practnr. 19:247-256.

Moore, J.N., and C.W. McIlwraith. 1977. Osteochondrosis of the equine stifle. Vet. Rec. 100:133-136.

Nilsson, F. 1947. Hastens goniter. Sven. Vet. Tidskr. 52:1-14.

Nixon, A.J. 1987. Diagnostic and surgical arthroscopy of the equine shoulder joint. Vet. Surg. 16:44-52.

Nixon, A.J. 1990. Osteochondrosis and osteochondritis dissecans of the equine fetlock. Compend. Cont. Ed. Pract. Vet. 12:1463-1475.

Nixon, A.J., T.S. Stashek, C.W. McIlwraith, et al. 1984. A muscle-separating approach to the equine shoulder for the treatment of osteochondritis dissecans. Vet. Surg. 13:247-256.

Nyack, B., M.B. Morgan, R.R. Pool, et al. 1981. Osteochondrosis of the shoulder joint of the horse. Cornell Vet. 71:149-163.

O'Brien, T.R. 1973. Radiology of the equine stifle. In: Proc. Amer. Assoc. Equine Practnr. 19:271-287.

Pascoe, J.R., R.R. Pool, J.D. Wheat, et al. 1984. Osteochondral defects of the lateral trochlear ridge of the distal femur of the horse: Clinical, radiographic and pathologic examination and results of surgical treatment. Vet. Surg. 13:99-110.

Pettersson, H., and G. Ryden. 1982. Avulsion fractures of the caudoproximal extremity of the first phalanx. Equine Vet. J. 14:333-335.

Pool, R.R., and D.M. Meagher. 1990. Pathologic findings and pathogenesis of racetrack injuries. Vet. Clin. N. Amer. 6:1-30.

Poulos, P. 1986. Radiologic manifestations of developmental problems. In: McIlwraith, C.W. (Ed.) AQHA Developmental Orthopedic Disease Symposium. p. 1-2. American Quarter Horse Association, Amarillo, Texas.

Rejno, S., and B. Stromberg. 1978. Osteochondrosis in the horse. II. Pathology. Acta. Radiol. Suppl. 358-153-178.

Roneus, B., and J. Carlsten. 1989. Bone fragments in fetlock and hock joints in young Standardbred trotters. Sven. Vet. Tidskr. 41:417-422.

Rose, J.A., R.D. Sande, and E.M. Rose. 1985. Results of conservative management of osteochondrosis in the horse. In: Proc. Amer. Assoc. Equine Practnr. 31:617-626.

Sandgren, B. 1988. Bony fragments in the tarsocrural and metacarpo-metatarsophalangeal joints in the Standardbred horse: A radiographic study. Equine Vet. J. Suppl. 6:66-70.

Schmidt, G.B., R. Dueland, and J.T. Vaughan. 1975. Osteochondrosis dissecans of the equine shoulder joint. Vet. Clin. North. Amer. (Small Anim. Pract.)

70:542-547.

Shelley, J., and S. Dyson. 1984. Interpreting radiographs: V. Radiology of the equine hock. Equine Vet. J. 16:488-495.

Smith, J.B. 1990. Osteochondritis dissecans of the trochlea of the femur. Arthroscopy 6:11-17.

Spurlock, G.H., and A.A. Gabel. 1983. Apical fractures of the proximal sesamoid bones in Standardbred horses. J. Amer. Vet. Med. Assoc. 183:76-79.

Steenhaut, M., F. Verschooten, and A. DeMoor. 1982. Osteochondritis dissecans of the stifle joint in the horse. Vlaams Dierg. Tigdchrift. 5:173-191.

Steinheimer, D.N., C.W. McIlwraith, R.D. Park, and P.F. Steyn. 1996. Comparison of radiographic subchondral bone changes with arthroscopic findings in the equine femoropatellar and femorotibial joints: A retrospective study of 72 joints (50 horses). Vet. Radiol. 36:478-484.

Stromberg, C., and S. Rejno. 1978. Osteochondrosis in the horse: I. A clinical and radiological investigation of osteochondritis dissecans of the knee and hock joint. Acta. Radiol. Suppl. 358:139-152.

Trotter, G.W., C.W. McIlwraith, and R.W. Norrdin. 1983. Comparison of two surgical approaches to the equine femoropatellar joint for the treatment of osteochondritis dissecans. Vet. Surg. 12:33-40.

Wright, I.M. and A.C. Pickles. 1991. Osteochondritis dissecans (OCD) of the femoropatellar joint. Equine Vet. Educ. 3:86-93.

Wyburn, R.S. 1977. Degenerative joint disease in the horse. NZ Vet. J. 25:321-335.

Yovich, J.V., and C.W. McIlwraith. 1986. Arthroscopic surgery for osteochondral fractures of the proximal phalanx of the metacarpophalangeal and metatarsophalangeal (fetlock) joints in horses. J. Amer. Vet. Med. Assoc. 188:273-279.

Yovich, J.V., C.W. McIlwraith, and T.S. Stashak. 1985. Osteochondritis dissecans of the sagittal ridge of the third metacarpal and metatarsal bones in horses. J. Amer. Vet. Med. Assoc. 186:1186-1191.

RECENT ADVANCES IN OSTEOCHONDROSIS RESEARCH

ELWYN C. FIRTH
Institute of Veterinary, Animal and Biomedical Sciences, Massey University, Palmerston North, New Zealand

Introduction

This presentation outlines recent advances in osteochondrosis (OC) through interpretative summaries of papers in the last four years, which record research work undertaken up to seven years ago. Only about 15 peer-reviewed papers have been produced in that time, and many are either case reports or the earliest work in new approaches to investigating pathogenesis. The amount of work conducted on OC is relatively sparse and insufficient to motivate a group of researchers interested in the disease to hold a planned meeting on osteochondrosis in 2004. A large amount of information was obtained from the study referred to as the EXOC study, which sought to determine if exercise in young horses would affect the incidence and severity of OC in warmblood foals. Other papers that provide information on OC management are also cited.

Hock and Stifle OC Have Different Progression and Regression in the First 11 Months of Life

The EXOC study was completed in 1999, and most findings have been published. All of the foals' sires (a total of eight) and 11 of the 43 dams had OC in the stifle (lateral trochlear ridge) or hock (intermediate ridge of tibia). The foals were randomly divided into three groups: box confined (Group$_{box}$), pastured (Group$_{pasture}$), or box confined and gallop exercised 6 days per week in a yard from 7 days of age (Group$_{training}$). The latter group was given 12-16 sprints to 24 days old, 24 sprints from 25-38 days, then 32 and 16 sprints on alternate days until 5 months of age. Thereafter, 24 (eight from each group) of the foals were euthanized, and the remaining 19 were all kept in a loose box with free access to a paddock.

All foals were radiographed monthly until 5 months and the remaining 19 until 11 months, and radiographic appearance classified as normal (0) through minimal, mild, moderate, and severe (4) changes of OC. The prevalence at various times was compared longitudinally.

Sixty-seven percent of tibial intermediate ridges had abnormal appearance at 1 month, 37% at 5 months, and 18% at 11 months, with lower severity of lesion with age. Regression of abnormal appearance was marked, progression was uncommon, and normal appearance rarely became abnormal. Normal and abnormal appearances were permanent from 5 months on.

In the lateral trochlear ridge of the femur, abnormality was rare at 1 month, was present in 20% of stifles at 5 months, and then regressed to 3% at 11 months. Most abnormalities had become normal by 8 months, after which normal and abnormal appearances were permanent (Dik et al., 1999).

Exercise Did Not Cause OC Lesions

At 5 months of age, there was a mean of 5.5 lesions (a range of 1-14) in all foals, with tibiotarsal (1.9 lesions/foal), stifle (1.0), neck (1.0), and fetlock (0.6) joints being most affected. At 11 months, there were considerably fewer lesions (mean 3.7, range 0-7) in each foal, the most obvious decrease being in the stifle and the least in the hock. There was no statistically significant influence of exercise on the number of lesions, but lesions were more severe in Group$_{box}$. In the stifle, lesions were in the femoral condyle of boxed foals and in the trochlear ridge of exercised foals. It was concluded that, although exercise may affect the appearance and site of lesions, it does not appear to have an initiating role (van Weeren and Barneveld, 1999).

Altered Proteoglycan Metabolism in OC Cartilage is Result, Not Cause

Osteochondrotic and normal cartilage was harvested from foals at 5 and 11 months of age, and proteoglycan metabolism investigated by use of conventional techniques. Sulfur incorporation of OC was markedly less in osteochondrotic than normal cartilage in 11-month-old foals. Serum stimulation of proteoglycan synthesis was less in osteochondrotic than normal cartilage at 11 months, indicating reduced capability of chondrocytes from osteochondrotic cartilage, which was not due to the number of cells present as indicated by DNA content. Osteochondrotic cartilage from 5-month-old foals appears to be in a state of stimulation but chondrocytes are highly viable since they can be stimulated to similar metabolic levels as normal chondrocytes. Osteochondrotic cartilage from 11-month-old foals has a lower vitality and cannot be stimulated. The reduced and altered proteoglycan production at 11 months from lesions which have not regressed is likely to indicate that the changed synthesis reflects a result rather than cause of the OC lesions (van den Hoogen et al., 1999).

Horses Severely Affected with OC Have Lower Bone Mineral Density

In OC, the role of trauma is still contested. It has been suggested that normal forces on suboptimal bone, or higher than normal forces on normal bone, may lead to microfracture and subsequent retention of cartilage. Showing that this occurs in normal life is difficult. In the EXOC study, mineral density was determined in the third carpal bone and in the distal radius. The data were analyzed in relation to the OC score of each animal, which was the sum of the number and severity scores of OC lesions in each animal. Of the four groups of OC scores, the highest (i.e., the most severely affected group of animals) had a significantly lower bone mineral density (BMD) than the other three groups. The implication might thus be that horses with severe OC may indeed have lower mineral density, which is a large determinant of bone's resistance to deformation. Further, OC is rare in the third carpal bone, which may indicate that the lower BMD found there was not localized. Although low BMD might be expected if OC or its sequelae caused lameness or recumbency, absolutely no such signs were evident. A further explanation is that of the 7 animals in the group with an OC score >20, four came from the 5-month-old Group$_{box}$, two were from the 5-month-old Group$_{training}$, and one was from the 5-month-old Group$_{pasture}$. None was from the 11-month-old foal group.

This indicates that horses in the most severely affected OC group were young and had been confined, at least to some degree, possibly indicating a reason for lower BMD. Boxed horses would develop less muscle or use muscle less and exert less force on their limb column; thus they are likely to have lower BMD (Firth et al., 1999).

Comparison of Distribution, Severity and Number of OC Lesions in Various Studies

The lesions encountered in four crops of pasture-raised foals in New Zealand have revealed the same lesions originally found in one of them (Pearce et al., 1998a). No other manifestations of the DOD complex were observed. In 21 pasture-fed 5-month-old Thoroughbreds, there were 1.6-3.3 lesions/foal; the most commonly affected site was the talar condylar ridge followed by the proximal humerus, though the lesions were not severe and so small as to be apparently innocuous. No intervertebral lesions were noted. The lesions were more numerous, the site order was different, and the severity of the lesions was greater in studies in Ohio (Knight et al., 1990), Canada (Hurtig et al., 1993), and The Netherlands (van Weeren and Barneveld, 1999). It is unclear if the differences are due to the variances in management system, nutrition, breed, and exercise possibilities at pasture.

Different Patterns of Decline in Liver Copper Concentration in Thoroughbred Foals

Serial liver biopsies were taken from foals soon after birth to 160 days of age. In seven of the foals, the normal decline in liver copper concentration was evident, as previously documented (Pearce et al., 1998c), and declined from a high mean (+/- SD) liver copper concentration at birth (374 +/- 130 mg/kg DM) to adult values (21 +/- 6 mg/kg DM) by 160 days of age. In three foals the decline was slower than in the other seven and at 160 days of age the mean concentration was 162 +/- 32 mg/kg DM. The differences between each of eight biopsies (P < 0.01) and between "normal" and "accumulator" foals (P < 0.002) were significant (Gee et al., 2000).

IGF and Collagen Changes in Osteochondrotic Cartilage are Related to Healing

Specimens were harvested and snap frozen from OC-affected immature horses and age-matched controls, either at surgery or necropsy. PCR was used to determine expression of IGF-1, and TGF-ß1, which was greater in cartilage from horses with OC, significantly in the case of IGF-1. Using rabbit polyclonal antibodies against human IGF, the site of localization of IGF-1 was shown to be just beneath the tangential zone and in the deepest cartilage layers of osteochondrotic cartilage. In situ hybridization showed increased type I collagen in deep layer fibrocartilage repair tissue and fibrous tissue in the osteochondrotic cleft. The increased expressions are most likely to be a healing response and are not etiologically significant (Semevolos et al., 2001).

Copper May Contribute to Repair of Early OC Lesions

The possible role of copper in OC in pasture-raised Thoroughbred remains unresolved, despite the alteration of foal copper status by oral administration of copper to pregnant mares (Pearce et al., 1998b,c). The very fact that the lesions were few and subtle may reduce the ability of researchers to determine if copper status does or does not affect lesion number and severity.

Therefore, the concentration of copper in foals known to be prone to OC was examined. Liver biopsies were taken from warmblood foals at 4 days and 5 months after birth, and liver copper concentration determined. For each foal, the liver copper concentration was related to the OC status of the foals as determined by scoring of stifle and hock OC lesions in radiographs taken at 5 and 11 months of age. The liver copper concentration was similar to those in Thoroughbred foals in previous studies (Gee et al., 2000; Pearce et al., 1998c) and declined to adult levels by 5 months. The reduction in number and severity of radiographically detectable lesions was similar to that previously described (Dik et al., 1999). Radiographic score was not related to liver copper concentration at birth. The foals with the lowest liver copper concentrations had a worsening OC score between 5 and 11 months. Foals with the highest 50% of liver copper concentrations had an improvement in score by 11 months in OC of the stifle but not the hock. This evidence supports copper being less involved in the cause of OC, and more in the repair of early OC lesions (van Weeren et al., 2003).

Injectable Copper Does Not Alter Foal Copper Status

Oral copper administration to late pregnant mares at pasture is labor intensive, and parenteral administration was investigated. The effects of copper supplementation by two injections of copper edetate given to mares in late gestation were determined by assessing liver copper concentration of their foals at birth. The injections did not improve copper status as shown by no significant difference in liver copper concentration of foals from mares that had received copper injections compared to those that had received saline injections (Gee et al., 2000).

Body Composition in Thoroughbred Foals

High-energy diets, overfeeding, and high growth rates are often cited as associated factors in the pathogenesis of OC. However, there is little basic nutrition work in Thoroughbred horses on which to begin determining what nutritional factors may be directly related to developmental orthopedic disease. Therefore, body composition was examined in 5-month-old Thoroughbreds using ultrasound, condition scoring, and bioelectrical impedance. Of the partial empty bodyweight, fillies had significantly more fat and higher percentage fat than did colts. Live animal condition scores, particularly rib condition scores, were closely related to fat mass and concentration, but condition scores were only slightly higher in fillies than colts. Ultrasound measurement of rump fat thickness was significantly correlated with condition score and explained 71% of variation in body fat mass. Impedance is difficult to measure in vivo (Gee et al., 2003).

References

Dik, K.J., E. Enzerink, and P.R. van Weeren. 1999. Radiographic development of osteochondral abnormalities, in the hock and stifle of Dutch Warmblood foals, from age 1 to 11 months. Equine Vet. J. Suppl. 13:9-15.

Firth, E.C., P.R. van Weeren, D.U. Pfeiffer, J. Delahunt, and A. Barneveld. 1999. Effect of age, exercise and growth rate on bone mineral density (BMD) in third carpal bone and distal radius of Dutch Warmblood foals with osteochondrosis. Equine Vet. J. Suppl. 13:74-78.

Gee, E.K., P.F. Fennessy, P.C.H. Morel, N.D. Grace, E.C. Firth, and T.D. Mogg. 2003. Chemical body composition of 20 Thoroughbred foals at 160 days of age, and preliminary investigation of techniques used to predict body fatness. New Zealand Vet. J. 51:125-131.

Gee, E.K., N.D. Grace, E.C. Firth, and P.F. Fennessy. 2000. Changes in liver copper concentration of Thoroughbred foals from birth to 160 days of age and the effect of prenatal copper supplementation of their dams. Aust. Vet. J. 78:347-353.

Hurtig, M.B., S.L. Green, H. Dobson, and J. Burton. 1993. Correlative study of defective cartilage and bone growth in foals fed a low copper diet. Equine Vet. J. Suppl. 16:66-73.

Knight, D.A., S.E. Weisbrode, L.M. Schmall, S.M. Reed, A.A. Gabel, L.R. Bramlage, and W.I. Tyznik. 1990. The effects of copper supplementation on the prevalence of cartilage lesions in foals. Equine Vet. J. 22:426-432.

Pearce, S.G., E.C. Firth, N.D. Grace, and P.F. Fennessy. 1998a. Effect of copper supplementation on the evidence of developmental orthopaedic disease in pasture-fed New Zealand Thoroughbreds. Equine Vet. J. 30:211-218.

Pearce, S.G., N.D. Grace, E.C. Firth, J.J. Wichtel, S.A. Holle, and P.F. Fennessy. 1998b. Effect of copper supplementation on the copper status of pasture-fed young Thoroughbreds. Equine Vet. J. 30:204-210.

Pearce, S.G., N.D. Grace, J.J. Wichtel, E.C. Firth, and P.F. Fennessy. 1998c. Effect of copper supplementation on copper status of pregnant mares and foals. Equine Vet J 30:200-203.

Semevolos, S.A., A.J. Nixon, and B.D. Brower-Toland. 2001. Changes in molecular expression of aggrecan and collagen types I, II, and X, insulin-like growth factor-I, and transforming growth factor-beta1 in articular cartilage obtained from horses with naturally acquired osteochondrosis. Am. J. Vet. Res. 62:1088-1094.

van den Hoogen, B.M., C.H. van de Lest, P.R. van Weeren, L.M. van Golde, and A. Barneveld. 1999. Changes in proteoglycan metabolism in osteochondrotic articular cartilage of growing foals. Equine Vet. J. Suppl. 13:38-44.

van Weeren, P.R., and A. Barneveld. 1999. The effect of exercise on the distribution and manifestation of osteochondrotic lesions in the warmblood foal. Equine Vet. J. Suppl. 13:16-25.

van Weeren, P.R., J. Knaap, and E.C. Firth. 2003. Influence of liver copper status of mare and newborn foal on the development of osteochondrotic lesions. Equine Vet. J. 35:67-71.

THE ROLE OF NUTRITION IN THE MANAGEMENT OF DEVELOPMENTAL ORTHOPEDIC DISEASE

JOE PAGAN
Kentucky Equine Research, Versailles, Kentucky, USA

Nutrition may play an important role in the pathogenesis of developmental orthopedic disease in horses. Deficiencies, excesses, and imbalances of nutrients may result in an increase in both the incidence and severity of physitis, angular limb deformity, wobbler syndrome (wobbles), and osteochondritis dissecans (OCD).

Nutritional Factors as a Cause of Developmental Orthopedic Disease

MINERAL DEFICIENCIES

A deficiency of minerals, including calcium, phosphorus, copper, and zinc, may lead to developmental orthopedic disease. The ration of a growing horse should be properly fortified because most commonly fed cereal grains and forages contain insufficient quantities of several minerals. A ration of grass hay and oats would only supply about 40% and 70% of a weanling's calcium and phosphorus requirement, respectively, and less than 40% of its requirement for copper and zinc (Table 1). The best method of diagnosing mineral deficiencies is through ration evaluation. Blood, hair, and hoof analysis is of limited usefulness.

Table 1. Mineral requirements for weanlings.

	Nutrient concentration required in total diet (90% dry basis)		Grass hay	Alfalfa hay	Oats	Corn	Barley
	Moderate growth	*Rapid growth*					
Calcium (%)	0.62	0.70	0.35	1.25	0.08	0.05	0.05
Phosphorus (%)	0.40	0.45	0.20	0.22	0.34	0.27	0.34
Zinc (ppm)	65	65	9	16	6	4	8
Copper (ppm)	22	22	17	28	35	19	17

MINERAL EXCESSES

Horses can tolerate fairly high levels of mineral intake, but excesses of calcium, phosphorus, zinc, iodine, fluoride, and certain heavy metals such as lead and cadmium may lead to developmental orthopedic disease.

Mineral excesses occur because of overfortification or environmental contamination. Massive oversupplementation of calcium (>300% of required) may lead to a secondary mineral deficiency by interfering with the absorption of other minerals such as phosphorus, zinc, and iodine. Excessive calcium intake may be compounded by the use of legume hays as the primary forage source. Iodine and selenium oversupplementation occurs if supplements are fed at inappropriate levels. A ration evaluation is the best way to identify this type of mineral imbalance.

Environmental contamination is a more likely cause of developmental orthopedic disease because contamination may result in extremely high intakes of potentially toxic minerals. If a farm is experiencing an unusually high incidence of developmental orthopedic disease or if the location and severity of skeletal lesions are abnormal, environmental contamination should be investigated. Blood, feed, and water analysis should be performed. In addition, chemical analysis of hoof and hair samples may reveal valuable information in such a situation. Farms that are located near factories or smelters are the most likely candidates for this type of contamination, although OCD from a zinc-induced copper deficiency has been reported on farms using fence paint containing zinc or galvanized water pipes.

Table 2. Toxic mineral levels (NRC, 1989; Cunha, 1997).

Mineral	Level of mineral needed by young horse (ppm)	Level at which mineral is toxic (ppm)
Iodine	0.2-0.3	5.0
Fluoride	–	50
Lead	–	80
Selenium	0.2-0.3	5.0
Manganese	60-70	4000
Copper	20-30	300-500
Cobalt	0.1	400

MINERAL IMBALANCES

The ratio of minerals may be as important as the actual amount of individual minerals in the ration. High levels of phosphorus in the ration will inhibit the absorption of calcium and will lead to a deficiency, even if the amount of calcium present was normally adequate. The ratio of calcium to phosphorus in the ration of young horses should never dip below 1:1 and ideally it should be 1.5:1. Too much calcium may affect phosphorus status, particularly if the level of phosphorus in the ration is marginal. Calcium to phosphorus ratios greater than 2.5:1 should be avoided if possible. Forage diets with high calcium levels should be supplemented with phosphorus. The ratio of zinc to copper should be 3:1 to 4:1.

DIETARY ENERGY EXCESS

Excessive energy intake can lead to rapid growth and increased body fat, which may predispose young horses to developmental orthopedic disease. A recent Kentucky study showed that growth rate and body size may increase the incidence of certain types of developmental orthopedic disease in Thoroughbred foals (Pagan et al., 1996). Yearlings that showed osteochondrosis of the hock and stifle were large at birth, grew rapidly from 3 to 8 months of age, and were heavier than the average population as weanlings.

The source of calories for young horses may also be important, as hyperglycemia or hyperinsulinemia have been implicated in the pathogenesis of osteochondrosis (Glade et al., 1984; Ralston, 1995). Foals that experience an exaggerated and sustained increase in circulating glucose or insulin in response to a carbohydrate (grain) meal may be predisposed to development of osteochondrosis. In vitro studies with fetal and foal chondrocytes suggest that the role of insulin in growth cartilage may be to promote chondrocyte survival or to suppress differentiation and that hyperinsulinemia may be a contributory factor to equine osteochondrosis (Henson et al., 1997).

Recent research from Kentucky Equine Research (Pagan et al., 2001) suggests that hyperinsulinemia may influence the incidence of OCD in Thoroughbred weanlings. In a large field trial, 218 Thoroughbred weanlings (average age 300 ± 40 days, average body weight 300 kg ± 43 kg) were studied. A glycemic response test was conducted by feeding a meal that consisted of the weanling's normal concentrate at a level of intake equal to 1.4 g nonstructural carbohydrate (NSC) per kilogram body weight. A single blood sample was taken 120 minutes post feeding for the determination of glucose and insulin.

In this study, a high glucose and insulin response to a concentrate meal was associated with an increased incidence of OCD. Glycemic responses measured in the weanlings were highly correlated with each feed's glycemic index (GI), suggesting that the GI of a farm's feed may play a role in the pathogenesis of OCD. Glycemic index characterizes the rate of carbohydrate absorption after a meal and is defined as the area under the glucose response curve after consumption of a measured amount of carbohydrate from a test feed divided by the area under the curve after consumption of a reference meal (Jenkins et al., 1981). In rats, prolonged feeding of high GI feed results in basal hyperinsulinemia and an elevated insulin response to an intravenous glucose tolerance test (Pawlak et al., 2001). Hyperinsulinemia may affect chondrocyte maturation, leading to altered matrix metabolism and faulty mineralization or altered cartilage growth by influencing other hormones such as thyroxine (Pagan et al., 1996; Jeffcott and Henson, 1998).

Based on the results of this study, it would be prudent to feed foals concentrates that produce low glycemic responses. More research is needed to determine if the incidence of OCD can be reduced through this type of dietary management.

Ration Evaluations

In almost every circumstance of developmental orthopedic disease, the surest way of determining if nutrition is a contributing factor is to perform a ration evaluation, which compares the intake of several essential nutrients with the requirements of the horse. Gross deficiencies or excesses of key nutrients can then be identified and corrected.

TYPES OF EVALUATIONS

Ration evaluations can be approached in two ways. One way is to add up what is being fed and compare it to the horse's requirements. This is actually more difficult than it may first appear since most horsemen do not actually know exactly what their horses are eating. There are a number of checks that can be used to more accurately estimate feed intakes, and these checks will be reviewed later. Alternatively, a new ration may be developed.

THE PROTOCOL

Every nutrition evaluation should include a description of the horse, definition of nutrient requirements, determination of nutrients in feedstuffs, determination of intake of feedstuffs, calculation of nutrient intake, comparison of intake with requirements, and adjustments of the ration to correct deficiencies or excesses.

Describe the horse. Different classes of horses have different nutrient requirements, and each class may eat different amounts of forage and grain. Within each class of horse, it is important to know the horse's current body weight, its age and mature body weight if growing, and its rate of body weight gain or loss.

Define nutrient requirements. Ration evaluations are intended to compare a horse's daily nutrient intake to a set of requirements to determine how well the feeding program meets the horse's nutritional needs. This would seem to be a straightforward accounting exercise, but what nutrient requirements should be used? The National Research Council (NRC) publishes a set of requirements for horses, but NRC values represent minimum requirements for most nutrients. These are the levels of intake that are required to prevent frank deficiency symptoms. No allowances are included to account for factors that may increase the requirement of a nutrient. The bioavailability of nutrients may be different, and other substances within a ration may interfere with the digestibility or use of a nutrient.

Kentucky Equine Research has developed its own set of nutrient recommendations for young growing horses. These requirements are based on a combination of NRC numbers, research that has been conducted since publication of the most recent NRC recommendations, and experience in the field. Digestible energy and protein are two NRC requirements that fairly accurately describe the needs of horses maintained under practical management conditions. These two requirements were primarily developed from direct measurements of growth response and energy balance in a number of different experiments. Other requirements, such as those for calcium and phosphorus, were developed using more theoretical calculations involving estimates of endogenous losses and digestibility. Still others were based on values developed for other species or from single experiments that were far from conclusive. For most of the vitamins and minerals, KER requirements use values ranging from 1.25 to 3.0 times those recommended by NRC. All of these nutrient requirements are far from absolute, and they will continue to evolve as more data become available. For now, though, it is assumed that these requirements adequately reflect what is needed by the horse under a wide range of conditions.

Determine nutrients in feedstuffs. The accuracy of evaluating the diet depends on proper sampling of feedstuffs. The feeds should be thoroughly mixed and a representative sample taken. Pelleted feeds are fairly uniform, but sampling is more critical for textured feeds and home mixes. If an odd nutrient value is encountered, look to sampling error as a likely cause.

A hay core can be used to obtain a representative hay sample for analysis. Pasture analysis is more difficult. Should the entire pasture be systematically sampled or only those areas heavily grazed? Horses tend to be spot grazers; therefore sampling the heavily grazed areas is probably best.

When expressing feed intakes and nutrient composition, air dry values for hay and grain and 100% dry matter values for pasture are used. This is because hay and grain intakes are actually measured as fed and pasture intakes tend to be estimated. The moisture content of the pasture is not relevant to the evaluation and only complicates intake calculations.

A number of commercial laboratories analyze forages and feeds. For a typical ration evaluation for young growing horses, the following nutrients should be either analyzed or calculated for each forage and concentrate: digestible energy (megacalories [Mcal] or megajoule [MJ], typically estimated), crude protein (percent), lysine (percent, typically estimated), acid or neutral detergent fiber (percent), calcium (percent), phosphorus (percent), zinc (percent), copper (percent), and manganese (percent).

These nutrients are usually included on a standard panel analysis at a reasonable cost. Other minerals, such as selenium and iodine, are usually analyzed separately, and analysis can be quite expensive. Selenium and iodine are not essential for most evaluations that focus on identifying nutritional causes of developmental orthopedic disease.

Determine intake of feedstuffs. A common flaw in many ration evaluations is measuring intake inaccurately. A scale should be used to measure the amount of grain and hay offered. A certain degree of hay wastage usually occurs, and this should be taken into account when calculating intake. Table 4 lists expected feed consumption by various classes of horses. The amount of forage and grain consumed by a young horse can vary tremendously depending on its geographic location and forage availability. Typically, horses that are raised in more tropical environments will depend more heavily on grain in their ration. Yearlings raised in temperate areas with abundant forage eat rations that contain 80% forage.

Table 3. Expected feed consumption by horses.

Horse	% of body weight		% of diet	
	Forage	Concentrate	Forage	Concentrate
Maintenance	1.0-2.0	0-1.0	50-100	0-50
Pregnant mare	1.0-2.0	0.3-1.0	50-85	15-50
Lactating mare (early)	1.0-2.5	0.5-2.0	33-85	15-66
Lactating mare (late)	1.0-2.0	0.5-1.5	40-80	20-60
Weanling	0.5-1.8	1.0-2.5	30-65	35-70
Yearling	1.0-2.5	0.5-2.0	33-80	20-66
Performance horse	1.0-2.0	0.5-2.0	33-80	20-66

Calculate nutrient intake. Determining pasture intake is the most difficult part of conducting a ration evaluation. Two methods usually are employed to estimate pasture intake. The simplest method is to arbitrarily estimate intake at about 1% to 1.5% of a young horse's body weight. The obtained value is only fairly accurate, but it is representative of most young horses on pasture the majority of the day. A second and more accurate method is to calculate pasture intake energetically by subtracting the digestible energy intake from all other feedstuffs from the horse's daily energy requirement. Dividing this number by the pasture's calculated energy density yields daily dry matter intake. For example, a yearling that weighs 330 kg with an average daily gain of 0.55 kg/day should require 20.4 Mcal of digestible energy per day. If that yearling is eating 3.65 kg of sweet feed (10.8 Mcal digestible energy) and 2 kg of mature alfalfa hay (3.6 Mcal digestible energy), then it must be consuming around 6 Mcal of digestible energy from pasture. Most grass pastures contain about 2.2 Mcal of digestible energy per kilogram, so this yearling must consume about 2.73 kg of pasture dry matter per day. These intakes can then be used to evaluate the adequacy of the ration for other nutrients in addition to energy. This method of calculating pasture energy intake works well provided the horse is actually consuming the intakes of other feedstuffs and the correct energy requirements were selected.

Using the method described above for estimating pasture intake often yields a negative number. If this occurs, then either the digestible energy intake of the other feeds was too high or the calculated energy consumption was too low. Sometimes horse owners report higher intakes of feeds than are actually eaten. This is particularly true for forages because hay is rarely weighed and large quantities are often wasted. Grain intake can also be overestimated. At other times the hay and grain intake may be correct, but the horse may be consuming more energy than calculated. Increased energy intake can occur if the horse is expending extra energy to work or to keep warm in cold weather, or a young horse may be growing faster than assumed. For example, a yearling needs about 5 kg of additional grain (16.1 Mcal of digestible energy) per kilogram of gain. If average daily gain is higher than assumed, then the horse may be eating significantly more digestible energy than calculated.

Compare intake to requirements. Rarely will the nutrients supplied by a ration exactly match the horse's requirements, and it is unnecessary to balance rations with this type of precision. Instead, the key to interpreting a ration evaluation is to identify deficiencies, excesses, or imbalances of nutrients that may affect growth and skeletal soundness. For most nutrients, a level of intake in excess of 90% of required is not considered deficient. What is interpreted as excessive varies tremendously among nutrients. For instance, potassium plays only a minor role in skeletal development; a young horse at pasture may consume greater than 300% of its potassium requirement. Most of this potassium comes from the pasture and is perfectly harmless. Even small excesses of other nutrients, such as energy, may play a significant role in the development of skeletal disease. Energy intakes that are 115% of required might trigger mild developmental orthopedic disease, and levels above 130% almost certainly will cause problems in rapidly growing horses.

Feeding Practices that Contribute to Developmental Orthopedic Disease

Several feeding scenarios may contribute to developmental orthopedic disease. Once identified, most can be easily corrected through adjustments in feed type and intake. Several of the most common mistakes made in feeding young growing horses are explained.

OVERFEEDING

One of the most common problems of feeding young horses is excessive intake that results in accelerated growth rate or fattening. Both conditions may contribute to developmental orthopedic disease. Unfortunately, there are no simple rules about how much grain is too much, because total intake of both forage and grain determines caloric consumption. Large intakes of grain are appropriate if the forage is sparse or poor quality, as often is the case in tropical environments. For example, grain intakes as high as 2% to 2.5% of body weight may be necessary to sustain reasonable growth in weanlings that have access to no forage other than tropic pasture. Conversely, grain intakes higher than 1% body weight may be considered excessive when weanlings are raised on lush temperate pasture or have access to high-quality alfalfa hay.

Table 4. Growth rates of fillies and colts in central Kentucky.

Average days of age	Colts BW (kg)	Fillies BW (kg)	Colts ADG (kg/d)	Fillies ADG (kg/d)	Colts HT* (cm)	Fillies HT* (cm)	Colts BCS**	Fillies BCS**
14	77.7	76.1	-	-	107.3	106.3	5.7	6.0
43	116.3	115.1	1.38	1.34	115.7	115.5	6.2	6.4
72	149.5	148.5	1.20	1.19	122.6	121.8	6.2	6.3
99	182.1	178.6	1.14	1.11	127.3	127.1	6.0	6.5
127	208.8	207.9	1.01	1.01	129.8	130.3	5.8	5.9
155	233.6	230.2	0.89	0.84	133.5	132.5	5.5	5.7
183	255.9	250.7	0.80	0.75	135.8	134.7	5.4	5.6
212	277.1	271.0	0.75	0.71	138.2	137.4	5.5	5.5
240	295.1	287.3	0.68	0.60	140.0	139.4	5.4	5.5
267	309.1	300.6	0.55	0.48	141.8	140.7	5.4	5.4
296	322.0	311.0	0.43	0.40	144.2	142.5	5.3	5.4
323	335.1	322.5	0.40	0.35	145.4	144.0	5.4	5.4
350	349.2	335.2	0.43	0.39	147.0	145.5	5.3	5.4
378	362.5	350.1	0.45	0.51	148.3	146.7	5.4	5.5
406	378.9	367.9	0.52	0.60	150.2	148.2	5.5	5.7
435	396.2	388.9	0.62	0.65	150.8	149.6	5.5	5.8
462	414.2	407.9	0.59	0.60	152.5	151.5	5.6	5.8
490	427.8	418.0	0.55	0.54	153.4	151.8	5.7	5.8

*Height, **Body condition score

The surest way to document excessive intake is by weighing and using condition scoring in the growing horse. Growth rates and condition scores for Thoroughbred foals can be compared to the data presented in Table 3. Based on a system developed by Henneke et al. (1981), condition scoring measures fat deposition. Horses are scored from 1 to 9 with 1 denoting extreme thinness and 9 indicating obesity. In a Kentucky study, fillies tended to have higher condition scores than colts, and the difference was greatest at 4 months of age (fillies 6.48; colts 6.0). These condition scores are considered moderate to fleshy according to the Henneke scoring system. By 12 months of age, the condition scores of the colts and fillies had dropped to 5.3 and 5.4, respectively. Both sexes increased condition score slightly from 14 to 18 months.

If growth rate cannot be measured, excessive intake can often be assessed by ration evaluation. For example, a six-month-old Thoroughbred weanling (250 kg body weight, 500 kg mature body weight) was being fed 4 kg/day of a 16% protein sweet feed and 2 kg of alfalfa hay and had access to high-quality fall Kentucky pasture. To support a reasonable rate of growth (0.80 kg/d), this weanling required about 17 Mcal of digestible energy per day. The hay and grain intake of this foal alone would supply about 17.5 Mcal of digestible energy, which is slightly above the weanling's requirement. If a reasonable level of pasture intake is included (1% of body weight or 2.5 kg dry matter), this weanling would be consuming 135% of its digestible energy requirement, a level likely to cause problems.

To reduce intake, the alfalfa hay should be eliminated, if the pasture is indeed adequate. If hay were needed when the weanling is stalled, grass hay would be more appropriate. Secondly, grain intake should be reduced to a level of about 3 kg/d. At this level of grain intake, the weanling would need to consume about 3.3 kg of pasture dry matter to support a growth rate of 0.80 kg/d, and the ration would be nicely balanced.

INAPPROPRIATE GRAIN FOR FORAGE BEING FED

Occasionally, the concentrate offered to a growing horse is incorrectly fortified to complement the forage that is being fed. The problem occurs particularly when the forage is mostly alfalfa or clover. Most concentrates for young horses are formulated with levels of minerals and protein needed to balance grass forage.

For example, a 12-month-old yearling (315 kg body weight, 500 kg mature body weight, 0.50 kg/d ADG) is raised without access to pasture and the only forage available is alfalfa hay, which is fed at a level of intake equal to 1.5% of the yearling's body weight (4.72 kg/d). At this level of forage intake, the yearling would only require about 2.5 kg of grain per day. If a typical 14% protein sweet feed that was formulated to balance grass forage is used, the ration would be inappropriate for a number of reasons. Calcium would be 183% of the yearling's requirement, with a calcium to phosphorus ratio of 2.9:1. This would not be a problem except that phosphorus and zinc are marginal in the ration. Because calcium may interfere with the absorption of both of these minerals, the yearling may be at risk of developmental orthopedic disease from a zinc or phosphorus deficiency. The solution is to feed a concentrate that is more appropriately balanced for legume hay. For example, a 12% protein feed with 0.4% calcium, 0.9% phosphorus, and 180 ppm zinc would be more suitable.

INADEQUATE FORTIFICATION IN GRAIN

The most common reasons for inadequate fortification are using unfortified or underfortified grain mixes, using correctly fortified feeds at levels of intake that are below the manufacturer's recommendation, or using fortified feeds diluted with straight cereal grains. These errors in feeding can be corrected by the incorporation of a highly fortified grain balancer supplement.

For example, a 6-month-old weanling (200 kg body weight, 400 kg mature body weight, 0.60 kg/d ADG) is fed 3 kg/d of a 10% protein sweet feed that is intended for adult horses. To compound matters, the weanling is also fed grass hay with an estimated intake of 2.3 kg/d. This ration is deficient in protein, calcium, phosphorus, zinc, and copper. This foal would be prone to a rough hair coat and physitis. There are two ways to correct this problem. A properly formulated 14% to 16% protein grain mix with adequate mineral fortification could be used, or 1 kg of a grain balancer pellet can be substituted for 1 kg of the 10% sweet feed. This type of supplement is typically fortified with 25% to 30% protein, 2.5% to 3.0% calcium, 1.75% to 2.0% phosphorus, 125 to 175 ppm copper, and 375 to 475 ppm zinc. This is an extremely useful type of supplement to correct underfortified rations.

Feeding Systems to Prevent Developmental Orthopedic Disease

BROODMARES

The nutritional requirements of a broodmare can be divided into three stages. Stage one is early pregnancy, from conception through the first 7 months of gestation. Barren mares and pregnant mares without sucklings by their sides fit into this nutritional category. Stage two encompasses the last trimester of pregnancy, which is from around 7 months of pregnancy through foaling. Stage three is lactation, which generally lasts 5 to 6 months after foaling. The most common mistakes made in feeding broodmares are overfeeding during early pregnancy and underfeeding during lactation.

Early pregnancy. Proper feeding during pregnancy requires an understanding of how the fetus develops during gestation. Contrary to popular belief, the fetus does not grow at a constant rate throughout the entire 11 months of pregnancy. Figure 3 illustrates a typical growth curve for a fetus expressed as a percent of birth weight. As is plainly visible, the fetus is small during the first 5 months of pregnancy. Even at 7 months of pregnancy, the fetus equals only about 20% of its weight at birth. At this stage in pregnancy, the fetus equals less than 2% of the mare's weight, and its nutrient requirements are minuscule compared with the mare's own maintenance requirements. Therefore, the mare can be fed essentially the same as if she were not pregnant. Mare owners often increase feed intake after the mare is pronounced in foal, reasoning that she is now "eating for two." Increased feeding is unnecessary and may lead to obesity and foaling difficulties, especially if the mare has access to high-quality pasture during early pregnancy.

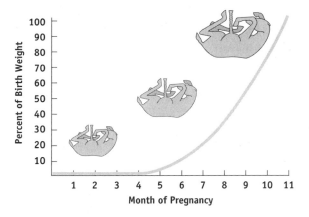

Figure 1. Typical growth curve for a fetus expressed as a percentage of birth weight.

Late pregnancy. The fetus begins to develop rapidly after 7 months of pregnancy, and its nutrient requirements become significantly greater than the mare's maintenance requirements; therefore adjustments should be made in the mare's diet. Digestible energy requirements only increase about 15 percent over early pregnancy. Protein and mineral requirements increase to a greater extent. This is because the fetal tissue being synthesized during this time is quite high in protein, calcium, and phosphorus. During the last four months of pregnancy, the fetus and placenta retain about 77 grams of protein, 7.5 grams of calcium, and 4 grams of phosphorus per day. Trace mineral supplementation is also very important during this period because the fetus stores iron, zinc, copper, and manganese in its liver for use during the first few months after it is born. The fetus has developed this nutritional strategy of storing trace minerals during pregnancy because mare's milk is quite low in these elements.

New Zealand researchers studied the effect of copper supplementation on the incidence of developmental orthopedic disease in Thoroughbred foals. Pregnant Thoroughbred mares were divided into either copper-supplemented or control groups. Live foals born to each group of mares were also divided into copper-supplemented or control groups. Copper supplementation of mares was associated with a significant reduction in the physitis (inflammation of the bone growth plates) scores of the foals at 150 days of age. Foals from mares that received no supplementation had a mean physitis score of 6, whereas foals out of supplemented mares had a mean score of 3.7. A lower score means less physitis. Copper supplementation of foals had no effect on physitis scores. A significantly lower incidence of articular cartilage lesions occurred in foals from supplemented mares.

However, copper supplementation of the foals had no significant effect on articular and physeal cartilage lesions. Mares in late pregnancy are often overfed energy in an attempt to supply adequate protein and minerals to the developing foal. If the pregnant mare becomes fat during late pregnancy, she should be switched to a feed that is more concentrated in protein and minerals so that less can be fed per day. This will restrict her energy intake while ensuring that she receives adequate quantities of other key nutrients.

Lactation. A mare's nutrient requirements increase significantly after foaling. During the first 3 months of lactation, mares produce milk at a rate equal to about 3% of their body weight per day. This milk is rich in energy, protein, calcium, phosphorus, and vitamins. Therefore, the mare should be fed enough grain to meet her greatly increased nutrient requirements. Mares in early lactation usually require from 4.5-6.5 kg of grain per day depending upon the type and quality of forage they are consuming. This grain mix should be fortified with additional protein, minerals, and vitamins to meet the lactating mare's needs. Trace mineral fortification is not extremely important for lactating mares because milk contains low levels of these nutrients and research has shown that adding more to the lactating mare's diet does not increase the trace mineral content of the milk. Calcium and phosphorus are the minerals that should be of primary concern during lactation. Grain intake should be increased gradually during the last few weeks of pregnancy so that the mare is consuming nearly the amount that she will require for milk production at the time that she foals. A rapid increase in grain should be avoided at foaling because this may lead to colic or founder. Milk production begins to decline after about 3 months of lactation, and grain intake can be reduced to keep the mare in a desirable condition.

SUCKLINGS

If the broodmare has been fed properly during late pregnancy, it is unnecessary to supplement the suckling with minerals until it reaches 90 days of age. At 90 days, moderate amounts of a well-fortified foal feed can be introduced and gradually increased until the suckling is consuming around 0.5 kg feed per month of age. It is critical that the suckling be accustomed to eating grain before it is weaned. If it is not, there is a very good chance that there will be a dramatic decrease in growth rate at weaning. When the weanling finally starts eating grain, a compensatory growth spurt will occur that may result in developmental orthopedic disease.

WEANLINGS

The most critical stage of growth for preventing developmental orthopedic disease is from weaning to 12 months of age, when the skeleton is most vulnerable to disease and nutrient intake and balance is most important. Weanlings should be grown at a moderate rate with adequate mineral supplementation. In temperate regions, the contribution of pasture is often underestimated, leading to excessive growth rates and developmental orthopedic disease.

YEARLINGS

Once a horse reaches 12 months of age, it is much less likely to develop several forms of developmental orthopedic disease than a younger horse. Many of the lesions that become clinically relevant after this age are typically formed at a younger age. Still, proper nutrient balance remains important for the yearling. It is best to delay the increased energy intakes that are required for sales prepping as long as possible because the skeleton is less vulnerable to developmental orthopedic disease as the yearling ages. Normally, increasing energy intake 90 days before a sale is enough time to add the extra body condition that is often expected in a sales yearling.

Physitis in the carpus is often a major concern with sales yearlings. To reduce the incidence of physitis in these horses, the level of trace mineral supplementation should remain high and a significant portion of the energy normally supplied from grain should be replaced with fat and fermentable fiber. Sales preparation grain mixes can contain as much as 10% fat. Sources of fermentable fiber include beet pulp and soy hulls.

Nutritional Management of Developmental Orthopedic Disease

The goal of a feeding program for young horses is to reduce or eliminate the incidence of developmental orthopedic disease. Unfortunately, developmental orthopedic disease will still occur in some foals. Nutritional intervention can help reduce the severity of many forms of developmental orthopedic disease, but not all of the damage resulting from developmental orthopedic disease is reversible. However, it is important to alter the feeding programs of foals with developmental orthopedic disease. The type of alteration will follow a similar pattern but will depend on the foal's age and the type of developmental orthopedic disease. In almost every instance, energy intake should be reduced while maintaining adequate levels of protein and minerals. The rationale for this type of modification is that skeletal growth should be slowed, but adequate substrate should be available to promote healthy bone development.

PHYSITIS

Grain intake should be restricted to a level supplying around 75% of the foal's normal energy requirement. This restriction, however, should not compromise protein and mineral intake, so a different type of feed formulation may be required. For instance, a six-month-old weanling (250 kg body weight, 500 kg mature body weight, 0.8 kg average daily growth) on a decent fall pasture would normally consume around 3.5 kg of a 16% protein foal feed. If this foal developed physitis, it would be confined and fed grass hay (3 kg/d). Reducing the grain intake to a level that was 75% of the foal's normal digestible energy would result in shortages of protein, lysine, calcium, and phosphorus. These shortfalls could be overcome by replacing 1 kg of the 16% percent sweet feed with a grain balancer pellet. This ration would supply 90% of the foal's normal protein requirement alone with a good supply of minerals. As the physitis resolves, intake of the 16% grain mix can be slowly increased and the supplement pellet intake slowly decreased until the foal returns to its normal ration.

WOBBLER SYNDROME

A feeding program like the one described previously is also appropriate for the horse with wobbler syndrome except that the degree of exercise and energy restriction may be more severe. In this case, a feeding program that combined grass hay (2 kg/d) with a moderate amount of alfalfa hay (2 kg/d) and 1 kg/d of balancer pellet would result in a reduction in energy intake equal to 65% of normal intake while maintaining adequate levels of protein and mineral intake.

OSTEOCHONDRITIS DISSECANS

Once a foal develops osteochondritis dissecans that is severe enough to produce clinical signs, the effect of diet is going to be minimal in solving the existing lesion. Again, reducing energy intake and body weight while maintaining adequate protein and mineral intake is advised. Conservative management of shoulder (humeral head) and stifle (lateral trochlear ridge) OCD lesions has been successful. Complete stall rest is recommended along with intra-articular hyaluronan and intramuscular Adequan. There have been anecdotal reports of improvement in lesions identified radiographically through the use of oral joint supplements containing glucosamine and chondroitin sulfate, but these findings have not been validated in a controlled study.

Summary

Nutrition may play a role in the pathogenesis of developmental orthopedic disease. Mineral deficiencies, excesses, or imbalances may be involved along with excesses in energy or carbohydrate intake. A computerized ration evaluation is the best method to identify potential problems. The feeding errors that most often cause developmental orthopedic disease are excessive grain intake, an inappropriate grain mix for the forage being fed, and inadequate fortification in the grain. Each of these can easily be corrected by selecting an appropriate grain mix and feeding it at the correct level of intake. Foals that already have developmental orthopedic disease should have their energy intakes reduced while maintaining adequate levels of protein and mineral intake.

References

Cunha, T.J. 1997. Horse Feeding and Nutrition (2nd Ed.). Academic Press, Orlando, Florida.

Glade, M.J., S. Gupta, and T.J. Reimers. 1984. Hormonal responses to high and low planes of nutrition in weanling Thoroughbreds. J. Anim. Sci. 59(3):658-665.

Henneke, D.R., G.D. Potter, and J.L. Kreider. 1981. A condition score relationship to body fat content of mares during gestation and lactation. In: Proc. 7th Equine Nutr. Physiol. Soc. Symp. 7:105-110.

Henson, F.M., C. Davenport, L. Butler, I. Moran, W.D. Shingleton, L.B. Jeffcott, and P.N. Schofield. 1997. Effects of insulin and insulin-like growth factors I and II on the growth of equine fetal and neonatal chondrocytes. Equine Vet. J. 29(6):441-447.

Jeffcott, L.B., and F.M. Henson. 1998. Studies on growth cartilage in the horse and their application to aetiopathogenesis of dyschondroplasia (osteochondrosis) Vet. J. 156(3):177-92.

Jenkins, D.J., T.M. Wolever, R.H. Taylor, H. Barker, H. Fielden, J.M. Baldwin, A.C. Bowling, H.C. Newman, A.L. Jenkins, and D.V. Goff. 1981. Glycemic index of foods: A physiological basis for carbohydrate exchange. Amer. J. Clin. Nutr. 34:362-366.

NRC. 1989. Nutrient Requirements of Horses (5th Ed.). National Academy Press, Washington, DC.

Pagan, J.D., R.J. Geor, S.E. Caddel, P.B. Pryor, and K.E. Hoekstra. 2001. The relationship between glycemic response and the incidence of OCD in Thoroughbred weanlings: A field study. In: Proc. Amer. Assoc. Equine Pract. 47:322-325.

Pagan, J.D., S.G. Jackson, and S. Caddel. 1996. A summary of growth rates of Thoroughbreds in Kentucky. Pferdeheilkunde 12:285-289.

Pawlak, D.B., J.M. Bryson, G.S. Denyer, and J.C. Brand-Miller. 2001. High glycemic index starch promotes hypersecretion of insulin and higher body fat in rats without affecting insulin sensitivity. J. Nutr. 131:99-104.

Ralston, S.L. 1995. Postprandial hyperglycemica/hyperinsulinemia in young horses with osteochondritis dissecans lesions. J. Anim. Sci. 73:184 (Abstr.).

THE RELATIONSHIP BETWEEN GLYCEMIC RESPONSE AND THE INCIDENCE OF OCD IN THOROUGHBRED WEANLINGS: A FIELD STUDY

JOE D. PAGAN
Kentucky Equine Research, Versailles, Kentucky, USA

Introduction

Hyperglycemia and hyperinsulinemia have been implicated in the pathogenesis of osteochondrosis (Glade et al., 1984; Ralston, 1995). More specifically, foals that experience an exaggerated and sustained increase in circulating glucose or insulin in response to a carbohydrate (grain) meal may be predisposed to development of osteochondrosis. In vitro studies with fetal and foal chondrocytes suggest that the role of insulin in immature cartilage may be to promote chondrocyte survival or to suppress differentiation and that hyperinsulinemia may be a contributory factor to equine osteochondrosis (Henson et al., 1997). Rutgers University was recently granted a United States patent for diagnosing a predisposition for equine osteochondritis dissecans (OCD) using an oral glucose tolerance test (United States Patent). This patent was based on the premise that foals exhibiting an exaggerated glycemic response to an oral glucose challenge were more susceptible to developing OCD. The purpose of the present study was to evaluate if there is a relationship between a glycemic response test and the incidence of OCD in Thoroughbred weanlings, and to determine if this test would be useful in identifying factors that may predispose young growing horses to OCD.

Materials and Methods

Two hundred eighteen Thoroughbred weanlings (average age 300 ± 40 d, average body weight 300 ± 43 kg) on six central Kentucky farms were studied during December 1999 and January 2000. A glycemic response test was conducted by feeding a meal that consisted of the weanling's normal concentrate at a level of intake equal to 1.4 g nonstructural carbohydrate (NSC)/kg body weight (BW). Two of the farms fed a pelleted concentrate, while the other four used a textured sweet feed mix. All of these concentrates were fortified with levels of protein and minerals deemed suitable for weanlings. The NSC content of the farms' feeds ranged from 40% to 50%, and the test meal size equaled 963 ± 170 g. A single blood sample was taken 120 min post feeding for the determination of plasma

433

glucose and insulin concentrations. The test meal was fed between 7:00-8:00 a.m. and the weanlings had not received any other grain for at least 12 h. Weanlings on five of the six farms spent the night before the test on pasture, whereas one farm confined the weanlings in box stalls with access to grass hay throughout the evening.

The glycemic index (GI) of each feed was also determined using four mature Thoroughbred geldings at the Kentucky Equine Research (KER) farm. These feeds were again fed in a single meal at a level of intake equal to 1.4 g NSC/kg BW. Blood samples were taken immediately pre-feeding and at 30-min intervals for 4 hours post feeding. GI was calculated from the area under the glucose response curves (AUC) for each feed. The overall incidence of OCD on these farms was recorded until the horses were sold as yearlings in July or September at ages ranging from 16-20 months. For the purpose of this study, OCD was defined as osteochondrotic lesions occurring in the fetlock, hock, shoulder, or stifle that were treated surgically. These lesions were either diagnosed after the foal showed clinical signs of lameness or joint effusion, or after routine radiographic examinations that were performed in January and February of the foal's yearling year. Weanlings with no evidence of lesions or with lesions that were identified radiographically but that did not require surgery were considered unaffected.

Results

Twenty-five of the 218 weanlings (11.5%) had OCD lesions that were treated surgically. There was a wide range in the incidence of OCD among farms (Table 1). Plasma glucose and insulin 2 h post feeding were significantly higher in weanlings with OCD than in unaffected foals ($p < .05$). Insulin/glucose ratios, however, were not significantly different (Table 2). The incidence of OCD was significantly higher in foals whose glucose and insulin values were greater than one standard deviation above the mean for the entire population (both OCD and unaffected) in the study (Table 3). Elevated insulin/glucose ratios did not appear to be correlated with an increased incidence of OCD. Each weanling's body weight was measured at the time of the glycemic response test and expressed as a percentage of a reference set of body weights collected from 350 fillies and 350 colts raised in Kentucky (Pagan et al., 1996). Each body weight was compared to the same age and sex in the reference data set. Overall, there was no difference between unaffected foals and OCD foals in relative body weight. However, affected foals from farm 2, which experienced a 32% incidence of OCD, averaged 115% of the reference weight whereas unaffected foals averaged 106%. Conversely, foals from farm 1, which reported no OCD, averaged 97% of the Kentucky average body weight.

There were strong positive correlations between mean glucose ($r = .84$, $p < .01$; Figure 1) and insulin ($r = .93$, $p < .01$; Figure 2) response on each farm and the incidence of OCD. Much of the difference in glycemic response among farms was probably due to the GI of the feed since there was also a strong positive correlation (r = .88, p < .05; Figure 3) between the GI of each farm's feed and the farm's weanling glucose response. GI was also positively correlated with the incidence of OCD on each farm (r = .74, p < .10; Figure 4).

Table 1. Incidence of OCD on individual farms.

Farm #	Total foals (n)	OCD foals (n)	OCD (% of foals)
1	24	0	0
2	19	6	32
3	27	2	7
4	51	4	8
5	74	9	12
6	23	4	17

Table 2. Plasma glucose, insulin, and insulin/glucose ratio two hours post feeding.

	Glucose (mg/dl)		Insulin (pmol/l)		Insulin/Glucose Ratio	
	OCD (n = 25)	Unaffected (n = 193)	OCD (n = 25)	Unaffected (n = 193)	OCD (n = 25)	Unaffected (n = 193)
Mean	150.1	134.2	130.3	106.0	0.846	0.779
SE	7.1	1.9	12.8	3.4	0.055	0.019
Significance	p < .01		p < .05		p > .10	

Table 3. Relationship between glucose, insulin, and insulin/glucose ratio and the incidence of OCD.

Standard deviations from mean	Glucose		Insulin		Insulin/Glucose Ratio	
	% Population	% OCD	% Population	% OCD	% Population	% OCD
< 1 SD	11.0	0.0	10.1	0.0	15.1	6.0
± SE	72.9	10.1	78.0	11.2	68.3	12.1
> 1 SD	16.1	25.7	11.9	23.0	16.5	13.9

Discussion

In this study, a high glucose and insulin response to a concentrate meal was associated with an increased incidence of OCD. Glycemic responses measured in the weanlings were highly correlated with each feed's GI, suggesting that the GI of a farm's feed may play a role in the pathogenesis of OCD. GI characterizes the rate of carbohydrate absorption after a meal and is defined as the area under the glucose response curve after consumption of a measured amount of carbohydrate

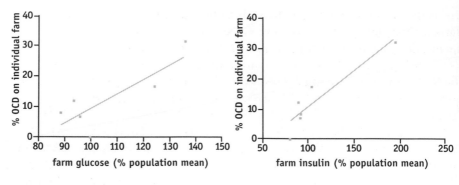

Figure 1. Relationship between farm glucose and incidence of OCD.

Figure 2. Relationship between farm insulin and incidence of OCD.

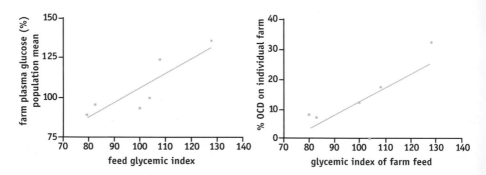

Figure 3. Relationship between glycemic index and farm glucose.

Figure 4. Relationship between feed glycemic index and incidence of OCD.

from a test feed divided by the area under the curve after consumption of a reference meal (Jenkins et al., 1981). In rats, prolonged feeding of high GI feed results in basal hyperinsulinemia and an elevated insulin response to an intravenous glucose tolerance test (Pawlak et al., 2001). In foals, hyperinsulinemia may affect chondrocyte maturation, leading to altered matrix metabolism and faulty mineralization, or altered cartilage growth by influencing other hormones such as thyroxine.

Within each farm, there was no significant difference in glycemic response between horses that had lesions and normal individuals. Therefore, using this type of glycemic response test in older weanlings to identify individuals that may be predisposed to OCD does not look promising. Perhaps diet-induced hyperglycemia or hyperinsulinemia predisposes every weanling to OCD, but other factors such as biomechanical stress or trauma are needed to produce a clinically relevant lesion. Body weight may have been a factor affecting the very high and low incidence of OCD in farms 2 and 1, respectively.

Based on the results of this study, it would be prudent to feed foals concentrates that produce low glycemic responses. More research is needed to determine if a glycemic response test using a more standardized oral glucose challenge (i.e., dextrose) can be used to identify younger individuals that are predisposed to OCD. This study was entirely funded by Kentucky Equine Research, Inc. which is the licensee of the patent (#5,888,756) discussed in this article. The authors wish to thank the owners and managers of the farms that participated in this study for allowing access to their weanlings. Also, thanks go to Dr. Rhonda Rathgeber of Hagyard-Davidson-McGee Assoc. for assisting in blood sampling, Dr. Sarah Ralston of Rutgers University for performing insulin assays, and KER interns Amanda Prince, Catherine Hudson, and Sonya Gardner for assistance with glucose assays and GI determinations.

This paper was first published as Pagan, J.D., R.J. Geor, S.E. Caddel, P.B. Pryor, and K.E. Hoekstra. 2001. The relationship between glycemic response and the incidence of OCD in thoroughbred weanlings: A field study. In: Proc. Amer. Assn. Equine Practnr. 47:322-325.

References

Glade, M.J., S. Gupta, and T.J. Reimers. 1984. Hormonal responses to high and low planes of nutrition in weanling Thoroughbreds. J. Anim. Sci. 59:658-665.

Henson, F.M., C. Davenport, L. Butler, et al. 1997. Effects of insulin and insulin-like growth factors I and II on the growth of equine fetal and neonatal chondrocytes. Equine Vet. J. 29:441-447.

Jeffcott, L.B., and F.M. Henson. 1988. Studies on growth cartilage in the horse and their application to aetiopathogenesis of dyschondroplasia (osteochondrosis). Vet. J. 156:177-192.

Jenkins, D.J., T.M. Wolever, R.H. Taylor, et al. 1981. Glycemic index of foods: A physiological basis for carbohydrate exchange. Amer. J. Clin. Nutr. 34:362-366.

Pagan, J.D., S.G. Jackson, and S. Caddel. 1996. A summary of growth rates of Thoroughbreds in Kentucky. Pferdeheilkunde 12:285-289.

Pawlak, D.B., J.M. Bryson, G.S. Denyer, et al. 2001. High glycemic index starch promotes hypersecretion of insulin and higher body fat in rats without affecting insulin sensitivity. J. Nutr. 131:99-104.

Ralston, S.L. 1995. Postprandial hyperglycemica/hyperinsulinemia in young horses with osteochondritis dissecans lesions. J. Anim. Sci. 73:184 (Abstr.).

United States Patent #5,888,756. Diagnosing a predisposition for equine osteochondrosis dissecans. Inventor: Sarah L. Ralston, Jackson, NJ; Assignee: Rutgers, The State University of New Jersey, New Brunswick, N.J.; Licensee: Kentucky Equine Research, Inc., Versailles, KY 40383.

LAMINITIS: CAUSES AND CURES

RIC REDDEN
International Equine Podiatry Center, Versailles, Kentucky

The word laminitis elicits fear among horsemen because many associate it with the end of the horse's career and sometimes the horse's life. Laminitis is a catastrophic syndrome that should always be treated as an emergency. Recent research and new techniques used to treat this condition now make it possible to save horses that might have died. A diagnosis of laminitis is no longer a death sentence.

What is laminitis? Simply put, laminitis is an inflammation of the laminae, the sensitive tissues that connect the hoof wall to the coffin bone and other structures of the horse's foot. The laminae play a major role in stabilizing the bones inside the foot. When inflammation occurs, the integrity of this crucial bond is often compromised, leading to serious damage to bones and soft tissues.

Laminitis can strike any horse regardless of its breed, use, or activity. It mostly occurs in mature horses and is rarely found in horses less than one year old. In my many years of practice, I have never seen a case in which laminitis is the primary disease; it has always been secondary to another disease process or trauma. Sometimes, the feet of a horse become involved as a result of another disease process, such as colic, Potomac horse fever, or salmonellosis.

Recent research has provided greater insights into what is actually happening to the blood supply within the foot and how that affects the integrity of the structure during acute and chronic laminitis.

Understanding the anatomy and physiology of the normal and laminitic foot gives the treatment team (consisting of a veterinarian, a farrier, and the owner) the means to reverse the damage incurred during a laminitic episode. Inflammation of the laminae leads to ischemia, which causes cell death. The cells die because they cannot obtain nutrients from the blood supply. The blood is shunted away from the foot by a mechanism that is not fully understood. However, it is known that reduced blood supply sets the stage for inflammation and subsequent cell death, which destroys the intricate network of laminae that suspends the horse's weight between the coffin bone and the hoof wall.

Laminae act like the tiny hooks and grippers in Velcro strips when they have been fastened together. One side is attached to the bone, the other side to the wall. If all of the laminae were placed flat, their surface area would approximately equal the size of a tennis court. For this reason, a horse can suffer from laminitis and have a very mild insult to a very small area of the total surface. Another laminitic horse might have a very severe insult that wipes out the majority of the laminae within hours, leading to a catastrophic situation in which the hoof wall separates from the foot.

Basic Steps of Progressive Disease

Laminitis can be triggered by a variety of factors. Careful attention to anything that might be a contributing factor and the presentation of this information to the veterinarian creates a history that may be essential in the diagnosis and treatment of the horse. A thorough history could have key implications on the diagnosis as well as the prognosis. Common primary problems that often precede laminitis are:

- Overeating grain or grass, especially by obese animals
- Prolonged high fever
- Severe colic
- Retained placenta for more than 12 hours
- Pneumonia
- Pleuritis
- Potomac horse fever
- Colitis caused by salmonella
- Stress brought on by constant movement, shipping, showing, loss of sleep, water deprivation, or dehydration
- Unilateral lameness brought about when a horse suffers a severe injury in one leg or foot and places excess weight on the opposite limb
- Road founder or excessive concussion for a prolonged period of time
- Accidents or mechanical trauma
- Black walnut shavings used as bedding
- Water founder or when an overheated horse is allowed to tank up with water
- Mastitis founder affecting lactating mares
- Enteritis/colitis or endotoxic absorption following surgery
- Postoperative colic laminitis

What Are the Signs of Laminitis?

The most common sign of laminitis is lameness. If the laminitic horse can be persuaded to walk, it moves with a shortened stride, with each foot quickly placed back on the ground. Standing still, the horse appears to have its feet "nailed to the floor" in the parlance of old-time horsemen. The characteristic stance of a laminitic horse includes hind feet brought forward under its belly in an effort to get most of its weight off the front feet, which are stuck out in front of its normal center of gravity. If all four feet are affected and the horse is in severe pain, it might lie down and be reluctant to rise.

Upon closer examination, the horse may have a bounding digital pulse. Always check the pulse before moving the animal, because even in a healthy horse, a few steps can increase the pressure within the blood vessels. There are cases of severe, acute laminitis in which the pulse is very faint or not detectable at all. Most have warmer than normal feet. In rare cases, however, they can be ice cold. Therefore, it is necessary to use other clinical signs if a case of laminitis is suspected. The most obvious sign is acute lameness or signs of pain. Even if the horse does not ultimately have laminitis, its pain requires prompt attention. A veterinarian and the horse's farrier should be asked to see the horse right away. The farrier should be included because he or she knows the horse's feet best and can be extremely helpful in telling the veterinarian what changes might be noticeable.

The quicker help is obtained for the horse, the greater the chances that the horse will recover. Help means treating the acute inflammatory stage as well as the inciting cause, and mechanically reversing the forces that are working to destroy the vital, sensitive areas inside the foot. It is crucially important for the vet and farrier to work together at this point to treat this potentially devastating disease. Therapy that is initiated the moment the horse shows the slightest sign of laminitis increases the window of response time so critical to the horse's recovery.

Establish the Grade of Lameness

Several published grading systems for general lameness have been published. However, it is helpful to differentiate the degree of lameness in the context of possible laminitis.

Grade 1 - Walks sound, trots lame, turns sore. All four feet can be readily elevated and handled.

Grade 2 - Walks sore, turns on hind feet, reluctant to trot. Reluctant to lift feet.

Grade 3 - Must to be persuaded to walk and refuses to trot. Very reluctant to lift feet.

Grade 4 - Stands with feet rooted to the ground. Reluctant to move even with strong persuasion. Refuses to lift feet. Very painful facial expression. If lying down, it is very difficult to make the horse get up.

Industry-wide statistics are not encouraging as far as prognosis is concerned, and many veterinarians worldwide consider complicated laminitis akin to a death sentence. A majority of laminitic cases recover using various means of treatment – some even without treatment – and seem to suffer no ill consequences. However, 20 to 30% of the across-the-board cases will have devastating insult, resulting in catastrophic damage to the laminae and costing either careers or lives.

A lackadaisical approach to this syndrome works well if there is a very mild insult. Unfortunately, it is impossible to differentiate between mild and complicated cases at the onset of the syndrome. If the complicated case is treated in a similar fashion as a mild case, the horse's chance of recovery can dwindle.

Looking for Clues

Early treatment is designed not only to attack the syndrome but to prevent secondary mechanical destruction. Review what might have prompted the onset of laminitis while waiting for the arrival of the veterinarian and the farrier. Consider what occurred during the previous 48 to 72 hours. Did the horse travel and have a stressful trip? Did it have a high fever or signs of stressful breathing? Has it been exposed to conditions that might precipitate pneumonia or some other respiratory disease? Has one or more of its limbs become swollen for no apparent reason? Has the horse recently received an influenza vaccination or any other kind of injection? Has the horse been given corticosteroids?

Although treating horses with corticosteroids can have very beneficial effects, caution should be taken. A small percentage of horses have developed laminitis within a few hours to a few days following corticosteroid therapy. Many veterinarians believe that there is a direct correlation. Even though the incidence is quite low, I am among the veterinarians who believe there is an inherent risk in such treatments and therefore advise caution to clients wishing to use corticosteroids.

In terms of steroid therapy, we basically have two: (1) corticosteroids (such as dexamethasone, Depo-Medrol, Vetalog, etc.) have potent anti-inflammatory properties indicated for numerous uses; and (2) anabolic steroids (including Winstrol-V, Equipoise, and others), which are used to increase appetite, stimulate muscle development, and are hormonal in nature. Anabolic steroids should not be confused with corticosteroids.

Has the horse inadvertently consumed a much larger amount of grain than it normally eats? Many horses require tremendous amounts of grain to maintain peak condition, whereas others might need only a handful. When a horse manages to break into a feed room, it might eat only what it needs while others will gorge until they have consumed all of the grain. Horses that devour too much grain can present a serious problem. A veterinarian should be called immediately as swift action cannot only prevent gastritis and subsequent laminitis, but it might also save the life of the animal.

Other Things to Consider

When was the horse last shod? Did the farrier have any problems or comments concerning the feet? The farrier most likely knows the unique characteristics of an individual horse's feet better than does the owner. This knowledge can be invaluable when assessing the degree of damage. Farriers might look for increased sensitivity around the coronary band itself, such as swelling, discharge, or moisture that might indicate serum leakage or a possible abscess; an abnormal ledge formation or an abnormally distinct margin to the hoof wall; or increased sensitivity over the sole and toe area detected through the use of a hoof tester.

Has the conformation of the sole changed? Is the sole sagging? Does it seem to be fuller? Is the sole bruised? The farrier might pull the shoe to better inspect the area under the shoe for hot nails and other shoe-related problems. Findings become invaluable in helping the veterinarian interpret the visual as well as radiographic evidence of a potential problem.

The veterinarian will assess the overall health of the animal in an effort to rule out underlying metabolic problems that could have precipitated the acute signs of pain. It is extremely important to address the seat of the problem if it can be diagnosed.

When nothing out of the ordinary has occurred, consider whether the horse has experienced stress. This could be stress from traveling, any change in routine, or changes in feed or water. Veterinarians have long acknowledged a link between stress and the onset of laminitis.

Certain disease syndromes can precipitate laminitis, but it is difficult to relate known causes to a particular case. Owners and trainers are sometimes distraught because they cannot pinpoint a precise cause for an episode of laminitis. Knowing the reason is not essential to resolving the problem. It can be a helpful indicator to what lies ahead, but close observation of the horse, radiographs, and response to therapy is more valuable than knowing what caused it.

Management and Prevention

Treating laminitis is one thing, but preventing it is quite another. The mechanism that triggers this devastating disease syndrome is unknown. However, being aware of several other clinical indications that usually precede laminitis helps in spotting high-risk patients. This knowledge gives some insight into prevention.

Laminitis that is directly associated with obesity is easy to prevent. The following is a great motto for maintaining healthy horses - "the fat ones get less and the thin ones get more."

How simple this might seem. There is a great tendency for owners to overfeed horses. The owners express their confidence that their heavy animals are not only the best of the breed, but the healthiest. Apparently, it is human nature to want to provide for our horses as we do for our children. Unfortunately, providing absolutely everything we think the horses might want is usually very different from what they actually need. It might give the owners a feeling of accomplishment to overprotect, but when they go overboard, they can harm their horses.

Maintaining horses on lush pastures with a balanced diet and adequate caloric intake poses a totally different problem than maintaining a proper diet for horses living in more arid areas. Lush pastures can yield up to 35% protein for several months of the year. Most people are totally unaware of the richness of their pastures. Even worse, there is no completely accurate means of knowing how much grass a horse eats in a 24-hour period.

I feel there is a worldwide tendency for people to overprovide food for their horses. Many broodmares and stallions routinely carry more than 200 pounds of excess weight, and these horses should be considered at high risk for laminitis. An unbiased view should be taken of every feeding program, and then each individual horse should be considered. Owners should be directed to work with nutrition specialists who are highly focused and dedicated to making a better tomorrow for them and their horses. Scales or body tapes, reasonably accurate for judging weight, are helpful, or the truck scales at the local feed dealer can be employed to keep a handle on the horse's weight so that changes can be caught early. Exercise programs should also be evaluated to determine if they match the feeding program for each horse.

Laminitis caused by opposing limb breakdown also can be prevented in many instances with proper management. The injuries that can trigger opposing limb founder, more correctly called unilateral laminitis, are:

- Any injury that will require more than two weeks to heal
- Deep puncture wounds to the navicular area
- Extensive fractures of the first, second, or third phalanx
- Fetlock breakdowns and shattered sesamoids
- Unilateral paralysis
- Complicated septic lower joints and/or tendon sheaths.

Any horse that is persistently lame for three to five days quickly becomes a high-risk candidate for laminitis. Septic joints, particularly hocks and stifles, seem to predispose the foot on the opposing limb to laminitis. It sometimes occurs in the previous "sound" leg within days of the first signs of pain or lameness in the "unsound" leg. In such cases of traumatic laminitis, the laminae become dysfunctional due to lack of blood flow. Venograms of normal feet have shown a marked absence of contrast throughout the lamellar vessels when the foot is bearing weight at the time the dye is injected. Apparently the weight of the horse is precariously balanced between the deep flexor tendon and the laminae. Once loaded, the laminae stretch to their normal physiological limit, which apparently restricts normal blood flow. When an injured horse stands planted on its sound foot for endless hours or days, its body weight shuts down delivery of adequate nutrients to the laminae of the good foot, which will soon become dysfunctional.

Horses that constantly shift back and forth from one leg to the other are much less likely to have laminitis than those that cock the unsound leg and stand like that all day. Proper management of such cases can prevent opposing limb laminitis in the majority of cases. Reducing tendon pull at the very onset of the injury can help prevent ischemia that causes lamellar death. Use of the Modified Ultimate Wedge provides the mechanics that can help prevent unilateral lameness. It is crucial to take into consideration the toe angle, heel angle, ventral angle, cup of foot, and overall quality and health of horn before beginning this corrective shoeing. Failure to do so can cause several problems.

I believe waiting until radiographic signs of laminitis are present before applying a mechanical aid seldom offers favorable results. The special shoeing mechanics can be too little, too late. Normally, the first six to eight weeks following an acute injury is the high-risk period, even if the original injury is responding quite favorably. Many times the foot balance on the injured leg goes off scale as well, putting these cases in double jeopardy.

After a shattered fetlock has been repaired surgically, the horse will have a tendency to develop a very low heel and tipped up coffin bone on the injured limb (caudal rotation), which often predisposes the horse to further problems as P1, P2, and P3 luxate. The severe luxation, or misalignment of these bones, can create abnormal stress on the supporting tendon. Unfortunately, this simply adds insult to injury, especially if the good foot has developed traumatic laminitis. On the bright side, however, caudal rotation in the leg in which the surgery was performed can be prevented with proper therapeutic shoeing when addressed at the onset.

Most traumatic unilateral cases are classic sinkers. Seldom do they have more than a few degrees of rotation. They often have two centimeters of sinking.

Summary

Once laminitis is evident, treat it accordingly. Reverse the forces at play. Unfortunately, most horses that develop unilateral laminitis have severe damage when they are diagnosed. Swift, aggressive mechanics can pull many through, but treatment is risky and costly. Frequent radiographs and constant monitoring of the sound foot is quite important for a successful preventative program.

CUSHING'S DISEASE AND OTHER PROBLEMS OF THE OLDER HORSE

RAY GEOR

R and J Veterinary Consultants, Guelph, Ontario, Canada

Introduction

In recent years, great strides have been made in the nutritional management of the older horse. Changes in digestive function (e.g., poor teeth) and the development of chronic illnesses such as Cushing's syndrome can alter dietary needs and dictate a change in dietary management. This paper will review what is known regarding problems of the older horse, with an emphasis on (1) known alterations in nutrient requirements and/or metabolism, and (2) dietary management to improve body condition and quality of life.

Demographic information suggests that older horses (e.g., more than 15 to 20 years of age) now comprise a much larger proportion of the overall horse population. More than ever, the horse is a treasured companion, and we strive to ensure that this rewarding relationship lasts for as long as is reasonably possible. Just what do we mean by old? There are no hard-and-fast rules. We do know that few horses survive into their 30s or 40s, but many horses do quite well until their late 20s. Geriatric and senior are terms frequently used to describe horses in this elderly age bracket. However, geriatric really refers to old humans or animals with problems and diseases. Old but otherwise healthy horses are just that – old.

Effects of Aging

The adage "you are only as old as you feel" perhaps also applies to horses. Some horses may begin to "slow down" in their late teens, while others may remain quite vigorous in their mid-20s. In many different athletic disciplines, there are numerous examples of horses remaining highly competitive until their late teens or even beyond. The reason for this difference is unknown. As in humans, it is possible that genetics, diet, and exercise history play some role in determining life span. In many horses, signs of aging are evident after 20 years of age. These signs include graying of the hair, particularly around the eyes, temples and nostrils, development of a sway back, increased prominence of the backbone, and poor dental health.

Dental problems are common in old horses and frequently result in loss of body weight and an inability to maintain condition. The most common dental problems include excessive wear, missing teeth, and abnormal wear patterns such as "wave mouth." Tooth decay and gum infections (periodontal disease) are also more common in older horses. The most obvious effect of dental problems is a decrease in feed intake. Decreased feed intake can be attributed to pain and an inability to properly chew dietary fiber. The latter is frequently manifest as "quidding" the feed; partially chewed wads of hay are dropped out of the mouth. Poorly chewed hay and fiber can also predispose the horse to choke because of lower than normal saliva production during mastication (the chewing of food). With decreased saliva production, there is less lubricant to aid the passage of ingesta through the esophagus.

Aging may adversely affect digestive function. In one study, the digestibility of protein, fiber, and phosphorus were lower in mares over 20 years of age compared to mares less than 10 years of age (Ralston et al., 1989). As the digestive profile of the old mares was similar to that reported for horses that had undergone resection of the large bowel (90% removed), these changes in digestibility were attributed to large intestinal dysfunction. However, more recent studies by the same investigator have largely refuted these earlier findings (Ralston et al., 2000). The authors hypothesized that poor dentition and/or the effects of parasitic larval migration in the large intestine were responsible for the lowered fiber, protein, and phosphorus digestibility observed in the earlier study (Ralston et al., 2000). More research is required to clarify these issues.

Some authors have suggested that decreased liver and kidney function is common in old horses. Although chronic liver and kidney failure are occasionally diagnosed in old horses, these problems are much less common than, for example, dental disease. More research is necessary to characterize the effects of aging on liver and kidney function in horses and the role of diet in the management of these problems. Chronic inflammatory respiratory disease is more common in older compared to younger horses, and this condition is discussed elsewhere in this proceedings. Another relatively common problem of older horses, Cushing's disease, is discussed later.

Feeding the Old Horse

Dietary fiber is the most important consideration when designing a diet for the old horse, particularly in circumstances where there are dental problems. Horses with moderate to severe dental abnormalities will do poorly on a predominantly hay diet, particularly when the hay is of low quality. Imperfect mastication will impair assimilation of energy and other nutrients from the feed, the result being progressive weight loss. Ideally, the older horse should have daily access to pasture as grass is easily chewed and digested and even horses with poor dentition can do reasonably well during the spring and summer months when given plenty of grazing time. An exception would be the horse who has damaged or missing incisor teeth.

Horses with poor dentition will require alternative fiber sources to ensure adequate fiber intake (e.g., hay cubes, hay pellets, chaff, beet pulp, soy hulls). Some horses will still have difficulty chewing hay cubes. In some cases, presoaking the cubes will aid mastication. Horses with very poor teeth are sometimes unable to properly digest the fiber contained in hay cubes or chopped hay, simply because they cannot adequately chew the ingested material. Mushy feeds such as soaked hay pellets or beet pulp can be used in these situations.

An easy method for provision of dietary fiber is the feeding of a complete "senior" feed. Most of the senior feeds on the market contain a fiber source such as alfalfa meal, soy hulls, beet pulp, or a combination of these ingredients. These feeds also contain grains which have either been extruded or processed into other highly digestible forms (e.g., rolled, steam flaked). These pelleted or extruded feeds are easy to chew, thus helping to prevent problems associated with poorly chewed feeds. For horses with very poor teeth, it is recommended that these feeds be soaked in water prior to feeding.

A well-formulated senior feed should contain, at the minimum, 12% dietary fiber and a protein percentage between 12 and 16%. The latter is often achieved by including soybean meal in the formulation. If there is evidence of decreased renal function, protein content should not exceed 12% and excess calcium should be avoided. Yeast and other digestive aids are also included to improve fiber and phosphorus digestion. Mineral and vitamin fortification should be higher than that for a standard maintenance horse feed to account for a possible age-related decline in digestive efficiency. Although these diets can be fed without other forage, it is always preferable to provide the horse access to some high-quality forage in the form of pasture or first-cut hay with a high leaf to stem ratio.

As weight loss and failure to maintain body condition are common problems in older horses, increasing the energy density of the diet by the addition of fat is a logical strategy. Oils such as corn, canola, and linseed are often added to commercial senior feeds, providing a 4 to 6% fat ration. If more calories are required, additional oil (e.g., 100-150 ml) or 1-2 lb of rice bran (20% fat) may be fed. Rice bran (and oil) contains gamma-oryzanol, a steroid-like compound that is purported to have anabolic effects in muscle.

It is generally necessary to feed older horses by themselves; in group situations, the younger, more dominant horses will often drive the older horse away from feed, contributing to weight loss problems.

Cushing's Disease (Equine Hyperadrenocorticism)

A reasonably common disorder in older horses is Cushing's disease or equine hyperadrenocorticism. This condition is caused by a tumor of the pituitary gland, specifically a pituitary pars intermedia adenoma (PIA). The disease is primarily attributed to an overproduction of pro-opiomelanocortin (POMC) peptides by the pituitary, including adrenocorticotrophic hormone (ACTH), ß-endorphin, and α-melanocyte stimulating hormone (MSH). In normal horses, the secretion of these peptides is under negative feedback control. For example, ACTH stimulates the adrenal glands to synthesize and secrete the glucocorticoids (cortisol and corticosterone). An increase in circulating cortisol, in turn, signals the pituitary to stop secretion of ACTH. In this manner, the body is able to regulate cortisol concentrations within a fairly narrow range. Other endocrine problems can arise when the PIA encroaches the neighboring tissues, particularly the hypothalamus and neurohypophysis.

Cushing's disease has been reported in horses and ponies. Although affected horses and ponies are typically greater than 15 years of age, there are reports of cases in horses as young as 7 years. In four reports, the mean age of affected horses ranged between 18 and 21 years (Boujon et al., 1993; Heinrichs et al., 1990; Hillyer et al., 1992; van der Kolk et al., 1993). There is no apparent sex or breed predilection, although an increased prevalence in ponies has been reported (Hillyer et al., 1992).

The onset of clinical signs can be very gradual (e.g., over a period of 1-4 years). The most remarkable clinical sign in horses and ponies with Cushing's syndrome is hirsutism, an excessively long and curly hair coat. Frequently, the owner will report that the horse or pony failed to shed out in the spring. Black and dark brown hair can lighten in color (usually to a golden brown). The other common clinical signs are weight loss and muscle wasting (frequently with a potbellied appearance), lethargy, hyperhidrosis (excessive sweating), and bulging of the orbit due to an increase in fat deposition around the eyes. Some horses will have increased appetite (polyphagia) and thirst (polydipsia) and an increase in urine production (polyuria). It is important to note that horses with Cushing's disease can present with any combination of these clinical signs; it is rare that an individual horse will display all of the common abnormalities.

There are two major secondary complications of PIA: laminitis and diabetes mellitus with concurrent weight loss. In one case series, 38% of affected horses had signs consistent with diabetes mellitus and 24% were laminitic (van der Kolk et al., 1993). The cause of laminitis in Cushing's disease horses is unknown. Some have proposed that elevated cortisol concentrations results in constriction of the digital blood vessels. Another theory proposes that insulin dysfunction is an underlying mechanism. As insulin is a vasodilator, insulin resistance could also result in peripheral vasoconstriction and laminitis. Regardless of the cause, chronic laminitis is a major problem in horses with Cushing's disease. Recurrent episodes often lead to rotational changes in the distal phalanx and a predisposition to development of sole abscesses. Abnormalities in hoof growth can also occur; affected ponies can develop very long overgrown toes ("pixie shoes").

Diabetes mellitus is attributed to insulin resistance and results in hyperglycemia and, in most cases, polyuria and polydipsia. Other complications include recurrent bacterial or fungal infections, delayed wound healing, blindness, seizures, and diabetes insipidus. Because persistently high cortisol can suppress the immune system, it is thought that the increased susceptibility to infection is a sequelae to immunosuppression.

Diagnosis of equine hyperadrenocorticism is a challenge. Routine hematology and blood chemistry can reveal abnormalities characteristic of the syndrome (e.g., hyperglycemia, increased plasma triglycerides), but these alterations are not present in every case. Some form of dynamic endocrine testing is required for a definitive diagnosis. The dexamethasone suppression test (DST) is commonly used. In normal horses, a small dose of dexamethasone results in a marked suppression (>60-70%) in plasma cortisol 24 hours later (Dybal et al., 1994). However, horses with PIA are usually unresponsive to the dexamethasone (i.e., cortisol concentrations remain unchanged). Another useful test is the measurement of the ratio of urine to plasma cortisol concentrations; this ratio is markedly increased in many horses with PIA.

There is no cure for PIA, and the prognosis is guarded to poor depending on the number of complications present at the time of diagnosis. However, medical therapy can result in clinical improvement in some affected horses. Currently, the drug pergolide is the treatment of choice for horses with PIA. Pergolide, a dopamine agonist, suppresses the secretion of ACTH by the pituitary, thereby decreasing the stimulus for cortisol production. Clinical improvement can be seen in as little as 3-4 weeks.

Given the increased susceptibility of PIA horses to infections, a top-notch preventive health program is necessary. Vaccination and deworming programs must be adhered to and minor ailments, such as skin infections, should be aggressively treated. Regarding nutritional management, a case-by-case approach is necessary when making recommendations. Some PIA horses are overweight, necessitating a restriction in dietary energy while ensuring provision of adequate protein, minerals, and vitamins. Others are thin and require a more energy-dense diet.

High starch diets may exacerbate diabetes mellitus and increase the risk for further episodes of laminitis. Therefore, a low starch diet is usually indicated for horses with PIA. Although fat can be a useful substitute, it should be recognized that dietary fat is associated with development of mild insulin insensitivity. For this reason it is preferable to feed a diet that emphasizes highly digestible fibers (e.g., non-molassed beet pulp, alfalfa meal) rather than fat. A chromium supplement is also recommended. Chromium has been demonstrated to improve insulin "effectiveness." Therefore, chromium supplementation may help in the control of diabetes mellitus in PIA horses. Supplemental vitamins (E and C) and zinc may be useful to ensure optimal function of the immune system.

References

Boujon CE, Bestetti GE, Meier HP, Straub R, Junker U, Rossi GL. Equine pituitary adenoma, a functional and morphological study. J Comp Path 109: 163-178, 1993.

Dybal NO, Hargreaves KM, Madigan JE, Gribble DH, Kennedy PC, Stabenfeldt GH. Diagnostic testing for pituitary pars intermedia dysfunction in horses. J Am Vet Med Assoc 204: 627-632, 1994.

Heinrichs M, Baumgärtner W, Capen CC. Immunocytochemical demonstration of pro-opiomelanocortin peptides in pituitary adenomas of the pars intermedia of horses. Vet Pathol 27: 419-425, 1990.

Hillyer MH, Taylor FGR, Mair TS, Murphy D, Watson TDG, Love S. Diagnosis of hyperadrenocorticism in the horse. Equine Vet Educ 12: 35-39, 1992.

Ralston SL, Malinowski K, Christensen R, Breuer L. Apparent digestion of hay/grain rations in aged horses – revisited. In Proceedings 2000 Equine Nutrition Conference for Feed Manufacturers, Kentucky Equine Research Inc., pp 193-195.

Ralston SL, Squires EL, Nockels CF. Digestion in the aged horse. J Eq Vet Sci 9: 203-205, 1989.

van der Kolk JH, Kalsbeek HC, Garderen Evan, Wensing T, Breukink HJ. Equine pituitary neoplasia: a clinical report of 21 cases (1990-1992). Vet Rec 133: 594-597, 1993.

LOSING CONTROL: NUTRITION-RELATED DISEASES OF THE CENTRAL NERVOUS SYSTEM

JONATHAN H. FOREMAN
University of Illinois, College of Veterinary Medicine, Urbana, Illinois

Introduction

Neurological diseases can be some of the most devastating and dangerous clinical problems seen in horses. Due to their size, strength, and temperament, neurological horses can become a danger to themselves or to those around them. Several neurological diseases of the horse have nutritional origins. Large, fast-growing young horses which are overfed can sometimes become wobblers. Equine protozoal myelitis is caused by organisms which are transmitted to the horse orally, via grain, hay, pasture, or water. Equine degenerative myelopathy and equine motor neuron disease are both rarer conditions which have been linked to dietary vitamin E deficiencies. Some of these neurological diseases are treatable, but most are preventable with proper, balanced nutrition in appropriate daily amounts.

Equine Cervical Vertebral Malformation

DEFINITION AND HISTORY

Equine cervical vertebral malformation (CVM) is a developmental defect of the cervical vertebrae. As a result of abnormal growth, two adjoining vertebrae articulate abnormally, resulting in compression of the spinal cord as it traverses those two vertebrae. The most commonly affected joint is between the third and fourth cervical vertebrae (designated C3-C4).

These horses are often termed "wobblers" because they wobble or walk as if drunk or uncoordinated. Other synonyms for the condition include true wobblers, wobbles, cervical vertebral instability (CVI), and cervical vertebral stenosis (CVS). Many of these horses may be from families which typically produce large, fast-growing racehorses. These families may have a tendency to produce young horses with other signs characteristic of osteochondrosis (abnormal cartilage maturation into bone) such as a tendency toward rapid growth compared to their cohorts (age-matched pasturemates); osteochondritis dissecans (OCD) of the hock, shoulder, or stifle; and epiphysitis (asymmetry or overactivity in one or more of the growth plates of the long bones such as the distal radius at the level just above the carpus [knee] and the distal cannon bone just above the fetlock).

rate can be slowed and the already abnormal vertebrae can be afforded time to remodel until no cervical compression is apparent. This technique has been described twice in unrefereed literature but has not gained wide acceptance due to its possible humane aspects and due to it not having been evaluated in a controlled experimental setting. Young Thoroughbred horses were observed with very early, mild neurological deficits (Donawick et al., 1989, 1993). They then were fed poor quality grass hay, no grain, and no pasture, and they received strict stall rest over several months. The result was that most eventually had minimal neurological deficits, and most went on to perform adequately as racehorses. Their marketability was diminished by severely slowing their growth rate, but their neurological signs were minimized without surgical intervention.

PROGNOSIS

Many horses which survive the immediate postoperative period improve as a result of the ventral fusion surgery. However, few if any are normal afterward; there are nearly always residual neurological deficits. From a liability standpoint, one must question the wisdom of having these horses, previously diagnosed as neurological, ridden and raced in the company of other horses.

PREVENTION

Preventive measures primarily involve careful breeding and feeding programs with slower dietary pushing for fast growth. Breedings observed to produce wobblers in the past should be avoided. Mares which have produced wobblers previously should be monitored carefully for level of milk production, as heavily milking mares may be predisposed to producing faster growing foals. This phenomenon has been most apparent to this observer in Thoroughbred foals raised on nurse mares of draft heritage. Creep feeding must be done judiciously to prevent overfeeding by a greedy suckling or weanling which pushes its pasturemates away from the feeder. Feeding for the commercial market may be necessary but again must be done wisely to prevent creation of a large, well-muscled but ataxic yearling. Allowing individuals to mature at a more natural rate of growth results in adults of similar size; however, some may develop as athletes later if allowed to mature more naturally.

Equine Protozoal Myeloencephalitis

DEFINITION AND HISTORY

Equine protozoal myeloencephalitis (EPM) is a sporadic and sometimes fatal neurological disease of horses (but not donkeys or mules) caused by *Sarcocystis neurona*, a protozoan parasite which invades the central nervous system. EPM is not contagious because the parasite stages in the infected horse do not produce protozoal stages which are infective to other horses. Synonyms for EPM include equine protozoal myeloencephalopathy, equine protozoal myelitis, equine protozoal encephalitis, EPM, and protozoal.

EPM was first reported as a clinical disease in horses in Kentucky in 1970 (Rooney et al., 1970). In 1974, an unidentified protozoal parasite was first associated with spinal cord disease in horses (Cusick et al., 1974). Initially, the organism was thought to be *Toxoplasma gondii* (Cusick et al., 1974) but was later shown to be a *Sarcocystis* species (Simpson and Mayhew, 1980). *Sarcocystis neurona* was first isolated from infected equine spinal cord and identified as the causative agent of EPM in 1991 (Dubey et al., 1991). In 1996, another protozoal parasite, *Neospora*, was also found to be associated with abnormal clinical signs of spinal cord disease in horses in California (Marsh et al., 1996).

LIFE CYCLE

Although the definitive life cycle is not completely known at this time, *Sarcocystis neurona* is believed to have a classic two-host predator-prey life cycle similar to all other *Sarcocystis* species. The opossum (*Didelphis virginiana*) is the definitive host (Fenger and Granstrom, 1995). Extrapolating from the known life cycle of another intramuscular parasite of opossums, *Sarcocystis falcatula*, it has been proposed that the organism normally lives in the muscles of cowbirds (*Molothrus ater*), pigeons, grackles, some finches, and other birds (the prey). Opossums (the predators) eat these birds. The organism then escapes from the bird muscle and sets up new life cycle stages in the intestine of the opossum. Recent work has shown that *Sarcocystis* spp. organisms (collected from infected bird muscle) can be given to naïve opossums, and *Sarcocystis* oocysts eventually can be collected from those opossums as the life cycle is completed (Cutler et al., 1999). The opossum excretes the parasite in its feces and possibly in its urine. Normally, the parasite is then ingested by another bird (the intermediate host), and the life cycle continues in a circular or cyclical manner.

The North American opossum is a definitive host for at least three species of *Sarcocystis*: *S. neurona* (Dubey et al., 1991), *S. falcatula* (Box et al., 1984), and *S. speeri* (Dubey and Lindsay, 1999). Genetic testing has shown that *S. neurona* and *S. falcatula* are >99.5% identical (Dame et al., 1995; Fenger and Granstrom, 1995). Combined with >99.5% genetic similarity with the parasite isolated from cowbird muscle, these data have been cited previously as evidence that *Sarcocystis neurona* and *Sarcocystis falcatula* are the same organism (Dame et al., 1995; MacKay, 1997). However, more recent work has disproven the identity problems between *S. neurona* and *S. falcatula* (Cutler et al., 1999). *S. falcatula* oocysts from naturally infected cowbirds were fed to naïve opossums. The infective opossum feces were then administered to naïve horses. There were no clinical signs in the horses and no conversion in *S. neurona* antibodies in either serum or

These horses usually deteriorate quickly and have a poor prognosis. The severity of their signs means that they should be considered dangerous, and clients are encouraged to handle them with caution.

Sometimes signs may be mild and may be confused with lameness (Foreman et al., 1990). With these neurological lamenesses, the source of the lameness cannot be determined through routine diagnostic testing such as nerve blocks, radiographs, and scintigraphs. There may be a history of stifle locking. Some performance horses are reported not to bend as well as previously or to misbehave at odd times (perhaps an early sign of brain disease).

DIAGNOSIS

Diagnosis of EPM may be presumed from the history and neurological signs, especially if lateralizing. EPM testing may be performed on blood samples, but there is a 50% chance that even a normal horse will test positive on an EPM blood test. One EPM scientist has stated that "positive results of a serum immunoblot test have no value in ruling in a diagnosis of EPM" (MacKay, 1997). Practitioners often use serum screening as a method to rule out EPM as a possible diagnosis because EPM is unlikely to be the cause of the neurological signs if the serum is negative for EPM exposure.

The current standard for positive clinical diagnosis of EPM is testing of CSF. This fluid must be obtained in a sterile manner from one of two sites, the atlantooccipital (AO) space directly behind the head or the lumbosacral (LS) space found at the highest point of the horse's hindquarters. The LS tap is frequently performed on standing horses under tranquilization. The AO space is sometimes sampled under general anesthesia in nervous horses, horses with conformation preventing successful LS taps (preexisting LS subluxations), and horses undergoing anesthesia for another reason, such as elective surgery. Appropriate and adequate restraint followed by meticulous spinal fluid collection are critical to the value of the results because even microscopic amounts of blood introduced into the CSF may cloud the results (Miller et al., 1999). Blood contamination makes interpretation difficult and introduces the likelihood of false positives (Miller et al., 1999).

CSF is tested for EPM in two ways, a Western blot or immunoblot test for EPM antibodies (proteins which fight the EPM organism), and a polymerase chain reaction (PCR) test specific for the DNA or RNA of the EPM organism. There is a high correlation (>90% agreement) between a positive immunoblot spinal fluid test and the presence of the parasite at postmortem (Granstrom and Saville, 1998). There is a similarly high correlation between a negative CSF test and a lack of organism at postmortem. There is a poor correlation between being seropositive and finding the organism or its associated changes at postmortem (MacKay, 1997). The PCR test is less accurate when negative but is quite specific for the presence of the EPM organism when positive. The current interpretation of these false negative PCR tests is that the organism may be present, causing antibody to be formed (and a positive Western blot result), but the organism is present in the spinal cord, not the CSF, making the CSF PCR-negative. Obtaining and properly testing CSF costs approximately $250-400 and more if general anesthesia is required.

TREATMENT

The conventional method of treatment for EPM is oral administration of drugs classified as folic acid inhibitors (sulfonamides and pyrimethamine) for a minimum of 90-120 days. These drugs prevent folic acid production within the protozoa, resulting in their death. They usually do not cause folic acid deficiency in the horse because horses absorb considerable dietary folic acid from their intestine as long as they are eating a good quality diet with either grass or green hay. Gastrointestinal absorption of pyrimethamine may be delayed by simultaneous feeding (MacKay et al., 2000), so it is recommended that hay not be fed for 30-120 minutes after drug administration. In many management situations this delay is impractical, and there are no data to prove that simultaneous feeding and drug administration decrease the chances of successful treatment. To further complicate matters, if folic acid is to be supplemented, it should be given separately, several hours apart from drug administration intervals, to prevent drug interference with gastrointestinal absorption of the supplemented folic acid.

Treatment rarely has adverse side effects. Some horses develop soft stools, probably due to the antibacterial effects of the sulfonamide, but this diarrhea is mild and self-limiting. Very rarely, foals born to mares treated during pregnancy may show signs of folic acid deficiency (Toribio et al., 1998). These signs include low red and white blood cell counts leading to weakness and inability to fight off infections, severe renal hypoplasia, and ultimately death in only a few days. Most of these foals were born to mares that received folic acid supplementation while undergoing EPM treatment. Folic acid requirements in mares may be 5-10 times higher in pregnancy than when not pregnant, but investigators have suggested that additional dietary folic acid given with pyrimethamine actually may inhibit absorption of most or all of the dietary folic acid, resulting inadvertently in folic acid deficiency despite folic acid supplementation (Toribio et al., 1998). If there is concern over possible toxicity, weekly blood counts and/or folic acid determinations can be made on blood samples, but these tests cumulatively can become expensive. Horses already eating good quality grass or green hay are thought to consume sufficient dietary folic acid to prevent folic acid deficiency during treatment.

Recent epidemiological research has shown that "the likelihood of clinical improvement after diagnosis of EPM was lower in horses used for breeding and pleasure activities. Treatment for EPM increased the probability that a horse would have clinical improvement. The likelihood of survival among horses with EPM was lower among horses with more severe clinical signs and higher among horses that improved after EPM was diagnosed" (Saville et al., 2000b). In other words, conventional treatment works, improvement is a good prognosticator, and severity of clinical signs correlates with likelihood of response to treatment.

Most horses are treated for a minimum of 30 days, at which time they are reexamined to determine whether or not they have improved with treatment. If improved, treatment is continued for another 60-90 days in most cases. If unimproved within the first 30 days, it is unlikely that improvement will be seen with further treatment. Ideally, testing of CSF for EPM antibodies should be repeated, and the results should be negative before treatment is discontinued.

Newer drugs are currently being tested, but their efficacy is unproven, their toxicity remains undocumented, they are not yet widely available, and they can be quite expensive. Diclazuril (Clinacox, Pharmacia and Upjohn) is used twice daily for 21-28 days as a grain top-dressing (Granstrom et al., 1997; Cohen, 1998). It has a long half-life (>50 hours) and seems to be similar in treatment efficacy to conventional therapies (about 75% positive results) (Tobin et al., 1997). One disadvantage is that the volume of powder may make the grain unpalatable. Toltrazuril (Baycox, Bayer) is available as a 5% suspension which is administered daily for 28 days. It also has a long half-life (>50 hours) and approximately 75% efficacy compared to conventional therapy (Tobin et al., 1997). Nitazoxanide (NTZ) is available as an oral paste formulation which is administered in an increasing dose over a 28-day period. Initial reports indicate 75% efficacy even in horses which have proven refractory to conventional treatment. Some possible side effects from NTZ include self-limiting febrile episodes early in treatment, worsening of clinical signs about two weeks into treatment, discoloration of urine, lethargy, diarrhea, and increased digital pulses (suspicious of laminitis).

In acute and severe presentations, other supportive treatments may be necessary. Intravenous fluids are important if the horse is not drinking or eating. Analgesics (e.g., phenylbutazone) are given if trauma is suspected. In acute cases with brain signs, rabies cannot be ruled out easily, so gloves are mandatory when handling the horse while awaiting the results of EPM testing. Corticosteroids (prednisone, dexamethasone) are contraindicated since they may actually make the infection worse due to their ability to suppress the immune system.

PROGNOSIS

Fewer than 1% of horses which are seropositive actually develop clinical signs of EPM. Early detection and treatment of EPM increases the chances of complete recovery (Saville et al., 2000a). Approximately 60-70% of treated horses return to their previous athletic function with no further abnormal signs. Approximately 10% of treated horses relapse after treatment is discontinued. At the first sign of a relapse, the horse should be reexamined and treatment should be reinstituted. Horses will rarely continue to test positive on CSF. In these horses, treatment may have to be continued for months or even years. Residual clinical signs after treatment may include varying degrees of ataxia, muscle atrophy, paresis, and focal cranial abnormalities such as facial nerve paralysis or dysphagia (difficulty in swallowing).

Treatment of pregnant mares is sometimes necessary. The real risk of treatment is to the fetus, although some studies have shown this risk to be minimal especially early in pregnancy (Brendemuehl et al., 1998). Supplementation with folic acid during pregnancy may actually increase risk to the fetus (due to impaired gastrointestinal absorption of folic acid after administration of both folic acid inhibitors and folic acid) (Toribio et al., 1998). Supplementation is not necessary if the mare is eating good quality grass or green hay routinely.

PREVENTION

The obvious method of prevention of EPM is to limit horses' exposure to opossums and their feces. Opossums should be kept out of the barn and especially away from sources of hay, feed, and water. It may even be necessary to keep cats or dogs loose in the barn to discourage midnight raids by opossums on the feed. Bagged feed may be safer than bulk feed, especially if the top of the bulk feed bin is open. However, the organism probably survives transport in bagged feed if the feed was contaminated before processing. Any shipment of feed or hay that may be contaminated with animal feces should be rejected. Extruded feeds are likely to be most protective since the heat exposure during the extrusion process seems to kill the parasite before it is ingested by horses.

Preventative treatment of a normal horse which is in the same barn as another horse with a definitive EPM diagnosis is not recommended. It should be remembered that an infected horse cannot infect a normal horse; the parasite must come from the opossum, not from an infected horse. Unnecessary use of the medications to treat EPM may lead eventually to development of parasite drug resistance, making it more difficult to treat all EPM cases.

Recently an EPM vaccine (Fort Dodge Animal Health) has received conditional licensure by the USDA. This restricted category of licensing means that the company has demonstrated product purity and safety; that there is a reasonable expectation of efficacy but it has not yet been demonstrated; that there is a clear need for the product in the community (a "special need" provision); and that individual states still have the right to refuse to allow its use within their borders. Approval is therefore on a state-by-state basis. The license must be renewed annually, and the company must demonstrate efforts to prove efficacy for the conditional license to be renewed. One example of a vaccine which was provisionally licensed in this manner is the rotavirus vaccine from the same manufacturer.

The EPM vaccine consists of inactivated whole *Sarcocystis neurona* merozoites from infected equine spinal cord. The merozoites are chemically inactivated, with that inactivation tested by three blind passages in tissue culture followed by cell fixation and fluorescent antibody examination to ensure that no living merozoites remain. The vaccine has an adjuvant (MetaStim, Fort Dodge Animal Health) added to help to stimulate immunological response to the merozoites. This adjuvant has been shown to be effective in enhancing the response to an eastern and western equine encephalitis vaccine given to 9-11 month old foals (n=10). The adjuvant's safety was demonstrated in the equine rotavirus vaccine given to pregnant mares (n=235). Vaccine safety has been demonstrated in horses (n=897) in California, Illinois, Indiana, Kansas, Kentucky, Minnesota, and Oklahoma. Only four horses had adverse reactions consisting of localized swelling (n=4), stiffness (n=3), and lethargy (n=1). Vaccination elicited demonstrable serum neutralizing (SN) antibody titer against *S. neurona* merozoites. The question then becomes one of clinical efficacy because it is not agreed upon scientifically that SN antibody is protective against EPM. Use of the vaccine under field conditions followed by demonstration of efficacy in the form of decreased EPM incidence will be required for full licensure by the USDA.

Equine Degenerative Myeloencephalopathy

DEFINITION AND HISTORY

Equine degenerative myeloencephalopathy (EDM) is a progressive, symmetrical disease of neuronal degeneration first described in 1977 (Mayhew et al., 1977). The disease is familial and dietary in origin. Neuraxonal dystrophy (NAD) is a similar but less diffuse disease of Morgan horses (Beech, 1984; Beech and Haskins, 1987) and is included for discussion here because the causes of both diseases are similar, varying primarily in severity. It is thought that certain families of horses may have a predisposition to poor dietary absorption of vitamin E, so that when a diet is lacking in vitamin E, minimal amounts may be absorbed. Vitamin E is critical to normal neuronal health in its role as a scavenger of free radicals produced in most metabolic processes.

EPIDEMIOLOGY

A familial predisposition for EDM has been described in Appaloosas (Blythe et al., 1991), Standardbreds, Arabians, Paso Finos, and Grant's zebras (Mayhew et al., 1987), and for NAD in Morgans (Beech and Haskins, 1987). Affected horses are routinely young, growing horses (sucklings, weanlings, and yearlings), although some aged horses have been described. There is no sex predilection. One report indicated that horses in the northeastern U.S. were more commonly affected with EDM than horses in other regions (Dill et al., 1990).

No specific heritable mode has been described, but it is clear that some families are affected more than others (Mayhew et al., 1987). In one report (Mayhew et al., 1987), one Standardbred farm had a 40% incidence of EDM in farm-raised yearlings two consecutive years prior to dietary intervention. Eventually, 19 EDM-affected young horses were observed in three crops (1983-1985), with 14 of the 19 sired by one Standardbred stallion. Progeny of that stallion raised on other farms were not affected. After the supplementation of pregnant and nursing mares with daily vitamin E (1500 IU/horse/day), the incidence of EDM in progeny from those same stallions was <5%. Similar responses have been observed in specific families of Morgans, Appaloosas, and Paso Finos (Mayhew et al., 1987).

One report also implicated other risk factors for EDM (Dill et al., 1990), including application of insecticide to affected foals, exposure of foals to wood preservatives, and foals housed primarily on dirt lots when turned outside. Affected foals were born more often to affected mares than to non-affected mares. Foals spending time outside on green pastures had decreased risk for developing EDM, lending further credence to the argument that affected foals have been deprived of sufficient vitamin E found in good-quality green grass and hay.

CLINICAL SIGNS

Onset of clinical signs is usually slow and insidious. Mild symmetrical hind limb ataxia progresses to involve the forelimbs. The initially mild ataxia worsens over time, and paresis, spasticity, and hypometria become evident. In later stages, EDM horses become recumbent and unable to rise without assistance. In terms of neurological signs, these horses may be indistinguishable from horses with CVM, but the size (perhaps smaller) and breed (perhaps Paso Fino, Arabian, and Morgan) may be an indication that CVM is not the most likely cause of the neurological disease. EDM horses are often remarkably weaker (more paretic) than CVM horses.

DIAGNOSIS

Testing for CVM and EPM are negative. EDM is essentially a rule-out diagnosis in that no antemortem test exists. Serum vitamin E concentrations may be measured and if low, are considered evidence for a presumptive diagnosis of EDM. Breed and familial history may also be important in making a diagnosis.

TREATMENT

Vitamin E supplementation has been cited as beneficial in treating EDM, especially if begun while signs are early and mild (Mayhew et al., 1987). Signs may only arrest but not reverse in severity (the affected horse may never be normal). It should be noted that the units "IU" and "mg" are the same for vitamin E but not for other vitamins, so conversion from one to another is not necessary in dosing. Recommended dosages of vitamin E range from 2000-9000 IU orally daily, with 6000-7000 IU/day commonly given to affected animals and 1500-2000 IU/day commonly used as a preventative. In acute cases, intramuscular injection of 1500-2000 IU in oil every 10 days has also been used (Mayhew et al., 1987). Follow-up measurements of serum vitamin E concentration may be used to assess efficacy of the dose. Supplementation has also been used as a preventative.

PROGNOSIS

EDM is a progressive disease, usually with an unrelenting course resulting in death. Horses affected at younger ages usually progress to recumbency and death, while the sporadic cases of horses affected at older ages often plateau and fail to progress to recumbency. Some of these horses have been used successfully as brood animals, but supplementation of progeny with vitamin E may be warranted.

PREVENTION

Feeding good-quality green grass or hay is the easiest and least expensive way to ensure that horses are ingesting sufficient vitamin E. If pasture is unavailable, or hay or pasture quality is suspect, then dietary vitamin E supplementation may be indicated. Heat-extruded feeds, oats stored for lengthy periods, and sun-bleached hays should be considered suspect with respect to available vitamin E concentrations (Matthews, 1998). Farms with large EDM problems have benefited from farm-wide vitamin E supplementation (Mayhew et al., 1987).

Equine Motor Neuron Disease

DEFINITION AND HISTORY

Equine motor neuron disease (EMND) is a progressive, debilitating, usually fatal neurological disease of horses first described in New England in 1990 (Cummings et al., 1990). An association between vitamin E deficiency and EMND has been described (De La Rúa-Domènech et al., 1997). The dramatic paresis in EMND is due to its affectation primarily of lower motor neurons (LMN), those nerves which supply the direct neurological input into all muscles. Without the normal trophic influence of the LMN, the associated muscles atrophy, resulting in the remarkable paresis and weight loss characteristic of this disease. This symmetrical wasting distinguishes the disease from CVM, EPM, and EDM as these diseases frequently occur in horses with good body condition. The disease in horses is similar to one in humans known as amyotrophic lateral sclerosis (ALS), or Lou Gehrig's disease. As found in familial ALS, it has recently been shown that EMND horses have abnormally high copper concentrations in their spinal cords (Polack et al., 2000), providing further evidence that oxidative spinal cord injury in EMND may be related to high copper and low vitamin E concentrations.

EPIDEMIOLOGY

EMND is sporadic and rare. Since the original 1990 description of EMND in New York, more than 200 cases have been reported in many states, Canada, Europe, Japan, and Brazil (Divers et al., 1997). Cases are clustered, however, in the northeastern United States and Canada (from Pennsylvania north through Prince Edward Island and west through Ohio). Seldom is more than one horse in a stable affected, although there are rare reports of multiple cases at a single site.

EMND more commonly affects middle-aged adult horses, with a mean age of onset of signs of 9 years (range 2-23 years)(Mohammed et al., 1993). Many breeds have been affected, but Standardbreds are underrepresented. Quarter Horses are overrepresented, perhaps owing to the non-pasture conditions under which they are often housed (Mohammed et al., 1993). Horses with EMND are nearly always housed in boarding stables with minimal or no turnout or turnout only on drylots with no grass (Mohammed et al., 1993; Divers et al., 1994; De La RúaDomènech et al., 1997). Affected horses generally receive large amounts of pelleted or sweet feed, no vitamin E supplements, no pasture, and poor-quality hay (described consistently as light green or brown or even sun-bleached grass hay with no alfalfa).

CLINICAL SIGNS

Horses affected with EMND have dramatic weight loss, muscle atrophy, paresis, recumbency, trembling, and hind limb treading when standing. Some of these signs may be easier initially to attribute to laminitis or colic than to neurological disease. Muscle atrophy is most commonly observed in the quadriceps, triceps, and gluteal areas (Divers et al., 1997). More than half of these horses carry their heads in a lowered posture with obvious neck muscle atrophy. Ataxia is not seen since the upper motor neurons are not affected, thus distinguishing this disease from CVM, EPM, and EDM. Horses may look better when walking than when standing, since the LMN supplying postural muscles are more commonly affected. Despite the weight loss, the affected horse's appetite is normal to ravenous. In approximately 50% of the cases, coprophagia is observed even though these are adult horses (Divers et al., 1997).

DIAGNOSIS

Diagnosis is based on history (no pasture exposure and a poor-quality hay diet), clinical signs, mild to moderate elevated serum muscle enzymes, and measurably low serum or plasma vitamin E concentrations. Electromyography reveals denervation atrophy but is best done in affected horses under general anesthesia because they tread so much when required to stand still (Divers et al., 1997).

Retinal abnormalities also have been described (Riis et al., 1999). Muscle biopsy has a high sensitivity but an unproven specificity for diagnosis of EMND (Divers et al., 1997).

TREATMENT

The only known treatment for EMND is supplementation with vitamin E (5000-7000 IU/horse/day orally). Good quality hay and/or pasture should also be provided whenever possible. If a response to therapy is seen, it takes a minimum of 3-6 weeks for observable improvement in trembling, followed eventually by increased weight and strength (Divers et al., 1997).

PROGNOSIS

The prognosis even with vitamin E supplementation remains guarded for life and poor for return to function (Divers et al., 1997). Most EMND horses are euthanized, but some reach plateaus in clinical signs where they can be comfortable even if they are unable to return to work.

PREVENTION

Proper balanced diet with less confinement and greater exposure to green pasture should be preventative. Daily vitamin E supplementation is recommended whenever diet or management considerations render the diet suspect in vitamin E intake.

References

Beech, J. 1984. Neuraxonal dystrophy of the accessory cuneate nucleus in horses. Vet. Pathol. 21:384-393.

Beech, J. and M. Haskins. 1987. Genetic studies of neuraxonal dystrophy in the Morgan. Am. J. Vet. Res. 48:109-113.

Bentz, B.G., D.E. Granstrom, and S. Stamper. 1997. Seroprevalence of antibodies to *Sarcocystis neurona* in horses residing in a county of southeastern Pennsylvania. J. Am. Vet. Med. Assoc. 210(4):517-518.

Blythe, L.L., B.D. Hultgren, A.M. Craig, L.H. Appell, E.D. Lassen, D.E. Mattson, and D. Duffield. 1991. Clinical, viral, and genetic evaluation of equine degenerative myeloencephalopathy in a family of Appaloosas. J. Am. Vet. Med. Assoc. 198(6):1005-1013.

Blythe, L.L., D.E. Granstrom, D.E. Hansen, L.L. Walker, and S. Stamper. 1997. Seroprevalence of antibodies to *Sarcocystis neurona* in horses residing in Oregon. J. Am. Vet. Med. Assoc. 210(4):525-527.

Box, F.D., J.L. Meier, and J.H. Smith. 1984. Description of *Sarcocystis falcatula*

Stiles, 1893, a parasite of birds and opossums. J. Protozool. 31:521-524.

Brendemuehl, J.P., B.M. Waldridge, and E.R. Bridges. 1998. Effects of sulfadiazine and pyrimethamine and concurrent folic acid supplementation on pregnancy and embryonic loss rates in mares. Proc. 44th Annual Conv. Am. Assoc. Equine Practnr., pp. 142-143.

Cummings, J.F., A. De La Hunta, C. George, l. Fuhrer, B.A. Valentine, B.J. Cooper, B.A. Summers, C.R. Huxtable, and H.O. Mohammed. 1990. Equine motor neuron disease: A preliminary report. Cornell Vet. 80:357-379.

Cusick, P.K., D.M. Sells, D.P. Hamilton, and H.J. Hardenbrook. 1974. Toxoplasmosis in two horses. J. Am. Vet. Med. Assoc. 164:77-80.

Cutler, T.J., R.J. MacKay, P.E. Ginn, E.C. Greiner, R. Porter, C.A. Yowell, and J.B. Dame. 1999. Are *Sarcocystis neurona* and *Sarcocystis falcatula* synonymous? A horse infection challenge. J. Parasitol. 85(2):301-305.

Dame, J.B., R.J. MacKay, C.A. Yowell, T.J. Cutler, A. Marsh, and E.C. Greiner. 1995. *Sarcocystis falcatula* from passerine and psittacine birds: Synonomy with *Sarcocystis neurona*, agent of equine protozoal myeloencephalitis. J. Parasitol. 81:930-935.

De La Rua-Domenech, R., H.O. Mohammed, J.F. Cummings, T.J. Divers, A. De La Hunta, and B.A. Summers. 1997. Association between plasma vitamin E concentration and the risk of equine motor neuron disease. Vet. J. 154:203-213.

Dill, S.G., M.T. Correa, H.N. Erb, A. De La Hunta, F.A. Kallfelz, and C. Waldron. 1990. Factors associated with the development of equine degenerative myeloencephalopathy. Am. J. Vet. Res. 51(8):1300-1305.

Divers, T.J., H.O. Mohammed, and J.F. Cummings. 1997. Equine motor neuron disease. Vet. Clin. No. Am. Equine Pract. 13(1):97-105.

Divers, T.J., H.O. Mohammed, J.F. Cummings, B.A. Valentine, A. De La Hunta, C.A. Jackson, and B.A. Summers. 1994. Equine motor neuron disease: Findings in 28 horses and proposal of a pathophysiological mechanism for the disease. Equine Vet. J. 26:409-415.

Donawick, W.J., I.G. Mayhew, D.T. Galligan, J. Osborne, S. Green, and E.K. Stanley. 1989. Early diagnosis of cervical vertebral malformation in young Thoroughbred horses and successful treatment with restricted, paced diet and confinement. Proc. 35th Annual Conv. Am. Assoc. Equine Practnr., pp. 525-528.

Donawick, W.J., I.G. Mayhew, D.T. Galligan, S.L. Green, E.K. Stanley, and J. Osborne. 1993. Results of a low-protein, low-energy diet and confinement on young horses with wobbles. Proc. 39th Annual Conv. Am. Assoc. Equine Practnr., pp. 125-127.

Dubey, J.P., S.W. Davis, C.A. Speer, D.D. Bowman, A. De La Hunta, D.E. Granstrom, M.J. Topper, A.N. Hamir, J.F. Cummings, and M.M. Suter. 1991. *Sarcocystis neurona* n. sp. (Protozoa: Apicomplexa), the etiological agent of equine protozoal meyloencephalitis. J. Parasitol. 77:212-218.

Dubey, J.P. and D.S. Lindsay. 1999. *Sarcocystis speeri* n. sp. (Protozoa: Sarcocystidae) from the opossum (*Didelphis virginiana*). J. Parastiol. 85:903-909.

Dubey, J.P., W.J.A. Saville, D.S. Lindsay, R.W. Stich, J.F. Stanek, C.A. Speer, B.M. Rosenthal, C.J. Njoku, O.C.H. Kwok, S.K. Shen, and S.M. Reed. 2000. Completion of the life cycle of *Sarcocystis neurona*. J. Parasitol. 86(6):1276-1280.

Fayer, R., I.G. Mayhew, J.D. Baird, S.G. Dill, J.H. Foreman, J.C. Fox, R. Higgins, S.M. Reed, W.W. Ruoff, R.W. Sweeney, and P. Tuttle. 1990. Epidemiology of equine protozoal myeloencephalitis in North America. J. Vet. Intern. Med. 4:54-57.

Fenger, C.K. and D.E. Granstrom. 1995. Identification of opossums (*Didelphis virginiana*) as the putative definitive host of *Sarcocystis neurona*. J. Parasitol. 81:916-919.

Foreman, J.H., T.E. Goetz, M.J. Boero, D.A. Wilson, S.M. Austin, and R.S. Pleasant. 1990. Evaluation and treatment of neurologic lameness. Proc. 36th Annual Conv. Am. Assoc. Equine Practnr., pp. 289-295.

Granstrom, D.E. and W.J. Saville. 1998. Equine protozoal myeloencephalitis. In: Equine Internal Medicine, S.M. Reed and W.M. Bayly (eds.). W.B. Saunders, Philadelphia, pp. 486-491.

MacKay, R.C. 1997. Serum antibodies to *Sarcocystis neurona*—half the horses in the United States have them! J. Am. Vet. Med. Assoc. 210(4):482-483.

MacKay, R.C., D.E. Granstrom, W.J. Saville, and S.M. Reed. 2000. Equine protozoal myeloencephalitis. Vet. Clin. No. Am. Equine Pract. 16(3):405-425.

Marsh, A.E., B.C. Barr, J. Madigan, J. Lakritz, R. Nordhausen, and P.A. Conrad. 1996. Neosporosis as a cause of equine protozoal myeloencephalitis. J. Am. Vet. Med. Assoc. 209:1907-1913.

Matthews, H.K. 1998. Equine degenerative myeloencephalopathy. In: Equine Internal Medicine, S.M. Reed and W.M. Bayly (eds.). W.B. Saunders, Philadelphia, pp. 483-486.

Mayhew, I.G., C.M. Brown, H.D. Stowe, A.L. Trapp, F.J. Derksen, and S.F. Clement. 1987. Equine degenerative myeloencephalopathy: A vitamin E deficiency that may be familial. J. Vet. Intern. Med. 1:45-50.

Mayhew, I.G., A. De La Hunta, and R.H. Whitlock. 1977. Equine degenerative myeloencephalopathy. J. Am. Vet. Med. Assoc. 170:195-201.

Miller, M.M., C.R. Sweeney, G.E. Russell, R.M. Sheetz, and J.K. Morrow. 1999. Effects of blood contamination of cerebrospinal fluid on western blot analysis for detection of antibodies against *Sarcocystis neurona* and on albumin quotient and immunoglobulin G index in horses. J. Am. Vet. Med. Assoc. 215(1):67-71.

Mohammed, H.O., J.F. Cummings, T.J. Divers, A. De La Hunta, G.C. Fuhrer, B.A. Valentine, B.A. Summers, B.R.H. Farrow, K. Trembicki, and A.

Mauskopf. 1993. Risk factors associated with equine motor neuron disease: A possible model for human MND. Neurology 43:966-971.

Polack, E.W., J.M. King, J.F. Cummings, H.O. Mohammed, M. Birch, and T. Cronin. 2000. Concentrations of trace minerals in the spinal cord of horses with equine motor neuron disease. Am. J. Vet. Res. 61(6):609-611.

Rantanen, N.W., P.R. Gavin, D.D. Barbee, and R.D. Sande. 1981. Ataxia and paresis in horses. Part II. Radiographic and myelographic examination of the cervical vertebral column. Comp. Cont. Educ. Pract. Vet. 3(4):S161-S171.

Reed, S.M. and B.R. Moore. 1993. Pathogenesis of cervical vertebral stenotic myelopathy. Proc. 39th Annual Conv. Am. Assoc. Equine Practnr., pp. 113-115.

Riis, R.C., C. Jackson, W. Rebhun, M.L. Katz, E. Loew, B. Summers, J. Cummings, A. De La Hunta, T. Divers, and H. Mohammed. 1999. Ocular manifestations of equine motor neuron disease. Equine Vet. J. 31:99-110.

Rooney, J.R., M.E. Prickett, F.M. Delaney, and M.W. Crowe. 1970. Focal myelitis-encephalitis in horses. Cornell Vet. 60:494-501.

Saville, W.J., P.S. Morley, S.M. Reed, D.E. Granstrom, C.W. Kohn, K.W. Hinchcliff, and T.E. Whittum. 2000b. Evaluation of risk factors associated with clinical improvement and survival of horses with equine protozoal myeloencephalitis. J. Am. Vet. Med. Assoc. 217(8):1181-1185.

Saville, W.J., S.M. Reed, P.S. Morley, D.E. Granstrom, C.W. Kohn, K.W. Hinchcliff, and T.E. Whittum. 2000a. Analysis of risk factors for the development of equine protozoal myeloencephalitis in horses. J. Am. Vet. Med. Assoc. 217(8):1174-1180.

Saville, W.J., S.M. Reed, D.E. Granstrom, K.W. Hinchcliff, C.W. Kohn, T.E. Wittum, and S. Stamper. 1997. Prevalence of serum antibodies to *Sarcocystis neurona* in horses residing in Ohio. J. Am. Vet. Med. Assoc. 210(4):519-524.

Simpson, C.F. and I.G. Mayhew. 1980. Evidence for *Sarcocystis* as the etiologic agent of equine protozoal myeloencephalitis. J. Protozool. 27:288-292.

Tanhauser, S.M., C.A. Yowell, T.J. Cutler, E.C. Greiner, R.J. MacKay, and J.B. Dame. 1999. Multiple DNA markers differentiate *Sarcocystis neurona* and *Sarcocystis falcatula*. J. Parasitol. 85:221-228.

Toribio, R.E., F.T. Bain, D.R. Mrad, N.T. Messer, R.S. Sellers, and K.W. Hinchcliff. 1998. Congenital defects in newborn foals of mares treated for equine protozoal myeloencephalitis during pregnancy. J. Am. Vet. Med. Assoc. 212(5):697-701.

Wagner, P.C., B.D. Grant, A. Gallina, and G.W. Bagby. 1981. Ataxia and paresis in horses. Part III. Surgical treatment of cervical spinal cord compression. Comp. Cont. Educ. Pract. Vet. 3(5):S192-S202.

MUSCLE DISORDERS: UNTYING THE KNOTS THROUGH NUTRITION

STEPHANIE J. VALBERG[1], RAY GEOR[2] AND JOE D. PAGAN [3]
[1]University of Minnesota, St. Paul, Minnesota [2]R and J Veterinary Consultants, Guelph, Ontario, Canada [3]Kentucky Equine Research, Inc., Versailles, Kentucky

Some unfortunate horses develop stiffness, painful muscle contractures, profuse sweating, and elevated respiratory rates during or following exercise. The term "tying-up" is used to describe horses with these clinical signs. In severe cases, horses may be unable to move their hindquarters after exercise, and muscle breakdown results in dark urine due to the release of myoglobin. Horses may be so painful with tying-up that they will paw and roll resembling colic. Other terms for this syndrome include azoturia, Monday morning disease, exertional rhabdomyolysis, and chronic intermittent rhabdomyolysis. It has been implied or assumed that there is one underlying cause for tying-up in horses. In 1917, Dr. Steffin commented on tying-up, saying "no one disease in the horse has been subject to so many theories and hypothetical suggestions as this one." This statement remains true. Veterinarians and owners have noted improvement in their horses' signs of tying-up with various new diets or supplements. The variable response of horses to these treatments has fueled the controversy regarding tying-up and its actual basis. In this article, we provide a brief review of the history of tying-up with regard to a nutritional basis and a summary of some of the most recent advances with regard to nutritional management of this syndrome.

A Search for a Nutritional Basis for Tying-Up

Tying-up was first described in draft horses during the preceding century. When some horses were rested from routine work on Sunday and fed their usual grain ration, they developed signs of tying-up on Monday morning when they resumed their work. A study performed in 1932 showed that draft horses given high amounts of nonstructural carbohydrates such as molasses were more likely to develop muscle damage with exercise (Carlstrom, 1932). As a result it became common to recommend a low-grain diet for all horses with tying-up. Carlstrom believed that the high-carbohydrate diet given while horses were resting resulted in loading of muscle glycogen that in turn precipitated lactic acid accumulation during exercise. While decreasing grain appears helpful for many horses with tying-up, this mechanism for rhabdomyolysis has never been substantiated. In fact, most horses tie-up when exercising at slow speeds when lactic acid is not produced (MacLeay et al., 2000). There are no clearly documented cases of horses that develop severe lactic acid accumulation with tying-up following exercise.

As the automobile replaced the draft horse for transportation, race and pleasure horses became increasingly popular. Veterinarians began to note a milder syndrome of tying-up in these lighter breeds of horses. It was suggested that, similar to other species, a dietary vitamin E and selenium deficiency might cause muscle damage in tying-up horses. Vitamin E and selenium act to protect muscles from toxic products called oxygen free radicals that can be generated with exercise. Documented cases of a selenium-responsive muscle disease were reported in foals from several countries with low selenium soil content in the 1970s. The association with muscle disease led to the recommendation that horses with tying-up should be given a selenium and vitamin E supplement. When the selenium and vitamin E status was studied in tying-up horses, most adult horses had normal to high levels of selenium and vitamin E, likely because they were being supplemented in their diet (Roneus and Hakkarainen, 1985). Although selenium deficiency may not be the primary cause for tying-up, many practitioners report a decrease in the severity of tying-up when horses receive vitamin E and selenium supplementation. This may be due to the fact that horses generate more toxic free radicals with the tying-up syndrome and therefore have a greater need for supplementation.

A subsequent focus of investigation into tying-up was the role of an imbalance in dietary electrolytes (Harris and Snow, 1991). Electrolytes are body salts that maintain an electrical gradient across muscle cell membranes. During exercise, muscles contract when nerves stimulate a change in the electrical gradient and electrolytes move across the cell membrane. Muscle cells contain high concentrations of the electrolytes potassium and phosphate and low concentrations of sodium, chloride, and calcium. Electrolytes are obtained in the feed, and the concentrations in the body are regulated by uptake by the intestinal tract and elimination in sweat and urine. Endurance horses lose large amounts of fluids and electrolytes during competition, creating major electrolyte imbalances. Some of these horses may develop tying-up and exhaustion from dehydration, electrolyte losses, and high body temperatures. Endurance horses need to be on a daily electrolyte supplement and may need additional supplementation during endurance rides.

Subtle electrolyte imbalances are believed to have an important role in causing tying-up in some pleasure and racehorses. Studies by Harris and Snow (1991) in the United Kingdom have focused on determining electrolyte balance in horses with tying-up. Blood samples do not accurately reflect electrolyte balance in horses so a technique that checks the balance of salts between urine and blood was used to study tying-up. Commercial diets were found to be too low in salt (sodium chloride) and most horses needed an additional 1-2 ounces of salt to maintain proper balance. While some horses improved dramatically by adding electrolytes in the form of table salt (sodium chloride), lite salt (potassium chloride), or epsom salt (magnesium chloride), other horses showed no improvement.

Perhaps one of the major roadblocks in interpreting research into tying-up is the assumption that all horses that show evidence of muscle pain and cramping following exercise have the same disease. Many studies group a small number of horses of many breeds and athletic types together to find one unifying cause. As a result, a great deal of controversy and confusion has developed regarding the cause and approach to treatment of this condition. Tying-up or exertional rhabdomyolysis likely represents a description of several muscle diseases that have common clinical signs. By applying clinical protocols that include muscle biopsies and exercise testing, a number of specific disorders recently have been identified.

Classification of Tying-Up

Occasionally, horses diagnosed with tying-up actually have strained a specific muscle group. Tying-up from a clinical standpoint can be divided into two syndromes: 1) sporadic rhabdomyolysis following exercise in horses that have a previous history of satisfactory performance, or 2) chronic exertional rhabdomyolysis in horses with repeated episodes of tying-up from a young age.

Sporadic Tying-Up

LOCAL MUSCLE STRAIN

Local muscle strain is a common injury in performance horses. Several factors may predispose horses to muscle strains, such as an inadequate warm-up, pre-existing lameness, exercise to the point of fatigue, and insufficient training. Muscles over the back are frequently injured in jumpers, dressage, and harness horses. The hamstring muscles on the back of the rear limbs are more frequently damaged in working Quarter Horses. Affected muscles are painful upon deep palpation and may feel warm. In chronic cases, hardened areas within the muscle may represent fibrosis and ossification. The stride has a short anterior phase with a characteristic hoof-slapping gait.

CLINICAL SIGNS OF SPORADIC TYING-UP

More generalized muscle damage often results in overall muscle soreness, reluctance to move, sweating, and rapid respiratory rates. A diagnosis of sporadic tying-up is made on the basis of a horse with no previous signs of tying-up, signs of muscle cramping and stiffness following exercise, and moderate to marked elevations in blood markers for muscle damage such as creatine kinase (CK) and aspartate transaminase (AST). Horses with signs of tying-up should stop exercising and be moved to a well-bedded stall with access to fresh water. A veterinarian should be called to assess whether horses need intravenous or oral fluids, tranquilizers, or pain relievers. Rest with a few minutes of hand walking once the initial stiffness has abated is of prime importance. The diet should be changed to good-quality hay with little grain supplementation, salt, and a vitamin/mineral mix. The amount of rest a horse should receive is controversial. Horses with chronic problems with tying-up appear to benefit from an early return to a regular exercise schedule. Horses that appear to have damaged their muscles from overexertion may benefit from a longer rest period with regular access to a paddock. Training should be resumed gradually and a regular exercise schedule, which will match the degree of exertion to the horses underlying state of training, should be established. Endurance horses should be encouraged to drink electrolyte-supplemented water during an endurance ride and monitored particularly closely during hot, humid conditions.

The most common cause of sporadic tying-up is exercise that exceeds the horse's underlying state of training. The incidence of muscle stiffness also has been observed to increase during an outbreak of respiratory disease. Deficiencies of sodium, calcium, vitamin E, and selenium in the diet may also contribute to muscle cell damage. Since the inciting cause is usually temporary, most horses respond to rest, a gradual increase in training, and diet adjustments. The ease of treating horses with overexertion may account for the myriad of treatments guaranteed to cure tying-up in horses. Skeletal muscle shows a remarkable ability to repair within 4-8 weeks following injury.

Chronic Exertional Rhabdomyolysis

A number of horses, predominantly fillies, will have recurrent episodes of rhabdomyolysis even with light exercise. Chronic exertional rhabdomyolysis is seen in many breeds of horses, including Quarter Horses, Paints, Appaloosas, Thoroughbreds, Arabians, Standardbreds, and Morgans. Several causes for chronic rhabdomyolysis have been proposed. These include electrolyte imbalances, hormonal imbalances, lactic acidosis, and vitamin E and selenium deficiencies. Many of these proposed causes do not have a sound scientific basis. As such we recommend that a complete battery of diagnostic tests be used to identify the cause of tying-up whenever possible.

Further diagnostic tests to try to determine the cause of chronic tying-up include a complete blood count, serum chemistry panel, blood vitamin E and selenium concentrations, urinalysis to determine electrolyte balance, exercise testing, muscle biopsy, and dietary analysis. A muscle biopsy may be useful in determining the basis for chronic rhabdomyolysis. Two forms of chronic tying-up have been identified using various forms of muscle biopsies. **Polysaccharide storage myopathy (PSSM)** is a form of tying-up in Quarter Horse-related breeds, warmbloods, and drafts. Biopsies of PSSM horses reveal many muscle fibers with subsarcolemmal vacuoles, dark p-aminosalicylic acid (PAS) staining for glycogen, and most notably abnormal complex polysaccharide accumulation in muscle fibers (Valberg et al., 1992). **Recurrent exertional rhabdomyolysis (RER)** is a disorder of Thoroughbreds and likely Standardbred and Arabian horses. Muscle biopsies are characterized by numerous mature muscle fibers with centrally located nuclei and moderately dark PAS stains for muscle glycogen without any complex polysaccharide accumulation (Valberg et al., 1999a). In some horses, the specific cause of tying-up is not known at this time.

Recurrent Exertional Rhabdomyolysis

RER is most common in fit young fillies at the racetrack. It has a more equal sex distribution after four years of age and is found most commonly in horses with a nervous temperament (MacLeay et al., 1999a). Factors that trigger episodes of rhabdomyolysis include excitement with exercise, rest prior to exercise, galloping or breezing exercise, and any lameness even if it does not interrupt the exercise regime. Many fillies with tying-up are in intense training, have trouble maintaining body weight, and are therefore fed at least 12 lb of grain or more. The reason why certain horses are prone to tying-up and others that are managed identically are not may be related to inheritance. Studies of equine lymphocyte antigens provide support for a familial basis for RER in Standardbred horses (Collinder et al., 1997). Genetic studies in Thoroughbreds suggest that susceptibility is inherited as a dominant trait (MacLeay et al., 1999b). That is, if one parent had RER, there is a 50% chance of the foal being susceptible to RER no matter who the other parent is. Whether the offspring expresses the disease depends on the diet, management, and training regime. A diagnosis of RER is based on the history and clinical signs as well as documented elevations in muscle proteins (serum AST and CK) that leak into the bloodstream when muscle is damaged. Muscle biopsy findings in affected horses include varying stages of muscle necrosis and regeneration with centrally located myonuclei.

THE BIOCHEMICAL BASIS FOR RER

A specific cause for the form of tying-up in many Thoroughbreds has recently been identified. It appears that the mechanism by which muscle contraction is regulated can be disrupted by excitement and exercise in some susceptible horses (Lentz et al., 1999). This discovery was based on the observation that intercostal muscle biopsies from RER horses readily develop contractures when exposed to agents (halothane and caffeine) that increase intramuscular calcium release. The threshold for developing a contracture is much lower for RER horses compared to normal horses and is similar to a muscle disease in people and swine called malignant hyperthermia. Every time a muscle contracts, calcium is released from muscle storage sites and then taken back up into storage sites for muscle relaxation. The altered contraction and relaxation of muscle suggests that abnormal intracellular calcium regulation is the cause of this form of RER. These intramuscular calcium concentrations are extremely small compared to the amount of calcium in the rest of the body and are completely independent of dietary calcium concentrations.

DIETARY MANAGEMENT OF RER

Obviously any diet for equine athletes needs to have a proper balance of vitamins, minerals, electrolytes, protein, fiber, and starch. Particular attention should be given to providing adequate electrolytes, vitamin E, and selenium. One of the problems with diets for nervous horses with RER in race training is that they often need to contain at least 28 MCal of digestible energy per day. To provide this energy, the starch content of the diet has traditionally been very high (>12 lb of grain/day) and this further exacerbates the excitability of the horse. Recent research suggests that replacing much of the grain in the diet with a fat supplement such as vegetable oil or rice bran is beneficial and will significantly decrease the amount of muscle damage. In a recent dietary trial, we exercised 5 Thoroughbred horses with RER on a treadmill for 5 days a week while they consumed hay and a variety of energy supplements for 3 weeks at a time. We found that keeping the caloric density at the calculated daily requirement of 21 MCal/day resulted in lower serum CK post exercise than when the amount of a corn/oat-based pellet was increased to provide 28 MCal/day (MacLeay et al., 2000). In contrast, if extra calories were provided with a fat supplement rather than a grain supplement at 28 MCal/day, no increase in post-exercise serum CK activity occurred. This research led to the development of a high-fiber, low-starch, high-fat diet called Re-Leve that is ideally suited to the management of RER in racehorses. No significant differences in muscle glycogen or lactate concentrations were apparent in our original studies as a result of feeding fat (MacLeay et al., 1999c). The effect of fat may lie in the ability to remove starch, which will decrease a key triggering factor for RER, excitability, in susceptible horses.

OTHER MANAGEMENT STRATEGIES FOR RER

Prevention of further episodes of RER in susceptible horses should also include standardized daily routines and an environment that minimizes excitement. The daily management of the horse including time of feeding, position in the stable, order of exercise, pasturemates, etc. should be evaluated to provide the lowest stress in the horse's day to day routine. The use of low doses of acepromazine before exercise is believed to help some excitable horses. Daily exercise is essential, whether in the form of turnout, longeing, or riding. In the past, horses have been box stall rested for several weeks following an episode of RER. It is the author's opinion that this is counterproductive and increases the likelihood that the horses will develop RER when put back into training. The initial muscle pain usually subsides within 24 hours of acute RER, and daily turnout in a small paddock can be provided at this time. Subsequently, a gradual return to performance is recommended once serum CK is within normal range.

Dantrolene (2-4 mg/kg orally) given one hour before exercise may be effective in preventing RER in some horses. Dantrolene is used to prevent malignant hyperthermia in humans and swine by decreasing the release of calcium from the calcium release channel. Phenytoin (1.4-2.7 mg/kg orally twice a day) has also been advocated as a treatment for horses with RER (Beech et al., 1988). Therapeutic levels vary, so oral doses are adjusted by monitoring serum levels to achieve 8 ug/ml but not exceed 12 ug/ml. Phenytoin acts on a number of ion channels within muscle and nerves including sodium and calcium channels. Unfortunately, long-term treatment with dantrolene or phenytoin is expensive.

Acknowledgement: Funding for studies in Thoroughbred horses has been provided by the Grayson Jockey Club Equine Research Foundation, Southern California Equine Research Foundation, and the Minnesota Equine Research Center.

Polysaccharide Storage Myopathy in Quarter Horses and Related Breeds

Polysaccharide storage myopathy (PSSM) has been identified in Quarter Horses, warmbloods, and draft horses (Valberg et al., 1992, 1997; Valentine et al., 1998). It is an uncommon occurrence in other equine breeds. The disease is characterized by the accumulation of phosphorylated glucose, glycogen, and abnormal polysaccharide in skeletal muscle.

CLINICAL SIGNS OF PSSM

Horses with PSSM often develop episodes of rhabdomyolysis at a young age when longed or broken to ride. Rest for a few days prior to exercise is a common triggering factor. Horses may have one episode per year or be affected at every exercise session. Episodes are characterized by a tucked-up abdomen, fasciculations, a camped-out stance, sweating, gait asymmetry, hind limb stiffness, and reluctance to move. Some horses paw or roll resembling colic. Myoglobinuria and recumbency occur occasionally with severe episodes. Serum CK and AST are increased during an episode (usually >10,000 U/L), and unlike other forms of rhabdomyolysis, subclinical episodes characterized by persistently abnormal CK are common (Valberg et al., 1997). Draft horses may be affected by a related disorder that has slightly different clinical signs. These include loss of muscle mass, difficulty standing with one hind leg raised, difficulty in backing without shaking a hind limb, progressive weakness, and recumbency. Elevations in CK and AST are often less than 10,000 U/L in drafts with this syndrome. Equine polysaccharide storage myopathy (EPSM) has been used to characterize the draft syndrome (Valentine et al., 1998).

DIAGNOSIS OF PSSM

A definitive diagnosis of PSSM should be based on the presence of PAS positive inclusions in scattered fast twitch muscle fibers in a muscle biopsy. An open surgical biopsy to remove a 1.5"x 1.5"x 2" sample of the semimembranosus is readily performed in the field, and samples can be shipped chilled or on dry ice overnight to specialized laboratories (Valberg et al., 1997). PAS positive inclusions are readily distinguishable in frozen sections, and these samples can also be used for other biochemical assays, thereby making frozen tissue more useful than for-malin-fixed muscle. Using the diagnostic criteria of abnormal PAS positive polysaccharide inclusions, PSSM is seen in particular Quarter Horse bloodlines, warmbloods, and draft horses. Pedigree analysis of Quarter Horses, Paints, and Appaloosas with PSSM supports a familial basis for this condition. Other laboratories have diagnosed PSSM solely on the basis of an apparent increase in muscle glycogen staining, and this has unfortunately resulted in the application of the term PSSM to a wide variety of breeds with various symptoms (Valentine et al., 1998). Complex polysaccharide is a rare finding in the Standardbred, Thoroughbred, Arabian, or other breeds of horses evaluated by our laboratory for exertional rhabdomyolysis.

PATHOPHYSIOLOGY

Because muscle glycogen concentrations in PSSM horses are 1.5 to 4 times those of normal horses or other breeds of horses with exertional rhabdomyolysis, this disorder is classified as a glycogen storage disease (Valberg et al., 1992). Glycogen storage diseases can result either from impaired utilization and breakdown of glycogen by tissues or increased and abnormal glycogen synthesis. No limitations in the ability of skeletal muscle to metabolize glycogen have been identified in PSSM horses. In fact, PSSM horses have higher glycogen utilization rates than healthy horses during anaerobic exercise (Valberg et al., 1999a). As such the metabolic defect responsible for marked glycogen accumulation appears to involve abnormal regulation of glycogen synthesis rather than a defect in utilization. We have found that horses with PSSM clear glucose from the bloodstream after an IV bolus or oral meal much faster than normal horses. It appears they do this because of increased insulin sensitivity (De La Corte et al., 1999a). When insulin is given to PSSM horses it causes a profound drop in blood sugar relative to normal horses which lasts for twice as long. Thus, it appears that one of the abnormalities in PSSM is that when fed a starch meal, these horses store a higher proportion of the absorbed glucose in their muscle compared to normal horses. The mechanism of glucose transport into muscles of PSSM does not appear to be regulated in the same fashion as healthy horses. Why this in itself causes muscle cells to become damaged with exercise is not clear at this time. The specific inherited cause of PSSM in horses remains unknown. PSSM can naively be seen as the opposite of type 2 diabetes.

PREVENTION

Diet. The research performed by our group on PSSM would suggest that one of the ways to manage this condition is to decrease the amount of starch in the diet. In contrast to Thoroughbreds with RER, breeds of horses with this disorder are often very easy keepers and therefore do not need many additional calories over and above hay. In addition, horses with PSSM are rarely performing at exercise intensities and durations that require a high caloric input. We have found, however, that even a small amount of fat added to the hay ration can have a beneficial effect on decreasing muscle glycogen concentrations (De La Corte et al., 1999b). This effect is likely due to the ability of dietary fat to decrease blood glucose and insulin concentrations. Adding 2 lb of rice bran per day to grass hay resulted in a significant decrease in muscle glycogen and glucose 6 P concentrations in PSSM horses within 3 weeks. Feeding fat has been shown to decrease insulin-sensitive glucose transport in other animals, and this may be a further reason that fat supplementation is beneficial to PSSM horses.

The diet of PSSM horses is best adjusted to eliminate grain or sweet feed and provide a diet of roughage with a fat supplement. In our experience, rice bran is a convenient mechanism of providing fat. Fussy eaters, warmbloods in heavy training, and draft horses may benefit from Re-Leve, a very palatable high fat diet developed by Kentucky Equine Research. Corn oil on alfalfa pellets provides another fat source without having to feed grain but tends to be messy for owners to feed. Horses receiving corn oil should also receive a supplemental 600-1000 IU/day of vitamin E. Some veterinarians suggest that PSSM horses should be fed a diet consisting of 25% fat. It may be that draft breeds benefit from such high fat diets; however, in our experience it is difficult to reach these levels of dietary fat intake, and it is unnecessary in Quarter Horse-related breeds with PSSM.

Training. Horses with PSSM will not improve if the only change made is the addition of dietary fat (De La Corte et al., 1999b). Prevention of further episodes of rhabdomyolysis requires a very gradual increase in the amount of daily exercise horses experience. Minimizing stress and providing regular routines and daily exercise are highly beneficial. Turnout each day with other horses in as large an area as possible will keep the horse active and is the single most important thing that can benefit these horses in my experience. If there has been a recent severe episode of tying-up, I recommend turning the horse out for two weeks on the diet recommended above. After switching the horse's diet for two weeks, the horse can begin longeing once a day for five minutes at a walk and trot. Gradually increase the time by two minutes a day. If the horse seems stiff, stand the horse for one minute and then see if the stiffness persists when walking. If stiffness is present, stop there; if not, continue after a two-minute walk. When the horse can trot 15 minutes, provide a five-minute break at a walk and gradually increase walking and trotting after this. Once the horse has reached 30 minutes of trotting on a longe line (with a break at 15 minutes), then begin to ride for 20 to 30 minutes and gradually increase the length and intensity of exercise. It should take at least three weeks of exercise before the horse is ridden. Keeping horses with PSSM fit increases oxidative metabolism and glycogen utilization, and this seems the best prevention against further episodes of tying-up.

Acknowledgment: We wish to thank the American Quarter Horse Association for funding research on PSSM.

References

Beech J, Lindborg S, Fletcher JE, et al. Caffeine contractures, twitch characteristics and the threshold for Ca^{2+}-induced Ca^{2+} release in skeletal muscle from horses with chronic intermittent rhabdomyolysis. Res Vet Sci 54:110, 1993.

Beech J, Fletcher JE, Lizzo F, et al. Effect of phenytoin on the clinical signs and in vitro muscle twitch characteristics in horses with chronic intermittent rhabdomyolysis and myotonia. Am J Vet Res 49(12):2130-2133, 1988.

Carlström B. Uber die atiologie und pathogenese der kreuzlahme des pferdes (Haemaglobinaemia paralytica). Scandinav Archiv 62:1-62, 1932.

Collinder E, Lindholm A, Rasmuson M. Genetic markers in Standardbred trotters susceptible to the rhabdomyolysis syndrome. Equine Vet J. 29(2):117-20, 1997.

De La Corte FD, Valberg SJ, Williamson S, MacLeay JM and Mickelson JR. Enhanced glucose uptake in horses with polysaccharide storage myopathy (PSSM). Am J Vet Res 60;458-462, 1999a.

De La Corte FD, Valberg SJ, MacLeay JM and Mickelson JR. The effect of feeding a fat supplement to horses with polysaccharide storage myopathy. Journal World Equine Health 4,2:12-19, 1999b.

Harris PA and Snow DH. Role of electrolyte imbalances in the pathophysiology of the equine rhabdomyolysis syndrome. In: Equine Exercise Physiology 3 ed. SGB Persson, A Lindholm and LB Jeffcott. ICEEP Publications, Davis CA 1991, pp 435-442.

Lentz LR, Valberg SJ, Balog E, Mickelson JR and Gallant EM. Abnormal regulation of contraction in equine recurrent exertional rhabdomyolysis. Am J Vet Res 60:992-999, 1999.

Lentz LR, Valberg SJ, Mickelson JR and Gallant EM. In vitro contractile testing of Quarter Horses with exertional rhabdomyolysis. Am J Vet Res 60:684-688, 1999.

MacLeay JM, Sorum SA, Valberg SJ, Marsh W and Sorum M. Epidemiological factors influencing exertional rhabdomyolysis in Thoroughbred racehorses. Am J Vet Res 60(12) 1562-1566,1999a.

MacLeay JM, Valberg SJ, Geyer CJ., Sorum SA and Sorum MD. Heritable basis for recurrent exertional rhabdomyolysis in Thoroughbred racehorses. Am J Vet Res 60:250-256, 1999b.

MacLeay JM, Valberg SJ, Pagan J, Billstrom JA and Roberts J. Effect of diet and exercise intensity on serum CK activity in Thoroughbreds with recurrent exertional rhabdomyolysis. Am J Vet Res 61:1390-1395, 2000.

Roneus B and Hakkarainen J. Vitamin E in skeletal muscle tissue and blood glutathione peroxidase activity from horses with azoturia-tying-up syndrome. Acta Vet Scand 26:425-428, 1985.

Valberg S, Cardinet III, GH, Carlson GP and DiMauro S. Polysaccharide storage myopathy associated with exertional rhabdomyolysis in the horse. Neuromusc Disorders 2:351-359, 1992.

Valberg SJ, Geyer C, Sorum SA and Cardinet III GH. Familial basis for exertional rhabdomyolysis in Quarter Horse-related breeds. Amer J Vet Res 57:286-290, 1996.

Valberg SJ, MacLeay JM and Mickelson JR. Polysaccharide storage myopathy associated with exertional rhabdomyolysis in horses. Comp Cont Educ 19(9)10:1077-1086, 1997.

Valberg SJ, MacLeay JM, Billstrom JA, Hower-Moritz MA and Mickelson JR. Skeletal muscle metabolic response to exercise in horses with polysaccharide storage myopathy. Equine Vet J, 31:43-47, 1999a.

Valberg SJ, Mickelson JR, Gallant EM, MacLeay JM, Lentz L and De La Corte FD. Exertional rhabdomyolysis in Quarter Horses and Thoroughbreds: one syndrome, multiple etiologies. International Conference on Equine Exercise Physiology Equine Vet J Suppl. 30: 533-538, 1999b.

Valentine BA, Hintz HF and Freels KM. Dietary control of exertional rhabdomyolysis in horses. J Am Vet Med Assoc 212:1588-1593, 1998b.

CHRONIC RESPIRATORY DISEASE: IS THERE A NUTRITION LINK?

RAY GEOR

R and J Veterinary Consultants, Guelph, Ontario, Canada

Introduction

Chronic respiratory disease is common in horses. The best known condition is chronic obstructive pulmonary disease (COPD), a disease characterized by chronic cough, increased respiratory rate, forced abdominal breathing, and exercise intolerance. Feeding and housing management play a critical role in the perpetuation of COPD. Specifically, dusts and molds contained within feed and bedding can trigger the allergic responses within the lung that ultimately result in development of COPD. Therefore, management of affected horses is heavily reliant on measures that minimize exposure to these airborne irritants.

"My horse has allergy problems" is not an uncommon statement by horse owners. Nutritionists are frequently put on the defensive by this statement because, in many situations, diet is identified as the most likely cause for these problems. Allergy or, more correctly, hypersensitivity refers to an altered state of immunoreactivity resulting in self-injury. Stated another way, an allergic reaction occurs when the immune system "overreacts" to a specific stimulus. Clinical signs of hypersensitivity reactions will vary depending on the severity of the reaction, the body system(s) involved, and whether the reaction is localized or generalized.

In the horse, the skin and the respiratory tract are frequently affected by hypersensitivity reactions. Urticaria, contact dermatitis, and insect hypersensitivity are examples of hypersensitivity-induced skin disease. Some authors and, in particular, commercial laboratories that offer allergy testing services believe that food allergy (to feed ingredients such as oats, corn, alfalfa, beet pulp, and barley) is an important cause of these skin reactions. The infamous "protein bumps" is an example of an urticarial reaction. In reality, skin hypersensitivity reactions are very rarely due to diet. More commonly, these reactions are due to insects, parasites (e.g., *Onchocerca* spp.), bedding, tack, drugs, and various other agents that, upon contact with the skin, may trigger a hypersensitivity reaction.

The most common equine disease with an allergic basis is chronic obstructive pulmonary disease (COPD), also known as recurrent airway obstruction, small airway disease, or heaves. Inflammatory airway disease (IAD) is a term used to describe a milder clinical syndrome that is frequently observed in younger horses.

Currently, there is no consensus whether IAD progresses to the more severe syndrome in the older horse. The remainder of this paper discusses these chronic airway diseases.

Chronic Obstructive Pulmonary Disease

COPD is a common respiratory tract disease of horses in temperate climates where horses are stabled; the condition is quite rare where horses are kept outside year-round. The exception is summer pasture-associated obstructive pulmonary disease. This condition, which is mostly a problem in the southern states, develops during the summer months when horses are at pasture. The cause of the pasture-associated disease is not known, although a hypersensitivity reaction to pollens is suspected.

The clinical signs of COPD are usually observed after exposure to hay and straw dust during stabling. In this sense, nutrition does play a role in the development of COPD. However, this author has also seen the clinical signs of COPD (e.g., cough, increased respiratory rate, exercise intolerance) attributed to a true "food allergy." This diagnosis is often based on the results of a RAST test, a blood test that measures concentrations of immunoglobulin E (IgE) specific to various allergens (inhaled and food). However, these tests are notoriously unreliable for the diagnosis of hypersensitivity conditions, mostly because the IgE measurements are nonspecific. Typically, both normal and diseased horses will have "positive" blood tests for the various IgE types assayed, reflecting a level of exposure rather than susceptibility to COPD or other hypersensitivity reactions. Therefore, the RAST test is not useful for differentiating normal horses from those prone to hypersensitivity reactions. Unfortunately, some veterinarians and owners interpret these "positive" test results as proof of a food hypersensitivity and proceed to remove various ingredients from the diet. Similarly, no relationship has been demonstrated between skin and lung airway reactivity. Therefore, there is no justification for the use of skin testing procedures, wherein tiny amounts of various purported allergens are injected into the skin, for the identification of culprit allergens.

The main cause of COPD is an allergic response to organic dusts, including molds in feed and bedding. In this respect, equine "heaves" resembles those human occupational lung diseases caused by inhaled organic dusts. Dust in horse stables contains over 50 types of molds, large numbers of forage mites, endotoxins, and other inorganic factors. The primary source of organic dust is hay and straw. Many of the molds contained in hay and straw are sufficiently small to reach and deposit in the small airways of the lungs when breathed in by the horse.

Water content at the time of baling is the most important factor in determining the mold count of hay or straw (Clarke and Madelin, 1987). Baling at 15 to 20% water content is associated with little heating. However, baling at 20 to 30% water may result in heating and moderate mold contamination, while baling at 35 to 50% water leads to spontaneous heating to 50 to 60° C and very heavy mold counts.

The concentration of molds and other organic dusts in the horse's breathing zone, the airspace around the nose, is a critical factor in the development of disease exacerbation in COPD-susceptible horses. Although horses can and do inhale organic dusts present in straw, hay is the major source of these aeroallergens. Characteristic feeding behavior, such as eating hay for long periods and shaking the hay, results in dust concentrations in the breathing zone that are much higher than in the rest of the stable (Woods et al., 1993). Therefore, while bedding and barn ventilation are considerations in improving the environment of COPD-affected horses, it is more important to remove the offending hay. This helps to explain the occurrence of COPD episodes in horses even when kept outdoors such as a susceptible horse given access to large round bales that contain significant mold contamination.

COPD is very similar to human asthma. Exposure of COPD-susceptible horses to hay and straw dust initiates inflammation in the lower airways (Robinson et al., 1996). This inflammatory response results in the accumulation of mucus in the airways, edema or thickening of the airways, and bronchospasm (airway narrowing). During clinical episodes, the airways are also hyperresponsive to nonspecific stimuli such as ammonia and other air pollutants, resulting in severe bronchoconstriction. Importantly, these lung changes are reversible after removal of the offending allergens.

In mild cases, the horse may appear normal at rest. However, during exercise, the horse may cough and discharge mucus from the nostrils. Horses with more severe COPD have obvious clinical signs at rest; these include frequent coughing, nasal discharge, increased respiratory rate, and increased effort of breathing. These horses will be exercise intolerant. Forced expirations eventually result in overdevelopment of the abdominal muscles, recognized as a "heave line." In individual horses, clinical signs often wax and wane, with more severe disease when the horse is stabled. Sudden changes in management or feeding (e.g., a new batch of hay or straw) can precipitate very severe clinical episodes. In most cases the severity of the clinical disease worsens with time unless prevented by treatment and management changes.

It is important to recognize that there is no cure for COPD. However, in all but the most severe cases, management and treatment measures can result in marked clinical improvement and minimize the number of further episodes. The most important component of treatment is environmental control to reduce exposure of the horse to the aeroallergens and other pollutants that cause the airway inflammation (Mair and Derksen, 2000; Jackson et al., 2000). Keeping the horse at pasture, without exposure to hay and straw, is by far the most effective means of environmental control. Indeed, in horses with signs of COPD, significant improvement in lung function can occur within three days of changing from a stable to a pasture environment (Jackson et al., 2000).

If the horse must be stabled, removing dry hay from the diet is the most important aspect of environmental control (Vandenput et al., 1998). In mild cases, soaking the hay prior to feeding is often effective in reducing dust levels in the horse's breathing zone. The hay must be thoroughly soaked, preferably by immersing the hay in a large tub of water for a 10-15 minute period. Dry areas in a poorly soaked hay portion can release enough mold spores to cause an allergic reaction. This process should be done no sooner than 20 to 30 minutes before feeding to avoid leaching of water-soluble nutrients from the hay.

A much less labor intensive approach involves use of alternative forages such as hay cubes, haylage, or complete pelleted feeds. Clinical experience has shown that these hay alternatives are necessary in severely affected horses. Haylage and silage are becoming more popular in the industry. Owners should be advised not to use broken or damaged haylage/silage bags and to use open bags within two to three days of opening; mold counts in haylage or silage can increase rapidly after exposure to air.

Bedding is the other major source of dust and mold spores in a barn. COPD horses should not be bedded on straw. Shredded paper, wood shavings, rubber mats, or peat moss should be used. It is also preferable to bed the stalls adjacent to the one used by the affected horse with the same bedding, although recent studies have demonstrated that clinical improvement occurs even when management changes are made only in the stall of the affected horse (Jackson et al., 2000). Horses should be turned outdoors during stall cleaning and re-bedding to minimize exposure to respirable dust. Barn ventilation is another consideration in optimizing the horse's environment. The build-up of ammonia, endotoxins, and other noxious agents can worsen the disease and delay recovery, even when other treatment measures have been instituted.

In mild cases, environmental management alone may effectively control the disease. However, horses with moderate to severe signs of COPD will also require medical treatment, at least initially. Treatment will often involve combined use of bronchodilator and corticosteroid drugs. Bronchodilator drugs (e.g., clenbuterol) are particularly indicated for horses experiencing an acute "heaves" attack – relief of bronchospasm will result in marked clinical improvement. However, this relief is short-lived and longer term drug therapy must be directed at reducing airway inflammation. This is achieved through use of corticosteroid drugs. Although environmental management will always be the most important factor in the control of COPD, some horses will require long-term treatment with corticosteroids to control the underlying airway inflammation.

Inflammatory Airway Disease

As mentioned, IAD is a term used to describe a much less severe form of chronic lower airway disease that is commonly diagnosed in young racehorses in training (Moore, 1996; Hoffman et al., 1998). These horses exhibit clinical signs of low-grade airway obstruction, including cough and mild nasal discharge. Furthermore, this syndrome is regarded as an important cause of poor exercise performance. At present, the relationship between IAD and COPD is unknown; however, it is possible that IAD can progress to the more severe syndrome of COPD with advancing years. The cause of IAD is also uncertain. Preceding viral infection, the inflammatory effects of repeated episodes of exercise-induced pulmonary hemorrhage ("bleeding") and hypersensitivity responses to inhaled environmental pollutants (including organic stable dusts, ammonia, and endotoxin) all may play a role in the development of this condition. Regardless of cause, the therapeutic measures recommended for the management of COPD, particularly environmental control, are also indicated in the treatment of IAD.

References

Clarke AF, Madelin T. Technique for assessing respiratory health hazards from hay and other source materials. Equine Vet J 19: 442-447, 1987.

Hoffman AM, Mazan MR, Ellenberg S. Association between bronchoalveolar lavage cytologic features and airway reactivity in horses with a history of exercise intolerance. Am J Vet Res 59: 176-181, 1998.

Jackson CA, Berney C, Jeffcott AM, Robinson NE. Environment and prednisone interactions in the treatment of recurrent airway obstruction (heaves). Equine Vet J 32: 432-438, 2000.

Mair TS, Derksen FJ. Chronic obstructive pulmonary disease: a review. Equine Vet Educ 12: 35-44, 2000.

Moore BR. Lower respiratory tract disease. Vet Clin Nth Am: Equine Pract 12: 457-477, 1996.

Robinson NE. International workshop on equine chronic airway disease, Michigan State University, 16-18 June 2000. Equine Vet J 33: 5-19, 2001.

Robinson NE, Derksen FJ, Olsweski MA, Buechner-Maxwell VA. The pathogenesis of chronic obstructive pulmonary disease of horses. Br Vet J 152: 283-306, 1996.

Vandenput S, Duvivier D, Votion D, Art T, Lekeux P. Environmental control to maintain stabled COPD horses in clinical remission: effects on pulmonary function. Equine Vet J 30: 93-96, 1998.

Woods PSA, Robinson NE, Swanson MC, Reed CE, Broadstone RV, Derksen FJ. Airborne dust and aeroallergen concentration in a horse stable under two different management systems. Equine Vet J 25: 208-213, 1993.

CHEMICAL ARTHRODESIS OF THE DISTAL TARSAL JOINTS USING SODIUM MONOIODOACETATE IN 104 HORSES

BRAD DOWLING AND ANDREW J. DART

University Veterinary Centre, Department of Veterinary Clinical Sciences, The University of Sydney, Australia

Introduction

Degenerative joint disease of the tarsometatarsal (TMT) and distal intertarsal (DIT) joints is the most common cause of hind limb lameness in performance horses (Gabel, 1983; Sonnichsen, 1985; Wyn-Jones and May, 1986; Sullins, 2002). While medical management of degenerative joint disease of the distal tarsal joints often results in temporary improvement in lameness, approximately 50% of horses treated conservatively remain lame (Stashak, 1987; Bohanon, 1998, 1999). The aim of medical management is to ameliorate pain and allow continued exercise, promoting progressive cartilage deterioration and disruption of subchondral bone. The proposed end point of medical management is spontaneous ankylosis of affected joints and soundness; however, results are variable and convalescence prolonged (Stashak, 1987).

Drilling of the distal intertarsal joints is the current recommended technique for surgical arthrodesis (Edwards, 1982; McIlwraith and Turner, 1987; Dechant et al., 1999; Adkins et al., 2000). Complementary surgical techniques appear to be of little benefit over drilling alone (Wyn-Jones and May, 1986; Dechant et al., 1999; von Salis et al., 2000). Chemical arthrodesis using sodium monoiodoacetate (MIA) has been described as an alternative to surgery and has been shown to produce radiographic evidence of ankylosis but variable degrees of soundness (Bohanon et al., 1991; Bohanon, 1995a,b; Bohanon, 1998; Schramme et al., 1998). In two studies, soundness and evidence of radiographic fusion were reported in 22% (5/23) and 93% (27/29), and 92% (21/23) and 97% (28/29) of horses, respectively, 12 months after MIA injection (Bohanon, 1995a,b; Schramme et al., 1998). However, comprehensive studies, detailed description of technique, and complications associated with this procedure are not presently available.

The purpose of this study is to report the technique used, outcome, and complications of chemical arthrodesis of the distal intertarsal joints in 104 horses with degenerative joint disease of the TMT and/or DIT joints using MIA.

Materials and Methods

Horses included in the study were presented or referred to the University Veterinary Centre for lameness evaluation, poor performance, or chemical fusion of the distal intertarsal joints based on examination and diagnosis by the referring veterinarian. A complete history was obtained from the owners. All horses underwent a lameness examination, including flexion tests and, if considered necessary to confirm the diagnosis, intra-articular anesthesia of the DIT and TMT joints. Lameness grade was recorded at admission and subsequent examinations using a standard grading system (Pasquini et al., 1995). All horses underwent radiographic examination of the TMT and DIT joints. A diagnosis of degenerative joint disease of one or more of the distal tarsal joints was made based on the history, lameness examination, and radiographic findings consistent with degenerative joint disease (Butler et al., 2000). Horses were included in the study if owners elected to proceed with arthrodesis using MIA in preference to other treatment options.

Sodium monoiodoacetate (Sigma-Aldrich, Castle Hill, Aust.) was prepared as a 100 or 200 mg/ml solution and sterilized by passing through a 0.2-μm filter as previously recommended (Bohanon, 1998). All solutions were prepared and used on the same day. Phenylbutazone (4.4 mg/kg, IV) was administered prior to chemical arthrodesis and all horses were sedated with detomidine hydrochloride (0.01 mg/kg, IV) and butorphanol tartrate IV (0.01 mg/kg, IV). Additional sedative was administered if required. The DIT and TMT on both limbs were injected at the same time irrespective of clinical and radiographic findings.

Tarsal joint injections were performed under aseptic conditions using a standard technique (Sack and Orsini, 1981; Kraus-Hansen et al., 1992). Contrast arthrography of the DIT joints was attempted in all horses. A 23-gauge, 2.5-cm needle was inserted into the DIT joints and 1 to 2 ml of iohexol (Omnipaque® 300 mg/Iml; Nycomed Pty Ltd, Aust.) was injected until resistance was encountered. The needles were capped and standard dorsopalmar and lateromedial radiographic views obtained. Radiographs were examined for correct needle placement. Radiographs were also examined for any evidence of communication between the DIT and the PIT (proximal intertarsal) joint, tarsocrural joint, or tarsal sheath (Bohanon, 1994). In horses where there was no suspicion of communication, needles were uncapped and the iohexol and any remaining joint fluid was aspirated. MIA was then injected through the same needle. The injection was stopped when there was resistance. The needle was then removed and digital pressure applied over the injection site. A maximum of 2 ml of MIA was injected into each joint. Contrast arthrography of the TMT joints was not performed. Needle placement in the TMT joints was confirmed by aspiration of joint fluid and low injection pressure. If there was any question about correct placement of the needle into any joint, the procedure was not performed on that joint. A second attempt was made 48 hours later or the injection was not performed.

Horses were monitored during the first 6 hours after injection for signs of pain. Each horse was assigned a comfort score (CS) of 0-4 (Table 1) (Johnson et al., 1993; Raekallio et al., 1997). Additional analgesia was provided using detomidine hydrochloride IV (0.01 mg/kg) and butorphanol tartrate IV (0.01 mg/

kg) if required. Phenylbutazone (4.4 mg/kg, PO, every 12 hours) was continued for 24 hours, and then the dose was reduced (2.2 mg/kg, PO, every 12 hours) for 10 to 14 days. Horses were allowed free exercise for the first 7 days. A graded exercise program was commenced after 7 days and incrementally increased to 30 to 45 minutes walking and trotting per day over the first 3 months and increasing to full work by 6 months post injection. When possible, a lameness evaluation including flexion tests and a radiographic examination was performed at 3, 6, 12, and 24 months.

Results

A total of 104 horses met the criteria for inclusion in the study. There were 27 warmbloods, 24 Thoroughbreds, 19 Quarter Horses, 7 Arabians, 19 Standardbreds, 5 Australian Stockhorses, 2 Andalusians, and 1 pony. Forty-four horses were used for dressage, 21 for racing (3 Thoroughbreds and 18 Standardbreds), 3 for endurance, 19 for western performance, 2 for showing, 8 for jumping, and 7 for pleasure riding. The mean age of treated horses was 7.2 years (range 2 to 17 years). Mean lameness grade on presentation was 2.9 out of 5 (range 1 to 4). Intra-articular anesthesia of all four distal tarsal joints was performed in 61 (60%) horses.

A total of 401 joints were injected with MIA. One hundred and ninety-five positive contrast arthrograms were successfully performed. In 12 horses (11.5%) communication was identified between DIT and TMT joints in one or both legs. No communication was identified between DIT joints and the tarsal sheath, PIT joint, or tarsocrural joint. The mean dose of MIA injected per joint was 192 mg (range 50-400 mg). The mean dose of MIA injected per DIT and TMT joint was 144 mg and 238 mg (range 50-400 mg), respectively.

The CS for each horse is recorded in Table 1. Horses assigned CS of 1 or 0 were treated with detomidine hydrochloride IV (0.01 mg/kg) and butorphanol tartrate IV (0.01 mg/kg) 4-6 hours after MIA injections. Five horses required only one treatment, and two horses required an additional injection 1-2 hours following the first. The mean MIA dose per joint in these 7 horses was 250 mg compared with a mean dose per joint of 187 mg in all other horses. Post-injection complications included transient, diffuse peri-articular swelling (57 horses), persistent peri-articular swelling and lameness (1 horse), focal temporary hair loss at injection site (2 horses), skin sloughing alone (2 horses), and skin sloughing and septic arthritis (4 horses). Six horses had focal swelling at one or more injection sites that resolved within 6 months of treatment. Three horses were euthanized, two due to septic arthritis of the DIT and one due to persistent peri-articular swelling and lameness. Two horses with septic arthritis survived. One is paddock sound, and the other is being ridden but not used for competition.

Table 1. The comfort scores used for assessing post-injection pain in horses undergoing chemical arthrodesis of the distal hock joints using MIA.

Score	Description	Observations	No. of horses
4	No discomfort	Normal. Bright, alert, and responsive. Eating normally. No tachypnea or sweating. Lameness grade 0-1. Heart rate = 40 bpm.	27
3	Mild discomfort	Bright, alert, and responsive. Eating normally. No tachypnea or sweating. Shifting weight on hind limbs. Lameness grade 2-3. Heart rate 41-60 bpm.	64
2	Moderate discomfort	Reduced appetite. Slight tachypnea and sweating. Lifting hind limbs. Lameness grade 3. Heart rate 41-60 bpm.	6
1	Considerable discomfort	Not eating. Moderate tachypnea and sweating. Pawing at ground. Lifting hind limbs. Lameness grade 4. Heart rate > 60 bpm.	5
0	Marked discomfort	Pawing at ground. Profuse sweating and tachypnea. Intermittently recumbent. Lameness grade 4. Heart rate > 80 bpm.	2

Where possible horses were radiographed and examined for lameness 3, 6, 12, and 24 months after treatment (Table 2). Twelve and 24 months following injection, 82% and 85% of horses examined were sound, respectively. Twenty-one horses were <3 months post treatment and had not been re-examined. A total of 12 horses were lost to follow-up. Twelve horses were ultimately retired due to lameness localized in another site, and three were euthanized for unrelated reasons.

Table 2. Results of lameness examination and radiographic evaluation of horses 3, 6, 12, and 24 months after injection of TMT and DIT joints with MIA.

Time post MIA (months)	No. of horses examined	Lameness evaluation results		No. of horses with radiographic evidence of fusion ≥1 joint (%)
		No. of sound horses (%)	Mean lameness grade (No. of horses)	
3	57	0	2.3 (57/57)	4/55 (8%)
6	55	14/55 (25%)	1.5 (41/55)	24/38 (63%)
12	50	41/50 (82%)	1.5 (9/50)	29/34 (87%)
24	34	29/34 (85%)	1.5 (5/34)	18/18 (100%)
>24	10	10/10 (100%)	-	10/10 (100%)

Thirteen DIT joints in 12 horses were not treated due to difficulty in confirming needle location, pre-existing fusion of joint space, or inconclusive contrast arthrograms. Radiographic evidence of ankylosis was evident in 4 of these horses 12 months after treatment. Three horses had progressive but incomplete radiographic evidence of ankylosis of the untreated joint at 6 months post treatment. Four horses were less than 3 months post treatment and had not been re-examined. One horse was lost to follow-up.

Owner satisfaction was recorded for 62 horses. Fifty-six owners (90%) were pleased with the outcome, and 6 owners (10%) were disappointed with the outcome.

Discussion

MIA causes an increase in intracellular concentration of adenosine triphosphate resulting in inhibition of glycolysis and cell death (Bohanon et al., 1991). It causes dose-dependant cartilage degeneration characterized by cartilage fibrillation, chondrocyte death, and glycosaminoglycan and proteoglycan depletion (Bohanon et al., 1991; Gustafson et al., 1992). MIA has been shown to produce reliable radiographic and histological ankylosis of the distal tarsal joints, and this technique for chemical arthrodesis has been recommended as an alternative to surgical techniques (Bohanon et al., 1991; Bohanon, 1995a,b; Bohanon, 1998, 1999). The results reported for soundness and evidence of radiographic evidence of ankylosis at 12 and 24 months in the study here compare favorably with previous reports (Bohanon et al., 1991; Bohanon, 1995a,b; Bohanon, 1998). In a recent study, in contrast, only 18% (7/38) and 22% (5/23) of horses were sound 6 and 12 months, respectively, after intra-articular injection of MIA into the distal tarsal joints (Schramme et al., 1998). Lameness was present despite a similar percentage of horses with radiographic evidence of ankylosis as reported in the present and previous studies (Bohanon et al., 1991; Bohanon, 1995a,b; Schramme et al., 1998). There was no explanation offered for the poor outcome in this study (Schramme et al., 1998). However, possible differences between studies may reflect differences in injection technique, in exercise regimen after injection, or differences in techniques for lameness evaluation and grading.

Exercise has been advocated to increase the rate of fusion after surgical and chemical arthrodesis (McIlwraith and Turner, 1987; Bohanon et al., 1991; Sammut and Kannegieter, 1995). Bohanon et al. (1998) recommended up to 1 hour of exercise per day, 6 days per week beginning 2 days after MIA treatment. In the present study, graded exercise commenced 7 days after injection, increasing to 30 to 45 minutes walking and trotting per day by 3 months, and increasing to full work by 6 months after treatment. Even though no horses were sound at 3 months and the incidence of radiographic ankylosis was low, most owners reported that horses were willing to work during this period. Previous reports have found MIA to cause acute synovial inflammation lasting for approximately 3 weeks after injection (Bohanon et al., 1991). Synovial inflammation may lead to disruption of synovial neural function and temporary analgesia, which may account for the improvement in demeanor and lameness (Bohanon, 1995a,b). Typically from 3 to

6 months post MIA, the degree of lameness is reportedly variable and may be related to mechanical failure of deposited woven or lamellar bone across the joint as the joints try to ankylose (Bohanon et al., 1991). Progressive ankylosis is associated with increased joint stability and subsequent resolution of lameness once approximately 70% of the articular surface is fused (Bohanon et al., 1991). In the present study, despite similar results for 12 and 24 months after injection, at 3 and 6 months soundness and evidence of radiographic ankylosis were comparably lower than reported in other studies (Bohanon et al., 1991; Bohanon, 1995a,b). This difference may reflect differences in the exercise programs following injection. While it would appear ankylosis and soundness can be achieved as early as 6 months post MIA treatment with more intensive exercise programs (Bohanon et al., 1991), we suggest progressive ankylosis may occur beyond 6 months such that maximal soundness may not be achieved until 12 or 24 months post MIA treatment in some horses.

Acute pain is reported to occur in approximately 30% of horses following drilling of the distal tarsal joints and is thought to be related to joint instability, surgical technique, and diameter of drill bit (Adams, 1970; Gabel, 1978; von Salis et al., 2000). Anecdotal reports of severe post-injection pain have contributed to a reluctance in using MIA for chemical arthrodesis of the distal tarsal joints. However, in the present study only 6.7% (7/104) of horses experienced severe discomfort (CS of 1 or 0). This discomfort was adequately managed with the use of additional analgesic drugs. The mean MIA dose used per joint in these 7 horses was 250 mg with 4 horses receiving a mean dose $\geq$ 300 mg. This was compared to a mean dose per joint of 187 mg in horses with a CS of 2, 3, or 4 suggesting a dose-related pain response.

Some authors have suggested the pain is associated with irritant effects on soft tissue, synovium, and plantar metatarsal nerves (Bohanon et al., 1991; Sammut and Kannegieter, 1995); however, to date the effects of MIA on soft tissue have not been investigated. It is reasonable to assume that in high enough concentrations MIA is detrimental to soft tissue viability. Peri-articular leakage, soft tissue inflammation, and subsequent pain is likely to be related to injection volume, the final pressure within the joint, gauge of needle, and the number of needle punctures required to correctly place the needle in the joint.

Other complications reported with the use of MIA include skin and soft tissue necrosis, septic arthritis, serous exudation at injection site, persistent lameness, and peri-articular swelling (Bohanon, 1995a,b; Schramme et al., 1998). In the present study, complications included transient peri-articular swelling (57 horses), persistent peri-articular swelling and lameness (1 horse), focal temporary hair loss at injection site (2 horses), skin sloughing alone (2 horses), and skin sloughing and septic arthritis (4 horses). These complications were most likely related to peri-articular leakage of MIA.

Previous investigations reported that intra-articular doses of 0.16 mg/kg (80 mg of MIA/500-kg horse) did not induce significant subchondral bone damage;

however, it is possible that at higher concentrations subchondral bone necrosis will occur (Gustafson et al., 1992). In all 4 horses that developed septic arthritis, the DIT joint was involved. Injection of the DIT joints in some horses is more difficult due to marked narrowing of the medial joint space, partial ankylosis, or medial osteophytosis. Repeated injection attempts combined with higher concentrations of MIA to compensate for lower volumes of injection may have contributed to soft tissue necrosis, septic arthritis, subchondral necrosis, and joint instability in some horses.

Based on our experience, we recommend using 23-gauge needles, a maximum volume of 2 mL of 100 mg/ml MIA, and stopping injection when resistance is felt on the syringe plunger. We suggest pain can be managed by using suitable analgesics administered prior to and following chemical arthrodesis and using the recommended technique to minimize injection-related complications.

In contrast to previous studies, communication occurred between the DIT and TMT joints in only 11.5% (12/104) of horses, and no communication was identified between the DIT joint and PIT joint or tarsal canal (Kraus-Hansen et al., 1992; Dyson and Romero, 1993; Bohanon, 1994). In a previous report, degenerative joint disease of the PIT joint is reported to have developed in 10% (4/39) of horses between 1 to 4 years after MIA treatment (Bohanon, 1998). Because no arthrograms were performed in this study, it was presumed that MIA had leaked into the PIT joint. To date no horses in the present study have developed degenerative joint disease of the PIT or tarsocrural joints. However, differences in injection volume and techniques make direct comparisons between studies difficult. Correct needle placement, use of radiographic control when injecting the DIT joint, and optimizing injection volume, in the absence of complications associated with joint injection, will minimize inadvertent leakage into synovial structures (Bohanon, 1994).

Numerous techniques have been described for surgical arthrodesis with success rates varying from 57-80% (Adams, 1970; Mackay and Liddell, 1972; Edwards, 1982; Barber, 1984; Sonnichsen, 1985; Wyn-Jones and May, 1986; McIlwraith and Turner, 1987; Archer et al., 1989; Dechant et al., 1999; Adkins et al., 2000; Hague et al., 2000; von Salis et al., 2000). Surgical techniques require general anesthesia and specialized instrumentation, and are associated with a variety of complications including sepsis, postoperative pain, and prolonged convalescence (Edwards, 1982; Barber, 1984; McIlwraith and Turner, 1987; Archer et al., 1989; Bohanon, 1998; von Salis et al., 2000). Chemical arthrodesis using MIA can be performed under standing sedation with minimal equipment. This technique appears to provide a more reliable outcome than surgical techniques with a low incidence of complications. PIT joint involvement or synovial communication between the tarsocrural joint, PIT joint, or tarsal sheath with the distal tarsal joints preclude the use of MIA.

The present study demonstrates that MIA is an effective treatment for degenerative joint disease of the distal tarsal joints and results are comparable to those achieved by surgical arthrodesis. Resolution of lameness may take up to 12 months and occasionally longer. Soundness can be achieved in 82% and 85% of horses at 12 and 24 months, respectively. Significant complications are uncommon but may occur and are likely related to peri-articular injection, leakage of MIA, or use of higher concentrations or volumes. Post-injection pain can be marked in a small number of horses but is transient and can be managed effectively with analgesic drugs.

References

Adams, O.R. 1970. Surgical arthrodesis for treatment of bone spavin. J. Amer. Vet. Med. Assoc. 157:1480-1485.

Adkins, A.R., J.V. Yovich, and C.M. Steel. 2000. Surgical arthrodesis of distal tarsal joints in 17 horses clinically affected with osteoarthritis. Aust. Vet. J. 79:26-29.

Archer, R.M., R.K. Schneider, W.A. Lindsay, and J.W. Wilson. 1989. Arthrodesis of the equine distal tarsal joints by perforated stainless steel cylinders. Equine Vet. J. Suppl. 6:125-130.

Barber, S.M. 1984. Arthrodesis of the distal intertarsal and tarsometatarsal joints in the horse. Vet. Surg. 13:227-235.

Bohanon, T.C. 1994. Contrast arthrography of the distal intertarsal and tarsometatarsal joints in horses with bone spavin. Vet. Surg. 23:396 (Abstr.).

Bohanon, T.C. 1995a. Chemical fusion of the distal tarsal joints with sodium monoiodoacetate in 38 horses clinically affected with bone spavin. Vet. Surg. 24:421 (Abstr.).

Bohanon, T.C. 1995b. Chemical fusion of the distal tarsal joints with sodium monoiodoacetate in horses clinically affected with osteoarthrosis. In: Proc. Amer. Assoc. Equine Practnr. 41:148-149.

Bohanon, T.C. 1998. Tarsal arthrodesis. In: N.A. White and J.N. Moore (Eds.) Current Techniques in Equine Surgery and Lameness. (2nd Ed.) p. 433-440. Saunders, Philadelphia.

Bohanon, T.C. 1999. The tarsus. In: J.A. Auer and J.A. Stick (Eds.) Equine Surgery (2nd Ed.) p. 848-862. Saunders, Philadelphia.

Bohanon, T.C., R.K. Schneider, and S.E. Weisbrode. 1991. Fusion of the distal intertarsal and tarsometatarsal joints in the horse using intra-articular sodium monoiodoacetate. Equine Vet. J. 23:289-295.

Butler, J.A., C.M. Colles, S.J. Dyson, S.E. Kold, and P.W. Poulos. 2000. The tarsus. In: Clinical Radiology of the Horse (2nd Ed.) p. 247-284. Blackwell Science, London.

Dechant, J.E., L.L. Southwood, G.M. Baxter, and W.H. Crawford. 1999. Treatment of distal tarsal joint osteoarthritis using 3-drill tract technique in 36 horses. In: Proc. Amer. Assoc. Equine Practnr. 45:160-161.

Dyson, S.J., and J.M. Romero. 1993. An investigation of injection techniques for local analgesia of the equine distal tarsus and proximal metatarsus. Equine Vet. J. 25:30-35.

Edwards, G.B. 1982. Surgical arthrodesis for the treatment of bone spavin in 20 horses. Equine Vet. J. 14:117-121.

Gabel, A.A. 1978. Lameness caused by inflammation in the distal hock. Vet Clin. North Amer. 2:101-124.

Gabel, A.A. 1983. Prevention, diagnosis and treatment of inflammation of the distal hock. In: Proc. Amer. Assoc. Equine Practnr. 28:287-298.

Gustafson, S.B., G.W. Trotter, R.W. Norrdin, R.H. Wrigley, and C. Lamar. 1992. Evaluation of intra-articular administered sodium monoiodoacetate-induced chemical injury to articular cartilage of horses. Amer. J. Vet. Res. 53:1193-1202.

Hague, B.A., A. Guccione, and O.K. Edmond. 2000. Clinical impressions of a new technique utilizing a Nd:YAG laser to arthrodese the distal tarsal joints. In: 10th Annual ACVS Symposium 464 (Abstr.).

Johnson, C.B., P.M. Taylor, S.S. Young, and J.C. Brearley. 1993. Postoperative analgesia using phenylbutazone, flunixin or carprofen in horses. Vet. Rec. 133:336-338.

Kraus-Hansen, A.E., H.W. Jann, and G.E. Fackelman. 1992. Arthrographic analysis of communication between the tarsometatarsal and distal intertarsal joints in the horse. Vet. Surg. 21:139-144.

Mackay, R.C.J., and W.A. Liddell. 1972. Arthrodesis in the treatment of bone spavin. Equine Vet. J. 4:34-36.

McIlwraith, C.W., and A.S. Turner. 1987. Arthrodesis of the distal tarsal joints. In: Equine Surgery Advanced Techniques. p. 185-190. Lea and Febiger, Philadelphia.

Pasquini, C., S. Pasquini, R. Bahr, and H. Jann. 1995. Lameness diagnosis. In: Guide to Equine Clinics. p. 68. Sudz, Texas.

Raekallio, M., P.M. Taylor, and R.C. Bennett. 1997. Preliminary investigations of pain and analgesia assessment in horses administered phenylbutazone or placebo after arthroscopic surgery. Vet. Surg. 26:150-155.

Sack, W.O., and P.G. Orsini. 1981. Distal intertarsal and tarsometatarsal joints in the horse: Communication and injection sites. J. Amer. Vet. Med. Assoc. 179:355-359.

Sammut, E.B., and N.J. Kannegieter. 1995. Use of sodium monoiodoacetate to fuse the distal hock joints in horses. Aust. Vet. J, 72:25-28.

Schneider, R.K., L.R. Bramlage, R.M. Moore, L.M. Mecklenburg, C.W. Kohn, and A.A. Gabel. 1992. A retrospective study of 192 horses affected with septic arthritis/tenosynovitis. Equine Vet. J. 24:436-442.

Schramme, M.C., D. Platt, and R.K.W. Smith. 1998. Treatment of osteoarthritis of the tarsometatarsal and distal intertarsal joints of the horse (spavin) with monoiodoacetate: Preliminary results. Vet. Surg. 27:296 (Abstr.).

Sonnichsen, H.V., and E. Svalastoga. 1985. Surgical treatment of bone spavin in the horse. Equine Pract. 7:6-9.

Stashak, T.S. 1987. The tarsus. In: T.S. Stashak (Ed.) Adams' Lameness in Horses. (4th Ed.) p. 694-725. Lea and Febiger, Philadelphia.

Sullins, K.E. 2002. The tarsus. In: T.S. Stashak (Ed.) Adams' Lameness in Horses. (5th Ed.) p. 930942. Williams and Wilkins, Philadelphia.

von Salis, B., J.A. Auer, and G.E. Fackelman. 2000. Small tarsal joint arthrodesis. In: G.E. Fackelman, J.A. Auer, D.M. Nunamaker (Eds.) AO Principles of Equine Osteosynthesis. p. 269-279. Thieme, New York.

Wyn-Jones, G., and S.A. May. 1986. Surgical arthrodesis for the treatment of osteoarthrosis of the proximal intertarsal, distal intertarsal and tarsometatarsal joints in 30 horses: a comparison of 4 different techniques. Equine Vet. J. 18:59-64.

INDEX

A

Aflatoxin 146
Allergy 142
Anabolic steroids 349
Antioxidants 172, 242
Arabian horses 3, 181
Australian horse management 185, 322

B

Beet pulp 5, 271
Biotin 27
Body condition 187
  and osteochondrosis 415
  of broodmares 206
Bone development 219-224, 289-293,
  295-304, 365
  methods of assessing 296
Bone disease 365-371
  diagnosis of 373-380
Broodmare management 193-214,
  426-428

C

Calcium 197, 304
  requirements of young horses 315,
  361-364
Cervical vertebral malformation 453
Chelated minerals 201
Chronic obstructive pulmonary disease
  142, 485-488
Colic 122
Computed tomography 374
Conformation and soundness 327-330
  in Quarter Horses 328
  in Thoroughbreds 327
Copper
  and osteochondrosis 413
  requirements of broodmares 199
  requirements of young horses 315
Corn oil 8, 38
Cushing's disease 447-451

D

Degenerative joint disease 491-500
Developmental orthopedic disease 292,
  295-296, 365
  role of nutrition 417-431
Digestion 107, 229, 250
Digestive tract 121, 129, 250
Disease 130, 139
Dry matter
  intake 13-14
  production 12-13
  requirement 13-14

E

Electrolytes 73, 113, 173
  and exercise 267, 273
  and tying-up 474
  during endurance training 114
Endurance riding 181
  and immune function 236
Energy 227, 249, 256
  and developmental orthopedic
    disease 419
  requirements of broodmares 194
  requirements of young horses 311-
    314, 359-360
Equine degenerative
  myeloencephalopathy 464
Equine motor neuron disease 466
Equine protozoal myeloencephalitis 456
Exercise 219
  and electrolytes 267, 279
  and immune function 235
  and injuries 412
  and stress 265
  and water 267
  effect of growth hormone 352

F

Fat 37-50
  and endurance exercise 117, 183

501